THE
Neighborhood™
2.0
Faculty Navigation Guide

Jean Foret Giddens, RN, PhD

Dean and Professor, School of Nursing

Virginia Commonwealth University

Richmond, VA

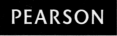

PEARSON

Boston Columbus Indianapolis New York San Francisco Upper Saddle River
Amsterdam Cape Town Dubai London Madrid Milan Munich Paris Montréal Toronto
Delhi Mexico City São Paulo Sydney Hong Kong Seoul Singapore Taipei Tokyo

Publisher: Julie Levin Alexander
Publisher's Assistant: Regina Bruno
Executive Acquisitions Editor: Kelly Trakalo
Editorial Assistant: Kevin Wilson
Developmental Editor: Rachel Bedard
Program Manager: Melissa Bashe
Project Manager: Michael Giacobbe
Interior Design: Maria Guglielmo Walsh
Cover Design: Mary Siener
Marketing Specialist: Michael Sirinides
Media Project Manager: Karen Bretz & Tanika Henderson
Composition: Integra Software Services Pvt. Ltd.

Notice: Care has been taken to confirm the accuracy of information presented in this book. The authors, editors, and the publisher, however, cannot accept any responsibility for errors or omissions or for consequences from application of the information in this book and make no warranty, express or implied, with respect to its contents.

The authors and publisher have exerted every effort to ensure that drug selections and dosages set forth in this text are in accord with current recommendations and practice at time of publication. However, in view of ongoing research, changes in government regulations, and the constant flow of information relating to drug therapy and drug reactions, the reader is urged to check the package inserts of all drugs for any change in indications of dosage and for added warnings and precautions. This is particularly important when the recommended agent is a new and/or infrequently employed drug.

Library of Congress Cataloging-in-Publication Data
Giddens, Jean.
   The neighborhood 2.0 : faculty navigation guide / Jean Foret Giddens, RN, PhD, Dean and Professor, School of Nursing, Virginia Commonwealth University, Richmond, VA.
      pages cm
   Includes bibliographical references and index.
   ISBN-13: 978-0-13-341640-4 (alk. paper)
   ISBN-10: 0-13-341640-2 (alk. paper)
   1. Nursing—Study and teaching—Audio-visual aids.   I. Title.
RT73.5.G53 2014
610.73076—dc23

                                                                                    2013040829

PEARSON

www.pearsonhighered.com

ISBN-10:   0-13-341640-2
ISBN-13: 978-0-13-341640-4

ABOUT THE AUTHOR

Jean Foret Giddens

Jean Foret Giddens, RN, PhD, is Dean and Professor at the Virginia Commonwealth University School of Nursing in Richmond, Virginia. A nurse educator for nearly 30 years, she is considered an expert in curriculum, conceptual learning, educational research, and innovative teaching strategies. She has authored and contributed to numerous nursing textbooks, media products, and peer-reviewed journal articles. In addition, Dr. Giddens has extensive experience as a nursing education consultant and has presented her work at multiple national and international meetings. She initially developed *The Neighborhood* for students attending the University of New Mexico nursing program.

ACKNOWLEDGMENTS

The Neighborhood 2.0 represents a huge collaborative effort. This revision includes efforts from those involved in the original project as well as current users of *The Neighborhood*. We thank Dr. Jean Giddens for continuing to support and develop *The Neighborhood* and incorporating so much of the feedback we received from our users into the 2.0 version. Special thanks go to Dr. Laura Gonzalez, Dr. Michelle Aebersold, and Dr. Cindy Fenske. Representing three of the early adopters of *The Neighborhood*, and active in research around virtual communities, these faculty conducted faculty training and consultation and contributed extensively to the 2.0 version of *The Neighborhood*. Many of the special features, the exemplar activities found in the course, and the new videos and photos are a direct result of their involvement. Thanks to South University, Tampa campus, for graciously allowing use of their school for our extensive video and photo shoots. A special thanks to Laurie Stark, PhD, RN, CNE for her technical assistance and support and to the numerous faculty and students who participated in the production of *The Neighborhood* 2.0. Special thanks also go to Rachel Bedard, our extraordinary developmental editor. Rachel held this complex project together. Without her fearlessness, commitment to excellence, and organizational skills this project would never have been completed on time!

In addition, a special thanks to Total Project Management for agreeing to undertake the massive video project, and to Rick Brady for all of the new and wonderful photos. Thank you to Mary Siener, our designer, who continually went above and beyond to make sure everything was just right. Also to Sarah South for always doing what was asked and working to bring all the supplemental pieces together. Our deepest thanks and appreciation to the eCollege development team of Remi Ajao, Steven Archibald, Jason Bell, Wayne Burton, Kyle Coberly, Christian Flanagan, Tim Laushman, Nicholas Lopez, Jay Lynch, Katherine McCool, Adam Meek, and Hani Park. Their contributions, enthusiasm, commitment to schedule, professionalism, and sense of humor kept us on track and delivered a beautiful interface and functionality.

Finally, thanks to the person who orchestrated the entire team for *The Neighborhood* 2.0, Kelly Trakalo. Kelly never took her eyes off the goal of a visually rich, smoothly interactive course with practically unlimited tools for nursing instructors and students. Through all phases of development, Kelly guided the team so that the end product looks right and is user friendly.

Contributors

Many thanks to the 2.0 contributors who developed website features in this new updated version:

Michelle Aebersold, PhD, RN, University of Michigan (scripts, simulations, videos and photography, course activities)
Tonya Chapin, RN, MSN, Colorado Mesa University (simulations)

Cindy Fenske, DNP, RN, CNE, University of Michigan (scripts, simulations, videos and photography, journals, course activities)
Laura Gonzalez, PhD, ARNP, CNE, University of Central Florida (scripts, simulations, videos and photography, course activities)
Laura Huisking (news)
Martha Olson, MSN, MS, RN, Iowa Lakes Community College (journals, news, course activities)
Cindy Parsons, DNP, PMHNP-BC, University of Tampa (simulations)
George Byron Smith, DNP, ARNP, GNP-BC, NP-C, CNE, South University, Tampa, FL (scripts, video)

Faculty Workshop Participants

Dr. Michelle Aebersold, PhD, RN
University of Michigan
Ann Arbor, MI

Ken Armstrong, MS, RN, CNE, CNOR
Prince George's Community College
Largo, MD

Tonya Chapin, RN, MSN
Colorado Mesa University
Grand Junction, CO

Cindy Fenske, DNP, RN, CNE
University of Michigan
Ann Arbor, MI

Jean Giddens (Neighborhood Author),
PhD, RN
Virginia Commonwealth University
Richmond, VA

Dr. Laura Gonzalez, PhD, ARNP, CNE
University of Central Florida
Orlando, FL

Amy Herboldsheimer, MSN, RN
University of Nebraska Medical Center
Omaha, NE

Dr. Barbara Limandri, DNSc, MSN, RN
Linfield College
Portland, OR

Martha Olson, MSN, MS, RN
Iowa Lakes Community College
Emmetsburg, IA

Reviewers

Michelle Aebersold, PhD, RN
University of Michigan
Ann Arbor, MI

Mike Aldridge, MSN, RN, CNS, CNE
Concordia University Texas
Austin, TX

Kathleen Brewer, PhD, ARNP, BC
St. Luke's College
Kansas City, MO

Tonya Chapin, RN, MSN
Colorado Mesa University
Grand Junction, CO

Conni DeBlieck, DNP
New Mexico State University
Las Cruces, NM

Patricia Duckworth, RN, MSN, CNE
Mildred Elley College
Pittsfield, MA

Cindy Fenske, DNP, RN, CNE
University of Michigan
Ann Arbor, MI

Janice Kaye Fuson, MSN, RN
Briggs Technology
Thomasville, NC

Laura Gonzalez, PhD, ARNP, CNE
University of Central Florida
Orlando, FL

Lynne Hancock, RN, MSN
Montgomery Community College
Troy, NC

Wende Heckert, RN, MSN, MFS, DNP, APRN-NP
J. Paul & Eleanor McIntosh College of Nursing
Omaha, NE

Yanick Joseph, RN
South University
Savannah, GA

Karen Lea, RN, MN
Saint Luke's College
Kansas City, MO

Barbara J. Limandri, DNSc, PMHNP, BC
Linfield College
Portland, OR

Shelly Noe, RN, DNP
New Mexico State University
Las Cruces, NM

Martha Olson, MSN, MS, RN
Iowa Lakes Community College
Emmetsburg, IA

Laurie Parks, RN, MSN/Ed
Guilford Technical Community College
Jamestown, NC

Nancy M. Peifer-Neil, BSN, MSN, PhD
Palm Beach State College
Lake Worth, FL

Laura Sescilla, RN, MSN
Randolph Community College
Asheboro, NC

Teresa Denk Smajda, RN, MSN
Saint Luke's College
Kansas City, MO

George Byron Smith, DNP, ARNP, GNP-BC, NP-C, CNE
South University
Tampa, FL

CONTENTS

SECTION I   **INTRODUCTION**   1

Description of *The Neighborhood*   2
   Theoretical Linkage and Basis for Learning   2
     Storytelling   3
     Longitudinal Case Study   3
     Interpretative Pedagogy   3
     Standardized Patients   3
Features   4
   Featured Characters   4
     Biography and Stories   4
     Content Links   4
     Neighborhood Connections   4
     Photographs and Video Vignettes   4
     Health Records   4
     Related News   5
   Supporting Characters   5
   News   5
   Community   5

Visual Map of *The Neighborhood* Characters   5
Instructional Tips and Techniques   6
Exemplary Teaching Strategies   9
   Featured Character Case Study   9
   Role-Play   9
   Simulation   9
   Concept or Topic Analysis   10
   Games   10
   Comparing and Contrasting   10
   Policy Analysis   10
   Family History/Genogram   11
   Concept Map   11
   Small Group Discussion   11
   Developing a Care Plan or Teaching Plan   11

SECTION II   **SPECIALTY COURSE USE AND SUGGESTED CHARACTERS**   13

Course Use Overview   14
Nursing Fundamentals—Basic Nursing Skills   14
   Fundamental Concepts   14
   Basic Nursing Skills   19
Adult Health Nursing   21
   Respiratory System   21
   Cardiovascular System   22
   Neurologic System   23
   Musculoskeletal System   23
   Gastrointestinal System   24
   Urologic System   24
   Metabolism and Nutrition   24
   Immune System   25
   Acid Base/Fluid Electrolyte Disturbances   25
   Visual and Auditory Systems   26
   Neighborhood Hospital Links   26
Maternity and Women's Health   26
   Pregnancy   26
   Women's Health Issues   27
Pediatric and Family Nursing   28
   Health Promotion and Wellness   28

   Health-Related Problems   29
   Family and Social Issues   31
   School Nurse Topics   32
Mental Health Nursing   33
   Psychotic Disorders   33
   Cognitive Disorders   34
   Mood Disorders   34
   Other Mental Health Issues   35
Geriatric Nursing   37
   Health-Related Conditions   37
   Family and Social Issues   39
   Senior Center Nurse Topics   40
Community Health   42
   Common Community Health Topics   42
Health Promotion   47
   Health Promotion   48
Nursing Leadership and Professional Concepts Course   49
   Professional Practice Issues   49
   Roles of the Professional Nurse   53

SECTION III   FEATURED CHARACTER OVERVIEWS AND STORIES   57

Allen Household   58
Clifford Allen   59
Season 1 Information   59
Season 2 Information   61
Season 3 Information   63
Pam Allen   66
Season 1 Information   66
Season 2 Information   68
Season 3 Information   70
Gary Allen   72
Season 1 Information   72
Season 2 Information   74
Season 3 Information   75
Bley Household   78
Jimmy Bley   79
Season 1 Information   79
Season 2 Information   81
Season 3 Information   83
Cecelia Bley   85
Season 1 Information   85
Season 2 Information   87
Season 3 Information   88
James Household   91
Norma James   92
Season 1 Information   92
Season 2 Information   95
Season 3 Information   97
Johnson Household   99
Yvonne Johnson   100
Season 1 Information   100
Season 2 Information   102
Season 3 Information   105
Randall Johnson   107
Season 1 Information   107
Season 2 Information   109
Season 3 Information   110
Martin & Ames Household   112
Gilbert Martin   113
Season 1 Information   113
Season 2 Information   115
Season 3 Information   117
Helen Martin   119
Season 1 Information   119
Season 2 Information   121
Season 3 Information   123
Mary Martin   125
Season 1 Information   125
Season 2 Information   128
Season 3 Information   129

Anthony Martin   131
Season 1 Information   132
Season 2 Information   133
Season 3 Information   135
Kristina Martin   137
Season 1 Information   137
Season 2 Information   139
Season 3 Information   141
Tracie Ames   143
Season 1 Information   143
Season 2 Information   145
Season 3 Information   146
Mark Martin   148
Season 1 Information   148
Season 2 Information   148
Season 3 Information   150
Tyler Martin   152
Season 1 Information   153
Season 2 Information   153
Season 3 Information   154
Ocampo Household   156
Danilo Ocampo   157
Season 1 Information   157
Season 2 Information   160
Lydia Ocampo   162
Season 1 Information   162
Season 2 Information   164
Season 3 Information   166
Reyes Household   168
Angelo Reyes   169
Season 1 Information   169
Season 2 Information   171
Season 3 Information   173
Rachel Reyes   175
Season 1 Information   175
Season 2 Information   177
Season 3 Information   179
Peter & Marissa   181
Season 1 and 2 Information   181
Season 3 Information   181
Riley Household   183
Evelyn Riley   184
Season 1 Information   184
Season 2 Information   186
Season 3 Information   188
Jenna Riley   191
Season 1 Information   191
Season 2 Information   193
Season 3 Information   194

Jason Riley   197
Season 1 Information   198
Season 2 Information   199
Season 3 Information   201
Riley & Holmes Household   203
Jessica Riley   204
Season 1 Information   204
Season 2 Information   206
Season 3 Information   209
Casey Holmes   212
Season 1 Information   212
Season 2 Information   214
Season 3 Information   215
Ryan Riley   217
Season 1 Information   217
Season 2 Information   219
Season 3 Information   220
Carrie Holmes   222
Season 1 Information   222
Season 2 Information   222
Season 3 Information   223
Ross & Jaramillo Household   225
Greg Ross   226
Season 1 Information   226
Season 2 Information   228
Season 3 Information   230
Benito Jaramillo   233
Season 1 Information   233
Season 2 Information   235
Season 3 Information   236
Young Household   239
Steve Young   240
Season 1 Information   240
Season 2 Information   242
Season 3 Information   243
Angie Young   245
Season 1 Information   245
Season 2 Information   247
Season 3 Information   249
Kelsey Young   252
Season 1 Information   252
Season 2 Information   254
Season 3 Information   255
Marcus Young   257
Season 1 Information   257
Season 2 Information   259
Season 3 Information   260

Eric Young   262
Season 1 Information   262
Season 2 Information   263
Season 3 Information   263
Health Connections Clinic   265
Shawn Jacobs   266
Season 1 Information   266
Season 2 Information   269
Season 3 Information   272
Hospital   276
Patrick Richman   277
Season 1 Information   277
Season 2 Information   279
Season 3 Information   281
Zainah Kattan   283
Season 1 Information   283
Season 2 Information   286
Season 3 Information   288
Bobby Schofield   290
Season 1 Information   290
Season 2 Information   292
Season 3 Information   294
Public School   296
Violet Brinkworth   297
Season 1 Information   297
Season 2 Information   300
Season 3 Information   302

Senior Center   305
Karen Williams   306
Season 1 Information   306
Season 2 Information   310
Season 3 Information   312
Women's Health Services   315
Carol Ramsey   316
Season 1 Information   316
Season 2 Information   318
Season 3 Information   320
Neighborhood News   323
Season 1 News   323
Season 2 News   332
Season 3 News   340

Appendix   349

References   371

Index   373

INTRODUCTION

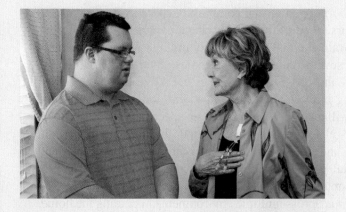

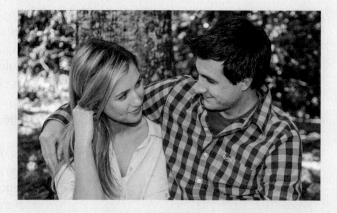

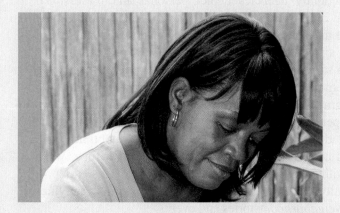

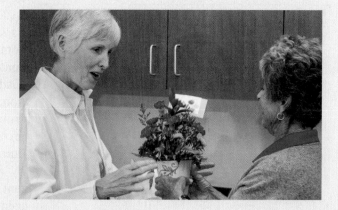

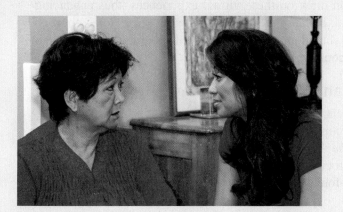

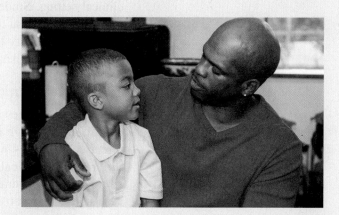

Welcome to *The Neighborhood,* an online virtual community that supports learning throughout the nursing program. This Faculty Navigation Guide introduces you to *The Neighborhood* and provides suggestions for incorporating this new way of learning into the nursing curriculum and your classroom.

Please access *The Neighborhood* at www.pearsonneighborhood.com. Information on getting started and on technical support is available online.

DESCRIPTION OF *THE NEIGHBORHOOD*

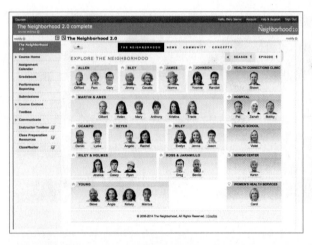

The Neighborhood, a virtual community specifically designed to enhance nursing education, represents a paradigm shift in teaching and learning. This Web-based community features 11 households and several community agencies. Interacting within the households and community agencies are 41 featured characters, representing individuals from various cultural groups across the age, health-illness, and socioeconomic spectrums.

Health-related issues are depicted through the household characters and represent acute and chronic biophysical and psychosocial problems correlating to the incidence and prevalence in population groups. Health care is represented in *The Neighborhood* across multiple environments, including the home, community agencies (such as schools and a senior center), outpatient offices, clinics, and a hospital. Nurse characters featured in the community agencies depict personal and professional issues faced by nurses in a variety of roles, including hospital nurse, nurse manager, advanced practice nurse, school nurse, and community agency nurse. *The Neighborhood* is presented in the context of a story; character stories evolve per episode over three academic terms and are supplemented with biographical information, photographs, video clips, medical records, and related news articles. Depending on the access requested by your school for the program, students may be able to see all stories at all times (full, unrestricted access) or the stories may unfold over time, week by week, with access limited to specific seasons. This is important for faculty to keep in mind when planning learning activities using *The Neighborhood* stories and events.

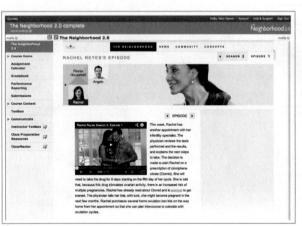

Students may well be exposed to concepts within the stories before formally studying them in didactic courses or encountering them in the clinical setting. Students can draw on these virtual experiences, thus enhancing didactic and clinical learning. Because the virtual community links to all courses, students and faculty have a shared experience through the stories, enabling them to link within and between courses.

Theoretical Linkage and Basis for Learning

Virtual communities represent an emerging technological application for nursing education. Although many computer-based learning programs exist, there are no direct comparisons with *The Neighborhood. The Neighborhood* is significantly different pedagogically in focus, depth, scope, function, and application. It has strong links to several well-founded teaching strategies: storytelling, longitudinal case study, interpretive pedagogy, and standardized patients. These strategies represent multicontextuality (Iberra, 2001), as well as constructivist, humanistic, and neurophysiologic learning theories.

Storytelling. The primary basis of learning in *The Neighborhood* is through character stories. Storytelling in this context focuses on the lived experiences of the characters, enabling students to gain an appreciation for personal issues and competing variables that are often not captured by journal articles and textbooks. *The Neighborhood* stories have the potential to grab and hold the interest and attention of students in a way that is similar to a good novel or television series. Milton (2004) describes storytelling as a "coming-to-know process" that provides a mechanism for learning concepts in a meaningful context. The multiple benefits of storytelling as a teaching strategy are described in the literature, including role modeling and enhancement of cultural sensitivity, empathy, ethical insight, self-esteem, critical thinking, and communication (Charon, 2004; Davidhizar & Lonser, 2003; Durgahee, 1997; Hodge, Pasqua, Marquez, & Geishirt-Cantrell, 2002; Milton, 2004).

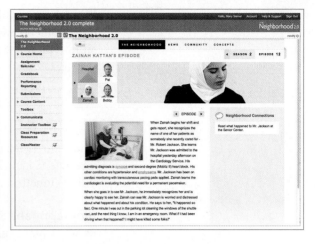

Longitudinal Case Study. Case study involves the analysis of a clinical situation or incident. This widely used teaching strategy includes the presentation of a patient (usually in a clinical context) with specific questions or problems for learners to analyze and address. Case-based learning has been used in nursing education for several years in a variety of applications and educational settings, including the traditional classroom, Web-based courses, clinical courses, and simulations. Benefits of case-based learning include acquisition of skills in critical thinking, clinical reasoning, organization and interpretation of information, and enhancement of student confidence (Thomas, O'Connor, Albert, Boutain, & Brandt, 2001).

The Neighborhood represents a unique form of case-based learning. The longitudinal application (over multiple academic terms), the interrelationship among the characters and community, and the fact that cases are told from the perspective of the characters represent significant differences from the traditional case-based approach.

Interpretative Pedagogy. *Interpretative pedagogy* is a process of drawing meaning from situations or experiences through reflection. In nursing education, interpretative pedagogy stimulates and develops thinking and cultivates a deep understanding of the lived experiences of individuals (Diekelmann, 2005; Ironside, 2005). The character stories provide a virtual experience that enables students to think critically and analyze circumstances in the context of realistic situations, thus enhancing affective learning. These opportunities are extended to all students, as opposed to a select few students who might encounter such experiences in a clinical setting.

Standardized Patients. Standardized patients are paid individuals who assume the identity of patients and accurately portray these patients in specific clinical scenarios (Ebbert & Connors, 2004). Standardized patients have been successfully used in medical education as well as graduate nursing education, particularly advanced practice education, for several years. The reported benefits of standardized patients include improvement of assessment and communication skills, knowledge development, and cultural competency (Ebbert & Connors, 2004; Rutledge, Garzon, Scott, & Karlowicz, 2004; Seibert, Guthrie, & Adamo, 2004; Vessey & Huss, 2002). The use of standardized patients has also been reported as a way to measure learning outcomes through performance of assessment and differential diagnosis (Shawler, 2008).

The Neighborhood essentially incorporates the use of standardized patients, but in a virtual context. Although there is no direct interaction between the student and the characters, all students and faculty are exposed to the same experiences through the character stories, providing for many of the same benefits (knowledge development, assessment skills, and cultural competency) and remaining accessible at all times—unlike traditional standardized patients.

FEATURES

Featured Characters

There are 41 featured characters who live and work in *The Neighborhood*. Featured characters include several elements website biography and stories, photos and video vignettes, medical records, and content links.

Biography and Stories.   Each featured character is introduced by a brief overview or windshield survey, followed by episode stories for each season (45 episodes). It is important to note that *The Neighborhood* does not correlate to real time; that is, the time frame between story updates might represent one or more episodes. In most cases, the stories in each episode are limited to one paragraph, so students will not feel overwhelmed by keeping up with the stories. However, when a major event occurs, the episode story is longer. Supplemental text (journals, texts, blogs, etc.) ▼ add more depth to characters' stories.

Content Links.   Embedded within the stories and biography are content links. Select medical terms, pharmacologic agents, and diagnostic tests are linked with brief content (definitions or descriptions) to provide real-time access to information enhancing students' understanding. Content links are accessed by clicking on the links within the stories.

***Neighborhood* Connections.**   Within episodes of individual stories are *Neighborhood* Connections, links between one character and/or family and another. A "click" on one of these links carries the reader to the other character's story, illustrating the complex web of relationships among *Neighborhood* characters.

Photographs and Video Vignettes.   Photographs and video vignettes are included throughout the website to enhance the stories. Over a thousand photographs and more than 150 videos are associated with the stories. The photographs and videos are embedded within the story. Most video clips are less than two minutes long. In this Faculty Navigation Guide, symbols embedded in each episode's stories (video clip ▶) alert faculty to supplements for that story.

Health Records.   For many of the characters who experience health-related events that require health care visits, a portion of a medical record is included with the story. More than 50 medical records that detail inpatient or outpatient care are available; some of them are updated over time to reflect follow-up visits (e.g., prenatal care, pediatric office visit, outpatient chemotherapy). Within the stories a link lets the user know when a medical record

Key: ▶ = video clip   ☰ = medical record   ▼ = journal entry   [NEWS] = news article

can be accessed; these records can be downloaded and printed, if desired. In this Faculty Navigation Guide, a symbol (▤) embedded in each episode's stories alerts instructors to medical record supplements for that story.

Related News. A News Article link in *Neighborhood* episodes brings the reader instantly from a story to a news article, announcement, or letter to the editor. This provides a broader perspective on the life of *The Neighborhood* as students read about particular characters. In the Guide, an icon [NEWS] indicates a related News Article.

Supporting Characters

Several characters are considered "supporting" characters, because their stories are not followed on a week-to-week basis. They are, however, important characters who appear frequently and have roles in the stories of several featured characters. Examples include Dr. Gordon in the emergency department; Dr. Rowe, a family practice physician; Dr. Jacobe, a psychiatrist; Carolyn Marquette, a pediatric nurse practitioner; Terry Clark, a pregnant teenager; a series of war veteran characters (Robert Jackson, Eloise Saunders, Matt Nolan, Vincent Matsui, others), Rebecca and Victoria Patterson, and nursing students Jacob McCain, Jennifer Porter, and Kayla Sharif.

News

The community news [NEWS] features announcements and portions of health-related articles that correlate with events in *The Neighborhood* character stories. Like the character stories, the news is updated in each episode. Common news features include community events (e.g., a forest fire, a hospital strike), health promotion topics (e.g., nutrition, exercise, child safety seats, prenatal care), health concerns of older adults, issues involving substance abuse, domestic violence, elder abuse, and issues within the schools. The news is enhanced by dozens of photographs.

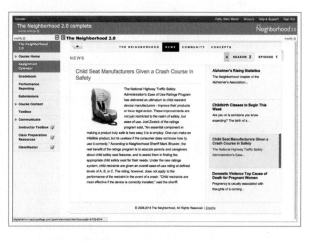

Community

Like most real communities, *The Neighborhood* has a Community link that acts as a community home page. Within this link, users will find a message from Neighborhood mayor Nathan Brice, along with links for population demographics, weather, income data (employment and average wages, unemployment and poverty rates, and cost-of-living data), and health-care information (inpatient and outpatient services, as well as health care organizations).

VISUAL MAP OF *THE NEIGHBORHOOD* CHARACTERS

One of the unique characteristics of *The Neighborhood* is the interrelationships of characters. Not only are character stories within families interrelated, but the stories connect with those of other characters outside the family setting. This interrelatedness

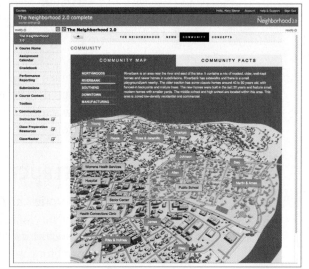

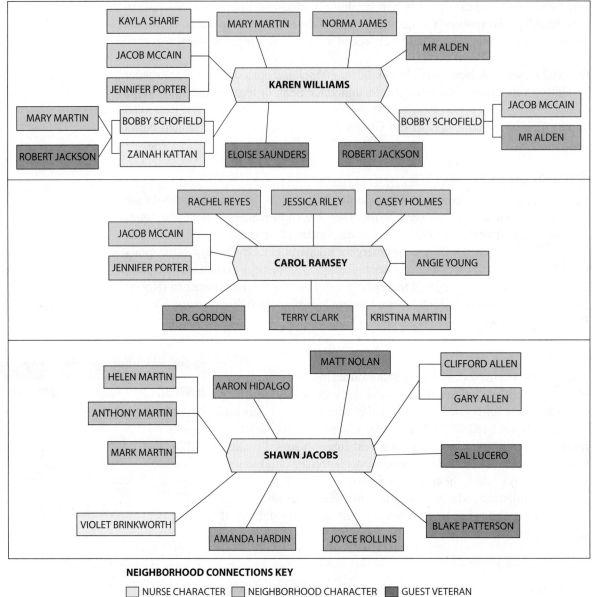

NEIGHBORHOOD CONNECTIONS KEY

- NURSE CHARACTER
- STUDENT NURSE
- NEIGHBORHOOD CHARACTER
- HEALTHCARE PERSONNEL
- GUEST VETERAN
- OTHER GUEST

becomes more complex in each of the seasons as the stories unfold, and it is an essential feature in creating the feel of a community. The following diagrams show various featured healthcare and community characters in each of the three seasons.

INSTRUCTIONAL TIPS AND TECHNIQUES

The stories in *The Neighborhood* represent many of the common health-related problems, social issues, and nursing practice issues that affect health care today. As such, they apply to most nursing courses, regardless of the curriculum. The instructor can determine how and to what extent the stories are applied in a course

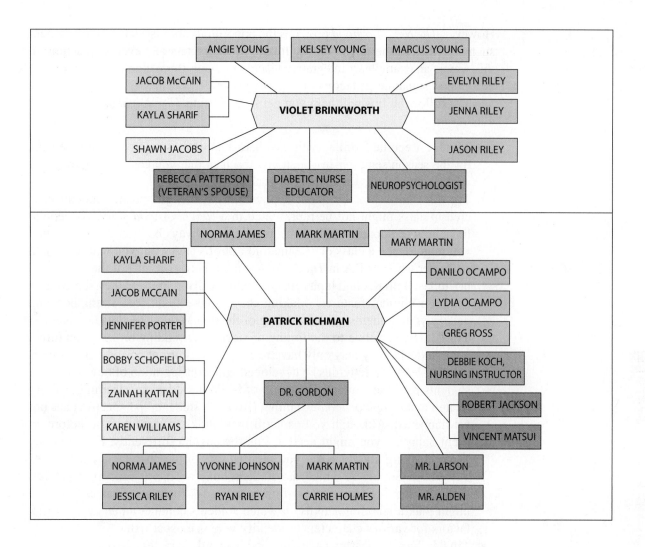

based on the course content and the placement (season) at which the course is offered in the curriculum. Activities, case studies, and other questions that have been compiled by other faculty users can be found within The Neighborhood 2.0 course and Class Preparation Resources Instructor Tool. *The Neighborhood* serves as a platform for the instructor to develop relevant and purposeful student-centered learning activities. *The Neighborhood* is not designed to replace classroom, online, or clinical instruction; it enhances student learning because it provides clinical and situational contexts for the content.

Faculty members who are new users may initially struggle with how to use *The Neighborhood* to enhance learning. This is not so much a reflection on the creativity or talent of faculty members as it is a reflection of current educational practice. Using *The Neighborhood* requires instructors to think differently about learning. One helpful suggestion is to think about teaching from the standpoint of what you want your students to be able to do. *The Neighborhood* provides a platform for practical application. For example, it is expected that students can write a care plan, prepare a teaching plan, prepare a health promotion activity, analyze risk factors, prepare discharge instructions, make a home visit, analyze effectiveness of care, and compare and contrast expected outcomes with actual outcomes. For the most part, these are practical applications only taught in clinical settings.

However, *The Neighborhood* provides the opportunity for instructors to implement such activities in the classroom by linking to characters and events. Teaching in this way is an example of integrative teaching, which Benner and Sutphen (2007) describe as signature pedagogy of expert teachers.

The following tips will help you get started using *The Neighborhood* in your classroom:

- **Tip #1:** Become familiar with the characters, stories, and community events for the season/semester in which you teach so that you can identify the most appropriate links to the content in your class.

- **Tip #2:** Think broadly about applications. Although specific content covered in class might not be represented in a *Neighborhood* story, conceptual links between content and stories can almost always be made. For example, you might teach a class on rheumatoid arthritis (RA), but you will not find a character who has RA in *The Neighborhood*. However, one of the characters has lupus; both RA and lupus are autoimmune disorders, and they share many common clinical features. Making these connections will strengthen and deepen your students' understanding of the underlying concepts involved.

- **Tip #3:** Be sensitive to the timing of stories. Depending on how you direct your students, they may only have read up to the current episode. It is important that learning activities be developed with consideration of how and when students read the content. In other words, do not develop a learning activity related to a *Neighborhood* event that (from the students' perspective) has not yet happened. Although you can still make links to class content before an event happens, you might need to link the content differently. For example, while teaching about stroke, you see that one of the characters experiences a stroke in Season 2, which the students may not be assigned to read yet. However, the character shows all the classic risk factors in Season 1, so you might plan a learning activity in which students conduct an analysis of risk factors for various characters to identify who is most at risk.

- **Tip #4:** Vary the learning activities and featured characters. No one likes to do the same thing over and over again, so it is important to modify the activities to keep learning interesting. Types of learning activities can range from those completed during class time to major course projects and assignments. It is most important that activities be purposeful. The beauty of *The Neighborhood* is that it is truly adaptable to almost any nursing course.

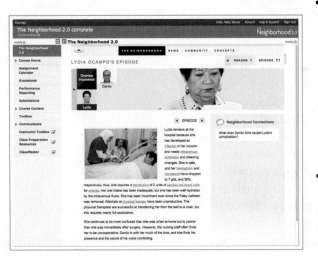

- **Tip #5:** Use *The Neighborhood* regularly. Student evaluations have shown that students become frustrated when they are asked to read *The Neighborhood* stories without application in class. Although it is not necessary to use the application in every class session to be successful, regular use is the perceived student benefit. Even during weeks when you do not have a specific class assignment, take a few minutes to reference *The Neighborhood* and give students a chance to share what is going on. This will help to keep them returning to *The Neighborhood* each week.

- **Tip #6:** Think about various ways you can use *The Neighborhood* characters/storylines. This should not be limited to just lecture or lab. Look for ways to help student make linkages between theory and clinical using *The Neighborhood* characters. If you are studying heart disease, ask students to compare a *Neighborhood* character with someone they cared for in clinical, or relate how a *Neighborhood* character is similar to or different from a patient during clinical debriefing sessions.

EXEMPLARY TEACHING STRATEGIES

Several instructional strategies can be used to teach using *The Neighborhood* characters and events, including the following learning activities: featured character case study, role-play, simulation, concept or topic analysis, games, comparing and contrasting, policy analysis, family history/genogram, concept map, small group discussion, and developing a care or teaching plan.

Featured Character Case Study

Perhaps the most obvious application of *The Neighborhood* is featuring the characters in a case study. This can be accomplished with any of the characters in any course; the possibilities for application of this type are endless. Case studies, particularly when done in small groups as an in-class assignment, provide a mechanism for dialog within the groups. Figure 1 (located in Appendix I) illustrates an example of a featured case study. You can use this or create your own.

Role-Play

Role-play is a learning strategy in which learners assume the roles of other individuals and act out specific situations. The situation may be unstructured or semistructured. Other students watch the interactions during the role-playing session, offer feedback, and critique the students. *The Neighborhood* stories provide multiple opportunities for role-playing. Because students know the characters, it is simple for them to assume the role and act in a way that is consistent with the personality of the character.

There are three phases to a role-play learning activity:

1. An overview or prebriefing, so students understand the objectives of the role-playing activity
2. The actual role-playing, which should take between 5 and 15 minutes
3. A debriefing, which usually involves a discussion regarding what was learned

Figure 2 (located in Appendix I) is one example of a role-play learning activity. You can use this or create your own.

Simulation

Simulation involves the imitation of a clinical situation that a student might encounter. Over the past decade, human patient simulation has become a prominent teaching strategy used in nursing education programs. Multiple benefits of human simulation have been identified; the most important include learner engagement and the opportunity to provide a safe environment in which to learn.

Simulation is an ideal way to infuse *The Neighborhood* characters into learning activities, through either actual character events or what-if scenarios. Because of the breadth of situations within the stories, simulation activities can range from simple (e.g., focusing on communication and wound care in Season 1) to complex (e.g., management of life-threatening illnesses in Seasons 2 and 3). Figure 3

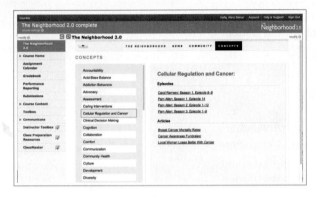

(located in Appendix I) shows one example of a simulation learning activity. Ten simulation scenarios have been provided for you in The Neighborhood 2.0 course.

Concept or Topic Analysis

A concept or topic analysis can be done in the form of a written assignment, a group project presentation, or an in-class assignment. In this activity, both a character and a problem are selected. Students are asked to analyze the character and the topic as they relate to the literature. Students gain a deep understanding of the topic as it presents in a clinical situation and how the character story is similar to and different from the presentation in the textbook or selected journal articles. Figure 4 (located in Appendix I) shows one example of a concept analysis learning activity. You can use this or create your own.

Games

The use of games to trigger active learning in the classroom and for independent learning is well described in the literature. There are multiple types of games that can be developed for instructional use; so many, in fact, that entire textbooks, sections of instructional textbooks, and websites are devoted to this topic alone. An important point about games is that they must be purposeful. A game that is fun but has no obvious purpose adds little value to the learning experience and can be perceived as a waste of time by students. Figure 5 (located in Appendix I) shows one example of a Jeopardy game linked to *The Neighborhood*. You can use this or create your own.

Comparing and Contrasting

Another effective learning strategy is to compare and contrast a selected topic across multiple characters. This enables students to develop an enhanced understanding of similarities and differences in presentation, effects, and outcomes related to the topic. Several topics addressed in *The Neighborhood* link to this activity, including hypertension, diabetes, oxygenation, and substance abuse. Figure 6 (located in Appendix I) shows one example of a comparing and contrasting learning activity. Use this or create your own.

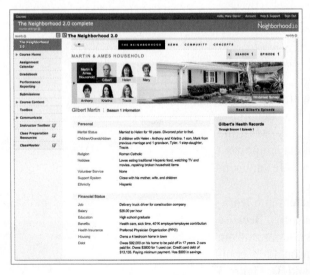

Policy Analysis

The Neighborhood provides the ability to analyze policy initiatives as they relate to professional nursing practice and community events. Community events are included in the character stories and featured in *The Neighborhood* news. A learning activity in which students study a specific policy or group of policies as they relate to characters or events in *The Neighborhood* helps students understand such initiatives as they apply to real-life situations. Figure 7 (located in Appendix I) features an example of a policy analysis learning activity involving injury prevention and protection; you can use this or create your own.

Family History/Genogram

An effective way to help students understand the benefits of taking a complete family history is by using information provided in *The Neighborhood*, specifically the biographical information of any of the characters. The complexity of the learning activity can be increased by enhancing existing content with additional information. With this additional information, students can draw a genogram for a given character or characters and use this information to identify risk factors for disease. Figure 8 (located in Appendix I) features an example of a genogram learning activity involving the Martin family; you can use this or create your own.

Concept Map

Concept maps have become popular as teaching strategies because they allow for the presentation of multiple primary concepts, interrelated concepts, and related linkages. They can be done as an independent learning assignment or as part of a group learning activity. There is significant variability with concept maps; therefore, there is no single correct way to use them. Learners identify the primary problems experienced by a *Neighborhood* character. Then, using a concept map, they show how the problems are interrelated. Figure 9 (located in Appendix I) features an example of a concept map activity; you can use this or create your own.

Small Group Discussion

Small group discussion involves an exchange of ideas about a situation or a specified topic. This approach fosters active student engagement, particularly when learning groups are small. (Between four and six learners is ideal.) Small group discussion is most effective when questions are interesting and thought provoking. Small group discussion can be geared for very short periods (5–10 minutes) or longer periods, depending on the learning goals. This application is useful for traditional classroom and online learning environments. Figures 10 and 11 (located in Appendix I) feature examples of small group discussion activities featuring *Neighborhood* characters; you can use these or create your own.

Developing a Care Plan or Teaching Plan

Learning to develop a care plan or a teaching plan can be challenging for students initially. Instructors can enhance this experience using the shared understanding of problems experienced by *Neighborhood* characters. Because data are already embedded in the stories, students and faculty have access to the same information, enabling instructors to provide more precise clarification and feedback to students. Figure 12 (located in Appendix I) shows an example of a care plan learning activity featuring a *Neighborhood* character, and Figure 13 is an example of a teaching plan learning activity. You can use these or create your own.

SPECIALTY COURSE USE AND SUGGESTED CHARACTERS

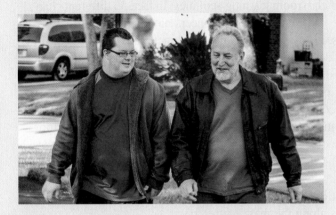

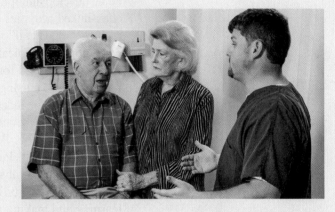

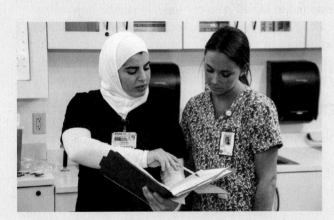

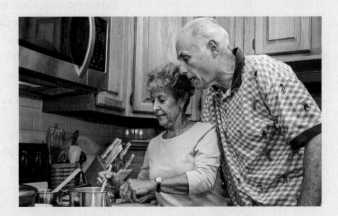

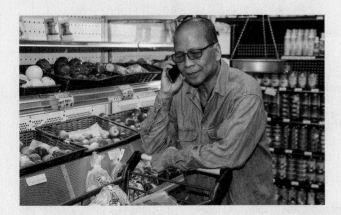

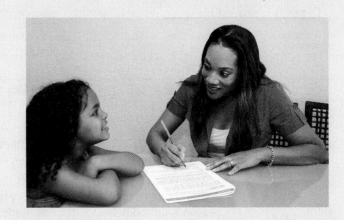

COURSE USE OVERVIEW

This section of the Faculty Navigation Guide links *The Neighborhood* character stories to content typically found in nursing courses. It is important to recognize that this section does not identify *all* possible linkages, because the extension of "what if" applications are not captured here. In addition, note that all of the teaching strategies described in Section I can be applied to most of these links. So, for example, an instructor who is interested in identifying different ways to teach the concept of elimination will find six characters who specifically experience problems related to elimination (see "Nursing Fundamentals—Basic Nursing Skills"). For each of these characters, the instructor could develop multiple types of classroom learning activities. In fact, 50 different character-linked activities could be generated from this concept alone—and this does not include the "what if" scenarios. In addition, a notation ▤ is included to indicate that a corresponding medical record is available for the episode and characters. A video link icon ▶ is included for each video. A news link table [NEWS] is provided for each of the courses to lead nursing faculty to additional story enhancements for learning. A journal notation ▼ is included for selected journal entries.

In this edition, three nursing students have been woven into the story as minor characters. Jennifer Porter, Jacob McCain, and Kayla Sharif are students who interact with Hospital, Public School, Senior Center, and Women's Health Services nurses. Like normal students, they learn, make mistakes, and begin to take on the roles and responsibilities that define nurses. Their mentors provide training, also learning and making mistakes along the way.

The potential applications of *The Neighborhood* stories to learning activities in nursing courses are truly endless, and to list all possible links would be impossible. However, this section is a helpful place to start. *The Neighborhood* Faculty User Forum is envisioned to be a repository of teaching strategies developed by faculty who are willing to share their work with others. Make sure to check this site periodically for newly added learning activities, and consider posting some of your own.

NURSING FUNDAMENTALS—BASIC NURSING SKILLS

Basic nursing principles and skills are featured throughout the stories in all three seasons of *The Neighborhood*. However, because these courses are typically taught in the first semester or term of most nursing programs, the most likely focus is on Season 1 stories. The following tables outline links to fundamental nursing concepts and basic nursing skills.

FUNDAMENTAL CONCEPTS

Concept Focus	Character Season/Episode	Comments	Additional Assets
Anorexia	Pam Allen S1E14-15 Season 2	As a consequence of chemotherapy and radiation therapy	▤s: S1E14, S2E5, S2E8; S1E15 ▶, S2E4 ▶; S2E4 ▼
Communication	Norma James Season 2, Episodes 6–10	Aphasia after stroke	S2E6 ▤
Elimination	Pam Allen, Season 1, Episodes 9–15	Oddly colored and shaped stools; constipation ends up being colorectal cancer; new colostomy and Foley catheter in postoperative period	S1E14 ▤
	Clifford Allen Season 1, Episodes 1–11	Urinary retention associated with benign prostatic hyperplasia (BPH); holmium laser enucleation of the prostrate (HoLEP)	S1E6 ▶, S1E8 ▶; S1E9 ▤ S1E8 [NEWS]: HoLEP Procedure for Senior Men

Key: ▶ = video clip   ▤ = medical record   ▼ = journal entry   [NEWS] = news article

FUNDAMENTAL CONCEPTS *continued*

Concept Focus	Character Season/Episode	Comments	Additional Assets
		Season 1, Episode 9: Foley catheter insertion and bladder irrigation	S1E9 ▤
	Greg Ross Season 1, Episode 14 Season 3, Episode 4	Diarrhea associated with acute exacerbation of colitis	S3E4 ▤
	Jessica Riley Season 2	Constipation associated with pregnancy	▤s: S2E1, S2E4, S2E7, S2E9, S2E11, S2E12
	Norma James Season 2, Episodes 6, 7	Problems with fecal and urinary incontinence after stroke; Foley catheter insertion	S2E6 ▤
	Eric Young Season 3, Episode 3	Infant diarrhea	
End of life	Pam Allen Season 3, Episodes 6–9	End stages of cancer; hospice nurse is involved	S3E6 ▶, S3E7 ▶, S3E8 ▶ S3E9 [NEWS]: Local Woman Loses Battle With Cancer
	Danilo Ocampo Season 2, Episodes 6–10	Danilo's deterioration as he attempts to care for Lydia alone at home Danilo having an MI and calling 911	S2E10 ▶; S2E10 ▤; S2E10 [NEWS]: Local Pathologist Dies
	Lydia Ocampo Season 3, Episode 10	Lydia dies in a nursing home	S3E10 [NEWS]: "Queen of Roses" Dies
	Shawn Jacobs Season 1, Episode 11 Season 3, Episode3	Reading about death of homeless person like a woman he treats Death of his patient, a veteran named Matt Nolan	S1E11 [NEWS]: Homeless Man Found Dead S3E3 [NEWS]: Local Vet Dies Outside Bar
Fatigue	Pam Allen Season 1, Episodes 12–15 Seasons 2, 3	Fatigue associated with cancer and cancer treatment	▤s: S2E5, S2E8, S3E2, S3E4
	Danilo Ocampo Seasons 1, 2	Fatigue and activity intolerance associated with chronic condition of heart failure and associated with stress of caregiver role	S1E12 ▶ S2E10 ▤
	Yvonne Johnson All Seasons	Yvonne complains about being tired. Fatigue as a symptoms of systemic lupus erythematosus (SLE) S3E6 to S3E15 debilitating fatigue and its consequences Effects of fatigue on family dynamics	S1E3 ▶, S1E13 ▶ Randall S3E6 ▶
	Jimmy Bley All Seasons	Fatigue and activity intolerance associated with chronic obstructive pulmonary disease (COPD)	▤s: S1E8, S2E10, S3E7, S3E10 S3E4 ▶
Infection	Norma James Season 1, Episodes 1–4 Season 2, Episode 7	Wound infection (diabetic ulcer); links with Karen Williams at the Senior Center Urinary tract infection from indwelling catheter	S1E3 ▶, S1E6 ▶ S2E6 ▤

continued

FUNDAMENTAL CONCEPTS *continued*

Concept Focus	Character Season/Episode	Comments	Additional Assets
Infection (cont.)	Lydia Ocampo Season 1, Episodes 10–12	Incision infection after open reduction with internal fixation (ORIF); links with nurses at Neighborhood Hospital	S1E10 ▤
	Pam Allen Season 1, Episode 14 Seasons 2, 3	Infection risk postoperatively in Season 1, Episode 14; infection risk in Seasons 2 and 3 associated with chemotherapy	▤s: S1E14, S2E2, S2E5, S2E8, S3E2, S3E4
	Ryan Riley Season 1, Episodes 14, 15	Respiratory syncytial virus (RSV)	
	Carrie Holmes Season 3, Episode 8	Seen in emergency department for otitis media	
	Marcus Young Season 1, Episode 9	Conjunctivitis—acute, one-time event	
Mobility	Lydia Ocampo Season 1, Episodes 10–15	Mobility problems after hip fracture; issues continue in other seasons; links with nurses at Neighborhood Hospital	S1E10 ▶, S1E10 ▤
	Norma James Season 2, Episodes 6–10	Mobility issues associated with stroke; rehabilitation	S2E6 ▤
	Ben Jaramillo Season 2, Episode 15	Ben has developed a stress fracture and has to wear a plastic boot for a few weeks.	S2E15 ▶
	Mark Martin Season 3, Episodes 4–15	Mobility issues associated with paraplegia after motor vehicle crash	S3E4 ▤ S3E04 [NEWS]: Auto Accident Leaves Local Man In Critical Condition; Nursing Staff Insensitive
	Marcus Young Season 3, Episodes 5–11	Bicycle accident, multiple fractures; acute care through home care/rehabilitation; links to	Season 3, Episode 5 [NEWS]: 7-Year-Old Hit by Car, Remains in Hospital
Nausea/ Vomiting	Jessica Riley Season 1, Episodes 10, 11	Nausea associated with pregnancy	S1E11 ▶
	Pam Allen All Seasons	Nausea in Season 1 related to postoperative nausea after colectomy; in Seasons 2 and 3, related to chemotherapy and radiation	▤s: S1E14, S2E5, S2E8; S1E15 ▶, S2E4 ▶; S2E4 ▽,
	Helen Martin Seasons 1, 2	Nausea in Season 1 related to cholelithiasis; Season 2 nausea/vomiting are associated with postoperative status	
Nutrition	Ryan Riley Season 1	Failure to thrive evolves over Season 1	
	Jenna Riley Seasons 1, 3	Adolescent obesity; ongoing story	S2E4 ▶
	Helen Martin Season 1	Adult obesity; cholelithiasis; attempts to manage condition through dietary modification	

Key: ▶ = video clip ▤ = medical record ▽ = journal entry [NEWS] = news article

FUNDAMENTAL CONCEPTS *continued*

Concept Focus	Character Season/Episode	Comments	Additional Assets
	Norma James Season 2, Episodes 7–10	Swallowing difficulties after stroke lead to need for tube feeding	S2E6 ▤
	Pam Allen Seasons 2, 3	Anorexia, nausea, and vomiting as side effects of chemotherapy and radiation lead to nutritional deficits	S2E4 ▶, ▤s: S2E5, S2E8
	Lydia Ocampo Season 1, Episode 10 Season 3	Dementia and nutrition problems begin after hip fracture and hospitalization; problems accelerate when placed in a nursing home in Season 3	S1E10 ▤
	Yvonne Johnson Season 1, Episode 3	Dr. Rowe suggests she loss weight and reduce her salt intake.	S1E3 ▶
	Violet Brinkworth All seasons	Violet monitors nutrition information and works to bring more nutritious foods into the schools	S1E13 [NEWS]: Childhood Obesity Rises S2E4 [NEWS]: Studies Show Inadequate Diets in Americans S2E14 [NEWS]: Vending Frustration S2E15 [NEWS]: Vending Viewpoints S3E2 [NEWS]: Changing Eating Habits S3E2 [NEWS]: Food Fight
Oxygenation	Jimmy Bley All Seasons	Advanced nursing skills in Season 3, Episodes 7–11 (respiratory failure, use of ventilator, sepsis)	S2E5 [NEWS]: Smoky Air Fills Healthcare Facilities with Patients COPD in Cecelia Bley S3E5 ▶; ▤s: S1E8, S2E10, S3E7, S3E10
	Ryan Riley Season 1, Episode 14	RSV	
	Kelsey Young Seasons 1, 2	Asthma	Angie Young S2E6 ▶ ▤s: S2E5, S2E6
	Zainah Kattan Season 2, Episode 5	Effects of forest fire on community and the hospital	S2E5 [NEWS]: Smoky Air Fills Healthcare Facilities with Patients
Pain	Ryan Riley Season 1, Episode 1	Infant pain from colic	
	Clifford Allen Season 1, Episode 9	Postoperative pain (bladder spasms)	S1E9 ▤
	Pam Allen Season 1, Episode 14	Postoperative pain (abdominal surgery)	S1E14 ▤
	Cecelia Bley All Seasons	Chronic pain from osteoarthritis	S1E9 ▶, S1E10 ▶; S2E2

continued

FUNDAMENTAL CONCEPTS *continued*

Concept Focus	Character Season/Episode	Comments	Additional Assets
Pain (cont.)	Yvonne Johnson Season 1, Episode 3	Yvonne sees Dr. Rowe complaining about being tired.	S1E3 ▶
	Helen Martin Seasons 1, 2	Intermittent pain associated with cholelithiasis	S1E2 ▶
	Gil Martin All Seasons	Chronic back pain in all seasons	
	Greg Ross Season 1, Episode 14 Season 3, Episode 4	Pain associated with acute exacerbations of colitis	S3E4 ▤
	Carrie Holmes Season 3, Episode 8	Infant pain from diarrhea	
Safety	Norma James Season 1, Episode 5 Season 2, Episode 15	Norma James is at risk for falls in home.	S2E15 ▶
	Lydia Ocampo All Seasons	Risk for injury in home; risk for injury while hospitalized due to exacerbated confusion; use of restraints in Season 1, Episode 10 due to combativeness in postoperative period; links with nurses at Neighborhood Hospital	S1E10 ▶; S1E10 ▤
	Anthony Martin	Risk for injury and suicide	▤s: S2E6, S2E13, S3E8
Self-care	Lydia Ocampo All Seasons	Dementia; functional limitations	S1E4 ▶
	Danilo Ocampo All Seasons	Limitations due to caregiver issues	S1E12 ▶
Sensory-perceptual	Jimmy Bley Seasons 1–3	Hearing deficits	▤s: S1E8, S2E10, S3E7, S3E10
	Mary Martin Seasons 1–3	Visual deficits; links with Karen Williams at Senior Center	
	Angelo Reyes Season 1, Episodes 12–14	Diabetic retinopathy; undergoes surgery for vitreous hemorrhage	
Skin integrity	Norma James Season 1, Episodes 1–4	Diabetic foot ulcer on leg; links with Karen Williams at Senior Center	S1E3 ▶, S1E6 ▶
	Lydia Ocampo Season 3, Episodes 2–10	Decubitus ulcer as a consequence of Alzheimer's disease, poor nutritional intake, and nursing home care	
	Mark Martin Season 3, Episodes 5–;10	Develops a decubitus ulcer as complication of paraplegia	S3E4 ▤
Sleep	Danilo Ocampo Seasons 1, 2	Problems sleeping due to poorly controlled heart failure; caregiver stress—particularly after Season 1, Episode 10	S1E12 ▶
	Lydia Ocampo Season 2, Episodes 8, 9	Dementia; tends to wander at night in Season 2	S2E8 ▶

Key: ▶ = video clip   ▤ = medical record   ▽ = journal entry   [NEWS] = news article

FUNDAMENTAL CONCEPTS *continued*

Concept Focus	Character Season/Episode	Comments	Additional Assets
	Jessica Riley All Seasons	Sleep deprivation associated with multiple roles	▤s: S1E15, S2E1, S2E4, S2E7, S2E9, S2E11, S2E12, S2E13
Spirituality	Pam Allen Season 1, Episode 1 Season 1, Episode 13 Season 2, Episodes 1, 4, 5, 6, 9, 11 Season 3, Episodes 4, 8, 9	Active member of church; receives support from members of church; anointing of sick; calls on parish priest (Father John) for spiritual comfort	▽s: S1E13 , S2E4, S3E4
	Mary Martin Season 3, Episodes 3, 5, 13	Prays for injured grandson	
	Evelyn Riley Season 1, Episode 2, 7, 11,13 Season 2, Episodes 3, 9, 10–14 Season 3, Episodes 9, 10	Prays for support and strength in helping her family	▽s: S1E2, S1E7, S1E11, S1E13, S2E3, S2E9, S2E10, S2E13, S3E9, S3E10

BASIC NURSING SKILLS

Featured Skill/Equipment	Character Season/Episode	Comments	Additional Assets
Blood transfusion	Lydia Ocampo Season 1, Episode 11	Transfusion to treat anemia (postoperative complication after ORIF)	S1E10 ▤
Documentation	Zainah Kattan Season 1, Episode 1	Describes difficulty finding time to chart; point-of-care charting	
	Carol Ramsey Season 1, Episode 2	Describes medical record transfer into a new system and the need to write office notes on a yellow pad	
Feeding tube	Norma James Season 2, Episodes 6–8	After stroke	S2E6 ▤
Foley catheter	Clifford Allen Season 1, Episode 9	Postoperative after HoLEP—has continuous bladder irrigation (CBI)	S1E9 ▤
	Pamela Allen Season 1, Episode 14	Postoperative after colectomy	S1E14 ▤
	Lydia Ocampo Season 1, Episodes 10–12	Postoperative after ORIF; links with nurses at Neighborhood Hospital	S1E10 ▤
	Norma James Season 2, Episodes 6–10	After stroke	S2E6 ▤
Injections (immunizations)	Karen Williams (Senior Center Nurse) Season 1, Episode 11	Supervises nursing students at immunization clinic	

continued

BASIC NURSING SKILLS *continued*

Featured Skill/Equipment	Character Season/Episode	Comments	Additional Assets
Intravenous (IV) therapy	Clifford Allen Season 1, Episode 9	Postoperative after HoLEP—has CBI	S1E9 🗐
	Pamela Allen Season 1, Episode 14 Seasons 2, 3	Postoperative after colostomy PICC line for chemotherapy	🗐s: S1E14, S2E2, S2E5, S2E8, S3E2, S3E4
	Lydia Ocampo Season 1, Episodes 10–12	Postoperative after ORIF	S1E10 🗐
	Norma James Season 2, Episodes 6–10	After stroke	S2E6 🗐
	Helen Martin Season 2, Episode 4	After cholecystectomy—IV therapy, including patient-controlled analgesia (PCA)	
	Angelo Reyes Season 2, Episode 8	IV therapy associated with Emergency Department (ED) visit for diabetic ketoacidosis	S2E8 🗐
	Danilo Ocampo Season 2, Episode 10	IV therapy associated with ED visit for acute myocardial infarction (AMI)/cardiac arrest	S2E10 🗐
	Jimmy Bley Season 3, Episodes 7–9	IV therapy associated with respiratory failure and sepsis	🗐s: S3E7, S3E10
Nasogastric (NG) tube	Pam Allen Season 1, Episode 14	Postoperative care after colectomy)	S1E14 🗐
Oxygen therapy	Jimmy Bley Season 3, Episodes 7–15	Intubation and subsequent oxygen therapy including oxygen therapy in home	🗐s: S3E7, S3E10
Positioning, transfers, body mechanics	Lydia Ocampo Season 1, Episodes 10–15 Seasons 2, 3	After ORIF Long-term care facility	
	Norma James Season 2, Episodes 6–10	Mobility issues associated with stroke; rehabilitation	S2E6 🗐
	Mark Martin Season 3, Episodes 4–15	Mobility issues associated with paraplegia after motor vehicle crash	S3E4 🗐
Postoperative care	Clifford Allen Season 1, Episode 9	After HoLEP	S1E9 🗐
	Lydia Ocampo Season 1, Episode 10	After ORIF link to nurses at Neighborhood Hospital	S1E10 🗐
	Pamela Allen Season 1, Episode 14	After colectomy	S1E14 🗐
	Helen Martin Season 2, Episode 4	After cholecystectomy	

Key: ▶ = video clip   🗐 = medical record   ▽ = journal entry   [NEWS] = news article

BASIC NURSING SKILLS *continued*

Featured Skill/Equipment	Character Season/Episode	Comments	Additional Assets
Restraints	Lydia Ocampo Season 1, Episode 10	Use of restraints due to combativeness in postoperative period; link to Bobby Schofield in Neighborhood Hospital	S1E10 📄 S1E10 ▶
	Anthony Martin Season 2, Episode 13	Psychosis, combative, restrained in ED and on unit to ensure safety	S2E13 📄
Wound care	Lydia Ocampo Season 1, Episodes 10–12 Season 3	Surgical incision decubitus ulcer	S1E10 📄
	Mark Martin Season 3, Episodes 4–11	Decubitus ulcer	S3E4 📄

ADULT HEALTH NURSING

Several character stories link closely to topics found in adult health nursing courses. Stories are found in all three seasons; therefore, it is important to remember that, depending on where your course falls in the curriculum, you can use stories from previous seasons. For example, if your course is a Season 2 course, you can use Season 1 and Season 2 stories.

Multiple household characters link directly to adult health concepts. Because the stories are all told from the perspective of the character, it is important to consider the stories of other household members to gain a perspective of the effects of an individual's health-related problem on other members of the household. In addition to the household characters, there are three featured characters in the Neighborhood Hospital and stories in the Neighborhood News that link to adult health course topics. The following tables present links to topics commonly addressed in adult health/medical–surgical nursing courses.

RESPIRATORY SYSTEM

Problem	Character Season/Episode	Comments	Additional Assets
Emphysema	Jimmy Bley All Seasons	Progression of disease from Season 1 to Season 3	📄s: S1E8, S2E10, S3E7, S3E10; S2E10 ▶, S3E5 ▶ S1E19 [NEWS] – Smoking Breaks a Thing of the Past? S2E5 [NEWS] – Forest Fire Continues to Burn S2E12 [NEWS] – Cutting Through the Smoke

continued

RESPIRATORY SYSTEM *continued*

Problem	Character Season/Episode	Comments	Additional Assets
Influenza	Kelsey and Marcus Young Season 1 Episodes 10 and 11	Kelsey and Marcus have the flu	S1E11 [NEWS]: Flu Shots Encouraged S1E11 [NEWS]: Flu Deaths Expected to Rise
Pneumonia	Jimmy Bley Season 3, Episodes 4–7	Evolution of a cough and upper respiratory infection to pneumonia	[医]s: S3E7, S3E10
Respiratory failure Acute phase through transition to home	Jimmy Bley Season 3, Episodes 7–11	Acute exacerbation of emphysema triggered by pneumonia; includes issues associated with transitioning to home and the rehabilitation process due to a deconditioned state after discharge	[医]s: S1E8, S2E10, S3E7, S3E10

CARDIOVASCULAR SYSTEM

Problem	Character Season/Episode	Comments	Additional Assets
Acute myocardial infarction (AMI)	Danilo Ocampo Season 2, Episode 10	As a complication of poorly managed heart failure	S2E10 [医]; S2E10 [▶]
Anemia	Lydia Ocampo Season 1, Episode 11	Links as a complication of ORIF	S1E10 [医]
	Pam Allen Season 1, Episode 14	Rectal bleeding from colorectal cancer	1E14 [医]
	Yvonne Johnson Season 3, Episode 10	Links as a complication of renal failure	
Atrial fibrillation	Norma James All Seasons	Links as a contributory factor to stroke	S2E6 [医]
Heart failure	Danilo Ocampo Seasons 1, 2	Presents typical symptoms and home management; acute exacerbation of symptoms in Season 1, Episodes 11, 14, 15 and in Season 2, Episodes 6–10	S2E10 [医]; S2E10 [▶]
Hypertension	Norma James All Seasons	As a comorbid condition	S1E6 [▶], S3E7 [▶]; S2E6 [医]
	Danilo Ocampo Seasons 1, 2	As a comorbid condition	S2E10 [医]
	Greg Ross All Seasons	New diagnosis in Season 1, Episode 7; focus is on side effects from antihypertensive medication	S2E13 [▶], S3E2 [▶]
Septic shock	Jimmy Bley Season 3, Episode 9	As a complication of pneumonia and respiratory failure	[医]s: S3E7, S3E10

Key: [▶] = video clip   [医] = medical record   [▼] = journal entry   [NEWS] = news article

NEUROLOGIC SYSTEM

Problem	Character Season/Episode	Comments	Additional Assets
Spinal cord injury Acute phase and rehabilitation hospital Transition and home care	Mark Martin Season 3, Episodes 5–10 Season 3, Episodes 11–15	Includes issues associated with common complications (depression, decubitus ulcer, autonomic dysreflexia) and impact on family; links to Neighborhood News in Season 3, Episode 4	S3E4 ▤ S3E4 NEWS: Auto Accident Leaves Local Man in Critical Condition; Nursing Staff Insensitive
Stroke Acute phase and rehabilitation hospital Home care	Norma James Season 2, Episodes 6–14 Season 3, ongoing	Includes issues with nonadherence to treatment plans in Season 1; multiple complications after stroke (speech, swallowing, incontinence, depression) and caregiving issues with transition home ; links to Karen Williams at Senior Center	S2E6 ▶ S2E6 ▤

MUSCULOSKELETAL SYSTEM

Problem	Character Season/Episode	Comments	Additional Assets
Chronic back pain	Gil Martin Season 1, Episodes 3, 6, 7, 9 Season 2, Episodes 3, 9	Coping mechanisms associated with ongoing chronic pain	
Hip fracture Acute phase rehabilitation after ORIF	Lydia Ocampo Season 1, Episodes 10–12 Season 1, Episodes 13–15 Season 2, Episodes 1, 2	Multiple related postoperative complications include delirium, anemia, mobility, and infection; multiple issues with rehabilitation and transition home	S1E10 ▤
Osteoarthritis	Cecelia Bley All Seasons	Story focus for Season 1, Episodes 2 and 6–10; in Season 2, concern regarding addiction to pain medication	S1E9 ▶, S1E10 ▶, S2E2 ▶
Osteoporosis	Mary Martin Season 1, Episodes 7–10	Screening, diagnosis, and treatment	Karen Williams S1E8 ▶
Pelvic fracture	Marcus Young Season 3, Episode 5	Read about Marcus's multiple fractures and laceration.	S3E05 NEWS: 7-Year-Old Hit by Car, Remains in Hospital
Spinal cord injury	Mark Martin Season 3, Episode 4	Read about Mark's spinal cord injury from his motor vehicle crash	S3E4 ▤; S3E04 NEWS: Auto Accident Leaves Local Man in Critical Condition; Nursing Staff Insensitive
Stress fracture	Ben Jaramillo Season 2, Episode 15	Ben develops a significant amount of pain and swelling in his leg	S2E15 ▶

GASTROINTESTINAL SYSTEM

Problem	Character Season/Episode	Comments	Additional Assets
Cholelithiasis	Helen Martin Seasons 1– through Season 2, Episode 4	Follows initial symptoms and diagnosis through surgery; postoperative pain and nausea	S1E2 ▶
Colorectal cancer	Pam Allen Season 1, Episode 14 through Season 3	Initial signs occur in Season 1, Episodes 12–14; issues associated with surgical procedure, body image, coping, nausea, vomiting, fatigue, nutrition, and neutropenia; end-of-life issues in Season 3	▤s: S1E14, S2E2, S2E5, S2E8, S3E2, S3E4; S1E13 ▶, S1E15 ▶, S2E4 ▶, S3E6 ▶ S2E3 [NEWS]: Cancer Awareness Fundraiser
	Clifford Allen Season 1, Episode 14	Clifford Allen talks with Pam's surgeon	S1E14 ▶
Crohn's disease	Greg Ross All Seasons	Exacerbations in Season 1, Episodes 13–15 and in Season 3, Episodes 4, 5	S3E4 ▤

UROLOGIC SYSTEM

Problem	Character Season/Episode	Comments	Additional Assets
Renal insufficiency and failure	Yvonne Johnson Season 3	As a complication of SLE; progression of renal insufficiency to renal failure	
Benign prostatic hyperplasia	Clifford Allen Season 1, Episodes 3, 5, 6, 7, 8, 9	Pharmacotherapy ineffective; symptoms progress to need for a HoLEP procedure	S1E5 ▶ S1E9 ▤ S1E8 [NEWS]: HoLEP Procedure for Senior Men
Urinary tract infection	Norma James Season 2, Episode 7	Associated with indwelling catheter	S2E6 ▤

METABOLISM AND NUTRITION

Problem	Character Season/Episode	Comments	Additional Assets
Inadequate nutrition	Violet Brinkworth Season 2, Episodes 4, 14, 15	Violet tries to bring healthier foods into school vending machines	S2E4 [NEWS]: Studies Show Inadequate Diets in Americans S2E14 [NEWS]: Vending Frustration S2E15 [NEWS]: Vending Viewpoints
Nausea and vomiting related to treatment for colorectal cancer	Pam Allen Season 2 Episode 4	Pam's nausea interferes with her getting the nutrition she needs	S2E4 ▶

Key: ▶ = video clip   ▤ = medical record   ▽ = journal entry   [NEWS] = news article

METABOLISM AND NUTRITION *continued*

Problem	Character Season/Episode	Comments	Additional Assets
Nutrition and type 2 diabetes	Violet Brinkworth Season 3, Episode 2	Violet sees Jenna Riley, who is showing some signs of type 2 diabetes; she reads articles on nutrition and fast food	S3E2 [NEWS]: Changing Eating Habits S3E2 [NEWS]: Food Fight
Obesity	Helen Martin All Seasons	Ongoing issue with weight; linked to gallbladder disease in Seasons 1 and 2	
Protein calorie malnutrition	Lydia Ocampo Season 3	Poor nutrition in nursing home	
Type 1 diabetes	Angelo Reyes All Seasons	Excellent adherence, well-controlled; complications featured: ketoacidosis and retinopathy	S2E9 ▶
Type 2 diabetes	Norma James All Seasons	Poor adherence and control; complications featured: foot ulcer, hypertension, and stroke	S1E3 ▶, S1E6 ▶; S2E6 ▤

IMMUNE SYSTEM

Problem	Character Season/Episode	Comments	Additional Assets
Systemic lupus erythematosus (SLE)	Yvonne Johnson All Seasons	Follows progression of disease from subtle to overt symptoms	S1E3 ▶, S1E13 ▶, S2E3 ▶
Immunization for influenza	Kelsey Young Season 1 Episodes 10 and 11	Influenza outbreak affects Kelsey and Marcus in Season 1 Episode 10	S1E11 [NEWS]: Flu Shots Encouraged
	Jimmy Bley Season 3 Episode 1	Jimmy refuses a flu shot	S1E11 [NEWS]: Flu Deaths Expected to Rise S3E1 ▶

ACID BASE/FLUID ELECTROLYTE DISTURBANCES

Problem	Character Season/Episode	Comments	Additional Assets
Dehydration/ hypernatremia	Angelo Reyes Season 2, Episode 8	Associated with ketoacidosis	S2E8 ▤
Hyperkalemia	Angelo Reyes Season 2, Episode 8	Associated with ketoacidosis	S2E8 ▤
Ketoacidosis	Angelo Reyes Season 2, Episode 8-9	Also has dehydration and hyperkalemia	S2E8 ▤; S2E9 ▶
Respiratory acidosis	Jimmy Bley Season 3, Episode 7	Associated with emphysema and respiratory failure	▤s: S3E7, S3E10

VISUAL AND AUDITORY SYSTEMS

Problem	Character Season/Episode	Comments	Additional Assets
Cataracts	Mary Martin All Seasons	Undergoes cataract surgery in Seasons 1 and 2	
Diabetic retinopathy	Angelo Reyes All Seasons	Experiences vitreous hemorrhage and undergoes vitrectomy in Season 1, Episode 12	
Glaucoma	Mary Martin All Seasons	Not the major focus of story, but part of health history	
Hearing loss	Jimmy Bley All Seasons	Contributes to communication issues with wife	S1E2 ▶; ▤s: S1E8, S2E10, S3E7, S3E10

NEIGHBORHOOD HOSPITAL LINKS

Topic	Season/Episode	Comments	Additional Assets
Colon cancer	Bobby Schofield Season 1, Episode 14	Links to Pam Allen	
Hip fracture care	Bobby Schofield Zainah Kattan Season 1 Episodes 10–13	Links to Lydia Ocampo	S1E10 ▤
Blood Supply	Season 1, Episode 2		S1E2 [NEWS]: Low Blood Supplies Alarm Medical Professionals

MATERNITY AND WOMEN'S HEALTH

Several featured characters in *The Neighborhood* represent women's health issues. The pregnancies of three characters (Jessica Riley, Angie Young, and Rachel Reyes) are followed from conception to birth, detailing prenatal and postpartum care. In all cases, a prenatal medical record is included. The stories of the nurse midwife (Carol Ramsey) provide further examples of pregnancy care and related practice issues. Other women's issues are reflected in the stories of Violet Brinkworth, Helen Martin, and Kristina Martin, and in the Neighborhood News. Because the stories are told from the perspective of the character, it is important to consider the impact on family members as well. The following tables present links to topics commonly found in maternity and women's health nursing courses.

PREGNANCY

Characteristic	Character Season/Episode	Comments	Additional Assets
High-risk pregnancy Cesarean section	Rachel Reyes Seasons 2, 3	Prenatal care; complications include preeclampsia in Season 3, Episode 4; hemolysis, elevated liver enzymes and low platelet count (HELLP) syndrome and premature delivery of twins in Season 3, Episode 5	▤s: S2E7, S2E9, S2E11, S2E13, S2E15, S3E1, S3E2, S3E4, S3E5; S3E2 ▶

Key: ▶ = video clip   ▤ = medical record   ▼ = journal entry   [NEWS] = news article

PREGNANCY *continued*

Characteristic	Character Season/Episode	Comments	Additional Assets
Unplanned teen pregnancy	Jessica Riley Seasons 1, 2	Prenatal care; links to domestic violence; abdominal trauma resulting in placental abruption; full-term, healthy infant links to Carol Ramsey, nurse midwife	📄s: S1E15, S2E1, S2E4, S2E7, S2E9, S2E11, S2E12, S2E13; S1E11 ▶, S1E13 ▶, S2E7 ▶, S2E9 ▶, S2E11 ▶,
Patient care provider— prenatal care, delivery, and postpartum care	Carol Ramsey Seasons 1–3	Nurse midwife; story reflects multiple patient and provider issues	S1E12 ▶, S2E7 ▶, S2E9 ▶, S2E11 ▶, S2E12 ▶
Planned pregnancy	Angie Young Seasons 1, 2	Prenatal care; full-term, healthy infant; no complications	S1E3 ▶, S2E1 ▶; 📄s: S1E10, S1E12, S1E15, S2E1, S2E4, S2E7 S2E1 [NEWS]: Childbirth Classes Begin This Week

WOMEN'S HEALTH ISSUES

Issue/Condition	Character Season/Episode	Comments	Additional Assets
Contraception	Carol Ramsey Season 1, Episodes 6, 7	Nurse midwife patient care provider	
	Jessica Riley Season 2, Episode 15	Contraception patch; postpartum anemia; links to Carol Ramsey, nurse midwife.	
	Kristina Martin Season 2, Episode 7	Oral contraceptives; links to Carol Ramsey, nurse midwife	S2E7 [NEWS]: Local Teen Pregnancy Numbers Down
Domestic Violence	Jessica Riley Season 1 Episodes 5, 13 Season 2	Jessica enters a relationship that becomes abusive	S1E13 ▶, S1E12 [NEWS]: Domestic Violence Hotline Established, S2E1 [NEWS]: Domestic Violence Top Cause of Death for Pregnant Women
Infertility	Rachel Reyes Season 1 Season 2, Episodes 1–6	Infertility workup and treatment; becomes pregnant in Season 2	S1E1 ▶
	Angelo Reyes Season 1, Episodes 1–2	Angelo discusses pregnancy and infertility with Rachel.	S1E1 ▶, S1E2 ▶
Menopause	Helen Martin All Seasons	Reference to menopause primarily in Season 1, Episodes 1–3 and Season 2, Episode 8	

continued

WOMEN'S HEALTH ISSUES continued

Issue/Condition	Character Season/Episode	Comments	Additional Assets
Sexuality, sexually transmitted infection (STI), and contraception in schools	Violet Brinkworth Season 3, Episodes 4–8	Attempting to provide adequate sex education and contraception in middle and high schools; principal in opposition	
Sexually transmitted infection	Kristina Martin Season 3, Episode 5	Chlamydia; links to Carol Ramsey, nurse midwife	

PEDIATRIC AND FAMILY NURSING

There are 13 featured infant, child, and adolescent characters in *The Neighborhood* stories. Infant through toddler-aged characters include Ryan Riley, Carrie Holmes, Eric Young, Peter and Marissa Reyes, and Tyler Martin. School-aged characters include Marcus and Kelsey Young and Jason Riley. Adolescent characters include Jenna Riley, Kristina and Anthony Martin, and Randall Johnson. Some of these characters (Eric Young, Carrie Holmes, Tyler Martin, and the Reyes twins) do not appear in *The Neighborhood* until Seasons 2 or 3. Most of these characters are healthy; their stories reflect well-child visits, typical episodic problems seen among children, or the effect of other situations occurring in the home. When possible, the stories of the younger children reflect their growth and development milestones.

In addition to these stories, stories involving the school nurse character (Violet Brinkworth) can be incorporated because of her interactions with children and adolescents. Finally, several links to pediatric and family nursing content are found in the Neighborhood News. Because the stories are told from the perspective of the character, it is important to consider the effects on other family members as well. The following tables present links to topics commonly found in pediatric and family nursing courses.

HEALTH PROMOTION AND WELLNESS

Featured Health Topic	Character Season/Episode	Comments	Additional Assets
Newborn care	Carrie Holmes Season 2, Episode 13	Full-term infant; describes after-birth care	S2E13 📋
	Eric Young Season 2, Episode 9	Full-term infant; describes after-birth care	
	Rachel Reyes	Rachel takes Peter and Marissa to see Carolyn Marquette for a follow-up visit.	S3E10 ▶
Well child visit and immunizations	Tyler Martin Season 2, Episodes 10, 14 Season 3, Episode 9	Information regarding height/weight, growth charts, vital signs, and immunizations are included	

Key: ▶ = video clip   📋 = medical record   🔽 = journal entry   [NEWS] = news article

HEALTH PROMOTION AND WELLNESS *continued*

Featured Health Topic	Character Season/Episode	Comments	Additional Assets
	Ryan Riley Season 1,Episode 3 Season 2, Episode 1 Season 3, Episodes 1, 14	Information regarding height/ weight, growth charts, vital signs, and immunizations are included	
	Carrie Holmes Season 3, Episode 14	Information regarding height/ weight, growth charts, vital signs, and immunizations are included	
	Eric Young Season 2, Episodes 9–11 Season 3, Episodes 2, 8, 15	Information regarding height/ weight, growth charts, vital signs, and immunizations are included	Angie Young S3E2 ▶
	Peter and Marissa Reyes Season 3, Episodes 3–13	Information regarding height/ weight, growth charts, vital signs, and immunizations are included	Rachel Reyes S3E13 ▶
	Randall Johnson Season 1, Episode 7	Sports physical examination; does not want mother in room during examination; nurse practitioner gets mother to agree to wait in the waiting room	S1E7 ▶
Screenings in school	Violet Brinkworth Season 1, Episode 4	Hearing and vision screening	

HEALTH-RELATED PROBLEMS

Problem	Character Season/Episode	Comments	Additional Assets
Allergic reaction	Tyler Martin Season 3, Episode 1	Allergy to peanuts	
Asthma	Kelsey Young All Seasons	Ongoing story; has acute exacerbation in Season 2, Episodes 5, 6 ; links to Violet Brinkworth	▤s: S2E5, S2E6
Attention deficit hyperactivity disorder	Jason Riley Seasons 1–3	Focus of story is problems in school and issues obtaining diagnostic workup and diagnosis; links to Violet Brinkworth	S2E6 ▶
Colic	Ryan Riley Season 1, Episode 1	ED visit; parent coping	
Conjunctivitis	Marcus Young Season 1, Episode 9	Acute, one-time event	
Dehydration	Ryan Riley Season 1, Episode 14	RSV and dehydration	
	Eric Young Season 3, Episode 3	Dehydration associated with diarrhea	Angie Young S3E3 ▶
Dental caries	Tyler Martin Season 2, Episodes 3, 8–14	As a result of poor hygiene and bottle mouth	Mary Martin S2E3 ▶

continued

HEALTH-RELATED PROBLEMS *continued*

Problem	Character Season/Episode	Comments	Additional Assets
Diabetes mellitus type 2	Jenna Riley Seasons 2, 3	Risk factors present in Season 1; early symptoms in Season 2; formally diagnosed in Season 3, Episodes 3–5	S3E5 ▶, S3E6 ▶, S3E14 ▶ S2E14; [NEWS]: Vending Frustration
Diarrhea	Eric Young Season 3, Episode 3	Infant diarrhea	Angie Young S3E3 ▶
Hyperbilirubinemia	Peter and Marissa Reyes Season 3, Episode 5	As a complication of prematurity	
Infant respiratory distress syndrome	Peter Reyes Season 3, Episode 5	As a complication of prematurity	
Nutrition	Ryan Riley Season 1, Episodes 7, 10, 15	Failure to thrive; poor infant weight gain	
	Kristina Martin All Seasons	Obsessed about being thin; excessive intentional weight loss	
	Jenna Riley All Seasons	Obesity	S2E4 ▶ S1E13 [NEWS]: Childhood Obesity Rises
Otitis media	Carrie Holmes Season 3, Episode 8	Seen in ED for otitis media	
Prematurity	Peter and Marissa Reyes Season 3, Episodes 5–15	As a complication of maternal preeclampsia	
Sexually transmitted infection	Kristina Martin Season 3, Episode 5	Chlamydia; links to Carol Ramsey	
Trauma	Marcus Young Season 3, Episodes 5–11	Bicycle accident, multiple fractures; story depicts acute care through home care/rehabilitation; links to Neighborhood News in Season 3, Episode 5	
Type 2 diabetes	Jenna Riley Seasons 2, 3	Risk factors present in Season 1; early symptoms in Season 2; formally diagnosed in Season 3, Episodes 3–5	S3E5 ▶, S3E6 ▶, S3E14 ▶ S2E14 [NEWS]: Vending Frustration
Upper respiratory infection	Eric Young Season 3, Episode 10	Mild case in infant	
Upper respiratory infection/RSV	Ryan Riley Season 1, Episode 14 Season 2, Episode 11	Required hospitalization in Season 1	

Key: ▶ = video clip   ▤ = medical record   ▽ = journal entry   [NEWS] = news article

FAMILY AND SOCIAL ISSUES

Problem	Character Season/Episode	Comments	Additional Assets
Domestic violence	Ryan Riley and Carrie Holmes All Seasons	Infant neglect in Season 1; mother is victim of domestic violence; social services follows well-being of children	Casey Holmes S1E4 ▶
Chronically ill parent	Randall Johnson All Seasons	Story addresses effect of mother's progressive illness on Randall	S3E6 ▶
	Tyler Martin Season 3	Story addresses effect of traumatic injury on Tyler's father	
Family in crisis	Martin family All Seasons	Story addresses effect on family in constant chaos	Helen S1E2 ▶ S2E8 ▶ Gil S3E7 ▶ Anthony S3E2 ▶, S3E11 ▶ Mary S3E12 ▶ Tracie S3E9 ▶
Gay/lesbian parenting	Carol Ramsey Season 2, Episodes 12 Season 3, Episodes 15	Carol sees Terry Clark who is thinking of giving her baby up for adoption to a gay couple.	S2E12 ▶, S3E15 ▶
	Greg Ross and Ben Jaramillo Season 2, Episodes 2 Season 2, Episodes 4 Season 3, Episodes 8 Season 3, Episodes 10	Greg and Ben go through the process of adoption.	S2E2 ▶, S3E10 ▶ Ben Jaramillo S2E4 ▶, S3E8 ▶
Parenting stress	Evelyn Riley All Seasons	Extreme stressors dealing with significant issues affecting welfare of all three children and grandchildren	S1E10 ▶
Potential Internet pedophile	Jenna Riley Season 3, Episodes 4–7	Story addresses Internet "boyfriend" and potential risks; links to Neighborhood News Season 2, Episode 10 and Season 3, Episode 10	S2E10 [NEWS]: Profile Site Appeal to Teens S3E10 [NEWS]: Sexual Predator Apprehended in Sting
Poverty and financial stress	Ryan Riley and Carrie Holmes All Seasons	Mother is single, works at restaurant and receives Medicare and WIC; boyfriend assists with finances at times	
	Johnson Family All Seasons	Yvonne loses job and benefits due to chronic illness; effect of change in socioeconomic status on teen	S3E13 ▶

SCHOOL NURSE TOPICS

Problem	Character Season/Episode	Comments	Additional Assets
Asthma	Violet Brinkworth Season 2, Episode 5	Kelsey Young has asthmatic attack; school nurse management	Kelsey Young 🗎s: S2E5, S2E6
Conjunctivitis outbreak management	Violet Brinkworth Season 1, Episode 9	Links to Marcus Young	S3E3 [NEWS]: Drug Rise Continues
Drug overdose, substance abuse, smoking	Violet Brinkworth Season 3, Episodes 13, 14	Monitors students rumored to be using drugs Student experiences overdose; principal criticizes school nurse for how she handles situation	S3E14 ▶ S3E7 [NEWS]: Teenage Girls Lead in Smoking, Drug Use
Hearing and vision screening	Violet Brinkworth Season 1, Episode 4	Links to Jason Riley	
Immunizations	Violet Brinkworth Season 3, Episode 10	Recordkeeping for children in Neighborhood Schools	S1E1 [NEWS]: Free Immunizations Peak Interests
	Zainah Kattan Season 1 Episode 1	Zainah volunteers at the immunization clinic	S1E1 [NEWS]: Immunizations Hit All-Time Low S1E1 [NEWS]: Medical Phobia Results in Tragedy
Learning problems	Violet Brinkworth Season 1, Episodes 2, 10 Season 2, Episodes 2, 3	Links to Jason Riley	
Nutrition in schools	Violet Brinkworth Season 1, Episodes 6, 12 Season 2, Episodes 8, 10, 15 (Kayla Sharif) S2E8 Season 3, Episode 1	Attempts to implement improved nutrition choices in schools and vending machines; encounters resistance from students and parents	S1E13 [NEWS]: Childhood Obesity Rises S2E4 [NEWS]: Studies Show Inadequate Diets in Americans S2E14 [NEWS]: Vending Frustration S2E15 [NEWS]: Vending Viewpoints S3E2 [NEWS]: Changing Eating Habits S3E2 [NEWS]: Food Fight
Safety	Marcus Young Season 2, Episode 14 Season 3, Episode 5	Marcus wants a bicycle	S2E14 [NEWS]: Pedaling to Safety S3E5 [NEWS]: 7-Year-Old Hit by Car, Remains in Hospital

Key: ▶ = video clip   🗎 = medical record   ▽ = journal entry   [NEWS] = news article

SCHOOL NURSE TOPICS *continued*

Problem	Character Season/Episode	Comments	Additional Assets
Sexuality, STIs, and contraception in schools	Violet Brinkworth Season 3, Episodes 4–8	Attempts to provide adequate sex education and contraception in middle and high schools; principal opposes	
Violence	Violet Brinkworth Season 1 Episode 8	Story addresses Internet predators	S1E8 [NEWS]: Gun Scare at Elementary School Ends in Expulsion S3E2 [NEWS]: Tragedy Strikes Family, Community
	Jason Riley Season 2 Episode 4	Jason is affected by bullying at school.	S2E4 [NEWS]: Neighborhood School Strikes Back at Bullying
	Jenna Riley Season 2, Episodes 10-15 Season 3, Episodes 4-10	Jenna becomes involved with an internet predator.	S2E10 [NEWS]: Profile Site Appeals to Teens S3E10 [NEWS]: Sexual Predator Apprehended in Sting

MENTAL HEALTH NURSING

Several mental health issues are featured in character stories and in the Neighborhood News. This edition offers a new nursing character, mental health practitioner Shawn Jacobs, DNP. Shawn works with established primary characters who experience mental health challenges: Clifford Allen and several members of the Martin family (Anthony, Helen, and Mark). Shawn also introduces new minor characters—such as several veterans, a homeless woman, a college-age addict—who come to the Health Connections Clinic for mental health care. Other primary characters experience mental health stresses related to behavior patterns, risk-taking, dementia, or substance dependency (Gil Martin, Kristina Martin, Lydia Ocampo, Jimmy Bley, and Bobby Schofield). Whether the stories are told from the perspective of the family member or the nurse, they highlight the fact that mental health issues affect both the individual and all those around them. The following tables present links to topics commonly found in mental health nursing courses.

PSYCHOTIC DISORDERS

Problem	Character Season/Episode	Comments	Additional Assets
Delirium	Lydia Ocampo Season 1, Episodes 10, 11	Delirium superimposed on dementia triggered by surgical procedure.	S1E10 ▤
Schizophrenia	Anthony Martin Seasons 1–3	Early symptoms in Season 1; psychotic break in Season 2, Episode 6	S3E4 ▶, S3E10 ▶ ▤s: S2E6, S2E8, S2E13, S3E4, S3E8, S3E10
	Links to Shawn Jacobs S3E10		S2E13 [NEWS]: Exposing Fears

COGNITIVE DISORDERS

Problem	Character Season/Episode	Comments	Additional Assets
Attention deficit hyperactivity disorder	Jason Riley All Seasons	Links to teasing, problems with social relationships, and behavioral issues	S2E6 ▶
	Evelyn Riley Season 2, Episode 8 Season 2, Episode 10	Evelyn takes Jason to the neuropsychologist.	S2E8 ▶, S2E10
Dementia	Lydia Ocampo All Seasons	Progressive dementia from Alzheimer's disease and caregiver issues	S1E4 ▶, S2E8 ▶ S2E1 [NEWS]: Alzheimer's Rising Statistics S2E6 [NEWS]: Laughing Away Alzheimer's
	Danilo Ocampo Season 1, Episodes 5	Danilo covers for Lydia when she does not recognize a neighbor.	S1E5 ▶

MOOD DISORDERS

Problem	Character Season/Episode	Comments	Additional Assets
Depression	Clifford Allen All Seasons	Primary diagnosis, exacerbated by death of spouse	S3E12 ▶
	Shawn Jacobs Season 3, Episodes 8–10; Season 3 Episodes 11, 13, 15	Shawn sees Clifford Allen for initial workup S3E8, follow up visits thereafter; grief counseling.	S3E12 ▶
	Mark Martin Season 3	Situational depression triggered by traumatic injury resulting in paraplegia; links to Shawn Jacobs Season 3, Episodes 6–8	S3E4 ▤
	Norma James Season 2, Episodes 6–15	Situational depression triggered by stroke resulting in hemiparesis	S2E6 ▤
	Anthony Martin Season 3, Episode 8	Dual diagnosis with schizophrenia	S3E8 ▤
	Shawn Jacobs Season 1, Episodes 5 and 11	Death of homeless man	S3E10 ▶ S1E11 [NEWS]: Homeless Man Found Dead
	Season 2, Episodes 4, 5, 10, 13	Shawn treats a vet (Blake Patterson) for major depression	
	Season 3, Episode 10	Shawn treats Anthony Martin for major depression and psychosis	

Key: ▶ = video clip   ▤ = medical record   ▼ = journal entry   [NEWS] = news article

OTHER MENTAL HEALTH ISSUES

Problem	Character Season/Episode	Comments	Additional Assets
Bipolar	Shawn Jacobs Season 1, Episode 5	Shawn treats woman with complex mental health and medical issues	
Anxiety	Helen Martin All Seasons	Overt symptoms begin Season 1, Episode 9	S1E9 ▶, S3E10 ▶
	Shawn Jacobs Season 3, Episodes 9, 10, 11, 13, 15	Treats Helen Martin; initial workup is S3E9	
Domestic violence	Jessica Riley and Casey Holmes All Seasons	Subtle initial indicators of domestic violence that escalates over time, especially with Jessica's pregnancy; links to Carol Ramsey	S1E13 ▶, S2E7 ▶, S2E9 ▶, S2E11 ▶, S3E5 ▶ Casey Holmes S1E4 ▶, S2E6 ▶ S1E12 NEWS: Domestic Violence Hotline Established S2E1 NEWS: Domestic Violence Top Cause of Death for Pregnant Women
	Evelyn Riley Season 3, Episode 5	She tells Jessica that she knows Casey is beating her and pleads with her to get away from him	S3E5 ▶
	Kelsey Young Season 1, Episode 12	Kelsey and her friends hear Victoria's parents arguing loudly and then hear Victoria's mother crying	S1E12 ▶
Eating disorder	Kristina Martin All Seasons	Obsession with thinness; begins excessive dieting in Season 1, Episode 11	
Pedophilia	Neighborhood News Season 3 Episodes 2–4 and 10 Zainah Kattan Season 3 Episodes 2–4	Sexual predation Ethical dilemma	S3E4 ▶ S3E2 NEWS: Tragedy Strikes Family, Community S3E3 NEWS: Suspect in Rape Case Injured During Chase S3E4 NEWS: Suspected Rapist Complains of Poor Medical Treatment S3E10 NEWS: Sexual Predator Apprehended in Sting

continued

OTHER MENTAL HEALTH ISSUES *continued*

Problem	Character Season/Episode	Comments	Additional Assets
Substance abuse	Neighborhood News	Drunk driving fatalities	S1E5 [NEWS]: Accident Ends in Death of Two
	Bobby Schofield All Seasons	Multiple substances; substance abuse as it affects professional nursing practice; diversion program	S3E11 [NEWS]: Robbing Spree Ends in Deadly Crash S1E9 [NEWS]: Drug Use Rise Continues S3E3 [NEWS]: Announcement: Conference Focuses on Substance Abuse
	Casey Holmes All Seasons	Multiple substances; links to domestic violence	S3E3 [NEWS]: Drug Use Rise Continues
	Mark Martin All Seasons	Alcohol; links to driving while intoxicated and traumatic injury	S3E4 [≣] S3E4 [NEWS]: Auto Accident Leaves Local Man in Critical Condition; Nursing Staff Insensitive S3E6 [NEWS]: March MADDness
	Clifford Allen Seasons 2, 3 Season 2 Episode 6	Alcohol; featured as ineffective coping Clifford's drinking problem	S2E6 [▶]
	Gil Martin All Seasons	Alcohol; featured as ineffective coping	
	Shawn Jacobs Season 1, Episodes 2, 4, 8, 10, 14, Season 2, Episodes 1 and 2 Season 3, Episodes 5	Shawn treats Amanda Hardin for substance abuse; initial workup S1E2	S1E2 [▶], S1E14 [▶], S3E5 [▶]
	Shawn Jacobs Season 1, Episodes 8, 9, 12,	Shawn Treats Aaron Hidalgo; initial workup Season 2, Episode 8	
	Shawn Jacobs Season 1, Episodes 1, 3, 11, 13, 14 Season 2, Episodes 5, 6 Season 3, Episode 3	Shawn treats Matt Nolan for substance abuse and anger issues; initial workup done S1E1	S1E13 [▶], S2E6 [▶]
Post-traumatic stress disorder	Shawn Jacobs Season 1, Episodes 6, 7, 15 Season 2, Episode 14 Season 3, Episode 1	Shawn Sees Sal Lucero; initial workup Season 1 Episode 6 Shawn listens to Sal Lucero describe his symptoms.	S1E7 [▶]
	Greg Ross Season 2, Episodes 3	Greg and Ben discuss how Sal would benefit from a therapy dog.	S2E3 [▶]
	Shawn Jacobs Season 2, Episodes 10	Shawn sees Blake Patterson about his relationship problems with his wife and daughter	S2E10 [▶]
	Steve Young Season 1, Episodes 10	Steve and Angie discuss Blake Patterson's return from military duty and his readjustment.	S1E10 [▶]

Key: [▶] = video clip   [≣] = medical record   [▽] = journal entry   [NEWS] = news article

OTHER MENTAL HEALTH ISSUES *continued*

Problem	Character Season/Episode	Comments	Additional Assets
Dog Therapy	Shawn Jacobs	Links to News	S1E9 [NEWS]: Therapy Dogs: Fur Therapy in Assisted Living
	Season 1 Episodes 9, 15		S1E15 [NEWS]: Funding Cuts to Therapy Dogs
	Season 2, Episodes 2, 3, 14		S2E2 [NEWS]: Furry Friends, Healers?
	Season 3, Episode 1		S2E3 [NEWS]: PTSD Veteran Seeks Therapy Dog

GERIATRIC NURSING

There are six featured geriatric household characters in *The Neighborhood*: Danilo and Lydia Ocampo, Jimmy and Cecelia Bley, Norma James, and Mary Martin. In addition, Karen Williams (the geriatric nurse specialist at the Neighborhood Senior Center) is a featured character whose story reflects multiple issues of concern among older adults. The Neighborhood News also includes multiple references to health-care concerns of older adults. Because the stories are told from the perspective of the character, it is important to consider the effects on other family members as well. The following tables present links to topics commonly found in geriatric nursing courses.

HEALTH-RELATED CONDITIONS

Problem	Character Season/Episode	Comments	Additional Assets
Acute myocardial infarction	Danilo Ocampo Season 2, Episode 10	As a complication of poorly managed heart failure)	S2E10 ▤, S2E10 ▤; S2E10 ▶
Anemia	Lydia Ocampo Season 1, Episode 11	Links as a complication of ORIF	S1E10 ▤
Atrial fibrillation	Norma James All Seasons	Links as a contributory factor to stroke	
Cataracts	Mary Martin All Seasons	Undergoes cataract surgery in Seasons 1, 2	
Delirium	Lydia Ocampo Season 1, Episodes 10, 11	Delirium superimposed on dementia triggered by surgical procedure	S1E10 ▤; S1E10 ▶
Dementia	Lydia Ocampo All Seasons	Progressive dementia from Alzheimer's disease; caregiver issues	S1E4 ▶, S2E8 ▶ Danilo Ocampo S1E5 ▶
Depression	Norma James Season 2, Episodes 6–15	Situational depression triggered by stroke resulting in hemiparesis	S2E6 ▤
	Clifford Allen All Seasons	Depressive disorder exacerbated by wife's illness and death	S3E12 ▶
Diabetes mellitus type 2	Norma James All Seasons	Poor adherence, poor control; complications featured: foot ulcer, hypertension, and stroke	S1E3 ▶, S1E6 ▶; S2E6 ▤

continued

HEALTH-RELATED CONDITIONS *continued*

Problem	Character Season/Episode	Comments	Additional Assets
Emphysema	Jimmy Bley All Seasons	Progression of disease from Seasons 1 to 3	📄s: S1E8, S2E10, S3E7, S3E10; S2E10 ▶, S3E4 ▶, S3E5 ▶
Glaucoma	Mary Martin All Seasons	Glaucoma is part of health history, but not major emphasis of stories; increased intraocular pressure as a result of nonadherence to eye drop regimen	
Hearing loss	Jimmy Bley All Seasons Season 1 Episode 2	Story focus is the effect of hearing loss on relationship and communication (particularly with his wife)	S1E2 ▶; 📄s: S1E8, S2E10, S3E7, S3E10
Heart failure	Danilo Ocampo Seasons 1, 2	Presents typical symptoms and home management; acute exacerbation of symptoms in Season 1, Episodes 11, 14, 15 and in Season 2, Episodes 6–10	S2E10 📄; S2E10 ▶
Hip fracture Acute phase through rehabilitation	Lydia Ocampo Season 1, Episode 10 Season 2, Episode 2	Multiple related postoperative complications, including delirium, anemia, mobility, and infection; story describes issues with rehabilitation, transitional care, and caregiving.	S1E10 📄
Hypertension	Norma James All Seasons	As a comorbid condition	S1E6 ▶, S3E7 ▶; S2E6 📄
	Danilo Ocampo Seasons 1, 2	As a comorbid condition	S2E10 📄
Osteoarthritis	Cecelia Bley All Seasons	Story focus for Season 1, Episodes 2 and 6–10; in Season 2, she has ongoing concern regarding addiction to pain medication	S1E9 ▶, S1E10 ▶, S2E2 ▶
Osteoporosis	Mary Martin Season 1	Screening in Season 1, Episode 7; diagnosis and treatment begin in Season 1, Episode 10	Karen Williams S1E8 ▶
Protein calorie malnutrition	Lydia Ocampo Season 3	As a consequence of progressive dementia and living in nursing home	
Pneumonia	Jimmy Bley Season 3, Episodes 4–7	Follows the evolution of a "cough" and simple upper respiratory infection to pneumonia	📄s: S3E7, S3E10
Respiratory acidosis	Jimmy Bley Season 3, Episode 6	Associated with emphysema and respiratory failure	📄s: S3E7, S3E10
Respiratory failure Acute phase, hospitalization, and transition home	Jimmy Bley Season 3, Episodes 7–11	Acute exacerbation of emphysema triggered by pneumonia; includes issues associated with transitioning to home and the rehabilitation process due to a deconditioned state after discharge	📄s: S3E7, S3E10

Key: ▶ = video clip   📄 = medical record   🔽 = journal entry   📰 = news article

HEALTH-RELATED CONDITIONS *continued*

Problem	Character Season/Episode	Comments	Additional Assets
Septic shock	Jimmy Bley Season 3, Episode 9	As a complication of pneumonia and respiratory failure	📄s: S3E7, S3E10
Stroke Acute phase through rehabilitation	Norma James Season 2, Episodes 6–14 Season 3, Ongoing	Includes issues with noncompliance with treatment plans in Season 1; multiple complications after stroke (speech, swallowing, incontinence, depression) and caregiving issues as she transitions to home	S2E6 📄

FAMILY AND SOCIAL ISSUES

Problem	Character Season/Episode	Comments	Additional Assets
Elder Abuse	Karen Williams (with Jacob McCain) Season 1 Episode 12 Season 2, Episode 7	Also links to Bobby Schofield Season 2, Episode 7	
Advance Directives	Clifford Allen Season 1, Episodes 14	Advance Directives are an important part of planning when Pam becomes ill again	S1E14 NEWS: Advance Directives Seminar Offered
	Cecelia Bley Season 3, Episodes 9	The physician asks Cecelia what she wants to do if Jimmy's heart stops.	S3E09 ▶
Caregiving	Norma James Season 2, Episodes 11–14 Season 3, Episodes 1–4	Son moves in to be mother's caregiver	S2E12 ▶, S2E15 ▶, S3E2 ▶
	Danilo Ocampo Seasons 1, 2	Managing care of wife with Alzheimer's disease and after hospital discharge; receives assistance from family member for a few episodes; after family member leaves, Danilo Ocampo is overwhelmed	S1E5 ▶, S1E12 ▶, S1E15 ▶, S2E5 ▶
	Cecelia Bley Season 3, Episodes 11–15	Managing care of husband after hospital discharge; receives assistance from family members	S3E11 ▶
	Mary Martin Season 3, Episodes 10–15	Mary becomes Mark's primary caregiver after discharge from spinal cord injury rehabilitation	
Financial concerns	Norma James All Seasons	Limited income; payment for medications a concern	S1E13 ▶
	Mary Martin Season 1, Episodes 3, 14	Widow with limited income; moves in with son; cuts corners with glaucoma medication to make it last longer	Gil Martin S1E2 ▶
	Karen Williams Season2	Karen continues to be aware of financial issues among seniors who visit the Center	S2E13 NEWS: Nest Eggs Hardly "Grade-A"
Functional status	Karen Williams Season 1, Episode 1 Season 3, Episode 7	Assessment of functional status in elderly clients	

continued

FAMILY AND SOCIAL ISSUES *continued*

Problem	Character Season/Episode	Comments	Additional Assets
Health promotion (elder)	Mary Martin Season 1, Episodes 7, 9, 10	Interest in participation at health fair; compliant with medication and walking to minimize osteoporosis	
	Cecelia Bley Season 1, Episode 7 Season 3, Episode 1	Interest in health fair and receiving flu shot; encourages Jimmy to receive flu shots and quit smoking	Jimmy Bley S3E1 ▶
	Jimmy Bley Season 3, Episode 1	Jimmy refuses the flu shot.	S3E01 ▶
	Karen Williams (with Jacob McCain) Season 1, Episode 11	Immunization clinic at Senior Center	S1E11 [NEWS]: Flu Shots Encouraged
	Karen Williams (with Jacob McCain) Season 1 Episode 9	Smoking Awareness	S1E9 [NEWS]: Smoking Breaks a Thing of the Past?
	Karen Williams (with Kayla Sharif) Season 1, Episode 7)	Health Fair	S1E7 [NEWS]: Health Fair Welcomes All
Power of attorney	Danilo Ocampo Season 1, Episode 6	Initial planning for wife's care in the event that he dies before she dies	
	Lydia Ocampo Beginning Season 2, Episode 10	No plans were finalized by husband before his death; family attorney has power of attorney over her care	
Transitional care	Lydia Ocampo Season 1, Episodes 12–15 Season 2, Episodes 1–3	Issues surrounding discharge coordination and care issues after arriving at home	Danilo S1E12 ▶; S1E15
	Norma James Season 2, Episodes 8–14	Issues surrounding discharge coordination and care issues after arriving at home	S2E12 ▶, S2E15 ▶, S3E2 ▶
	Jimmy and Cecelia Bley Season 3, Episodes 11–15	Issues surrounding discharge coordination and care issues after arriving at home	S3E11 ▶

SENIOR CENTER NURSE TOPICS

Topic	Character Season/Episode	Comments	Additional Assets
Elder abuse	Karen Williams (with Jacob McCain) Season 1, Episode 12 Season 2, Episode 7	Recognizes possible elder abuse; contacts social services; links to Neighborhood News in Season 2, Episode 7–9	S1E12 ▶ S2E7 [NEWS]: National Center on Elder Abuse Releases Warning Signs S2E8 [NEWS]: Rising Number of Elder Abuse Cases S2E9 [NEWS]: Nursing Home Abuse and Neglect Widespread

Key: ▶ = video clip   ▤ = medical record   ▽ = journal entry   [NEWS] = news article

SENIOR CENTER NURSE TOPICS *continued*

Topic	Character Season/Episode	Comments	Additional Assets
Independent living	Karen Williams Season 1, Episode 1	Family attempting to "force" man into moving to assisted living	
Health-care access	Karen Williams Season 1, Episodes 3, 10 Season 2, Episode 14	Facilitates and encourages seniors to obtain appointments for various conditions	S1E3 ▶ S2E2 [NEWS]: Senior Center Visits on the Rise
Health promotion	Karen Williams All Seasons	Smoking Awareness (with Jacob McCain) Episode, Season 1, Episode 9	S1E9 [NEWS]: Smoking Breaks a Thing of the Past?
		Flu Vaccinations, (with Jacob McCain) Season 1, Episode 11	S1E11 [NEWS]: Flu Shots Encouraged
		Senior Center Outing, Season 2, Episode 2	S2E2 [NEWS]: Members of Senior Center to Visit National Park
		Fitness for Elders, Season 3, Episode 13	S3E13 [NEWS]: Encouraging the Elderly to Exercise
		Health Fair (with Kayla Sharif) Season 1, Episode 7	
Health teaching	Karen Williams All Seasons	Karen talks with Norma about her medications and gives her information about managing her diabetes; Season1, Episode 14 (with Jacob McCain)	S1E3 ▶, S1E6 ▶, S1E8 ▶; S1E10
		Osteoporosis—Mary Martin, Season 1, Episode 8, 14 (with Kayla Sharif Episode 8)	S2E5 [NEWS]: Forest Fire Continues to Burn
		Forest fire—Season 2, Episode 5	
		Cataracts Mary Martin, Season 1, Episode 14 (with Jacob McCain); cataract surgery—Season 2, Episode 15	S3E5 [NEWS]: Senior Center Set to Host Talk
		Medication management (with Jennifer Porter)—Season 3, Episodes 3, 5	
Professional boundaries	Karen Williams Season 2, Episode 1	Sets limits with seniors who request special assistance and favors	S2E9 ▶, S2E11 ▶
	Season 2, Episode 9, 11	Karen talks with Eloise Saunders about what patient care she can perform.	
Professional behavior	Karen Williams with Kayla Sharif Season 1, Episode 3	Corrects inappropriate behavior of student.	S1E3 ▶
Social isolation	Karen Williams Season 1, Episode 10 Season 3, Episodes 1, 7	Recognizes social isolation among some residents	

COMMUNITY HEALTH

There are multiple opportunities to use and apply *The Neighborhood* stories in community health courses. Topics found in the character stories and the Neighborhood News span all types of community events. In the following table, various community topics that are commonly addressed in community health courses are described, along with the character or characters.

COMMON COMMUNITY HEALTH TOPICS

Topic	Character Season/Episode	Comments	Additional Assets
Battered women's shelter	Jessica Riley Season 2, Episodes 11	Carol Williams shares with Jessica shelter information.	S2E11 ▶
	Season 3, Episodes 9–11	Seeks protection from Casey with her two children	
Community assessment	Not applicable	Go to Community Facts link on home page for community health-care resources, demographics, jobs, income, and so on	
Community deaths reported in the News	Season 1, Episodes 4–14	Domestic homicide	S1 ongoing News: Police Report: Local Man Dies, Cause Unknown … to … Trial Report: Murder Trial Ends in Conviction
	Violet Brinkworth Season 1, Episode 5	Drunk driving crash	S1E5 [NEWS]: Accident Ends in Death of Two
	Season 1, Episode 11	Homeless man	S1E11 [NEWS] - Homeless Man Found Dead
	Danilo Ocampo Season 2, Episode 10	Danilo Ocampo has MI	S2E10 [NEWS]: Local Pathologist Dies
	Season 3, Episode 1	Worker at local factory	S3E1 [NEWS]: Local Man Dies in "Freak Accident"
	Season 3, Episodes 2	Child abduction, rape	S3E2 [NEWS]: Tragedy Strikes Family, Community
	Shawn Jacobs Season 3, Episode 3	Matt Nolan (patient of Shawn Jacobs)	S3E3 [NEWS]: Local Vet Dies Outside Bar
	Season 3, Episode 8	Infant murder	S3E8 [NEWS]: Teen Charged With Murder of Infant
	Pam Allen Season 3, Episode 9	Pam Allen dies of colorectal cancer	S3E9 Local Woman Loses Battle With Cancer
	Lydia Ocampo Season 3, Episode 10	Lydia Ocampo dies in nursing home	S3E10 [NEWS]: "Queen of Roses" Dies
	Casey Holmes Season 3, Episode 11	Casey Holmes and accomplice flee police, causing fatal crash	S3E11 [NEWS]: Robbing Spree Ends in Deadly Crash

Key: ▶ = video clip   ▤ = medical record   ▼ = journal entry   [NEWS] = news article

COMMON COMMUNITY HEALTH TOPICS *continued*

Topic	Character Season/Episode	Comments	Additional Assets
Community events (partial list)	Season 1, Episode 6	Rodeo	S1E6 [NEWS]: Mosey Down to the Rodeo Grounds
	Season 2, Episode 2 (links to Karen Williams)	Senior center trip	S2E2 [NEWS]: Members of Senior Center to Visit National Park
	Season 2, Episode 5	Science fair	S2E5 [NEWS]: Middle School to Host Science Fair
	Season 2, Episode 10	Cardiopulmonary resuscitation (CPR) class	S2E10 [NEWS]: Hospital to Offer Life-Saving Course
	Season 2, Episode 11	Music event	S2E11 [NEWS]: Event May Make People Play a Different Tune
	Season 2, Episodes 13–14 (links to Gary Allen)	Special Olympics	S2E13 [NEWS]: Special Olympics Golf Tournament Next Week
	Season 3, Episode 4	Running club	S3E4 [NEWS]: Run, Neighborhood, Run!
	Season 3, Episode 8	Macular degeneration lecture	S3E4 [NEWS]: Lecture to Help People See Danger
	Season 3, Episode 10	Swimming lessons	S3E10 [NEWS]: Swimming Classes to Be Offered
	Season 3, Episode 14	Gay/lesbian awareness	S3E14 [NEWS]: Pride Parade Addresses Inequities
Community health department	Kristina Martin Season 2, Episode 7 Season 3, Episode 5	Utilizes the community health department for oral contraceptives and for sexually transmitted infection workup	
	Mark and Tyler Martin Season 2, Episode 8, 14 Season 3, Episodes 2, 9	Community Health Clinic Free immunizations and dental care	S2E8 [NEWS]: Campaign Puts Smiles on Faces
Community services	Mary Martin and the Bley and Young families Season 1, Episode 7	Health Fair events and screening described within stories; links to Neighborhood News, Season 1, Episode 7	S1E7 [NEWS]: Health Fair Welcomes All
	Season 1, Episode 15	Cancer center	S1E15 [NEWS]: New Treatment Facility Planned
	Season 2, Episodes 3, 12 Season 3, Episodes 6	Retirement community	S3E6 [NEWS]: Forum Open to Discuss Proposed Community

continued

COMMON COMMUNITY HEALTH TOPICS *continued*

Topic	Character Season/Episode	Comments	Additional Assets
Community services (cont.)	Season 1, Episode 4	Poison control hotline	S1E4 [NEWS]: Hotline Puts Families at Ease
	Season 3, Episode 12	Homeless shelter	S3E12 [NEWS]: Homeless Shelters Running at Critical Capacity
Community support groups	Season 2, Episode 9	Support group	S2E9 [NEWS]: Group Wants to Hear Your Troubles
	Season 3, Episode 1	Grief and bereavement	S3E1 [NEWS]: Seminar Offers Closure
	Season 3, Episode 9	Meditation group	S3E9 [NEWS]:Meditation Group Forming
Environmental issues	Forest fire Season 2, Episode 5	Mentioned in several stories, most significant effect on Jimmy Bley and staff at Neighborhood Hospital	S2E5 [NEWS]: Forest Fire Continues to Burn S2E5 [NEWS]: Smoky Air Fills Healthcare Facilities with Patients
	Season 2, Episode 11	Noise control	S2E11 [NEWS]: Road Construction Woes
	Season 2, Episode 12	Smoking ban	S2E12 [NEWS]: Cutting Through the Smoke
	Season 3, Episode 11	Trash burning	S3E11 [NEWS]: Bin Burning Ban to Begin
	Season 1, Episode 3	Water pollution	S1E3 [NEWS]: Officials Confirm Pollution Worries
	Season 3, Episode 6	Water supply	S3E6 [NEWS]: Water Supply Breached— Broken Water Line?
Health fair	Mary Martin and the Bley and Young Families Season 1, Episode 7	Events and screening described within stories; links to Neighborhood News, Season 1, Episode 7	S1E7 [NEWS]: Health Fair Welcomes All
Healthcare issues	Season 3, Episode 13	Cancer mortality rising	S3E13 [NEWS]: Breast Cancer Mortality Rates
	Season 2, Episode 9 (links to Danilo Ocampo)	Caregiver issues	S2E9 [NEWS]: Group Wants to Hear Your Troubles
	Season 1, Episode 13	Childhood obesity	S1E13 [NEWS]: Childhood Obesity Rises

Key: ▶ = video clip   ☰ = medical record   ▼ = journal entry   [NEWS] = news article

COMMON COMMUNITY HEALTH TOPICS *continued*

Topic	Character Season/Episode	Comments	Additional Assets
	Season 2, Episodes 7 and 9	Elder abuse	S2E7 [NEWS]: National Center on Elder Abuse Releases Warning Signs
			S2E8 [NEWS]: Rising Number of Elder Abuse Cases
			S2E9 [NEWS]:Nursing Home Abuse and Neglect Widespread
	Season 1, Episode 1, Season 1, Episode 11	Immunizations	S1E1 [NEWS]: Free Immunizations Peak Interests
			S1E1 [NEWS]: Immunizations Hit All-Time Low
			S1E1 [NEWS]: Medical Phobia Results in Tragedy
			S1E1 [NEWS]: Local Immunization Protest Ends in Arrest
			S1E11 [NEWS]: Flu Shots Encouraged
			S1E11 [NEWS]: Flu Deaths Expected to Rise
	Season 3, Episode 12	Spider bites	S3E12 [NEWS]: Black Widow Outbreak Worries Residents
	Season 2, Episode 7	Teen pregnancies	S2E7 [NEWS]: Local Teen Pregnancy Numbers Down
	Season 3, Episode 7	Teen smoking increasing	S3E7 [NEWS]: Teenage Girls Lead in Smoking, Drug Use
Occupational health/injury	Season 1, Episodes 2, 9		S1E2 [NEWS]: Budget Cuts Increase Strike Concerns
			S1E9 [NEWS]: Smoking Breaks a Thing of the Past?
	Season 3, Episode 1		S3E1 [NEWS]: Local Man Dies in "Freak Accident"

continued

COMMON COMMUNITY HEALTH TOPICS *continued*

Topic	Character Season/Episode	Comments	Additional Assets
Public policy	Bobby Schofield Season 1, Episode 9	**Smoking ban** Links to Neighborhood News, Season 1, Episode 9	S1E9 [NEWS]: Kicking the Habit
	Season 2, Episode 12	Citywide smoking ban	S2E12 [NEWS]: Cutting Through the Smoke
	Season 2, Episodes 14, 15 (Violet Brinkworth)	Junk food ban	S2E14 [NEWS]: Vending Frustration S2E15 [NEWS]: Vending Viewpoints
	Season 2, Episode 7	MP3 player ban	S2E7 [NEWS]: Proposed Music Ban
	Season 1, Episode 12	Pit bull ban	S1E12 [NEWS]: Citizens Seek Pit Bull Ban
	Season 3, Episodes 11, 13	Speed bumps	S3E11 [NEWS]: Bumping Up Safety S3E13 [NEWS]: Safety Crusader Met With Mixed Reception
	Season 3, Episodes 3, 6	Substance abuse	S3E3 [NEWS]: Drug Use Rise Continues S3E6 [NEWS]: March MADDness
	Season 3, Episode 11	Trash burning ban	S3E11 [NEWS]: Bin Burning Ban to Begin
Public safety	Angie Young Season 3, Episodes 9–13	Attempts to lobby city to install speed bumps; links to Neighborhood News, Season 3, Episodes 11 and 13	S3E11 [NEWS]: Bumping Up Safety S3E13 [NEWS]: Safety Crusader Met with Mixed Reception
	Jenna Riley Season 2 Episode 12 to Season 3 Episode 9	A sexual predator stalks Jenna on Facebook	S2E10 [NEWS]: Sexual Predator Apprehended in Sting
	Season 2, Episode 14 (links to Young family)	Bicycle safety	S2E14 [NEWS]: Pedaling to Safety
	Season 2, Episode 1	Child safety seats	S2E1 [NEWS]: Child Seat Manufacturers Given a Crash Course in Safety
	Season 2, Episode 1	Domestic violence	S2E1 [NEWS]: Domestic Violence Top Cause of Death for Pregnant Women

Key: ▶ = video clip   ▤ = medical record   ▼ = journal entry   [NEWS] = news article

COMMON COMMUNITY HEALTH TOPICS *continued*

Topic	Character Season/Episode	Comments	Additional Assets
	Season 2, Episodes 7 and 9	Elder abuse	S2E7 [NEWS]: National Center on Elder Abuse Releases Warning Signs
			S2E8 [NEWS]: Rising Number of Elder Abuse Cases
			S2E9 [NEWS]:Nursing Home Abuse and Neglect Widespread
	Season 1, Episode 8	Gun scare at school	S1E8 [NEWS]: Gun Scare at Elementary School Ends in Expulsion
	Season 2, Episode 10 Season 3, Episode 10 (links to internet predator stalking Jenna Riley Season 2 Episode 12 to Season 3 Episode 9)	Internet predators	S2E10 [NEWS]: Profile Sites Appeal to Teens
	Season 1, Episode 10	Pit bull attack	S1E10 [NEWS]: Pit Bull Attacks Child
	Season 1, Episodes 5, 9 Season 3, Episodes 3, 4 (links to Mark Martin) Season 3, Episode 11 (links to Casey Holmes)	Substance abuse	S1E5 [NEWS]: Town Meeting Will Focus on Drunk Driving
			S1E9 [NEWS]: Drug Use on the Rise
			S3E34 [NEWS]: Accident Leaves Local Man in Critical Condition; Nursing Staff Insensitive
			S3E11 [NEWS]: Robbing Spree Ends in Deadly Crash
	Season 1, Episode 4	Terrorism	S1E4 [NEWS]: Terrorism Concerns Reach Community

HEALTH PROMOTION

Health promotion concepts are represented throughout the character stories and the Neighborhood News. For this reason, health promotion courses link well to *The Neighborhood* regardless of the placement of the course within the curriculum. Several characters make ongoing efforts to improve or enhance health, whereas others do not seem to give much thought to health promotion behaviors. The following tables summarize the links that can be made in character stories and the Neighborhood News.

HEALTH PROMOTION

Topic	Character Season/Episode	Comments	Additional Assets
Alzheimer's prevention	Lydia Ocampo All Seasons	Preventive measures can be taken in relation to dementia	S2E1 [NEWS]: Alzheimer's Rising Statistics S2E6 [NEWS]: Laughing Away Alzheimer's
Childbirth classes	Carol Ramsey Season 2, Episode 1 Angie and Steve Young Season 2, Episode 1 Rachel and Angelo Reyes Season 2, Episode 15	Describes plans to attend classes or teach classes	S2E1 [NEWS]: Childbirth Classes to Begin This Week
Dental screening and community-based dental care	Mark Martin, Tyler Martin , Tracie Ames Season 2, Episodes 8, 14 Season 3, Episode 2	Aunt Tracie takes Tyler to screening; follow-up dental work needed	S2E8 [NEWS]: Campaign Puts Smiles on Faces
Exercise and fitness (partial list)	Ben Jaramillo All Seasons	Exercise as a way of life	S3E4 [NEWS]: Run, Neighborhood, Run
	Zainah Kattan Season 1, Episode 3 Season 2, Episode 3 Season 3, Episode 13	Run for the Fish participant; having trouble finding time for exercise; Walk for Life organizer; aerobics class	S1E3 [NEWS]: Run—Not Swim—for Fish
	Karen Williams Season 3, Episode 13	Geriatric exercise	S3E13 [NEWS]: Encouraging the Elderly to Exercise
Health teaching	Mary Martin, Bley and Young Familes, Carol Ramsey Season 1, Episode 7	**Health fair** Events and screening described within stories	S1E7 [NEWS]: Health Fair Welcomes All
	Karen Williams (with Jennifer Porter) Season 3, Episode 5	**Medication management (elders)**	S1E6 [▶], S1E10 [▶], S3E5 [NEWS]: Senior Center Set to Host Talk
	Norma James Season 1, Episode 13 Season 2, Episodes 2, 11	Refilling prescription Hoarding medications	S1E6 [▶], S1E10 [▶], S1E13
	Jimmy Bley Season 1 Season 2	Smoking cessation	S2E10 [▶]
Hearing and vision screening	Violet Brinkworth (with Jacob McCain) Season 1, Episode 4	Screening at Neighborhood School; links to Jason Riley	
	Casey Holmes Season 1, Episode 4	**Hearing protection** Context of on-the-job ear protection	
Immunizations	See Pediatric and Family Nursing		

Key: [▶] = video clip   [≡] = medical record   [▽] = journal entry   [NEWS] = news article

HEALTH PROMOTION *continued*

Topic	Character Season/Episode	Comments	Additional Assets
Nutrition	Violet Brinkworth Seasons 1–3, ongoing	Efforts to improve nutrition at school	
Prenatal care	See Maternity and Women's Health		
Safe sex/sex education	Carol Ramsey Season 1, Episodes 6, 7 Season 2, Episode 7 Season 3, Episode 5	At health fair and with clients; links to Kristina Martin	
	Violet Brinkworth Season 3, Episodes 4, 6, 7	School-based education and resistance from principal	
Smoking cessation	Steve Young Season 1, Episodes 4–6 Season 2, Episode 12 through Season 3	Depicts one unsuccessful attempt to stop smoking, followed by success	
	Jimmy Bley Season 1, Episodes 8–12 Season 2, Episodes 3–6 Season 2, Episodes 10–14	Depicts three unsuccessful attempts to stop smoking	S2E10 ▶
Support groups	Shawn Jacobs Season 1, Episode 7 and Season 2, Episode 12 Season 2, Episode 9 Season 3, Episode 1 Season 3, Episode 9	Group theraapy Support group Grief and bereavement Meditation group	
Well infant and child care	See Pediatric and Family Nursing		

NURSING LEADERSHIP AND PROFESSIONAL CONCEPTS COURSE

The nurse character stories provide the basis for most of the links made to content that is typically taught in a leadership or professional nursing roles course. Concepts are divided between typical practice issues and roles of professional nurses. The Neighborhood News also presents stories that provide the basis for many learning activities. The following tables summarize the content, concepts, character stories, and news linkages that can be made.

PROFESSIONAL PRACTICE ISSUES

Topic/Issue	Character Season/Episode	Comments	Additional Assets
Bed control	Zainah Kattan Pat Richman Season 2, Episode 5	Bed control due to excessive hospital admissions and ED need associated with forest fire	S2E5 [NEWS]: Smoky Air Fills Healthcare Facilities with Patients
Budget	Karen Williams Season 2, Episode 2 Season 3, Episode 6	Budget restraints in clinic; must justify service for funding; writes letter to request additional funding	

continued

PROFESSIONAL PRACTICE ISSUES *continued*

Topic/Issue	Character Season/Episode	Comments	Additional Assets
Ethics	Lydia Ocampo Season 1, Episode 10	Placed in restraints; links to Bobby Schofield, who medicated her to keep her quiet	S1E10 ▤ S1E10 ▶ Bobby Schofield S1E10 ▶
	Violet Brinkworth Season 2, Episode 6 Season 3, Episode 1	Medical privacy issues; links to Health Insurance Portability and Accountability Act (HIPAA)	
	Zainah Kattan Season 3, Episodes 4 Pat Richman Season 3, Episodes 3, 4	Accused rapist and murderer on inpatient unit reporting poor care; links to Neighborhood News, Season 3, Episodes 2–4	S3E4 ▶ S3E4 ▧: Suspected Rapist Complains of Poor Medical Treatment
	Pat Richman Season 2, Episode 3	Pat has a meeting with Bobby this week to discuss the complaint filed by Dr. Ocampo.	S2E3 ▶
	Pat Richman Season 2, Episode 8–10	Mr Alden dies, and Pat wonder what how the abuse investigation is going.	S2E9 ▧: Nursing Home Abuse and Neglect Widespread
	Karen Williams (with student nurse Jacob McCain about elder abuse – Mr. Alden Season1E5, 12	Karen Williams (with student nurse Jacob McCain about professional obligation to report elder abuse with Mr. Alden)	S1E12 ▶
	Shawn Jacobs Season 1, Episode 10 Season 3, Episode 12	Privacy regarding treatment of family members	
Impaired nurse	Bobby Schofield All Seasons	Closely links to stories of Zainah Kattan and Pat Richman; story progresses from initial behavior to diversion program with the Board of Nursing	S3E1 ▶, S3E15 ▶ Zainah Kattan S2E4 ▶
Insurance and payment systems	Jessica Riley Biography page	WIC assistance and Medicaid	
	Mary Martin Season 1, Episode 14	Prescription assistance program	
	Gil Martin Season 2, Episode 15 Anthony Martin Season 3, Episode 8, 10,	Maxes out insurance coverage for mental health	S3E10 ▶ ▤s: S3E8, S3E10
	Yvonne Johnson Season 3, Episodes 8, 12–14	Loses job and insurance; COBRA insurance coverage, attempting to obtain social security disability	
Legal Issues	Karen William Season 2, Episodes 9, 11	Karen talks with Eloise Saunders about what patient care she can perform.	S2E9 ▶, S2E11 ▶

Key: ▶ = video clip ▤ = medical record ▼ = journal entry ▧ = news article

PROFESSIONAL PRACTICE ISSUES *continued*

Topic/Issue	Character Season/Episode	Comments	Additional Assets
Legal—power of attorney	Danilo Ocampo Season 1, Episode 6	When Danilo dies, Lydia has no family to care for her	
	Lydia Ocampo Season 2, Episodes 11, 12		
Mandatory reporting	Karen Williams Season 1, Episode 12 Season 2, Episode 7	Suspects elder abuse, notifies social services	S1E12 ▶ S2E7 NEWS: Is Elder Abuse on the Rise?
	Zainah Kattan Pat Richman Season 2, Episodes 5, 6	Suspects drug impairment of staff nurse; links to Bobby Schofield	
Medical records	Carol Ramsey Season 1, Episode 2	Describes difficulty associated with transferring old medical records into a new computerized system.	
	Violet Brinkworth Season 1, Episode 13 Season 3, Episode 10	Maintaining and updating medical records of students in Neighborhood Schools	
Nursing shortages, workload, and nursing strike	Pat Richman All Seasons	Ongoing theme in story	S1E8 NEWS: Health Career Fair This Weekend S2E6 NEWS: Mandatory Overtime Angers Nurses, Cite Unsafe Work Conditions S2E6 NEWS: The Myth of the Nursing Shortage? S3E5 NEWS: Nursing Strike Imminent? S3E8 NEWS: Nurses Walk Out, Cite Poor Working Conditions S3E10 NEWS: Hospital Strike Ends
	Zainah Kattan Season 1, Episodes 1–3, 6, 15 Season 2, Episode 3	Increased patient loads in context of hospital inpatient unit	
	Bobby Schofield Season 1, Episode 2	Staffing shortages in context of hospital inpatient unit	
	Violet Brinkworth Season 1, Episode 5	Shortage of help; issues associated with covering three schools	
	Karen Williams Season 2, Episode 2	Increasing number of senior visits to clinic despite reduced nursing hours	
	Carol Ramsey Season 1, Episodes 1, 14 Season 3, Episodes 1, 13	Increasing patient loads in context of advance practice nurse in group practice	

continued

PROFESSIONAL PRACTICE ISSUES continued

Topic/Issue	Character Season/Episode	Comments	Additional Assets
Nursing shortages, workload, and nursing strike (cont.)	Zainah Kattan Season 3, Episodes 8-10 Pat Richman Season 3, Episodes 5–10	Links to Neighborhood News, Season 3, Episodes 5–10	S3E10 ▶
Policy	Neighborhood Hospital nurses Season 2, Episodes 5, 6	Mandatory overtime policy announced; eventually leads to strike	
	Pat Richman Season 2, Episodes 13, 14	Employee policy for drug testing	
	Violet Brinkworth Season 3, Episodes 13, 14	School principal disciplines Violet for not following after-school policy regarding notification for health-care emergencies	S3E14 ▶
	Karen Williams Season 3, Episode 6	Letter writing for clinical financing	
Professional development	Pat Richman Season 3, Episodes 6-15	Pat and Debbie Koch discuss continuing education; Pat decides to go for advanced degree	S3E6 ▶
	Zainah Kattan Season 3, Episode 2	She joins a state level professional work group on nursing education.	
	Shawn Jacobs Season 2, Episode 11 Season 3, Episode 10	Presentations and professional meetings	
Recruitment	Karen Williams Season 2, Episode 10 Violet Brinkworth Season 3, Episode 9	Calls from nurse recruiter with job offer at Neighborhood Hospital	
	Pat Richman Season 1, Episodes 1, 7 Season 3, Episode 10	Recruitment and hiring of hospital nurses	S1E8 [NEWS]: Health Career Fair This Weekend
Referral/ collaboration of care	Violet Brinkworth Season 1, Episode 9 Season 1, Episode 14 Season 2, Episode 5 Season 3, Episodes 2, 13	Several examples of referral to another healthcare provider based on assessment and clinical judgment	S1E14 ▶
	Carol Ramsey Season 1, Episode 9 Season 2, Episodes 3, 12	Examples of referral to another healthcare provider based on assessment and clinical judgment	
	Karen Williams Season 1, Episode 3, 8 Season 3, Episode 12	Examples of referral to another healthcare provider based on assessment and clinical judgment	S1E3 ▶, S1E8 ▶
Social services	Jessica Riley Season 1, Episode 15 Season 2, Episodes 13, 14	Social services involved due to concern for child safety; links to Carrie Holmes and Ryan Riley, Season 3, Episodes 2, 6	▤s: S2E13

Key: ▶ = video clip   ▤ = medical record   ▼ = journal entry   [NEWS] = news article

PROFESSIONAL PRACTICE ISSUES *continued*

Topic/Issue	Character Season/Episode	Comments	Additional Assets
Workplace morale	Pat Richman All Seasons	Story from perspective of nurse manager	
	Zainah Kattan Season 2, Episodes 5-6	Story from perspective of staff nurse	

ROLES OF THE PROFESSIONAL NURSE

Role/Behavior	Character Season/Episode	Comments	Additional Assets
Advocate	Karen Williams Season 1, Episodes 3, 10–12 Season 2, Episodes 8, 14 Season 3, Episodes 7,11	Examples of patient advocacy in her practice	S1E3 ▶, S1E10 ▶,
	Carol Ramsey Season 1, Episodes 12 Season 2, Episodes 11, 12 Season 3, Episodes 2, 3,	Examples of patient advocacy in her practice	S1E12 ▶, S2E12 ▶
	Zainah Kattan Season 2, Episode 4	Zainah notices patients complaining about poor pain control when she follows Bobby's shift.	S2E4 ▶
	Bobby Schofield Season 1 Episodes 10 Zainah Kattan	See Bobby Schofield, Season 1, Episode 10 for example of lack of advocacy	S1E10 ▶
Boundary setting	Karen Williams Season 2, Episode 1	Role-modeling	
Care provider	Zainah Kattan All Seasons	Context of acute care in hospital, new graduate	
	Bobby Schofield All Seasons	Context of acute care in hospital	
	Karen Williams All Seasons	Context of community care in senior center	S1E3 ▶ S1E6 ▶, S1E8 ▶, S1E10 ▶, S1E12 ▶
	Violet Brinkworth All Seasons	Context of community-based care in schools	
	Carol Ramsey All Seasons	Context of advanced nursing practice	
Community service	Zainah Kattan Season 1, Episodes 1, 11	Volunteer at immunization clinic	
		Volunteer at senior center for flu shots	
	Season 2, Episode 3	Volunteer at Walk for Life event	
	Carol Ramsey Season 2, Episode 1	Teaches childbirth classes as community service	
Educator	Karen Williams Season 1, Episodes 3–12, 14 Season 2, Episodes 5, 15 Season 3, Episodes 3, 5, 10, 11	Multiple examples of teaching as a component of nursing practice	S1E3 ▶ S1E6 ▶, S1E8 ▶, S1E10 ▶, S1E12 ▶

continued

ROLES OF THE PROFESSIONAL NURSE *continued*

Role/Behavior	Character Season/Episode	Comments	Additional Assets
Educator (cont.)	Carol Ramsey Season 1, Episode 6 Season 2, Episodes 1, 7, 15 Season 3, Episodes 5, 7	Multiple examples of teaching as a component of nursing practice; teaches childbirth classes as community service	
	Violet Brinkworth Season 3, Episodes 4–8	Sex education classes in the middle school	
Empathy	Zainah Kattan Season 1, Episodes 10–13 Season 2, Episode 10	Empathy, attachment, and grief related to Mr. and Mrs. Ocampo; see Bobby Schofield, Season 1, Episodes 8, 14 for examples of lack of empathy	
Linking to community resources	Karen Williams	Mrs. James—transportation to physician office	S1E3 ▶
	Season 1, Episode 3	Mrs. James—properly fitting shoes	S1E10 ▶
	Season 1, Episode 10	Brian James—transitional care	
	Season 3, Episodes 1, 7	Senior Center Ride Service	
Manager/leader	Pat Richman All Seasons	**Bed control (inpatient)** – Nurse manager at Neighborhood Hospital	S1E7 [NEWS]: Emergency Department Sees Critical Capacities S2E5 [NEWS]: Forest Fire Continues to Burn S2E5 [NEWS]: Smoky Air Fills Healthcare Facilities with Patients
Orientation/mentor	Carol Ramsey Season 3, Episode 7	Begins process of orienting and mentoring a new midwife who has joined the practice	
	Violet Brinkworth Season 2, Episode 11	Begins process of orienting two new health aides to work at schools	
Practice improvement project	Shawn Jacobs Season 1, Episodes 7, 11 Season 2, Episode 3, 7, 9, 10, 15 Season 3, Episodes 2, 4	Barriers to access and patient satisfaction	
Professional behavior	Zainah Kattan Karen Williams All Seasons	These two characters are positive role models of professionalism (with a few exceptions on Kate's part)	
	Zainah Kattan Season 1, Episode 8	Zainah questions Bobby about his call lights being on when he is in the break room.	S1E8 ▶
	Pat Richman Season 1, Episode 5	Pat Richman discusses accountability with Zainah, Jennifer and Bobby in association with medication administration.	S1E5 ▶

Key: ▶ = video clip   ▤ = medical record   ▼ = journal entry   [NEWS] = news article

ROLES OF THE PROFESSIONAL NURSE *continued*

Role/Behavior	Character Season/Episode	Comments	Additional Assets
	Pat Richman Season 2, Episode 3	Pat and Debbie Koch discuss Bobby's behavior with student nurse Kayla.	S2E3 ▶
	Bobby Schofield Seasons 1–2	Bobby exhibits unprofessional behaviors towards his patients throughout the seasons	S1E8 ▶, S1E10 ▶
	Karen Williams (with Kayla) Season 1 Episode 3	Karen reminds Kayla that she should not talk about patients with other seniors at the center.	S1E3 ▶
	Zainah Kattan (with Kayla) Season 2, Episode 2	Flirting at work	
Advanced practice role	Carol Ramsey All seasons/episodes		
	Shawn Jacobs All seasons/episodes		
Evidence-based practice	Carol Ramsey (with Kayla) Season 3 Episode 2		

FEATURED CHARACTER OVERVIEWS AND STORIES

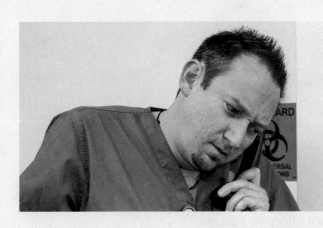

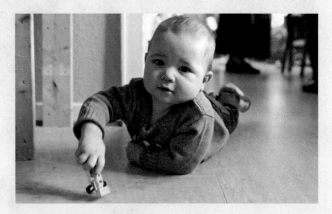

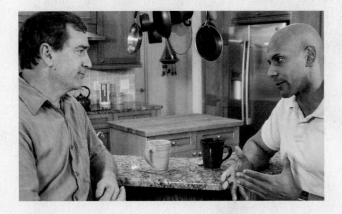

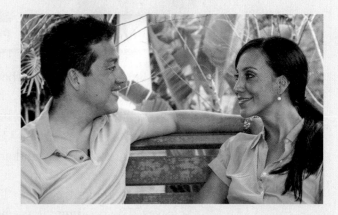

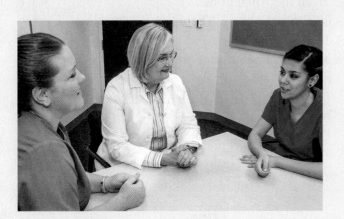

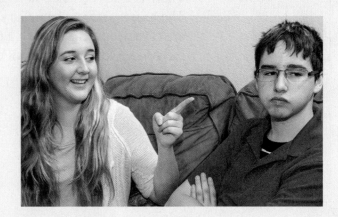

ALLEN HOUSEHOLD

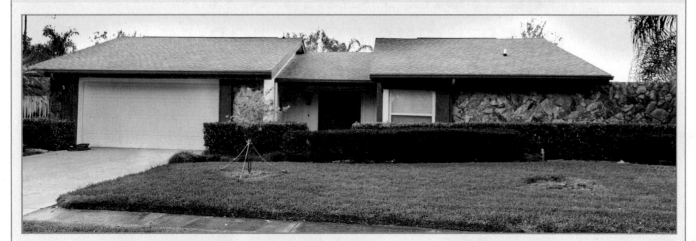

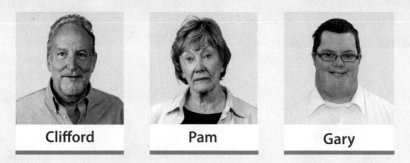

Clifford   **Pam**   **Gary**

Housing   The Allens live in the Riverbank area. They live in a 1-story, single-family, frame house. The house is 50 years old and has been well maintained. They have a small fenced yard.

Parks and Recreation   There is a large park about 3 blocks from the Allen's home. It has a children's playground and a track for running and walking. At the edge of the area there is a YMCA that has both an indoor and an outdoor pool. The Y also holds various exercise classes. The bowling alley where Clifford plays on a league is a short drive.

Services   There is a convenience store 2 blocks from the Allen home. The grocery store where Gary works is 12 blocks away. There are several churches within a 6-block radius of the home and the public elementary school is 7 blocks away. The hospital is 1-1/2 miles away.

Key: ▶ = video clip   ▤ = medical record   ▽ = journal entry   [NEWS] = news article

CLIFFORD ALLEN

Season 1	Season 2	Season 3
Clifford is generally well and has plans to retire in the next couple of years. During this season he is diagnosed with BPH and has a TURP after trying unsuccessful medical treatment. Shortly after this, his wife is diagnosed with colorectal cancer. When Pam has surgery, Clifford takes off work to care for Pam and Gary.	During this season, Clifford is overwhelmed as he takes care of Pam (while she undergoes chemotherapy and radiation) and Gary. He experiences insomnia and weight loss, and begins drinking alcohol in the evenings as a coping measure.	Pam has a recurrence of cancer. When she elects to stop treatment, Clifford becomes very depressed. After Pam dies, he struggles with grief, loss and depression. He makes a decision to retire and care for Gary on a full-time basis.

Clifford Allen Season 1 Information

Episode 1

Clifford is a 64-year-old male who has been married to his wife Pam for 40 years. Their only child, 24-year-old Gary, has Down syndrome and lives with them. Clifford is a middle manager for a small manufacturing company, where he has worked for the past 20 years.

Overall, Clifford is in good health, although he has recently been undergoing conservative treatment for benign prostatic hypertrophy. He has a history of depression and his brother committed suicide as a teenager. Clifford had a brief depressive episode during college, for which he did not seek treatment. He had another episode shortly after Gary was born. At that time, with encouragement from his wife, Clifford sought treatment, which consisted of counseling and antidepressant agents. He quit taking the medications after about 6 months and decided he would just learn to deal with depression on his own. Although he has had mild episodes of depression over the years since that time, Clifford has been unwilling to seek treatment because he fears the social stigma associated with being labeled as medically depressed. He is also concerned that his employer will find out about it through his use of the medical benefits. It is Clifford's opinion that his employer would perceive depression as a sign of weakness. Overall, he has done well without the medications.

Clifford has been thinking about retiring within the next few years. He and his wife have always planned to do some traveling, but mostly he looks forward to being able to escape the busy and stressful work environment. Clifford and Gary are involved with activities at their church; they also enjoy a walk each evening after supper. Clifford belongs to a bowling league and is at the bowling alley a few evenings each week.

This episode Clifford, Pam, and Gary enjoy a pizza for dinner on their backyard patio. As they eat, they discuss what kind of a trip they should plan for their upcoming vacation next month. Pam verbalizes an interest in going to Alaska someday but realizes they don't have enough time to plan a trip like that. Clifford suggests they should save Alaska for a retirement trip. Ultimately, they decide to take a trip to a national park in Colorado.

Episode 2

Clifford has felt tired, grumpy, and irritable at work all day due to waking up at night to use the bathroom and then not being able to go back to sleep. When one of his project managers reports to Clifford that they are behind on a job, he snaps at her and tells her she needs to get her act together. He later feels badly about how he reacted, but he has a hard time apologizing.

Despite being tired, Clifford and Gary go for a walk after dinner and then to a father-son bowling event with the Special Olympics group. While bowling Clifford experiences urinary frequency and has to go to the bathroom several times during the game. In the bathroom, he has a hard time starting his stream and has to strain to relieve himself.

At one point, Clifford spends so much time in the bathroom that when he returns to the bowling game, he learns that everyone has been waiting on him to take his turn. Clifford feels annoyed and embarrassed about this [NEWS].

Episode 3
Clifford calls to make an appointment to see his urologist for a follow-up examination for his benign prostatic hypertrophy (BPH) treatment. He has been taking finasteride (Proscar) for just over a year, but he doesn't feel that it's been particularly effective. He still has problems urinating and, in fact, believes his symptoms are worse than they were before he started taking the medication. Although Clifford reported the lack of improvement of his symptoms to his physician 6 months ago, he was asked to continue the medication regimen for 6 more months and then return for a reevaluation of his condition. When he calls the office, Clifford learns that the physician is booked through the end of the week, is out of town the following week, and Clifford plans to be out of town the week after that. It will be another 3 weeks before he can get an appointment [▼].

Episode 4
Clifford wakes up every night - sometimes more than once - to use the bathroom. He tries to reduce fluids in the evening to minimize the effects. He hates the fact that he is getting older and having to deal with annoying urinary problems.

Clifford joins Pam and Gary's vacation planning efforts by studying the hiking trails to select the ones Gary can enjoy and also physically manage [▼].

Episode 5
Clifford is in Colorado on vacation this week with Pam and Gary. He really enjoys the outdoors and spending time with Gary in this way, and Clifford wonders if he could afford to buy a small cabin in the mountains once he retires. Despite the beautiful surroundings, he does not find the week very relaxing because of his ongoing urinary symptoms. He wishes he could just pee normally and sleep through the night!

Episode 6
Clifford finally sees the urologist this week for a follow-up visit. He shares with the physician that he often feels as if

his bladder is full after voiding, he has a hard time starting his stream, and, when he does void, the urinary stream is weak. He also reports that he gets up frequently at night to void. His score on the American Urological Association Symptom Index is 28. Six months ago, his score was 18. Based on the current symptoms and findings from the digital rectal exam, the urologist confirms with Clifford that the medication has not been effective. He schedules Clifford for further tests, including an outpatient uroflowmetry test, a post-void residual test, prostate biopsy, a prostate-specific antigen (PSA) blood test, and a urinalysis. He also discusses the possibility of a surgical procedure known as a holmium laser enucleation of the prostate (HoLEP) [▶].

Episode 7
This week, Clifford undergoes the uroflowmetry test, the post-void residual test, an ultrasound prostate measurement, a prostate biopsy, and a Prostate specific antigen (PSA) test at the outpatient diagnostics clinic. Results from the uroflowmetry and post-void residual tests show a significant obstruction of urinary flow. The ultrasound prostate measurement was 112.4.

The PSA is negative, the biopsy shows no evidence of malignancy, and the urinalysis is consistent with bladder inflammation. In a follow-up visit, the urologist shares with Clifford the results of the tests and recommends a holmium laser enucleation of the prostate (HoLEP) procedure in the upcoming weeks [▼].

Episode 8
Even though Clifford's urologist provided detailed information about the upcoming procedure, Clifford spends time online reading information about the holmium laser enucleation of the prostate (HoLEP) procedure. Clifford is generally comfortable with the decision, but he feels anxious about the potential for incontinence and impotence, despite the low incidence of these complications. He finds Pam at the computer looking at information about the HoLEP procedure [▶] [NEWS].

Episode 9
This week, Clifford goes to the Neighborhood Hospital for a holmium laser enucleation of the prostate (HoLEP) procedure. Although he has been very anxious about having the procedure performed, the procedure goes smoothly, and he experiences no complications. In the immediate postoperative period, he has a three-way urinary catheter and notices his urine is a little bit bloody. He is allowed to eat dinner and has no pain other than generalized discomfort from the catheter. His catheter is removed the next morning and he goes home after he is able to urinate on his own. He is somewhat distressed when he gets home and experiences urgency, burning sensation when he urinates, and uncontrolled dribbling. Pam reminds Clifford

these were mentioned in the discharge instructions as common occurrences for a few days after the procedure. He performs Kegel exercises, as instructed by the discharge nurse .

Episode 10

Clifford decides to take a week off following his procedure but realizes he really could have gone back to work. He feels great and is thrilled he can actually urinate with ease. He is also very happy to be sleeping through the night again. Clifford still notices some blood in his urine and is trying not to be too concerned about the intermittent incontinence for which he wears a light pad .

Episode 11

Clifford is back at work this week and really enjoying the simple pleasure of urinating without difficulty. He listens to Pam as she shares her concerns regarding Gary and his occasional outbursts, and is so grateful for Pam's patience. He knows she has much a greater skill in managing Gary's needs.

Episode 12

It has been a month since Clifford had his HoLEP procedure. He has a follow-up visit with the urologist. Clifford reports that he is passing urine easily, his urine is completely clear, and he has no urgency or burning and just occasional urinary dribbling. The urologist assures Clifford that he is doing very well and should be able to resume all activities he did before - including sexual activity. The urologist asks Clifford to see him again in 6 months.

Episode 13

Pam tells Clifford that she is having routine follow-up tests at the physician's office this week. He does not think too much about this news and is focused on catching back up with work.

Episode 14

Clifford is shocked when he gets a phone call from Pam informing him that she is being admitted to the hospital and needs surgery because she has a mass in her abdomen. He immediately worries about the possibility of cancer. He leaves work at once to be with Pam.

The following day, Clifford and Gary stay at the hospital most of the day. Immediately after surgery, the physician talks with Clifford at length to explain Pam's condition. As soon as the physician says "colon cancer," Clifford is in such a state of shock that he does not hear anything else that is said. He has a hard time interpreting just what is going on .

Episode 15

Clifford takes the entire week off work to take care of Pamela and Gary after she is discharged from the hospital. He finds the colostomy bag on Pam's abdomen disgusting and avoids looking at it unless he must. Clifford refuses to believe that the prognosis is poor; he knows Pam was cured of cancer last time, and he is sure she can conquer it again. He is angry with her when she tells him that she is not sure she wants to go through with chemotherapy and radiation.

Clifford feels overwhelmed with the job of managing the home, taking care of Gary, and helping Pam. He is accustomed to Pam taking care of most things and has a hard time getting organized. In fact, he often finds himself sitting in a chair in the living room, staring at the walls, unable to get anything done. Clifford takes Gary to and from work all week and, although he shares with Gary that his mother is sick and had to have surgery, he does not elaborate on Pam's condition .

Clifford Allen Season 2 Information

Episode 1

Clifford's wife has recently been diagnosed with colon cancer, which has turned his world upside down. She is beginning chemotherapy and radiation therapy, and he finds this very stressful. He is trying to work, take care of his son, and support his wife. He does not have strong coping skills, and his history of depression further complicates matters. He has not been treated for depression for a number of years, partly because he fears the social stigma associated with being labeled as medically depressed and partly because he is concerned that his employer would find out through the use of the medical benefits. It is Clifford's opinion that depression would be perceived as a sign of weakness by his employer.

Before his wife became sick, Clifford was thinking about retiring within the next few years, but now he is concerned about medical bills and does not believe he can afford to retire anytime soon. Clifford and his son Gary are involved with church. Since Pam became ill, Clifford has not regularly gone for a walk with Gary, and he has also stopped bowling in his league.

Clifford has been trying to keep himself occupied so that he does not constantly think about Pam. Although he has been told that her prognosis is poor, he wants her to undergo the radiation and chemotherapy treatments. He takes Pam to outpatient surgery for a central line port insertion.

Episode 2

Clifford takes Pam to her chemotherapy treatments this week and drops Gary off at work. He is able to go in to the office by late morning and still get part of a day of work in, but he has a hard time focusing on his work.

Episode 3

Clifford is glad to see Pam feeling better this week. He decides that the oncology nurse was probably exaggerating the treatment side effects, because Pam is obviously doing fine. He continues to be very preoccupied and is having a hard time focusing on his work.

Episode 4

Clifford feels frustrated with Pam because, despite his best efforts, she does not want to eat anything that he makes. He is trying to prepare meals that she will eat, but she always tells him the food makes her nauseated. Clifford also feels more frustrated with Gary than usual. He is usually very patient with his son, but he finds himself being irritated when Gary continually interrupts him to find an object or to go for walks. Clifford feels guilty for getting angry with Pam and Gary.

Episode 5

Clifford is feeling overwhelmed. Pam is feeling very sick, and he has to work and take care of Gary. Pam is too weak to do anything. He feels sick to his stomach when he needs to help her empty her colostomy bag. He does not want to look at it, let alone smell it. He appreciates the help from people from church, but he still feels helpless. He is having a hard time sleeping at night and has lost his appetite. He has a couple of drinks of scotch each evening to help him relax ▼.

Episode 6

Clifford is feeling very down. He wants to believe that Pam is going to get better, but by the way she is acting, he thinks she is giving up. He thinks she should be more optimistic and just believe things will be okay. Clifford also is frustrated that Gary is increasingly irritable and dependent on him. He really had to hold his temper when Gary threw a pillow in his room and broke a lamp.

Clifford has been feeling increasingly stressed. He has a hard time being productive at work, avoids social interactions, and has begun to lose weight. His alcohol use in the afternoon and evenings as a coping mechanism has increased. He is surprised and angry when Pam confronts him about his drinking and tells him to get help for depression. He doesn't have time for that! ▶

Episode 7

Pam tells Clifford that she has asked some of their friends to help get Gary to and from activities. At first Clifford feels angry at Pam for doing this – after all, he should be able to manage things and asking for help is not something Clifford really wants to do. However, he does notice that Gary is much easier to manage after an outing, and having him gone periodically is a relief.

Episode 8

Clifford is glad that Pam has completed the chemotherapy regimen. He is hopeful that everything will get back to normal. He loves Pam, but this illness has changed things. Although he feels bad about it, he does not like to touch her, he does not like the way she smells, and he does not like the colostomy bag. He feels very tired from the ordeal.

Episode 9

Clifford is glad to see Pam begin to feel better—this makes him feel better as well. He realizes he has lost 15 pounds over the past several months. He vows to eat better and stop drinking in the evenings [NEWS].

Episode 10

While at work, Clifford receives a call from Pam informing him Gary is sick and he needs to go to a doctor. Clifford leaves work, takes Gary to the emergency department, and learns that he has pneumonia. Clifford takes the next several days off work to care for Gary in hopes of limiting Pam's exposure to his illness. While looking over medical bills one evening, Clifford wonders just how many more medical bills his family can absorb. At this rate he may have to work another five years to pay everything off ▼ [NEWS].

Episode 11

Clifford finds that caring for Gary in the evening has been surprisingly satisfying and has interrupted Clifford's evening drinking. Clifford also notices he has been sleeping better. In fact, he now realizes he had been in a fog for the last few months—existing without really living.

Clifford is glad Gary is feeling better again. He realizes how little time he has spent with Gary over the past few months. He takes his son fishing, which is the first activity they have done together in a very long time [NEWS].

Episode 12

Clifford takes Pam and Gary on a weekend vacation and has a wonderful time. After getting home he talks to Pam about taking a Caribbean cruise next year. He is disappointed that Pam is not enthusiastic about the idea and wishes she would think more positively. He decides to start looking at some travel plans anyway ▶

Episode 13

Clifford continues to look at travel options. He remembers Pam mentioning that she would like to go on an Alaskan cruise and considers booking a trip as a surprise for her. After calculating the total cost, he decides to wait until he can pay down the debt from all of the medical bills. He can't imagine what they would have done without medical insurance.

This week Clifford also goes on a church youth group bicycling outing with Gary. With the exception of Gary getting upset with him for not signing up for a 35-mile ride, Clifford enjoys the experience and thinks about the possibility of joining a cycle club for men. It would be a great way to get into better shape.

Episode 14

Clifford goes bowling this week and joins his friends for a card game. He is feeling rested and energetic; his friends tell him he looks better now than he has in months. He tells his friends he is so thankful that Pam has beaten the cancer again.

Episode 15

Clifford and Gary have resumed their nightly walks after dinner. While on the walk, Gary surprises Clifford when he tells him about his girlfriend at work. Clifford realizes how hard the past year has been on him and vows never to let family issues get in the way of meeting his own needs again. Clifford goes online to research his company's retirement requirements and evaluate his options.

Clifford Allen Season 3 Information

Episode 1

Clifford is a 65-year-old male who has been married to his wife Pam for 41 years. Their only child, 25-year-old Gary, has Down syndrome and lives with them. Clifford is a middle manager for a small manufacturing company, where he has worked for over the past 21 years.

During the past year, Pam was diagnosed with colorectal cancer, had a colectomy and colostomy, and underwent chemotherapy and radiation therapy. Following her treatments, the oncologist was optimistic, and Pam began feeling good again. However, a few weeks ago, Pam became ill again. They were told that her cancer had metastasized to her liver and pancreas, and her prognosis was very poor.

Clifford has a history of depression, although he has not undergone treatment for several years. While Pam was going through chemotherapy and radiation several months ago, he became depressed, but did not seek treatment. He has been feeling very angry since learning of Pam's metastatic cancer NEWS.

Episode 2

Clifford takes Pam to have a central line port reinserted for chemotherapy. He tells his employer that things might be rough for a while and he might need to take some time off. His boss at work is very understanding of the situation and lets him know he can take the time as he needs it. However, Clifford knows he has used up his family leave benefits.

Episode 3

This has been a bad week for Clifford. He tries to take care of Pam while she is nauseated, but he feels helpless. On top of this, Gary has had several angry outbursts the past few days. At one point he breaks several things in his room. Clifford can't seem to keep up with Pam's and Gary's needs. He cannot sleep and loses his appetite. Again, he feels as if he is in a fog and is almost nonfunctional. He makes arrangements for Gary to stay with the Marshalls, people he knows from church, for the next few weeks, because he knows he cannot cope with his son right now. He begins to drink alcohol heavily in the evenings again. He goes to work but just sits in his office and stares at the walls. He has quit going to church on Sundays because he does not see any point in going at this time ▼.

Episode 4

At the encouragement of his boss, Clifford completes the paperwork necessary for family medical leave so he can focus on taking care of Pam. He realizes he has been nonproductive at work anyway, and maybe the medical leave will help him do a better job taking care of Pam.

Clifford considers letting the Marshall family know that Gary can come back home since he is taking family medical leave but decides not to. He just does not want to try to manage Gary and Pam right now. Although he knows it is the right decision, he feels very guilty about not taking care of his son.

Episode 5

Pam continues her chemotherapy. Clifford has become almost nonfunctional. The people caring for Gary become very concerned about Clifford and suggest that Gary continue to stay with them until things improve at home. Clifford becomes very angry with them and says he feels as though he is losing his son and wife at the same time. Because of Clifford's actions, they notify the parish priest about what is going on ▼.

Father John visits with Clifford and asks him how things are going. Clifford shares with him that he does not understand why God is doing this to them. He also confides that he is afraid that Pam might not make it. Father John recommends that he get counseling or come back and talk with him again so that Clifford can better support his wife. He also tells Clifford he should cut back on the drinking - Clifford wonders how he knows about that. Clifford tells Father John he will think about the therapy but is not really interested in talking to anybody. He does not think he has time for therapy, even if he wanted to go.

Episode 6

Clifford has an angry outburst at the clinic this week when Pam refuses to have her chemotherapy treatment. The nurse at the clinic gradually calms him down and talks with him about changing the focus of care. When he gets home, he sobs uncontrollably, and he gets drunk later that evening. He has not slept well in a week and has eaten very little. He also has no energy and has been suffering from frequent headaches. Many people have come to the home to help out, but he refuses to speak with them. It is obvious to everyone that Clifford is not managing things well at all.

Episode 7

Early in the week Clifford meets the hospice nurse. He starts off being very angry. She allows him to express his anger and frustration about the events of the past year, and she does not try to "talk him into" anything. Once he has vented, he begins to acknowledge Pam's decline. Then the nurse shares with him the services that hospice can provide. Clifford feels a sense of relief that he can get help. He decides he likes the hospice nurse and believes that hospice will be helpful. The hospice nurse mentions that grief counseling is available to family members and hands Clifford a business card with contact information. He tells the nurse he doesn't need anything like that but puts the card in his wallet. He continues to be angry with Pam for stopping treatment and "giving up." He feels powerless and as if everything is out of his control. He continues to drink heavily. He refuses to talk to Pam about caring for Gary when she dies; he wants to talk with her about getting better, but he does allow hospice to begin visits.

Later in the week Father John, the parish priest, makes a visit to their home. Clifford shares with him that he doesn't think he can go on without Pam. Father John reminds him that he must go on—not only for himself, but also for Gary. He also reminds Clifford that he needs to put Pam's mind at ease. Clifford tells Father John there really is not much to look forward to. Father John recognizes that Clifford is deeply depressed and convinces Clifford to get counseling immediately. NEWS

Episode 8

Clifford is able to get an appointment to see Shawn Jacobs, the mental health DNP at the community-based clinic. On the first visit, he shares his previous history of depression some 20 years ago and the fact that his brother committed suicide when they were teenagers. He also shares his ongoing feelings about not wanting to go on without Pam, that he has been a worthless husband, and that he has nothing to look forward to. Shawn asks Clifford many additional questions that Clifford finds irrelevant and somewhat annoying (such as how he is sleeping and how his appetite has been, what his coping mechanisms are, if he is using drugs or alcohol to cope, and if he has contemplated ending his own life). At the end of the visit Shawn recommends that Clifford begin taking two new medications, bupropion (Wellbutrin) for depression and trazodone to help him sleep. Clifford actually feels better after his first session and decides to get the prescriptions filled.

On a second visit this week, Clifford is able to talk more about the possibility of his wife's death and feelings of anger, abandonment, and hopelessness. Shawn talks with Clifford about how to deal with those feelings and, most importantly, how to keep from taking them out on his wife and son.

Clifford also has benefited from the social worker who has been working with the family, specifically regarding how to talk to Gary about what is happening with Pam to prepare him for her death. Although Clifford struggles with these conversations, he has accepted the fact that Pam is dying and finally agrees to let Pam talk with Gary alone ✉.

Episode 9

Clifford can see that Pam is declining fast. She has had nothing to eat or drink for the past 5 days, and she is putting out very little urine. With the help of the hospice nurse, Clifford knows the medications well and has been able to take charge of managing her pain.

Clifford notices that Pam's respiratory rate has become more irregular and calls the hospice nurse for advice. He is told that it is likely that she will die soon and he should continue to manage her pain the way he has been. Clifford asks that she come to see Pam herself. When the hospice nurse arrives, she finds Pam resting comfortably and confirms the change in her breathing pattern. She reassures Clifford and he is finally able to accept fully that Pam is dying. He tells her that he will be okay and that he will take good care of Gary. He calls Father John and asks him to come. Clifford is at Pam's side when she dies peacefully early the following morning. Clifford has never experienced such pain.

Two days after she dies, Clifford keeps his appointment with Shawn Jacobs, the mental health nurse practitioner. It is a much-needed appointment, and he talks about his overwhelming sense of loss and grief. Clifford mentions that he has tremendous support from his church and friends but is worried because Gary has become withdrawn and won't talk with him. Shawn suggests Clifford and Gary attend grief counseling offered through hospice. He pulls out the card given to him by the hospice nurse and mentions he has already heard about this and wants to know if he really needs both. Shawn encourages Clifford to check it out and decide for himself ▼.

Episode 10

Clifford keeps his weekly appointments with Shawn Jacobs and continues to take the bupropion (Wellbutrin). The dose has been slowly increased, and Clifford thinks it has been helpful. He talks about his loss and grief and the overwhelming support from members of the church. Shawn asks Clifford to start thinking about his plans for taking care of Gary and for ongoing self-management. Clifford makes arrangements to attend grief counseling with hospice services. He is surprised when it is advised that he and Gary attend different sessions.

Episode 11

Clifford attends his first hospice grief counseling session. He finds that his experiences are similar to many others in the group and he finds it helpful to know he is not alone. At the meeting he feels a special connection with another man about his age who also recently lost his wife to cancer. He leaves the meeting thinking the two could perhaps become friends.

Episode 12

Clifford is now seeing Shawn Jacobs, the mental health nurse practitioner, just twice a month and has been making progress. He has attempted to establish a regular routine for Gary. Clifford knows how important it is for him to stay mentally and physically well for Gary's benefit, and he makes a commitment to see himself through this challenging period of his life. He tells Shawn he is seriously thinking about retiring so he can focus his efforts on Gary. Shawn points out that this represents another loss of identity and encourages him to hold off on any major decisions for now ▶.

Episode 13

It would have been Pam's birthday this week. Clifford cries off and on all day. In spite of his sadness and sense of loneliness, Clifford and Gary decide to make a birthday cake to honor her. This week, Clifford also officially announces his retirement, which will become effective at the end of the month. He tells his colleagues that he realizes he has an opportunity to do something positive with the remainder of his life- to give his full attention to Gary.

Episode 14

Clifford meets with Shawn Jacobs and tells him that he officially gave notice for his retirement. He mentions that he feels much better at this point – he is sleeping well, eating well, has given up alcohol completely, and has more energy now than he has had in months. He tells Shawn that he is sure this is the best decision he could possibly make and hopes Shawn is not angry with him for making this decision.

Episode 15

On Clifford's last day of work, his company gives him a retirement party and several nice gifts. During the party, he shares plenty of laughs and tears with his coworkers and feels grateful for their sincerity. As he leaves the office for the last time and gets into his car to drive home, Clifford experiences the emotion of multiple losses - the end of a career and the loss of his wife. He is struck with profound sadness and feels lonely. Despite this experience of grief and loss, Clifford remains hopeful and is receptive to the ongoing support of friends, church members, and his grief support group. He looks forward to meeting with Shawn Jacobs the next morning ▼.

PAM ALLEN

Season 1	Season 2	Season 3
Pam is a middle-aged woman who presumes to be in perfect health. She spends most of her time managing the home and caring for Gary. After experiencing rectal fullness and blood in her stool, Pam is diagnosed with advanced stage colorectal cancer. She has surgery and prepares for chemotherapy and radiation treatment.	Pam undergoes chemotherapy and radiation on an outpatient basis. She experiences stomatitis, nausea, diarrhea, and fatigue. She finds it difficult to keep up with home management and caring for Gary. Following chemotherapy, Pam feels pretty good for a while and begins to believe she has beaten the cancer.	At the beginning of Season 3, Pam learns that the cancer has metastasized to her liver and pancreas. She initially agrees to undergo chemotherapy again, but shortly after decides to stop treatment. The focus of story is around end-of-life care issues and family coping responses. Pam dies during this Season.

Pam Allen Season 1 Information

Episode 1

Pamela is a 65-year-old female who has been married to Clifford for 40 years. Their only child, 24-year-old Gary, has Down syndrome and lives with them. In the past, Pamela worked as an administrative assistant in a law firm. After Gary was born, Pam gave up her career to care for Gary. She is active at her church where she has been a member for a number of years.

Pam describes her health as excellent. She has no current medical conditions or problems for which she seeks treatment. She frequently experiences constipation, which she treats with over-the-counter agents. She considers the constipation more of an annoyance than anything else. The only medical condition she has ever had requiring treatment was endometrial cancer at age 50. The cancer was diagnosed at a very early stage, and she underwent a total hysterectomy and bilateral salpingo-oophorectomy. Because there was no evidence of lymph node involvement, Pam was considered cured and has been cancer-free ever since. Her last examination was 14 months ago.

Pam is very close and devoted to her son Gary. Her goal is to optimize his potential, despite his limitations. She provides almost everything he needs, including most of the transportation to and from his part-time job and to various activities. Her favorite hobby is quilting, and she belongs to a quilting group. Pamela regularly wins awards for her quilts, which are highly sought after. She sells a few each year for additional income.

This episode Pam and Clifford discuss vacation plans at dinner. Pam always looks forward to short trips because she can see how much Clifford and Gary enjoy their time together. The one place Pam really wants to go someday is Alaska. She hopes they can do a trip like that soon while they are young enough to enjoy it.

Episode 2

Pam enjoys an afternoon with her quilt club this week. She talks with the other women about the travel plans she and Clifford have after he retires. One of the other women in the quilting group, Mary Martin, recently lost her husband to cancer. She tells Pam and the other women she wishes they had traveled before her husband got sick. Pam listens to Mary talk about her plans to move in with her son and his family.

Episode 3

Pam receives a call from Gary's manager informing her that Gary bruised his fingers in a grocery cart, is very upset, and is having a hard time calming down. Pam is very well aware that when Gary gets upset, he can become very difficult to manage - especially for people who don't know him well and who don't understand Down syndrome. After picking Gary up from the store, Pam calms him by sitting with him and having him hold an ice pack on his injury.

Episode 4

Pam and Gary look online to learn about the national park they will soon be visiting. They create a list of things they will need for the trip and begin the process of packing.

Episode 5

This week Pam enjoys taking a few hikes, reading, and sightseeing while on vacation. In the past they camped out, but Clifford and Pam no longer enjoy sleeping on the ground in a tent. Instead, they opt for a "rustic cabin" in the national park.

Episode 6

Pam knows that Clifford is often uncomfortable when he is unable to urinate completely. She knows he tends to downplay his symptoms, not wanting to look like a complainer. She is glad that he has decided to go for some tests.

Pam arrives home from a hair appointment and wonders why Gary has not yet arrived home from work. She then receives a call from Gary who is upset and crying. She finally is able to figure out he is on the bus but does not know where he is. She uses a GPS location indicator from Gary's phone to determine where he is and tells him to get off at the next stop. As she drives across town to pick him up from a bus stop, she wonders how he will manage when she and Clifford get too old to help him. When she picks Gary up, she find he is agitated from the experience. She spends several minutes talking with him to calm him down.

Episode 7

Pam takes Clifford to the various diagnostic tests for his prostate problem. She is glad to hear about the procedure recommended by the urologist, because she has been very aware how uncomfortable Clifford has been. She just hopes he does not get too stressed out from the entire process.

Episode 8

Pam looks at medical websites with Clifford as he reads up on his upcoming procedure. They find a few articles written by doctors but have a hard time understanding the information. They did find information about the low incidence of incontinence and impotence; she knows Clifford seems most worried about that.

Pam takes Gary to the church to participate in the church cleaning. She feels unusually tired and feels bloated. She wonders if she needs to start taking vitamins.

Episode 9

Pam continues to keep Gary's routine as uninterrupted as possible while managing to be at the hospital with Clifford for his procedure. She is relieved that there were no complications from the surgery. Pam has been experiencing constipation all week and continues to feel unusually tired. She takes laxatives to relieve herself. The following day she experiences diarrhea with an odd reddish-brown color and odor ▼.

Episode 10

Pam is glad to see Clifford is feeling better and also glad he is getting some much-needed sleep. On the other hand, she continues to feel tired and constipated. She has been straining to have bowel movements and notices that her stools are thinner than usual.

Episode 11

Pam takes Gary to his annual exam this week. Dr. Rowe tells Pam things look great and also comments that Gary should have an echocardiogram at some point in the future and perhaps they can do that on his visit next year. Dr. Rowe gives Pam a new prescription for Gary's thyroid medication. Before they leave, Dr. Rowe comments to Pam she is looking pale and worn out. Pam confirms she has been tired and explains the recent stress with Clifford's surgical procedure.

On the way home Pam and Gary stop at the drugstore to get the new prescription filled. Feeling tired, Pam finds a chair to sit in and wait while Gary goes to the toy aisle. She later finds Gary on the floor of the store enjoying himself with an open package of cookies. When she interrupts the activity, Gary becomes very upset and smashes the cookies on the floor. Pam has to calm Gary before they can purchase the items he opened and go home ▶.

Episode 12

Pam continues to experience constipation and odd-shaped stools, and now she senses fullness in her rectum and pelvic areas, even after defecating. The appearance of reddish-brown in her stools has become more regular. She continues to feel very tired. On Friday afternoon, Pam finally decides to call for an appointment with Dr. Rowe to discuss the symptoms. She is told to come to the office on the following Monday morning. Given her past history of cancer, she has a feeling of dread and becomes worried that something serious may be wrong. Pam begins to worry about her son and wonders if Clifford could manage if she were to get sick and die. She decides it might be best to just wait and see what the physician has to say before sharing any of this with Clifford.

Episode 13

Pam sees Dr. Rowe on Monday morning. He again comments that she looks pale. After eliciting a history, Dr. Rowe conducts an examination, including a digital rectal exam. Dr. Rowe tells Pam there is a palpable mass and that her stool tested positive for occult blood. After consulting with a surgeon, Dr. Rowe arranges for additional diagnostic tests, including blood work and a computed tomography (CT) scan of the abdomen. These tests are performed on an outpatient basis over the next few days. Pam is very worried at this point. She tells Clifford that she is having some tests done, but she does not elaborate or show that she is concerned. She knows Gary can sense something is wrong and immediately comforts him to keep him from getting too upset ▶ ▽.

Episode 14

Pam follows up with the surgeon, Dr. Vigil, regarding her test results. Dr. Vigil tells Pam that she has a mass in her upper rectum and lower colon that extends into surrounding structures. A CBC confirms that she has anemia. He tells her that she needs to be admitted to the hospital for surgery. Pam calls Clifford to inform him that she is being scheduled for surgery the following day. Pam is sent to the preadmission clinic for a preoperative work-up and teaching.

The following morning, Pam is admitted to the hospital and taken to surgery for a colectomy and possible colostomy. When she wakes up in recovery, she is nauseated and experiences a tremendous amount of pain. She has tubes in her arms, bladder, and nose. She feels a bandage and a strange object on her stomach. After she is transferred to the surgical unit, she sees her surgeon, who confirms her worst nightmare. Pam is told she had a large cancerous tumor in her lower colon and upper rectum. The surgeon was unable to remove all of it because the tumor had adhered to the side walls of her lower abdominal cavity. The physician also biopsied lymph nodes in her groin, which were thought to contain cancerous cells ▤ ▽ NEWS.

Episode 15

Pam is discharged from the hospital this week. She is told that her condition is serious, and further treatment with chemotherapy and radiation therapy is recommended. These treatments would start in about one month, after she has healed from surgery. Pam tells Clifford that she is not sure she wants chemotherapy and radiation treatment. Clifford argues with her that she needs to go through the treatment.

At home, Pam is slowly learning to care for the colostomy. A home-care nurse makes a few visits to help her adjust to her colostomy and provide other aspects of support; Pam is grateful for the help. She is very aware that Clifford is disgusted with her colostomy ▶ ▽ NEWS.

Pam Allen Season 2 Information

Episode 1

Pamela is a 65-year-old female who has been married to Clifford for 40 years. Pam was recently diagnosed with advanced colorectal cancer. Last month, she had surgery (colectomy and colostomy), and she is still adjusting to having the colostomy. Because the tumor extended into the perineum and lymph nodes, she has been advised to start radiation and chemotherapy. She previously underwent treatment for endometrial cancer at age 50.

At this time, Pam is very concerned about not being able to take care of Gary. She also is worried about Clifford and his ability to cope with these changes.

Pam has begun to regain the strength she had before surgery and has resumed many of her regular routines with Gary. Although she was initially reluctant to begin chemotherapy, after talking to Clifford she decided to go ahead and begin treatment. Her first chemotherapy is scheduled to begin early next week. She goes to the outpatient clinic to have a central line port inserted. This will prevent frequent needle sticks and allow the infusion of medications and blood samples to be drawn through the line when needed. She thinks this will be an advantage, but she is a bit anxious about having one more thing to care for. She is feeling optimistic that the treatment will cure her cancer. Pam receives the Sacrament of Anointing of the Sick at her church and hopes that this will help her through her treatment.

Episode 2

Pam begins her chemotherapy treatment this week. Her treatment regimen includes leucovorin followed by 5-fluorouracil (5-FU) daily for 5 days every month for the next 4 to 5 months. The oncology nurse explains the common side effects of treatment, which could include mild to moderate nausea or changes in her interest in food.

To prevent nausea, she is given ondansetron (Zofran) before chemotherapy. In addition, she is told to watch for changes in her stool consistency, because 5-FU can cause loose stools. Pam experiences nausea, slight changes in her appetite, and a slight loosening of her stools, which is controlled with Diphenoxylate/atropine (Lomotil). She tries to drink plenty of fluids ▤.

Episode 3

Pam is feeling physically better this week. The nausea has subsided, and she has a good appetite. She decides to start working on a special quilt for Gary. This week she started external lymph node radiation therapy to her right groin. The radiation treatment schedule is Monday through Friday for 6 weeks. She takes Gary to and from work, just as she had before her surgery, and still takes care of most household chores. Caring for her colostomy and the central line port are daily reminders of her situation, which bring with them emotions and fears about the cancer. She is self-conscious of the colostomy bag and its contents, knowing that it is difficult for Clifford to deal with, and it has interfered with their intimacy. She has not told Gary how sick she is, but she knows he is aware that she is not feeling well. Pam worries about Gary's long-term care if she dies; she is not sure Clifford can handle it.

Episode 4

Pam does not feel very good this week. She is back to feeling nauseated and can't seem to find anything that tastes good. Even the sight of food makes her want to throw up. She is aware that Clifford is feeling frustrated. She also notices that Gary has been very demanding. She wishes she would feel better so she could help out ▶ ▽.

Episode 5

Pam recently completed another round of chemotherapy and is still undergoing radiation. This week, she feels as if she hit a wall. She is extremely fatigued and nauseated, has diarrhea, and has developed sores in her mouth. The diarrhea makes managing the colostomy bag a challenge. Her hair begins to fall out and she has redness and irritation of the skin in her right groin area from the radiation treatment. She doesn't feel like she has the energy to do anything—even Gary's routine care has become a huge task.

Fortunately, people from her church have come to help. Every day, somebody comes into the home to do housework and either brings or prepares meals. Mary Martin, a member of her church and quilting group, is especially generous with her time. Mary not only has helped with meals, but she also organized several people to transport Gary to and from work and other activities. Pam feels relieved to have the help, but she hates feeling so tired and helpless. It is difficult to explain to others just how tired she is. The one bit of good news she had from her doctor is that her white blood cell (WBC) count has remained above $3,000/mm^3$, and her platelets have remained above $100,000/mm^3$ during therapy. She has mild anemia, which explains part of her fatigue ▤.

Episode 6

Pam continues to feel completely exhausted. She had no idea she could ever feel so tired. She feels worse the longer she has the treatments. She continues to feel nauseated and never feels like eating. Pam continues to have sores in her mouth and diarrhea. She is beginning to wonder if she will even survive the treatments. She feels so tired, for example, that reaching for a glass of water on the coffee table is a huge effort. She receives a Blood transfusion this week because she has become progressively more anemic.

Pam feels badly about not being able to be a mother to her son or a wife to Clifford, but frankly she has little interest in doing anything right now. Although she has completed the radiation therapy, she is still getting the chemotherapy. Friends from the church continue to come in daily to help. She knows Clifford is not coping well with her illness, and she suggests that he get counseling for depression. She also is aware of his new pattern of drinking alcohol in the evening, which worries her ▽.

Episode 7

Being aware of how the change in routine is affecting her son, Pam asks several families who normally interact with Gary to help out by taking Gary to his normal activities. She is able to see a big difference in Gary. He comes home from his events and tells his mother all about what they did. Although she is too tired to be truly interested in what he has to say, she is grateful that he is preoccupied with his activities.

Episode 8

Pam has finally completed the chemotherapy and is looking forward to feeling better. She was happy to have the central line port removed. She knows she will continue to feel tired for a while, but the sores in her mouth, diarrhea, and her appetite have all improved. She has lost weight through this ordeal, and when she looks at herself in the mirror, she hates what she sees. She sees a bald, skinny woman with draping skin and a bag of stool on her abdomen. She feels as if she has lost all that she was. She does not look the least bit feminine or attractive and understands why Clifford seems to physically avoid her. Pam is soothed through her ongoing relationship with Gary, who continues to seek comfort from her ▤.

Episode 9

Pam continues to feel a little better and is slowly able to take care of more household tasks- although she still gets tired easily. She has started to go back to church services with Gary and Clifford and also has decided to start working on Gary's quilt again.

Episode 10

Pam gets a call from Gary's store manager asking her to take Gary home. He tells Pam Gary is acting angry and does not seem to be feeling well. When Pam picks Gary up, it is clear to her Gary is sick. She takes his temperature and he has a fever. Pam calls Dr. Rowe's office but is unable to get Gary an appointment. Pam calls Clifford and asks him to come home from work and take Gary to the emergency department. When Pam learns that Gary has a viral pneumonia, she is thankful that this did not happen while she was taking chemotherapy, but she is still very worried about catching his illness. She limits her exposure by spending most of her time in her bedroom, allowing Clifford to care for Gary. Fortunately, she does not get sick!

Episode 11

Pam goes to her quilting group for the first time since becoming sick. She is worried about what the women in her group will think when they see her, but she is very glad to get out and see some of her friends again. Pam listens to Mary Martin tell the quilting group all about the medical workups she is having and wonders if Mary has any idea how annoying she can be. Regardless, she enjoys the outside interaction. Pam also goes with Clifford and Gary to a volunteer service meeting at the church.

Episode 12

Pam actually feels good enough now to go with Clifford and Gary on an out-of-town trip for a weekend. It has been so long since she has felt well enough to enjoy herself and her family. Although she still tires easily, the fatigue is becoming less of an obstacle. Her appetite has returned, and she is gaining some of her weight back. Pam is relieved that Clifford seems to be back to his "old self" again and has stopped drinking in the evening. He suggests to Pam that they go on a cruise next year. She tells him she is not sure how things will be next year, and they should just take life one day at a time. Pam continues to work on Gary's quilt. She is thankful that she is better, but she is scared that it won't last [NEWS].

Episode 13

The women in Pam's quilting group rave about the quilt Pam has been working on. She can hardly believe herself what she has created – especially considering how poorly she has felt. Since it is an original design, she realizes others might be interested in this quilting pattern. She wonders how much a quilting pattern like this could be worth.

Episode 14

Pam is really regaining her energy and agrees to lead a volunteer group at the church. She is almost finished with Gary's quilt and decides to enter it in a quilting contest at the annual Neighborhood Arts and Crafts Fair [NEWS].

Episode 15

This week at the Neighborhood Arts and Crafts Fair, Pam wins the grand prize for her quilt and is awarded $2,500 for it. She has never been offered so much money for a quilt, but she also realizes she has never made a quilt so beautiful. She decides to sell it, aware that her family could use the extra money and that she can always make Gary another one. Pam feels guilty about it afterward—the quilt was part of her cancer therapy, and she made that quilt especially for Gary [NEWS].

Pam Allen Season 3 Information

Episode 1

Pamela is a 66-year-old female who has been married to his Clifford for 41 years. Their only child, 25-year-old Gary, has Down syndrome and lives with them. In the past, Pamela worked as an administrative assistant in a law firm. After Gary was born, Pam gave up her career to care for Gary.

During the past year, Pam was diagnosed with colorectal cancer, had a colectomy and colostomy, and underwent chemotherapy and radiation therapy. Following completion of her treatments, the oncologist was optimistic, and Pam began feeling good again. However, a few weeks ago,

Pam began experiencing intermittent right upper quadrant discomfort and a decline in her appetite again. More recently, she noticed a hint of yellow coloration to the sclera of her eyes and a dark color to her urine. She called her oncologist and was seen immediately. After a series of diagnostic tests, Pam is given very grave news: the cancer has metastasized to her liver and pancreas. Her prognosis is very poor. The oncologist outlines two treatment options: another course of chemotherapy with bevacizumab (Avastin) or palliative treatment.

Pam hates to even think about more chemotherapy, but she also knows that if she does not undergo chemotherapy, she will surely die. Part of her reluctance to get treatment is based on her understanding of the severity of side effects. Clifford is angry with her for considering any option other than chemotherapy, and the physician also strongly encourages Pam to undergo the chemotherapy. Pam has had time to think about everything. Deep down, she knows she will die - she just doesn't know if living longer while enduring the adverse effects of treatment outweighs having a shorter, better quality life. After talking with her priest, Father John, and despite the fact that she really does not want to go through chemotherapy again, Pam agrees to this treatment.

Episode 2

Pam has another central line port inserted and begins the chemotherapy. She will be receiving bevacizumab, 5 mg/m^2 every 2 weeks, at the outpatient chemotherapy unit. On her way to the first chemotherapy treatment, Pam experiences a high degree of nausea ▤.

Episode 3

Mouth sores, diarrhea, and vomiting have returned with the new chemotherapy agent. Pam can't get relief from the nausea and vomiting, even after trying several different anti-nausea medications. Her platelet count has also dropped due to the chemotherapy.

Episode 4

Despite various anti-nausea medications, Pam continues to have constant nausea and diarrhea. She has lost 15 pounds. Her muscles and joints ache, and she has persistent headaches. Lab results prior to her next treatment show her total white blood cell (WBC) count is 2,300/ mm^3. Treatment is delayed due to her symptoms and her WBC count ▤ ▽.

Episode 5

Pam feels worse than ever- in fact, she feels much worse than the last time she went through chemotherapy. She has decided this is not worth it, and she tries to tell Clifford she does not want to continue treatments.

Episode 6

Pam continues to feel terrible this week. When it is time for her next appointment, she tells Clifford—in no uncertain terms—that she does not want to continue with the chemotherapy treatments. However, he picks her up, carries her out to the car, and takes her to the clinic. She is too weak to refuse. At the clinic, Pam tells the nurse that she does not want any more treatments, but her husband made her come. The nurse talks with Clifford and tells him Pam has the right to stop treatment. Clifford explodes and yells at the nurse to stay out of their affairs. Pam is embarrassed by his reaction in the clinic and wishes he would just let it go. Once Clifford has calmed down, the nurse engages in a discussion about changing the focus of care and introduces the concept of hospice care to the couple ▶.

Episode 7

Pam and Clifford have elected to interview a hospice nurse and hear what the program has to offer them. During the home visit, the hospice nurse learns that Pam has not been eating well, has continued to lose weight, and has been experiencing a great deal of pain. Pam tells the hospice nurse she wants pain medication to make her comfortable. The hospice nurse increases her pain dosage to keep her comfortable. Later in the week, Pam tells Clifford she is ready to die and wants to talk with him about Gary. She is frustrated and angry that Clifford will not discuss this with her - when she attempts to have the conversation he refuses to listen and changes the subject ▶.

Episode 8

Pam and Clifford experience a good relationship with the hospice nurse and other team members. The agency has supplied them with a hospital bed, bedside commode, and a medication box to help organize her pills. Clifford is fond of the social worker who has begun working with them, specifically regarding how to talk to Gary about what is happening with Pam and to prepare him for her death. Although Clifford struggles with these conversations, he has finally accepted the fact that Pam is declining and agrees to let her talk to Gary.

Pam has had very little to eat or drink this week and is rarely urinating. The hospice nurse notices that she has abdominal fullness (ascites) due to the accumulation of fluid in the peritoneal cavity and appears more jaundiced. Her pain continues, but the nurse establishes a pain management plan that works for Pam. The hospice nurse is in phone contact nearly every day to assess Pam's pain and make adjustments to the medication.

Pam sleeps most of the day, but when she is awake, she is alert and able to engage in conversation. She talks with Clifford about all the things she wants taken care of before she dies, such as things she wants various people to have. During one of those moments, she tells Clifford that she regrets selling the quilt. Friends from the church continue to visit, bring food for Clifford and Gary, pray with Clifford, Gary, and Pam, and offer support in whatever ways they can ▶.

Episode 9

Pam has had nothing to eat or drink for the past 5 days. There has been no stool in the colostomy bag for several days. She now has a urinary catheter because she is too weak to get up to use the bedside commode; it only has small amounts of dark, concentrated urine. She is more alert in the mornings and talks to those around her. The hospice aide comes in every other day to bathe her and provide comfort care. The hospice nurse has implemented a good pain management regimen, and Pam is more comfortable this week.

When Pam's respiratory rate becomes irregular, Clifford calls the hospice nurse and asks her to come to the home. The hospice nurse finds Pam resting comfortably. When she approaches her, Pam wakes slowly but is quite weak and unable to talk. She offers a smile when she recognizes the nurse. When her breathing pattern changes, the nurse reassures Clifford. He is finally able to truly accept that Pam is dying. Clifford tells her that he will be okay and that he will take good care of Gary. Father John comes by the house to give Pam the Sacrament of Anointing of the Sick. Pam drifts off to sleep and does not wake again. She dies early in the morning the next day, peacefully, with her family at her side ▐NEWS▌.

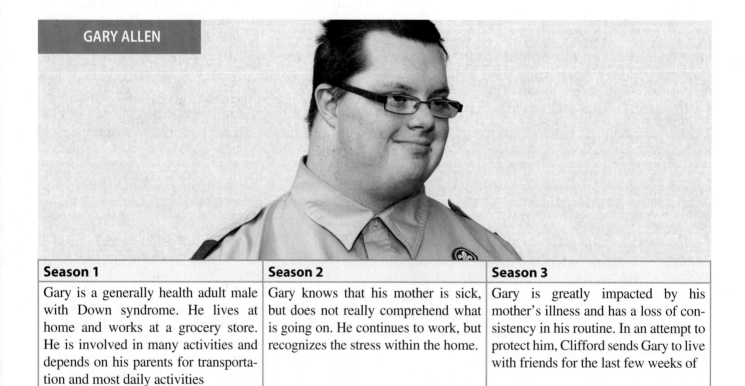

GARY ALLEN

Season 1	Season 2	Season 3
Gary is a generally health adult male with Down syndrome. He lives at home and works at a grocery store. He is involved in many activities and depends on his parents for transportation and most daily activities	Gary knows that his mother is sick, but does not really comprehend what is going on. He continues to work, but recognizes the stress within the home.	Gary is greatly impacted by his mother's illness and has a loss of consistency in his routine. In an attempt to protect him, Clifford sends Gary to live with friends for the last few weeks of

Gary Allen Season 1 Information

Episode 1

Gary is a 24-year-old male with Down syndrome. He lives with his parents, Clifford and Pamela. He is very close to his parents and has not been interested in living elsewhere. Gary has a part-time job as a courtesy clerk at a grocery store near their home. He is also given other duties as assigned, such as collecting baskets from the parking lot and helping customers carry groceries out. He works every afternoon from 1 pm to 5 pm. He has been doing this type of work for about 5 years now, and he loves having a job.

Gary has had only a few health-related problems during his life, including a congenital heart defect that was surgically corrected when he was a child and hypothyroidism since infancy. Gary also has poor vision due to nearsightedness and keratoconus in both eyes. Gary is unable to drive and usually relies on his parents for transportation. When they are unavailable to provide transportation, Gary rides the bus.

Gary helps his parents with many things around the house. He has learned to do laundry and help with the dishes and cleaning. Gary is able to make his own breakfast and lunch now (e.g., heat soup in a pan, make a sandwich, heat something in a microwave), but he is unable to interpret cooking directions or recipes. Gary does best when in controlled settings or in a routine setting with which he is familiar.

Gary enjoys a very active life. He is involved in various Special Olympics programs, including golf, swimming, and bowling; an Explorer Scout troop consisting of individuals with cognitive disabilities; and his church. Gary also rides his bike a couple miles three times a week, and he enjoys daily walks with his father. These various activities have afforded him multiple social connections and allowed him to enjoy friendships with a number of individuals.

Pizza is Gary's favorite food. He enjoys it when his father brings pizza home for dinner. While they eat, Gary listens to his parents discuss vacation options. When they settle on visiting a national park in Colorado, Gary asks if they will see bears.

Episode 2

Each day this week, Gary goes to work in the afternoon for 4 hours, comes home, and watches television until dinner time. After dinner, he takes a walk with his father. They talk about the fishing and hiking they will do while on vacation. Gary continues to ask his father about bears.

Episode 3

Gary becomes upset at work after getting his fingers caught in a grocery cart. It takes over 30 minutes for the store manager to calm him. Although he only sustains mild bruising, he is too upset to finish his shift. His mother is called to take Gary home for the rest of the day. Gary sits in front of the TV with an ice pack on his fingers when he gets home.

Episode 4

Gary missed two days of work last week after hurting his fingers while rounding up grocery carts. He is afraid of hurting his fingers again and is very leery of the grocery carts. Gary tells several of the customers he is going to Colorado to catch fish but does not know when.

Episode 5

Gary enjoys fishing and hiking with his father while on vacation this week. He also enjoys sleeping inside a log cabin instead of a tent. Although Gary is a bit worried about the bears, he does not see any ▼.

Episode 6

One day this week, Gary rides the city bus home from work because his mother has an appointment. While on the bus, Gary begins to talk to a man about his recent trip and all about fish and bears that live in Colorado. Unfortunately, Gary is not aware that he missed getting off at his stop until the man he is talking to gets off the bus. Gary becomes frightened because he does not recognize any of the stops. When Gary becomes upset and has a hard time communicating with those around him and has a hard time calming himself. He finally finds his cell phone and calls his mother who tells him to get off at the next bus stop and wait for her ▼.

Episode 7

Gary has been reluctant to take the bus home from work since his incident a week ago. Pam encourages him to take the bus home and reassures him that she will go to the bus stop to wait for him. He is happy to see her when he gets off the bus. As they walk to the house, Gary tells his mother that a lady fell down at the store and an ambulance came and took her to the hospital.

Episode 8

Gary and his mother go to church to participate in a church-cleaning activity. Gary loves to go to these activities because he likes to help with projects. He has many friends at the church, and he likes the fact that they talk to him. Gary also spends time riding his bike.

Episode 9

Gary's mother shares with him that his father will be going to the hospital to fix a problem with his bladder. Gary understands that you go to the hospital when you are sick or for tests or procedures, but he does not grasp what she means by "bladder problems." He stays at home alone for several hours in the afternoon while his parents go to the hospital. He is happy when Pam arrives home and tells him that his father is fine.

Episode 10

Gary enjoys having his father at home during the week. Every afternoon they watch a movie together and then take a short walk together. He also spends time in the swimming pool with his Special Olympics team.

Episode 11

Gary has his annual exam with Dr. Rowe this week. Gary loves Dr. Rowe because he is nice. On this visit Gary has vision, hearing, and screening checks done as well as a regular physical exam. There are no changes to Gary's vision or hearing, and all his exam findings are within normal limits. On the way home from his visit with Dr. Rowe, Gary and his mother stop at the drugstore to get a new prescription filled. While waiting, Gary helps himself to some cookies from a package and finds the toy aisle. He takes a toy off the shelf to play with. Gary becomes very angry a short time later when his mother tells him it is time to leave. He smashes the cookies on the floor in frustration. Gary yells and screams in anger - scaring some children in the aisle.

Episode 12

Gary goes on a bus trip with the youth group at church to a one-day church retreat. He has a great time with the members of the youth group. He gets home shortly after dinner time and is so excited that he has a hard time telling his mother and father what he did that day. He also has a hard time falling asleep that night .

Episode 13

Pam asks Gary to catch the bus home from work several days this week because she has appointments. Gary does not know what the term "appointments" means, but he can see that she is upset. Gary gets upset and confused when other people, particularly his mother or father, are upset. Pam reassures Gary everything is fine and suggests that they make a sandwich.

Episode 14

Gary is aware that his mother is at the hospital because she is sick. His father makes arrangements for friends from church to spend time with him in the evenings. Although Gary doesn't like the fact that his parents are not home, he is happy to talk with the people from church. He spends time playing games on his iPad .

Episode 15

When Pam arrives home from the hospital, Gary is sensitive to the fact that she does not feel well. He notices that she spends a lot of time lying around. He helps his father with chores around the house and wonders why his father spends so much time sitting in the living room chair and why they don't take their walk after dinner. On Sunday morning, he reminds his father that it's time for church, but he is told they will not go this week.

Gary Allen Season 2 Information

Episode 1

Gary has always relied on his mother for help with living skills. His mother, however, has recently been ill, and she has been unable to help him in the ways to which he is accustomed. His father has been helping him more, but his father seems so angry. Gary is aware of the changes going on around him, but he does not understand them.

This episode Pam shows Gary the dressings where the central line port is located under the skin on her upper chest. Pam tells him that she will be getting medicine to help her get well. Gary cannot quite understand how the medicine will get in the port. Later in the day, he goes to Poly Hockey with his Special Olympics group.

Episode 2

Gary can tell that his mother does not feel well this week and asks her if she is taking the medicine to get better. He goes on a camping trip with the Explorer Scout troop this week.

Episode 3

Gary's Mom takes him to and from work this week. He can tell she is feeling tired. He still wonders about the medicine tube and when she will take the medicine. He spends time in his room listening to his favorite music.

Episode 4

Gary is feeling frustrated but is not aware why. The entire household routine has changed and he does not adapt well to changes in the routine. He goes outside, finds a stick, and starts hitting things with the stick in anger and frustration. Why can't they go for a walk? Why can't they go bowling? Why is his father being mean?

Episode 5

Many people at Gary's church have been giving him rides to and from work and have been spending time at the house helping his mother. He is always happy to have them there because they talk to him and they are always very nice. They often stay long enough to cook dinner. He is glad to have dinner, but he likes the food his mother makes even better. When he gets tired of the extra people in the house, he retreats to his room to watch television.

Episode 6

Gary notices that his mother spends all of her time lying on the couch. He does not think his mother looks the same, and she smells different. He knows she is sick and he asks her when she is going to take her medicine. Pam tells him she is taking the medicine, but it just makes her feel tired. Gary does not understand any of this. The ladies from the church continue to come over, but his father has not taken him to church lately and has not been able to get him to all of his Special Olympics activities. He misses spending time with his friends. Frustrated, he throws a pillow at a lamp in his room and breaks it.

Episode 7

Many different people from church, Special Olympics and the scout troop have come over to the house this week to take Gary to his regular activities. Gary feels happy to see his friends. He tells his mother all about the things he has been doing.

Episode 8

Gary learns from his mother that she has finished taking all of her medicine. She tells him that she hopes to be able to start doing more things with him again. Gary loves his mother and has never complained about her lack of attention while she has been sick. He spends time in the garage sorting recyclables and then placing them by the curb for pickup ▽.

Episode 9

Gary goes back to church this week for the first time in a long time. He is so happy to see his friends there. He tells his mother they should not miss church any more.

Episode 10

Gary feels very tired at work. He goes upstairs to the break room and lies down on a couch and goes to sleep. Some of the other store employees wake him up and tell him to get back to work and Gary becomes very angry and tells them to leave him alone. The store manager sends Gary home for the day.

When Gary gets home all he wants to do is sleep. He does not feel good and is not hungry. He starts to cough and he feels hot. His father takes him to the hospital and he sees doctors and nurses, but he does not feel like talking to them.

When he gets home he is told by his father he needs to stay away from his mother so she does not get sick again. That is okay with Gary - all he wants to do is sleep and watch TV. His father brings him medication, food, and plenty of fluids to drink. Over the course of several days, Gary begins to feel much better.

Episode 11

Gary finally feels well again and his energy has returned. He is thrilled to go fishing with his Dad. Gary loves to fish.

He fails to catch anything, but he doesn't care, because he enjoys sitting with his Dad and throwing rocks in the water.

Episode 12

Gary goes with his parents on a short vacation. He loves to take trips and see new places and things. One of the visits they make is to the Museum of Natural History. Gary enjoys looking at the dinosaur bones and the mammal section ▽.

Episode 13

Gary participates in a cycling event with members of the youth group at his church to raise money for the neighborhood homeless shelter. Event participants could sign up for a 5-mile, a 10-mile, or a 35-mile ride. At the turn-around point of the short-distance ride, Gary tells his father he wants to complete the 35-mile ride. When Clifford tells Gary the distance is too far for him, Gary gets angry and takes his helmet off and throws it down to the ground. It takes Gary about 20 minutes to calm down before they can resume the ride [NEWS].

Episode 14

Gary plays in a Special Olympics golf tournament this week. He does not win the gold medal, but he shoots a personal best score. He is congratulated by his golf sponsor ▽ [NEWS].

Episode 15

Gary accompanies his mother to the arts and crafts fair and shows a few paintings he did that his family said were exceptional. To his delight, he sells one of them! His mother wins a prize. Later in the afternoon, a nice man named Greg spends time talking to Gary and his mother. Greg tells Gary that his name starts with the letter "G," just like Gary's name does. The man buys a quilt from his mother. Gary is happy to see his mother smile. Gary is also very happy that his Dad has been asking him to take walks in the evenings. While on a walk, he tells his Dad about his new girlfriend at work ▽.

Gary Allen Season 3 Information

Episode 1

Gary is a 25-year-old male with Down syndrome. He lives with his parents Clifford and Pamela. Gary has a part-time job as a courtesy clerk at a grocery store near their home. He works every afternoon from 1 pm to 5 pm. He has been doing this type of work for about 6 years now.

Gary helps his parents with many things around the house. Gary does best when in controlled settings or in a routine setting with which he is familiar.

Gary enjoys a very active life. He is involved in various Special Olympics programs, including golf, swimming, and bowling; an Explorer Scout troop consisting of individuals with cognitive disabilities; and his church. Gary also rides his bike a couple miles three times a week, and he enjoys daily walks with his father. These various activities have afforded him multiple social connections and have allowed him to enjoy friendships with a number of individuals.

Gary's mother tells him she is very sick again - even sicker than last time. Gary is very worried about this and feels sad. He asks his mother if she is going to get more medicine.

Episode 2
When Gary sees the bump where the central line port is on in his mother's chest, he tells her she is going to get medicine. Gary's mother confirms his understanding. Gary goes bowling with his Special Olympics friends this week.

Episode 3
Gary sees his mother and is worried about how sick she is. She keeps throwing up, and she tells his dad that she just can't eat anything. He gets upset when he sees his dad get angry. His dad tells Gary that he is going to stay with the Marshall family, their friends from church, for a little while until his mother is feeling better. He likes the Marshalls and willingly goes to stay with them, but he is worried about his mother. He takes his iPad and several movies to keep him busy.

Episode 4
Gary continues to stay with the Marshall family. He gets upset when one of the Marshall children changes the television channel from the cartoons Gary is watching to another program. To the shock of the Marshall family, Gary gets completely out of control and throws the TV controller at the TV and knocks a vase to the floor. They had no idea Gary had such a temper. They give Gary space and gradually he calms down. Mr. and Mrs. Marshall elect not to call Clifford, knowing it would upset him. Instead they decide to hang in there and do the best they can to support Gary.

Episode 5
Gary has been at the Marshall's house for several weeks now and, although he likes being with them, he misses his mother. He hears his dad yelling at the Marshalls and wonders why he is so upset. Gary visits his mother frequently and is worried about how sick she looks. He spends a lot of time in his room making models. The Marshalls take Gary to work and to as many of his activities as they can manage.

Episode 6
Gary remains with the Marshalls. They take Gary over to his house and find Clifford sitting in the living room crying and Pam in the bedroom crying. Gary is very sad and starts to cry, but he does not know what's wrong. He hugs his mother for a very long time ◣.

Episode 7
Gary goes to work every day this week and continues to stay with the Marshalls. He has come to feel very comfortable in their home and is actually pretty happy. He gets sad every time he sees his mother and father, and he wonders why the medicine his mother is taking is not helping her get well.

Episode 8
Gary's father picks him up from the Marshall's house and takes him for a pizza. They then drop by the house so he can see his mother. Gary misses being at home. His mother tells him she is very, very sick and she will soon be going to heaven. Gary knows what this means because his grandparents died a few years ago. He cries when he leaves to go back to the Marshalls.

Episode 9
The Marshalls learn that Pam will soon die. They talk to Gary and ask him if he wants to be with his mother and father. He says yes. When Gary gets to the house, he notices the house smells bad. Clifford holds him in his arms and tells him he is so sorry that he could not make his Mom well. Gary is shocked at how his mother looks. Her skin is yellow, and her face is hollow. She is breathing very fast, and her eyes are closed. Gary is comforted by Father John's presence. He talks to his Mom about going to heaven, but Gary is unsure if she hears him. After his mother dies, Gary goes back to the Marshalls' home, where they sit with him and let him talk about how he is feeling.

Episode 10
After his mother's funeral, Gary goes back to live at home with his Dad. He is glad the bad smells are gone. He checks all the rooms to be sure his mother is not there. Clifford tells Gary that they are on their own now, and they need to stick together.

Episode 11
Gary attends a hospice grief counseling session. He does not really know what it is about but meets several kids who have lost a parent or sibling to cancer. Gary tells them about his mother and that she got sick and died and is now an angel.

After the session Gary tells his father that the people were nice and he painted pictures and he had a brownie and he told the people there about his mother. When asked if he would like to go back for another session, Gary said he would like that ◣.

Episode 12
Gary learns from his dad that he is going to retire and stay home with him every day. Gary is very happy to hear this and asks him when they can go fishing again. While some friends from the church are over at the house, Gary proudly shows off the medals he has won over the years in Special Olympics.

Episode 13

Gary helps his dad bake a cake in honor of his mother's birthday. It makes him happy to do this because he likes cooking with his dad - and because he loves birthdays. After dinner, they talk a long walk together and talk about his mother living in heaven ▼.

Episode 14

Gary has settled into a comfortable routine with his father. He thinks about his mother and talks about her every day. He draws a picture of his mother as an angel in heaven and tells his father she has wings now.

Episode 15

Gary receives a package in the mail this week. He is very excited because he rarely gets a package. In the package is the quilt his mother had sold several months ago at the art fair. There is a card attached to the quilt, and it reads:

Dear Gary,

I was saddened to learn that your mother recently passed away. Your mother made this beautiful quilt. I would like you to have it to keep you warm at night.

Your friend,
Greg Ross ▼

BLEY HOUSEHOLD

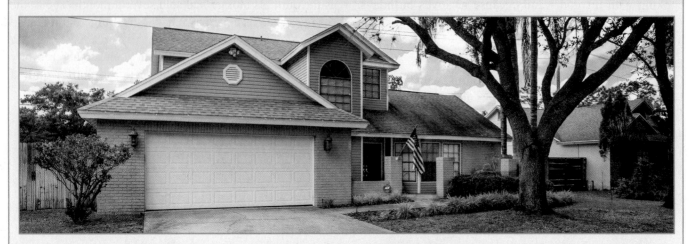

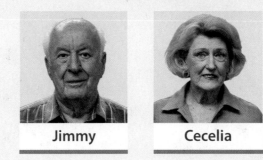

Jimmy   Cecelia

Housing The Bleys live in a newer two-story home in the Riverbank area. They live close to the river and have an open backyard with a small garden.

Parks and Recreation There is a soccer field close by where the Bley's grandson plays soccer.

Services The Neighborbood hospital and clinics are across town from where the Bleys live. Bus service does not extend into their area.

Key: ▶ = video clip ≣ = medical record ▽ = journal entry 🗞 = news article

JIMMY BLEY

Season 1	Season 2	Season 3
Jimmy is an 84-year-old man with emphysema and hearing loss. He is able to do most things needed around the house, but he needs to pace himself. He does not perceive that his breathing problems are all that bad. He is still a smoker, and he uses an inhaler when absolutely necessary, but he is not oxygen-dependent. He makes an unsuccessful attempt to quit smoking during this season.	Jimmy's story continues with a description of daily activities and another unsuccessful attempt to quit smoking.	During this season, Jimmy gets the flu, which leads to respiratory failure and sepsis. He is admitted to the ICU, requiring intubation and mechanical ventilation. He suffers from delirium during the acute illness. Following discharge, he has less oxygen capacity is oxygen-dependent at home. He becomes depressed and is given a prescription for Wellbutrin.

Jimmy Bley Season 1 Information

Episode 1

Jimmy is an 84-year-old male with moderate emphysema and hearing loss. He is a retired veteran who served as an electronics technician in the Army for his entire career. In his retirement, Jimmy has taken an interest in computers. He spends a great deal of time on the internet or playing games on the computer; he also likes to build computers. Jimmy has been married for 60 years to his wife Cecelia. They argue a lot, but they would not know what to do without each other just the same. They have several grown children, grandchildren, and great-grandchildren who live within the community. Jimmy and Cecelia also have 2 dogs, both of them strays that they just adopted. Jimmy often goes with his wife to the Neighborhood Senior Center for bingo night.

Jimmy considers himself healthy. He describes his hearing loss as mild. He has a hearing aid but does not like to wear it and thus does not make changing the batteries a priority. He does not perceive his hearing loss to be much of a problem. Likewise, Jimmy describes his emphysema as "not that bad." However, he becomes short of breath with most activities. He compensates by taking his time to do most things. He knows he must pace himself to avoid getting exhausted. When he over-exerts himself, it can take a few days to recover. Jimmy is very aware of his limits, yet he does not generally consider his illness to be very bad. Although he would not admit it, he recognizes that his breathing has become more of a problem during the past couple of years. He continues to smoke and knows he should quit, but he just can't seem to get interested in quitting because he enjoys smoking.

Jimmy goes shopping with Cecelia. He knows that she has more energy than he does when it comes to shopping, and that he has a tendency to become tired rather quickly. When she asks him if he's tired, Jimmy tells her he is not tired; he just gets bored with the shopping trips. He doesn't even consider staying home because their outings have been part of their routine for years. On the way home from shopping, Jimmy gets annoyed with Cecelia when she yells at him while he is driving, claiming that he does not hear an ambulance. He has been driving all of his life, and he thinks that he can hear well enough. He thinks to himself, "I don't drive with my ears!" ▼

Episode 2

The bathroom sink faucet breaks this week. Cecelia suggests that they ask one of their sons to fix it, but Jimmy wants to do it himself. It takes him three days to complete the repair. On the first day, he takes the faucet apart to see what is wrong with it. On the second day, he makes a trip to the hardware store for supplies, and on the third day, he replaces the faucet with the new supplies. Cecelia is annoyed that it takes him so long, but she is used to it ▶ ▽.

Episode 3

Jimmy notices a stray dog running around outside their home. He gets a little food and puts it in a dish outside the door. Watching from the window, he sees the dog carefully approach the food bowl and eat the food. He does this for a few days and then introduces the stray to his two dogs. Noting that his two dogs have accepted the stray into their pack, he decides to keep the dog – despite Cecelia's protest. He tells her that he is doing some good by taking in the dog.

Episode 4

Each week, Jimmy mows the lawn at their home. It usually takes him 3 to 4 days to do it, because he does just a little at a time. He refuses to have someone do it for him. This week Jimmy becomes very short of breath while mowing and needs to stop and rest. Because his shortness of breath does not subside, he uses his albuterol inhaler. Jimmy uses this only when absolutely necessary, and his current inhaler is 2 years old. He is aware that it is past the expiration date, but he doesn't want to get a new one. He considers that to be a waste of money ▽.

Episode 5

Jimmy hears a dog fight out in the backyard. He goes outside and sees all three of his dogs in a tangle. He tries to pull the new dog away, but he gets bitten on the hand in the process. Cecelia turns on a water hose and sprays the dogs to stop the fight. Jimmy goes to the Emergency Department at Neighborhood Hospital to have his dog bite treated. After irrigating the wound on his hand, Dr. Gordon (the ED physician), uses two loose sutures to hold the wound edges together and tells Jimmy that he does not want to close the wound up because it is likely to get infected. Jimmy is given a prescription for oral antibiotics and told to come back in 48 hours for a wound check. When he gets home, Jimmy notices that the new dog is gone but he does not ask about it ▽.

Episode 6

Cecelia tells Jimmy that the kids and grandchildren are going to be coming over during the weekend to celebrate a birthday. Jimmy does not hear her say this. Over the weekend, when the kids show up, he asks Cecelia why nobody told him they were all coming over.

The family stays at their home most of the day. During their visit, Jimmy enjoys himself with two of his grandsons by playing computer games with them. After the family leaves, he feels very tired and short of breath and needs to use his inhaler. Cecelia suggests to Jimmy that he quit smoking and get more exercise instead of sitting at the computer all day.

Episode 7

Cecelia asks Jimmy to come with her to the community Health Fair. Jimmy declines, telling her that he is too busy. He actually doesn't go because he knows it would just make him tired. Cecelia brings a smoking cessation flyer home for him to look at. He reminds her that the last time he tried to quit smoking it nearly killed him 📰.

Episode 8

Jimmy's daughter and Cecelia accompany Jimmy to his family physician, Dr. Rowe, for a routine visit for his emphysema. Dr. Rowe tells Jimmy that his lung capacity continues to decline and that he really needs to stop smoking. Jimmy agrees to try to quit. Dr. Rowe refers him to the Neighborhood Patient Education Center. He is told that success is highest with group classes. He agrees to give a smoking cessation class a try ▤.

Episode 9

Jimmy attends his first smoking cessation class. Although he likes the nurse who leads the class, he is not sure what to think or do. He feels awkward when asked to share with the group his experiences related to smoking and what smoking means to him. He finds one lady particularly annoying. She wears heavy perfume, laughs loudly, and always wants to dominate the discussion. After the class is over, he is not so sure about the class, but he decides it is worth going to for a while. In the meantime, he decides to cut back his smoking to about one-half his normal amount 📰.

Episode 10

Jimmy and his son accompany Cecelia to her x-ray tests and blood test at the diagnostic lab. Jimmy is uncomfortable because he has a serious craving for a cigarette. Later in the day, they go to play bingo at the Neighborhood Senior Center. Jimmy has a hard time concentrating on the game because he keeps thinking about smoking. He goes to the smoking cessation class again this week; the annoying lady is there, and once again she gets on his nerves ▽.

Episode 11

Jimmy is driving to his son's house to visit. Jimmy does not hear the sirens of an ambulance until it is right behind him with the horn blaring. Jimmy looks in the rear view mirror and is so startled he turns his car to the right and hits a curb and road sign. When he gets out to assess the damage, he can see that his right front wheel and rim are bent and the car is not drivable. Jimmy calls his son who arrives about the time the police respond to fill out a report. Jimmy's car is towed to a repair shop. He does not look forward to telling Cecelia about the accident.

Episode 12

Jimmy is not successful with his smoking reduction plan. Although he intended to cut back the amount he smoked by about one-half over the past few weeks, he has crept back up to almost the same number of cigarettes that he smoked before. He finds that he actually feels as though he can breathe better when he smokes. This week, he decides to stop going to the smoking cessation classes because he can't stand the lady with the perfume. He does not tell the nurse who leads the class because he doesn't want to disappoint her.

Episode 13

Jimmy and Cecelia are notorious for saving food - in many cases, for longer than they should. This week,

Jimmy experiences nausea, vomiting, and diarrhea. He believes he got sick from the leftover lasagna that had been in the refrigerator for a little over a week. Jimmy's daughter tells him that they should throw away leftovers after three days. There was one positive thing about his 24-hour illness: he did not crave cigarettes for a whole day ▾.

Episode 14

The nurse who leads the smoking cessation class calls Jimmy in response to his absence. Jimmy tells her that he couldn't come last week because of car trouble, but he might make it to the next class.

Jimmy wins $20 playing bingo this week.

Episode 15

Jimmy and Cecelia go to a school band concert to listen to their grandson play. Jimmy does not wear his hearing aid and is glad that he didn't. He thinks the music is awful, but, of course, he would never admit that he doesn't like it.

Jimmy Bley Season 2 Information

Episode 1

Jimmy is an 84-year-old male with moderate emphysema and hearing loss. He has been married for 60 years to his wife Cecelia. They argue a lot, but they would not know what to do without each other just the same. They have several grown children, grandchildren, and great-grandchildren who live within the community.

This episode Jimmy and his wife attend a granddaughter's soccer game. It is chilly outside, and Jimmy feels more short of breath than usual when walking back to the car. He never returned to the smoking cessation class because he just didn't believe it was worth it. He finds that he is okay just using his inhaler when needed, but he realizes that he should quit smoking. He uses his inhaler while walking to the car.

Episode 2

Jimmy has been cleaning out the garage for the past few days and notices that it takes him quite a while to catch his breath. He feels especially short of breath and uses his inhaler again. He also notices that the past several times he's mowed the grass, it's been more exhausting than usual. Cecelia has also noticed these changes and has been nagging him about how much better he would feel if he quit smoking. Jimmy and his daughter accompany Cecelia to the clinic ▾.

Episode 3

Jimmy makes a decision this week to quit smoking. He is not sure yet how he will do it, and decides *not* to tell anyone, just in case things don't work out. He reads about smoking cessation tips online to help him get motivated ▾.

Episode 4

Jimmy smokes outside so that Cecelia does not give him a hard time. He keeps thinking about a smoking cessation tip he read about online that he thinks might help: Every time he thinks about or really craves a cigarette, he will take one and place it in a jar. He decides he might give that a try when he is *really* ready ▾.

Episode 5

The local forest fire has kept Jimmy indoors. He knows that if he goes out, he will have problems breathing. Cecelia tells Jimmy that the dryer is broken "AGAIN!" Jimmy looks at it and determines that he needs to go to the store for parts to fix it. Cecelia also wants to go out, but he tells her they should stay home until the air clears ▾ [NEWS].

Episode 6

The air is clear enough for Jimmy to venture out with Cecelia again. They go to the Neighborhood Senior Center to play bingo and to the hardware store to buy parts for the dryer. Jimmy has made an effort to reduce the number of cigarettes he smokes a day. He feels better since he "cut down," but knows that he still needs to quit. Over the weekend, Jimmy enjoys having his family at the house. He spends most of his time playing computer games with his grandchildren.

Episode 7

Jimmy accompanies Cecelia and his daughter to the nurse practitioner to see about Cecelia's arthritis pain. While sitting in the waiting room, he notices another man come in with portable oxygen. The man appears to be short of breath from the walk into the office from the parking lot. Jimmy is glad he does not have to tote an oxygen tank around with him.

Episode 8

Jimmy receives word that his younger brother died after battling lung cancer for several years. He was very close to his brother and was glad he was able to visit him last year when he was still feeling good. Jimmy's nephew tells Jimmy not to worry about traveling because they are planning a very small memorial service and will scatter his ashes in the ocean. Jimmy does not like the idea of cremation but keeps his opinion to himself. He tells his nephew that he hopes to visit again soon.

Episode 9

Jimmy goes to his son's home to help him fix a computer. They have to move furniture in order to pull the computer out. In shifting the furniture, Jimmy becomes very short of breath and is without his inhaler. He panics and struggles to get air. He sits down for about 30 minutes to rest and catch his breath. His son is concerned and inquires about the last time his dad has talked to a doctor about his breathing. Jimmy tells his son his breathing is fine; he is just a little out of shape.

Episode 10

Jimmy sees Dr. Rowe for routine follow-up care. He has a routine chest x-ray taken to evaluate his condition. Jimmy tells Dr. Rowe that he's been feeling fine; he just gets short of breath on occasion. The physician talks with Jimmy about the progression of his disease and reinforces the need to stop smoking. He inquires about Jimmy's attempts at doing so. Jimmy starts telling Dr. Rowe about his idea to put cigarettes in jars, but Dr. Rowe isn't sure what he is talking about. Thinking about his experience last week and the words of his physician, Jimmy decides to learn more about nicotine gum. He reads about nicotine gum on the Internet and places an order online. He

also decides to try the cigarettes-in-a-jar technique as well.

Episode 11

Jimmy receives the nicotine gum and has been following the directions. He is down to chewing one piece every few hours and is proud of his progress. He also decides to place one cigarette in a jar every time he craves one. This really helps motivate Jimmy.

Cecelia has the flu this week. One of Jimmy's daughters and a granddaughter spend a lot of time at the house taking care of things for them.

Episode 12

Jimmy takes Cecelia to the Wednesday evening potluck and bingo game at their church. Cecelia never wins, despite the fact that they play frequently - and this has been a great source of friendly teasing. She finally has a change in luck and wins this week. He wonders what he can tease her about now.

Episode 13

While outside doing a little yard work, Jimmy sees the dogs fighting with a cat that has gotten into the yard. Jimmy scurries across the yard to break it up. The cat runs off, but one of his dogs has a big scratch across its nose. Jimmy becomes very upset and short of breath, and he badly wants a cigarette. To calm himself down, he reaches into his pocket and takes three pieces of nicotine gum, thinking more is better. It burns his tongue, and he feels dizzy and becomes sweaty.

Episode 14

Cecelia tells Jimmy she thinks nicotine gum is dangerous. After his recent experience with the gum, Jimmy decides she is probably right. He decides it is probably safer to smoke just a few cigarettes a day and use his inhaler when needed. He is glad Cecelia does not nag him when she sees him smoking. He coughs nearly every morning for a few minutes when he wakes up; he attributes this to his body readjusting to the cigarettes.

Episode 15

Cecelia "drags" Jimmy to the neighborhood arts and crafts fair. He really does not want to go, but it is an activity they go to each year. Jimmy gets tired and finds a bench to sit on while his wife and daughters walk around to each exhibit. A couple of other men who are also waiting for their wives begin to talk with Jimmy. He has a hard time hearing them because they don't talk very loud, and there are a lot of other people talking nearby.

Jimmy Bley Season 3 Information

Episode 1

Jimmy is an 85-year-old male with moderate emphysema and hearing loss. He has been married for 61 years to his wife Cecelia. They argue a lot, but they would not know what to do without each other just the same.

Jimmy considers himself healthy. He describes his emphysema as "not that bad." Recently, his episodes of shortness of breath have interfered with activities more than usual, and he has made efforts on two occasions to stop smoking. Both times, Jimmy was not successful. He is privately very aware of the fact that his breathing has worsened and that he is using his inhaler much more frequently.

This episode Jimmy's daughter hears an announcement on the radio that free flu shots are being offered at a local health clinic. She tells both of her parents, but Jimmy is sure it will just make him sick. He is already not feeling great and he does not want to take the vaccine. His daughter tells him that both of them are considered at high risk for getting the flu. Jimmy feels that he is basically fairly healthy and never gets sick anyway, so he will just take his chances ▶.

Episode 2

Although Jimmy has had less energy and a cough, he enthusiastically agrees to help his 13-year-old granddaughter research information about snakes on the Internet to help her find what she needs for a school science project. Feeling very tired, he takes a nap after she leaves ✉.

Episode 3

Jimmy has been doing very little the last several days. He wakes up, does a few things, takes a nap, gets up for lunch, takes care of some chores, and then naps again before dinner. He tells Cecelia he is just sleepy all the time, but otherwise he feels fine. He does not believe that he is in need of a physician visit.

Episode 4

Jimmy continues to feel very tired and has a nagging cough. He gets short of breath very easily while doing chores outside. Over the weekend, he has so much difficulty mowing the lawn that he lets his son finish the job for him. He goes into the house, lies on the couch to watch TV, and naps off and on for the rest of the afternoon. His son and daughter suggest that he go to his doctor. Jimmy tells them his appointment is in another month or so, and he can wait to see his doctor then. Jimmy's cough at night has become more frequent, although he tends to sleep through it ▶.

Episode 5

Jimmy has begun waking in the middle of the night with a persistent, productive cough. He finds himself needing his inhaler as soon as he is awake. Jimmy believes he has just caught a bad cold. To help him sleep, Jimmy props himself up on several pillows. Cecelia sets up a humidifier in the room at night, which seems to help. He spends most of the day resting and taking over-the-counter cold medicine in an effort to treat this "cold." Jimmy is resistant to Cecelia's suggestion that he see a doctor. "It is just a cold," he tells her ▶ ✉.

Episode 6

Jimmy feels a bit better this week. He still has a cough at night, but he feels like he has more energy and is sleeping a bit better. He feels good enough to accompany Cecelia on errands, but he is very tired by the time they get home. Jimmy's son comes by the house and takes care of the yard work. Jimmy does not object to this, believing that he should conserve his strength. He is sure that by next week he will feel up to doing the yard work. He has intermittent "coughing fits," and Cecelia tells Jimmy to quit the cigarettes.

This week there is also a disruption in water service for a couple of days. Jimmy finds the problem an inconvenience, but not a big deal. Cecelia and their daughter bring some water home from a water distribution center.

Episode 7

This week, Jimmy feels worse than before. He is surprised at how long the symptoms have lasted. He continues to have a persistent, productive cough. He finds that he becomes short of breath much more easily than he normally would, and it takes him twice as long to shower and get dressed in the morning. His appetite has dropped off, and he has not been drinking as many fluids as he needs, partly because of the effort involved in eating and drinking.

Jimmy wakes up suddenly in the middle of the night and is unable to catch his breath. He tries to use his inhaler, but this doesn't seem to help. He can't move air well enough to take a deep breath and get any medication into his lungs. He feels like he is suffocating and becomes very anxious. Cecelia wants to call for an ambulance, but Jimmy insists on going to the hospital in their car. Cecelia calls her daughter and son, and they take him to the Emergency Department. Walking from the house to the car is very difficult and compromises Jimmy further. Jimmy is seen and treated in the Emergency Department by Dr. Gordon and is admitted to the intensive care unit (ICU) with a diagnosis of pneumonia and acute respiratory failure ▤ ▽.

Episode 8
Jimmy has spent the past week intubated on a ventilator and is receiving antibiotics. He is very scared and anxious. Although he is unable to talk, he is comforted by having his family with him. When they are present, Jimmy is much calmer. A family member stays with him as long as the nursing staff allows a visitor. Although the pneumonia is resolving, the nurses in the ICU have not yet been successful in weaning Jimmy from the ventilator ▽.

Episode 9
Jimmy has taken a turn for the worse. He has become septic, and his blood pressure has dropped significantly. He remains on a ventilator, is receiving medications to maintain his blood pressure, and is on multiple antibiotics. He is confused and disoriented. The nurses keep him heavily sedated to manage his anxiety and control patient-ventilation asynchrony ▽.

Episode 10
Jimmy's condition stabilized at the end of last week, and he is now improving quickly. Jimmy is not confused, but he feels like he has just awakened from a bad dream. He cannot recall much of anything. The experience has left him very weak and frightened.

The ICU nurses successfully wean Jimmy off the ventilator, and he is moved to the step-down unit. He is on oxygen, and his oxygen saturation is monitored carefully. A nurse brings in a fan to help relieve Jimmy's sense of shortness of breath. It really makes him feel better ▤ ▽.

Episode 11
Jimmy's condition has improved. Because he is deconditioned, the respiratory, physical, and occupational therapists have been working with him to help him regain mobility and the ability to perform activities of daily living (ADLs). Case management is involved with assessing his discharge needs. Because his oxygen saturation falls below 90% when he is off oxygen and doing any kind of activity, it is determined that he will need supplemental oxygen at home. He also will need to continue with outpatient physical and occupational therapy after discharge. He is unable to ambulate without the use of a walker. A dietitian meets with Jimmy and Cecelia to talk about ways to improve Jimmy's nutritional status.

Because of this ordeal, Jimmy has become very depressed. He does not interact much with his family or

the staff. He does not like the idea of being dependent on oxygen, and his weak condition makes him feel helpless. The physician prescribes bupropion SR (Wellbutrin SR) for depression. He is started on an initial dose of 150 mg a day with a gradual increase to 150 mg twice a day. Jimmy just wants to go home. He believes that, if he could just get home, all of these problems would resolve. Jimmy is discharged at the end of the week.

Episode 12
Jimmy is very happy to be at home in his own bed and with his family. He prefers being cared for by Cecelia and his daughters rather than by the nurses at the hospital. He is happy to eat the food prepared by his family. He is very discouraged about the oxygen and doesn't want to be dependent. Cecelia places a fan in his room at night to help him rest. He goes to outpatient physical and occupational therapy three times a week, and he is slowly regaining his strength. He just can't believe how weak he became while in the hospital. He also goes to the pulmonary rehabilitation clinic this week.

Episode 13
Jimmy continues going to outpatient physical therapy and the pulmonary rehabilitation clinic this week. He hates being attached to the oxygen, but he realizes he cannot do without it. Sometimes, he takes it off and sneaks a cigarette, although the idea of smoking turns out to be better than the actual smoking. He begins to lose his desire for cigarettes ▽.

Episode 14
Jimmy is very surprised how long it is taking him to get better. He recognizes now that he was in bad shape and is lucky to be alive. He is so focused on his own condition that he fails to notice the toll his illness is taking on Cecelia.

Episode 15
Jimmy has completed his rehabilitation and is attempting to get back into his normal daily activities. However, he has had to redefine "normal routine." His energy is gradually improving, but he is unable to do many of his former activities. His son and daughters come by the house every day to help out with whatever needs to be done. Everyone notices that his spirits have improved significantly as well; he especially enjoys it when his grandchildren come to the house. Jimmy has finally been able to quit smoking and has vowed never to touch cigarettes again.

Cecelia suggests to Jimmy they go to the Senior Center for bingo, but Jimmy doesn't want to do this because he feels embarrassed about the oxygen. Instead, they decide to spend an evening at their daughter's home.

CECELIA BLEY

Season 1	Season 2	Season 3
Cecelia is a very mentally sharp 83-year-old who is in excellent health. She has osteoarthritis that causes pain in the morning, but feels better as the day progresses. She takes care of most of the routine home activities. She often is frustrated trying to communicate with her husband Jimmy.	Cecelia's story continues with a description of daily life with joint pain. When her pain increases, Cecilia sees a physician and is formally diagnosed with osteoarthritis.	When Jimmy becomes ill, Cecelia is very concerned for him; she stays with him at the hospital and has strong support from her family members.

Cecelia Bley Season 1 Information

Episode 1

Cecelia is a very healthy, mentally sharp 83-year-old female. She has been married to Jimmy for 60 years and has been a homemaker all her life. She and Jimmy raised eight children. All of their children are grown with families of their own and live in the area; they remain very close. Cecelia and Jimmy argue and bicker a lot, primarily because Jimmy can't hear well. The hearing loss frustrates Cecelia when she is trying to talk with Jimmy. At the same time, Cecelia does not know what she would do without him.

Cecelia's only health-related problem is joint pain, which she describes as an annoyance. The joint pain has become more noticeable over the past few years, but she has never had a medical evaluation for this. She wakes up very stiff and sore in the morning, but she usually feels better once the day gets going. Cecelia does most of the general housekeeping, grocery shopping, and cooking. Her primary hobby is painting. She is very skilled at this. When she was younger, she used to sell her paintings at shows and art galleries. Now that she has gotten older, she only paints on occasion and gives most of her paintings to her daughters to sell for her. Although she likes to spend time in the garden, she limits this activity because her knees hurt too much. She also enjoys reading and

watching television. She is very fond of their two dogs and is an active member of her church.

This episode Cecelia and Jimmy run errands and do their weekly shopping as they have for years. On the way home, Cecelia hears sirens approaching their car from behind and realizes that Jimmy is completely unaware. She has to yell at Jimmy to pull over. He responds to her, "I heard them! You don't have to yell!" She often feels frustrated with him because of his lack of concern about his hearing ▼.

Episode 2

Cecelia falls in the bathroom after slipping on water from a leaky faucet. She experiences considerable joint pain and hollers out for Jimmy. Because Jimmy is not wearing his hearing aid and is in another room working on the computer, he does not hear her yelling. Cecelia finally gives up yelling for him to help her and gets up slowly herself. She goes into the other room, yells at Jimmy for not helping her, and tells him to fix the leaky faucet ▼.

Episode 3

Jimmy tells Cecelia about a stray dog that he has seen the past few days and mentions that he is probably hungry. Cecelia tells Jimmy not to feed it because it will just encourage the dog to hang around more. A few days later Jimmy tells Cecelia he would like to keep the dog because it needs a home. Cecelia tells Jimmy they need to call the city shelter and have the dog picked up; the shelter will find the dog a home. The next thing Cecelia knows, the dog is in their backyard playing with their other two dogs. Cecelia tells Jimmy that she does not want anything to do with any of his dogs and that he needs to take care of them.

Episode 4
Cecelia's granddaughter asks her to come to her school to talk about being an artist and painter for career day. She is not sure the children will be interested, but she agrees to do it for her granddaughter. Cecelia gives a short presentation to the grade-school children and then lets them try painting. She enjoys having a chance to share her experiences with others ▾.

Episode 5
Cecelia hears the dogs fighting out in the backyard and sees Jimmy go out to take care of things. She follows him and sees Jimmy get bitten while trying to break up the fight. Cecelia turns on a water hose and sprays the three dogs; this quickly breaks up the fight. After looking at the wound on his hand, Cecelia tells Jimmy that he needs to go to the hospital. She calls her daughter, who takes her parents to the Neighborhood Hospital Emergency Department. Cecelia tells her daughter to get rid of the stray dog. She overhears her daughter calling her husband and telling him to go to the house to take the dog away.

Episode 6
One of Cecelia and Jimmy's granddaughters has a birthday this week; their entire family will have a party for her at their home over the weekend. Cecelia tells Jimmy about the plans on Wednesday. On Saturday, the family spends the entire day at their home. Jimmy asks Cecelia why he was not told about the party, and Cecelia tells him that he is an old fool for not wearing his hearing aid. Cecelia thoroughly enjoys having her family visit her, but by the time they all go home, her knees and hips are hurting quite a bit. She realizes that she has been on her feet nearly the entire day.

Episode 7
Cecelia goes to a community Health Fair with her daughter and granddaughter. At the fair, Cecelia has screenings for osteoporosis, blood pressure, and glucose, and she has her height and weight checked. At one of the stations, Cecelia talks with a nurse about her joint pain. The nurse encourages Cecelia to make an appointment with her healthcare provider to have this symptom evaluated, and gives her a patient-information flyer on osteoarthritis. After reading the flyer, Cecelia is pretty sure that osteoarthritis is what is causing her pain. Cecelia learns that several over-the-counter medications such as glucosamine, acetaminophen, and ibuprofen are effective for treating arthritic pain. Cecelia's daughter agrees to pick these medications up from the drug store for her to try.

Cecelia also picks up a flyer on smoking cessation from a table at the health fair. She takes the flyer home and gives it to Jimmy to read ▾ [NEWS].

Episode 8
After spending time in her garden this week, Cecelia experiences a great deal of pain in her joints. Her daughter helps her by massaging her joints. Cecilia tells her daughter that she is experiencing so much pain that she wants to see a physician to find out if she could benefit from other treatments. Cecelia's daughter calls and makes an appointment for next week ▾.

Episode 9
Cecelia's daughter and Jimmy accompany Cecelia to Dr. Rowe's office, where a history and examination are done. From the history, Dr. Rowe learns that Cecelia's primary symptoms are joint pain and joint swelling. He also learns that Cecelia has had joint pain since her early 40s, but it has become more noticeable and progressively worse since her 70s. Her pain is most severe in the knees and hips—often making walking very painful, especially in the early part of the morning. In the past, Cecelia could get relief by resting, but over the past several years, she has experienced pain both with activity and during rest. In fact, she often awakens at night with joint pain. She self-treats with ibuprofen and aspirin. Occasionally, she uses a heating pad over her joints and relates that her daughters help by massaging her joints. After an examination, the physician advises Cecelia to have some lab work and x-rays performed; she is scheduled for these tests in the upcoming week ▶.

Episode 10
Cecelia's son takes her to the outpatient radiology services to have x-rays taken of her knees, hips, and spine. She also goes to the outpatient lab to have blood tests done (complete blood count and erythrocyte sedimentation rate). Several days later, she returns to Dr. Rowe's office to get her results. She is told that she has joint space narrowing in her joints, a finding that is consistent with osteoarthritis. She is also told that her blood tests were all normal. Dr. Rowe tells Cecelia to do what she has already been doing; basically, she is told to use over-the-counter medications to treat her condition—acetaminophen, ibuprofen, and glucosamine. Additionally, she is advised to increase the period of rest between activities and avoid strenuous movement of her knee and hip joints. Cecelia wonders why she even bothered going to the doctor ▶ [NEWS].

Episode 11

Cecelia begins to worry about Jimmy because he has been gone all afternoon and should have been back hours ago. She calls her son's home and learns he is still there and will be home soon. When he is brought home by his son, she learns that Jimmy had a minor accident with their car after hitting a curb and bending the wheel rim. Cecelia is grateful that Jimmy was not hurt, but she wants to know how much it will cost to fix the car. Jimmy does not mention to Cecelia that the accident was caused by his failure to hear an ambulance [NEWS].

Episode 12

Cecelia has been spending a great deal of time painting the past few weeks, as she has agreed to go to an art show with her daughter out of town next week. Fortunately, painting is something she is able to do without causing joint pain [NEWS].

Episode 13

Cecelia shows her paintings at an arts and crafts fair with her daughter. She enjoys the show and realizes that she misses doing this, but she also recognizes the amount of work involved in preparing and doing the showing. She has a successful show but is quite tired from the experience.

Episode 14

Cecelia and her daughters spend two full days cleaning the house. It has been a long time since the kitchen cabinets have been emptied and cleaned, the refrigerator moved and cleaned beneath, the windows cleaned, and so forth. Cecelia is very happy to have this level of cleaning done, but she is very tired afterwards and her joints ache. She takes ibuprofen and aspirin to manage her symptoms [▼].

Episode 15

Cecelia attends her grandson's music concert at the school. He is thrilled that she and Jimmy have come to hear him play. After the concert, Cecelia and Jimmy go to their son's home to visit with family members.

Cecelia Bley Season 2 Information

Episode 1

Cecelia is a very healthy, mentally sharp 83-year-old female. She has been married to Jimmy for 60 years and they raised eight children. Cecelia and Jimmy argue and bicker a lot, primarily because Jimmy can't hear well, but at the same time, Cecelia does not know what she would do without him.

Cecelia's only health-related problem is osteoarthritis, which has become more noticeable over the last few years. She finally had a formal medical evaluation a few months ago. She was told to treat her condition with acetaminophen, ibuprofen, and glucosamine. Additionally, she was advised to increase the period of rest between activities and to avoid strenuous movement to her knee and hip joints.

This episode Cecelia and her husband attend a granddaughter's soccer game. It is chilly, and she gets cold sitting outside in the wind. Her arthritis makes walking and moving her hands painful. Jimmy needs to use his inhaler as they are returning to the car after the game because he is quite short of breath. The cold air bothers both of them. In the car, Cecelia takes an aspirin for her pain.

Episode 2

Cecelia has returned to Dr. Rowe to seek a different treatment, because the arthritis pain is getting worse. Dr. Rowe prescribes acetaminophen and oxycodone, 1 tablet orally every 6 hours as needed for pain. She is told to be careful and not to take too many, because the medication can be addictive and is constipating [▶] [NEWS].

Episode 3

Cecelia has been worried about what Dr. Rowe said regarding addiction and constipation from oxycodone. She is also very aware of her bowel habits and hates the idea of becoming constipated. For these reasons, she rarely takes the oxycodone, despite the fact that she has been experiencing a great deal of pain and joint stiffness.

Episode 4

Cecelia has a very physically active weekend and her joints are causing her to be in a great deal of pain. Cecelia decides to take the oxycodone and is amazed at how much better it makes her feel. She takes it several times over the next few days and is pleased with the results – until she becomes constipated.

Episode 5

Cecelia is frustrated because the dryer is not working properly again and she can't get her laundry dried. Jimmy can fix the dryer, but he does not want to leave the house until the smoky air from the forest fires clears. Cecelia's daughter comes by the house to pick up the laundry and she takes Cecelia to her home where they do the laundry together. Jimmy stays at home and watches a sports event on television all afternoon [▼].

Episode 6

Cecelia cooks a Sunday dinner for her entire family. Her daughters can tell that she is having pain and they insist that she sit down while they do the dishes. By the time everyone leaves, Cecelia is very tired and hurting from standing and preparing the meal. She decides to take the oxycodone and risk getting addicted and constipated.

Episode 7

Cecelia returns to a follow-up appointment with Dr. Rowe, taking her oxycodone bottle as requested. Dr. Rowe asks Cecelia about her pain and how often she has been taking the pills. Cecelia is reluctant to complain and embarrassed to admit her concerns about constipation and addiction. Dr. Rowe notices how few of the prescribed pills Cecelia has used and inquires further. Cecelia explains why she has not taken many of the pills. Dr. Rowe counsels Cecelia about appropriate use to minimize her fears about the medicine ✉.

Episode 8

Cecelia is saddened to hear of the death of her brother-in-law (Jimmy's brother). She was very close to him and had known him for more than sixty years. Cecelia knows that he died of lung cancer and was a smoker – just like Jimmy. She wonders if this will motivate Jimmy to stop smoking.

Episode 9

Now that some of her misunderstandings and fears about the pain medication have been addressed, Cecelia is much more willing to take her pain medicine when she needs it. She has begun to work in her garden more regularly again. Her daughter suggests that they do another art show. Cecelia would like to do it, but the show is out of town, and she is pretty sure that Jimmy would rather stay home.

Episode 10

Cecelia and Jimmy go to a grandson's soccer game. Cecelia takes some pain medication before she goes, anticipating having pain with the walking. She and Jimmy find a comfortable spot from which to watch the game and set up their lawn chairs. She becomes annoyed when some people decide to stand along the sidelines in front of where they are sitting. They pack up their things and

move to another part of the field. After the game, they go to their son's home for supper.

Episode 11

Cecelia comes down with the flu this week. She is very weak and tired, and she has a cough and fever. Cecelia's daughter and granddaughter come to the house to help take care of Cecilia and the household so that she can rest. Cecelia's daughter gives her plenty of fluids ✉.

Episode 12

Cecelia and Jimmy go to play bingo at their church this week. Cecelia actually wins for the first time. "It's about time I win," she tells Jimmy. "How many years have we being playing?" She wins a gift certificate to the Neighborhood mall. Cecelia is not interested in going shopping at the mall, so she gives the gift certificate to her daughter.

Episode 13

Cecelia hears the commotion of a dog and cat fight in the yard and goes outside. She sees that Jimmy is short of breath. She watches him take out some of his nicotine gum and is concerned a short while later when he becomes sweaty and a little pale. She tells Jimmy that the gum is probably not as good for him as he thinks and encourages him to throw it away.

Episode 14

Cecelia can see that the bird feeder is empty. She gets a step stool to reach the upper shelves of the pantry to retrieve bird seed. She loses her balance and falls from the step stool to the floor. Fearing that she may have broken her hip, she lies on the floor a few minutes and then decides she is not seriously hurt. She sustains bruises to her hips and has a lot of joint pain the next few days.

Episode 15

Cecelia, her daughters, and Jimmy go to the Neighborhood arts and crafts show. She and her daughters visit each booth and are particularly impressed with the quilts on display. Cecelia has never made a quilt and talks with her daughters about making one. They talk to Pam Allen, the grand prize winner, about quilting designs and the best place in town to shop for quilting supplies ✉ [NEWS].

Cecelia Bley Season 3 Information

Episode 1

Cecelia is a very healthy, mentally sharp 84-year-old female. She has been married to Jimmy for 61 years and has been a homemaker all her life. She and Jimmy raised eight children, all of whom live in the area; they remain very close. Cecelia and Jimmy argue and bicker a lot, primarily because Jimmy can't hear well. The hearing loss

frustrates Cecelia when she is trying to talk with Jimmy. At the same time she would not know what to do without him.

Cecelia's only health-related problem is osteoarthritis. A few months ago, the pain really interfered with her activities, and she went back to see her family physician, Dr. Rowe. Her pain medications were adjusted, and Cecelia has had some improvement.

This episode Cecelia's daughter tells her that she heard an announcement on the radio about free flu shots offered at the Neighborhood Health Department. She recommends that both of her parents get the vaccine, as they are older and considered to be at high risk for the flu. Cecelia agrees that this is a good idea and plans to go when the shot clinic is offered. Jimmy goes along but decides not to get the shot.

Episode 2

Cecelia and her daughters spend an afternoon working on their quilts. Cecelia finds the work enjoyable, but it causes her hands to be sore. She takes ibuprofen and feels a bit better.

Jimmy frequently coughs during the night lately, waking Cecelia. She gets annoyed, not only because it wakes her up, but also because Jimmy sleeps right through it. She figures he sleeps through it because he can't hear anything.

Episode 3

Cecelia notices that Jimmy has been napping a lot more. He tells her he is just sleepy but feels fine. She is concerned about his breathing problem but she is unable to get him to agree to see Dr. Rowe about his increased fatigue.

Episode 4

Cecelia attends an all-day function at the church, making lunches for the Neighborhood Homeless Shelter. One of the ladies comments to Cecelia that she looks tired. She shares with the ladies that her arthritis has been acting up (which is true). She does not mention that the real reason she is tired is because Jimmy's coughing wakes her frequently at night. After spending the entire day on her feet, she takes an oxycodone tablet and puts her legs up when she gets home ▽.

Episode 5

Cecelia continues to be kept awake at night with Jimmy's coughing. She knows he is not feeling like himself because of his limited activity. He can hardly do anything without waiting a long time to catch his breath. She has repeatedly tried to get him to see the doctor, but he does not think he is that sick.

Episode 6

Cecelia is glad to see that Jimmy finally seems to be feeling better – he has been so stubborn about going to see their family doctor.

There is a disruption in water service for two days in the community. Cecelia is very annoyed about the fact that they have no water service because it is a significant disruption to her routine. Her daughter comes by the house and they go to a water distribution center to pick up some bottles of water for the house. She is very glad when service is restored [NEWS].

Episode 7

This week Cecelia notices that Jimmy is eating and drinking very little, and he has shortness of breath with limited activity. Cecelia wakes from sleep hearing Jimmy coughing and gasping for air; he is very anxious and gets no relief with his inhaler. Jimmy does not argue with her when she tells him they must go see a doctor, but he refuses to go in an ambulance. He insists that they go in their car. She calls her daughter and her son to help her take Jimmy to the Neighborhood Hospital Emergency Department, where he is treated by Dr. Gordon and later admitted to intensive care ▽.

Episode 8

Cecelia is very distressed about Jimmy's condition. She and her family stay at the hospital and visit him whenever they are allowed into the ICU. She tries to get as much information as she can from the doctors and nurses, but everybody is so busy. She has a hard time understanding everything that is happening ▽ [NEWS].

Episode 9

Jimmy has taken a turn for the worse. The physicians tell Cecelia and her family that Jimmy's condition is very serious, and they want to know what she might want to do if his heart stops. She has not had this conversation with Jimmy before and is confused about what to do. In her family growing up, death was never discussed. She doesn't want to talk to her children about it either. She is angry that the doctors are discussing the possibility of Jimmy dying. She would rather they attend to him in every way and not speak of such things. She doesn't like being asked these questions. She prays often for his healing. Cecelia worries about the care Jimmy is receiving. She has read in the newspaper about the nursing strike and wonders if the nurses caring for Jimmy know what to do. She wonders if the reason he got worse is because of the nursing care ▶ ▽ [NEWS].

Episode 10

Cecelia continues to remain with Jimmy every day. She is relieved that her prayers have been answered. Although she is glad that he has improved enough to be moved to a step-down unit, she is worried that they will not monitor him as closely as they were able to in the ICU. She also does not know if the nurses will care for her husband the way they should. She is very tired from spending so much time at the hospital. Cecelia's daughter convinces her to go home and rest for part of the day while she and her husband stay with Jimmy [NEWS].

Episode 11

Cecelia worries about how low Jimmy's spirit is; he does not seem to care about getting better. She wishes there was something she could do to lift his spirits. Cecelia meets with the discharge planner to discuss Jimmy's needs once he leaves the hospital.

Cecelia shares her concerns with the staff about Jimmy's mood; she learns that the physician has prescribed an antidepressant. Cecelia and her family prepare to bring Jimmy home from the hospital. The medical supply company comes to the home to install grab bars in the showers and to deliver home oxygen. Cecilia and her sons and daughters are taught how to use the oxygen tanks. Cecelia is thankful for her children, who will help her take care of Jimmy once he comes home ▶.

Episode 12

Cecelia and her family are thankful to have Jimmy home, although caring for him is much harder than they anticipated. Cecelia is glad that the physical therapist taught them how to help Jimmy get up and is thankful that the nurses taught them about oxygen therapy and his medications. Cecelia's children and friends are at the house regularly and take Cecelia and Jimmy to all of his outpatient appointments.

Episode 13

Cecelia is encouraged by the progress that she sees Jimmy making with rehabilitation. His spirits seem to be better, and he is taking a greater interest in the activities around him. She also notices that Jimmy is not smoking much. She knows he tries to "sneak" a cigarette on occasion, but she doesn't let on that she knows.

Episode 14

Cecelia is really feeling worn down and is suffering from joint pain as a result of caring for Jimmy. Although her daughters and sons help a lot, she tries to do as much herself as possible. It takes a very stern but respectful discussion from her daughter to get her to slow down. She does not want to be so dependent on her children. She knows they have busy lives, but at the same time she is grateful for their help. Cecelia just hates to admit she and Jimmy are "dependent elders ▼."

Episode 15

As Jimmy's condition has improved, Cecelia has been able to get more rest. She finally has a chance to get back to the quilts that she and her daughters started months ago, and her daughter has talked about getting a few paintings done for an upcoming show. With all of the activity, Cecelia has let the garden go these past few months and is not sure she will get back to it this season.

JAMES HOUSEHOLD

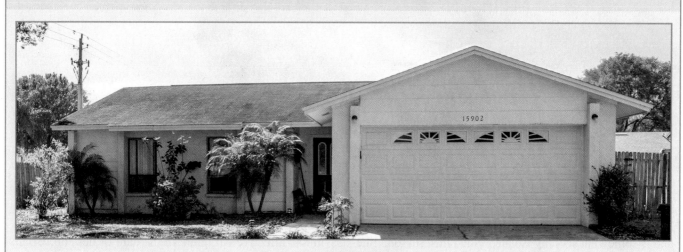

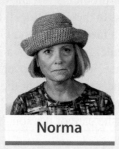

Norma

Housing	Mrs. James lives in a small one story home in the Southend. She lives close to the manufacturing area
Parks and Recreation	There are only a few parks in the area and some of them are in disrepair.
Services	The Senior Center is close to the James home and there is a grocery store within walking distance. There is bus service to the area also.

NORMA JAMES

Season 1	Season 2	Season 3
Mrs. James is a widow who lives alone and is somewhat socially isolated. She has type 2 diabetes, atrial fibrillation, and hypertension. She sees multiple physicians and takes multiple medications. Early in this season she has a diabetic ulcer on her foot. She becomes acquainted with Karen, a nurse at the local Senior Center, and begins to go there regularly.	Mrs. James has a mild stroke during this season. She has initial affective aphasia, problems swallowing, and weakness to the right side of her body. She has a feeding tube and Foley for a short while, and develops a UTI. She experiences depression over her situation. She spends time at the rehabilitation hospital and eventually returns home in the care of her son, Brian.	Mrs. James makes remarkable progress at home in the care of her son, Brian. Eventually she becomes independent enough that Brian is able to return to his home. The ordeal has resulted in the reestablishment of a positive relationship between Mrs. James and her son.

Norma James Season 1 Information

Episode 1

Norma James is a 65-year-old widow who lives alone. Although she has lived in the Neighborhood for years, she is somewhat socially isolated. She has two adult sons with whom she has limited contact; they live out of the state and rarely call. There are only a few individuals whom Mrs. James considers friends; she does not particularly like most people and prefers the company of her six cats. She has a long history of type 2 diabetes mellitus and hypertension. In recent years, she was diagnosed with atrial fibrillation. She has multiple physicians and takes multiple medications including:

- glipizide (Glucotrol), 10 mg twice a day
- captopril, 50 mg twice a day
- digoxin, 125 mcg once a day
- warfarin sodium (Coumadin), 5 mg once a day

Mrs. James has a known drug allergy to penicillin.

Mrs. James does not work; she has very limited savings and relies on Social Security benefits for income. She smokes about $1/2$ pack of cigarettes per day and has

been a smoker since she was in her twenties. She drinks alcohol "a couple times a year, usually a glass of wine at a special dinner." Mrs. James does not drive and relies on her friends, neighbors, or the city bus for transportation. She lives near a grocery store and prides herself on being able to get most things she needs without any assistance. She spends most of her time alone at home and occupies herself by watching television, reading, and doing crossword and jigsaw puzzles.

Mrs. James has a sore on her ankle that has been there for the past several weeks. It does not really hurt much, but she has been unable to get it to heal. The cashier at the convenience store tells Mrs. James that she should use butter to help heal wounds, because it keeps the wound moist and helps to enhance healing.

Episode 2

Mrs. James decided to follow the advice of her friend (the cashier at the convenience store) and has been applying butter to her wound for about one week. The wound does not seem to be getting any better. In fact, it looks a little worse, so Mrs. James stops the butter treatment. She knows that she should get an appointment with her primary care provider, but when she calls to make an appointment, she is told that the physician she likes is out of the office on vacation for the next 2 weeks. She has heard about a nurse clinic at the Neighborhood Senior Center not far from her home, but she has never been to the center because she does not perceive herself to be old. Mrs. James decides to continue treating the wound herself.

Episode 3

Mrs. James' wound continues to look progressively worse; it now has a yellowish drainage, and the skin around the wound has become red. Her foot also now hurts when she walks on it. She goes to the Emergency Department (ED) early in the morning. After sitting in the waiting room for 4 hours, Mrs. James tells the ED receptionist that she has better things to do than sit in a waiting room all day. She decides to go to the Senior Center just this once to see if the nurse at the clinic will look at her leg.

At the Senior Center Nursing Clinic, Mrs. James meets Karen, a geriatric clinical nurse specialist, and a student nurse by the name of Kayla. Kayla starts asking Mrs. James a number of questions that she finds very annoying. Mrs. James says, "Why are you asking me such stupid questions? Can't you see that my leg is hurting?" The other nurse, Karen, takes a short history and checks Mrs. James' vital signs and glucose levels. Mrs. James is unable to recall all of the medications that she takes. After looking at the wound, Karen tells Mrs. James that she must see her healthcare provider. Karen makes an appointment to see her physician for that day and arranges a ride for Mrs. James on the Senior Center shuttle. Before Mrs. James leaves, Karen suggests that Mrs. James come back to see her next week and bring a list of the medications that she takes. Mrs. James also learns from Karen that a free lunch is served at the Senior Center. Mrs. James does not care for Mr. Jackson, the shuttle driver. She is annoyed that he talks so much and she asks him to just be quiet.

At her physician's office, Mrs. James is told that her leg wound is infected and will require antibiotic treatment and dressing changes. The office staff arranges for Mrs. James to have a home health nurse make daily visits for IV antibiotic therapy and dressing changes for 10 days. The nurse and physician both note that her blood pressure and glucose level are somewhat elevated, but they assume that the change is related to the infection and pain ▶ ▼.

Episode 4

Mrs. James completes her 10-day course of antibiotic therapy. The wound is no longer painful and is beginning to heal. She has a follow-up visit at her primary care physician's office and is instructed to continue with daily wound care. The office nurse talks with Mrs. James about the need for medication adherence to limit the effects of her diabetes. The nurse asks her if she has any problems with her medications. Mrs. James says that she has no problems; she just doesn't always take her medications.

Episode 5

Noticing quite a collection of cat fur on the floor under the bench and in the corners of the living room, Mrs. James sets out to sweep and scrub the floors. In the process of cleaning, Mrs. James slips on the wet floor and falls, landing on her extended right arm. Despite the fact that it hurts, Mrs. James is not about to go back to the doctor. Her arm hurts with any movement for a few days, but by the end of the week, the pain is present primarily when she raises her arms over her head.

Episode 6

Mrs. James decides to go back to the Senior Center Nurse Clinic to see the nurse because she likes Karen and wants to show her that her leg is healing. Mrs. James can see that the student nurse, Kayla, is there again. Mrs. James completely ignores Kayla when she tries to talk with her, and only gives her attention to Karen. Karen checks her vitals (temperature 98.7, pulse 90, respiratory rate 18, blood pressure 140/90 mm Hg) and glucose level (234 mg/dL), noting the elevation in her blood pressure and glucose. Karen looks at the leg and can see that the wound is healing. Mrs. James forgets to bring the list of medications she is currently taking, so Karen talks with her about how she obtains her medications and how she keeps them organized. Karen gives Mrs. James a diabetes-and-foot-care brochure and asks her to bring a list of the medications she takes on her next visit. Mrs. James is in a hurry to leave so that she can get to the free Senior Center lunch ▶ ▼.

Episode 7

Mrs. James is planning to go back to the Senior Center this week to see the nurse, but she doesn't like what is on the lunch menu for that day. She is scheduled for another follow-up visit at her physician's office. However, she elects not to go because it is raining hard on the day of her appointment and she does not want to be out in bad weather.

Episode 8

As part of her normal routine, Mrs. James reads the Neighborhood newspaper every morning. She reads an article about a boy who brings a gun to school. Mrs. James wonders if the boys who wait at a nearby bus stop each morning carry guns. She thinks they look like the type of boys that would carry guns because of the way they dress and their shaggy hair style. She watches them closely from her living room window for a few days to see if she can see guns ▼ NEWS .

Episode 9

Mrs. James is on her way out the door to go to the Senior Center for lunch and to see the nurse, when one of her cats gets out. She spends the next hour waiting by the window for the cat to come back. She is worried that the cat will be killed by a car or a dog and is angry that she is going to miss the lunch that day. When the cat comes back to the front door, Mrs. James is relieved and decides that she needs to stay home the rest of the day to take care of her cats.

Episode 10

Mrs. James finally decides to go back to see Karen at the Senior Center Nursing Clinic. Remembering that she was asked to bring a list of medications with her but not wanting to take the time to make it, Mrs. James puts all the medications in a bag and takes them with her to the clinic.

At the clinic, Karen checks her vital signs (blood pressure 126/92 mm Hg; blood glucose 124 mg/dL) and asks Mrs. James about her medication list. Mrs. James opens her bag of medications and dumps them out on the table. A new nursing student by the name of Jacob sits down to look at the medications while Karen examines her feet. Karen notices that her shoes are in poor shape; the edges of her shoes have been cut down and covered with cotton balls and tape. Karen talks with Mrs. James about the need for shoes that fit and suggests that she check at the Senior Center for help obtaining properly fitting shoes. Karen also notes that the wound on her leg has almost completely healed. Jacob tells Karen and Mrs. James that many of the drugs are expired, and he can't tell which drugs Mrs. James is supposed to be using. Mrs. James grabs all of her pill bottles and puts them back in her bag. She says, "I know what these are all for and I don't have time to explain it all to you!"

Mrs. James goes to the Senior Center with the intention of getting lunch but instead wanders into a leather craft class. She sits down and begins to work with the leather. She listens to some of the other women in the class and is annoyed at all their chatter, especially that of one lady named Mary Martin. She likes the leather craft activity, but she does not like interacting with the women there ▶ ▽.

Episode 11

Mrs. James gets a notice in the mail from the city, stating that the bushes in her front yard are encroaching on the street and blocking the view. The notice states that she has 30 days to cut back the branches or pay the city to remove the brush and potentially face a city fine. This warning makes Mrs. James very upset. She attempts to cut the branches back with hedge clippers, but reinjures her shoulder in the process. She knows she can't just go out and cut down bushes at her age ▽.

Episode 12

Mrs. James continues to worry about the city notice to clean up her bushes and wonders if the city will try to evict her from her home. She tells her neighbor about the problem and asks if there is anybody who could do the work for her. A few days later she sees a teenager in her yard cutting back the bushes. Mrs. James does not go out to talk to him or thank him. She watches him work from her window and wonders if he is in a gang. She is not sure if he can be trusted.

Episode 13

Mrs. James runs out of her glipizide (Glucotrol) and when she calls the drugstore to get it refilled, she is informed that her prescription has expired. Mrs. James goes to the Senior Center Nurse Clinic the following day to see if Karen can help her. Mrs. James is annoyed when she sees the student nurse Jacob at the clinic again. He measures her blood glucose (192 mg/dL) and takes her vital signs, which are within normal limits. Karen calls the physician's office and arranges for a small refill to be made available to her until she comes in for an appointment. While on the phone with the physician's office, the nurse is able to get a list of Mrs. James' medications and dosages, as well as the names of her cardiologist and gynecologist. Karen also sees that Mrs. James is still wearing the same shoes she had on for the last visit.

Karen also talks with Mrs. James about her prescription drug benefits. Mrs. James indicates that she received something in the mail some time ago, but she did not understand what it said and threw it away ▶.

Episode 14

Mrs. James' son Brian calls her this week. She does not often talk with her son, and she is very happy to hear from him. She suggests that he come to visit. He responds that he has started a new job and is busy, and he really likes the new job. Mrs. James is not too interested in hearing about his new job and instead gets into an argument with him about the fact that he rarely visits.

Episode 15

Mrs. James has become a regular at the Senior Center on days when the nurse is in the clinic. She has come to trust Karen and, in fact, considers her a friend. Over time, she has become more open about discussing personal matters. Mrs. James talks to Karen in detail about her cats and some of her neighbors. When questioned about her sons and whether they are available to help, Mrs. James explains that her sons don't like her very much, but they would help her if she needed them. She goes on to mention that they are very busy and they know she does not need their help ▶.

Norma James Season 2 Information

Episode 1

In recent months, Mrs. James has been going to the Neighborhood Senior Center regularly.

The Senior Center is sponsoring a weekend trip by bus to a nearby national park. Although a fee is required, the cost is minimal. Karen (the nurse at the Senior Center) tells Mrs. James about the trip and suggests that she go on the outing. Mrs. James tells Karen that she has already seen all those parks before, and if she were to go on a bus trip, she would have to listen to all the women chatter. She tells Karen, "It's bad enough to listen to them at lunch. I can't imagine listening to them for days." Mrs. James also reminds Karen that she could never leave her cats alone for that length of time.

Episode 2

Mrs. James goes to the drugstore to get her prescriptions refilled. When she gets there, she is told that her co-payment for the prescriptions (Warfarin sodium (Coumadin) and digoxin) is $20. This makes Mrs. James very angry. She demands to know why the co-pay has changed and is told the extra charge is due to changes in the insurance plan. Although she has the money, Mrs. James decides not to pick up the prescriptions in protest. Instead, she goes to the grocery store to buy a new carton of cigarettes and then to the Senior Center for lunch. She dreads an encounter when she walks into the Senior Center and sees Mary Martin, the lady who talks too much. She glares at Mary as she walks past her and sits at a table by herself so that she doesn't have to listen to Mary talk.

Episode 3

Mrs. James loves all six of her cats, but her favorite cat is 12-year-old Millie. Mrs. James notices that Millie is less active than usual and is not eating much. She wonders if she is sick and actually contemplates taking Millie to the vet, but she decides against the trip because she worries about incurring a large vet bill that she couldn't afford. She hopes that whatever is ailing Millie is just a minor and temporary problem.

Episode 4

Mrs. James' favorite cat, Millie, does not act normally for several days, then seems to get better. But, when taking the trash outside, Mrs. James spots Millie lying dead on the patio. She is so devastated that she does not leave the house for several days. She buries Millie in her backyard near the graves of her other deceased cats. She covers up the area with rocks to prevent dogs from coming along and digging up her kitty ▾.

Episode 5

Mrs. James is still feeling very sad about the death of her pet, Millie. She goes to the local animal shelter to look at cats and sees one that reminds her of Millie. The adoption fee is more than she wants to spend right now, and she is unable to convince the animal shelter staff to let her have the cat for free. She is told to watch for the occasional free adoption events that are held when the shelters get too full.

Episode 6

On Tuesday morning, Mrs. James wakes up at about 7 a.m. She does not feel right, but she is not sure why. Her right arm feels tingly and somewhat numb. She feeds her cats and decides to go back to bed. At 9 a.m., she wakes up again. When she tries to sit up, her right arm feels very heavy. When she tries to stand up, her right leg also feels heavy, making it difficult to walk. She can't seem to get her leg to support her.

Mrs. James wonders if the diabetes has caused her blood glucose levels to drop. She navigates to the kitchen and checks her glucose, noting that it is 137. She decides to eat some breakfast, thinking that she will feel better soon. Mrs. James begins to get worried when her symptoms don't subside. At about 10:30 a.m., she calls her neighbor on the phone, explains the situation, and asks her to come over to help her. The neighbor tells Mrs. James that she should call 9-1-1 for an ambulance and that she will come over as soon as she can. Mrs. James does not want to call 9-1-1 because ambulances charge too much. She decides to wait for her neighbor to take her to the hospital.

The neighbor arrives at Mrs. James' home at about 10:50. By this time, Mrs. James is talking, but not making any sense. The weakness on her right side has worsened so that Mrs. James is now unable to walk. The neighbor (believing Mrs. James already called 9-1-1) is hopeful that the ambulance will show up soon. By 11 a.m., the neighbor decides to call 9-1-1 and ask about the ambulance. She learns that no previous call was made. An ambulance arrives shortly thereafter and takes Mrs. James to Neighborhood Hospital. She arrives in the emergency department about 11:35. She is treated by Dr. Gordon, who determines that she is having a stroke. Mrs. James is admitted to the medical-surgical unit ▤ ▶.

Episode 7

Mrs. James remains at Neighborhood Hospital. She has a difficult week. Because of swallowing problems, a feeding tube is placed and tube feeding is initiated. She has ongoing issues with nausea and abdominal fullness.

Additionally, she experiences diarrhea; she has two episodes of fecal incontinence because she is unable to get the nursing staff to answer her call light. She is unable to ambulate independently at this time.

Mrs. James also develops an elevated temperature and confusion before anyone notices that the urine in her Foley bag is cloudy. A urinalysis (UA) and Culture and Sensitivity (C&S) test confirm that she has a urinary tract infection.

She has become very depressed and has taken a very passive role in her care. She wants the nurses just to take care of all of her needs. She continues to experience expressive aphasia and is embarrassed about the way she sounds. Mrs. James' son Brian comes to see her at the hospital this week. She barely speaks to him while he is there. He only stays for a few days to take care of some things at her home. Brian leaves his contact information with the nursing staff in case they need to contact him for anything. Mrs. James feels angry about the entire situation, and she is unhappy with the general inconsistency in the care she has received. One of the nurses she really does not like is Bobby. She does not find him to be nice or caring at all ▾.

Episode 8

This week Mrs. James is transferred to the Neighborhood Rehabilitation Center. Because of ongoing swallowing difficulties, a percutaneous endoscopic gastrostomy (PEG) tube is inserted for continued tube feedings shortly before she is transferred.

At the Rehabilitation Center, she works with physical, speech, and occupational therapists. She continues to have little or no motivation for improvement. Mrs. James is pleased when Karen (the nurse from the Senior Center) comes to visit her. She tells Karen what a horrible experience she has had. Karen, who is aware that Mrs. James has been very passive, tells her she needs to work on getting better so she can go home to take care of her cats. If she fails to improve, she might be placed in a nursing home. Mrs. James tells Karen that the cats are probably all dead by now and that there is no point in going home. Karen assures Mrs. James that her son Brian placed them in a boarding facility and that they are being well cared for. This information provides a spark for Mrs. James. She now has a reason to get better: her cats need to be rescued from the inhumane treatment they are probably receiving at the boarding facility.

Episode 9

Mrs. James remains at the Neighborhood Rehabilitation Hospital. She is beginning to make progress and has regained some mobility. She continues to work with the staff with a goal of regaining enough activities of daily living (ADL) skills to go home. She is surprised to see that Mr. Jackson, the shuttle bus driver from the Senior Center, has come to see her. "What are you doing here?" she asks. "I miss hearing your crabby voice, woman," he tells her. Mrs. James cracks a smile and he sits to visit with her for a few minutes.

Episode 10

Mrs. James remains at the Neighborhood Rehabilitation Hospital and continues to progress in her mobility, speech, and swallowing ▾.

Episode 11

Arrangements are being made for Mrs. James to be transferred home. Because of her ongoing care needs, her son Brian has agreed to spend up to a month with his mother in the role of caregiver while she makes the transition home.

Brian returns to the Neighborhood and spends several days making the necessary arrangements for her discharge. The arrangements include making home modifications (such as rails and a seat for the shower), obtaining equipment (wheelchair, walker, and grab bars), making appointments for follow-up physician visits and ongoing outpatient physical therapy, and figuring out her medication regimen. Because Mrs. James has prescriptions from several physicians, it takes Brian several days to figure out which are current and which are not. Additionally, Brian finds a box of medications in her home. It seems that Mrs. James has been hoarding medications for years. Brian throws all the old medications away and buys a pill box to help his mother keep her medications organized.

Episode 12

This week Mrs. James finally returns home. She is very happy to be home and is thrilled to see her cats. She is so thankful that Brian rescued them. Although she is glad Brian has come to help her, she immediately begins to criticize many of the things that he has done. She really did not want those ugly bars placed in the shower; he should have asked her first. She is also angry when she learns that he threw her box of medications away and that he won't buy her cigarettes. At the same time, Mrs. James does not understand why her sons have ignored her for so many years ▶.

Episode 13

Mrs. James still needs a lot of assistance with walking because she has lost a lot of strength and has some balance issues. She has regained good swallowing coordination with thick-consistency foods that do not require much chewing (such as oatmeal, mashed potatoes, puddings, and applesauce). She enjoys the food Brian prepares much more than the meals she was getting at the Neighborhood Rehabilitation Hospital, so she begins to regain weight.

Episode 14

Mrs. James' son remains at her home, caring for her, taking her to her various appointments, and enduring a constant barrage of criticism. He is highly motivated to get his mother back to functional independence so that he can go home.

Episode 15

Mrs. James needs to use the bathroom and her son has left her at home for a few hours to run errands. She gets up from a chair, uses her walker, and heads toward the bathroom. Along the way, she is startled by one of her cats (who has darted between her legs and the walker), and Mrs. James falls down. Fortunately, she is able to get herself to a sitting position and she waits for Brian to come home. When he arrives back at the house a short time later, she tells Brian that he might have to move back to the Neighborhood permanently to be with her ▶.

Norma James Season 3 Information

Episode 1

Mrs. James is currently recovering from her stroke. Brian James, her son, has been helping her to regain basic living skills so that she can continue to live in her own home. Before her stroke, Mrs. James smoked $1/2$ pack of cigarettes per day. She has not smoked since the stroke, primarily because her son refuses to purchase cigarettes for her.

Up until this recent stroke, Mrs. James' contact with her sons was very limited. There are only a few individuals whom she considers friends; she does not particularly like most people and prefers the company of her five cats. She does not drive and relies on her friends, neighbors, or the city bus for transportation. She lives near a grocery store and has always been able to get most things done without assistance.

Mrs. James has become accustomed to having her son Brian help her with things around the house. He literally takes care of everything for her, and she has come to expect him to do so. Although she is very appreciative of his efforts, Mrs. James has a hard time openly acknowledging Brian's hard work and dedication to her care. Instead she usually praises him through the eyes of her cats. "My cats think you take good care of me," she tells him ▼.

Episode 2

Mrs. James has finished her outpatient physical therapy. Brian tells his mother that he will be leaving soon, but before he goes, he wants her to prove to him that she is safe living on her own. Brian levels with his mother and tells her that, if she is unable to live alone, they might have to consider assisted living options. Mrs. James is furious with this suggestion and is determined to show Brian that she is capable of being on her own and that she does not need him ▶.

Episode 3

Mrs. James, accompanied by her son Brian, walks to the grocery store to do some shopping. It is her first time at the store since her hospitalization. Brian evaluates her ability to get to the store, make purchases, and get home. He is impressed by her determination and stamina, despite changes in mobility. Mrs. James decides not even to try to buy the cigarettes that she craves; she figures that Brian will be leaving soon enough. Next, they go to the drugstore to get refills for all of her medications.

At home, Mrs. James makes all three meals for several days in a row, takes care of all the household chores, and is able to get to the toilet and to get dressed and bathed without any assistance. She has learned to keep her medications organized and checks her glucose twice a day. During this week, she gives hints to Brian that he could help out, but he just sits and watches her. Mrs. James wonders aloud how she ever raised such a lazy son.

Episode 4

Brian heads home this week after the long stay with his mother. Mrs. James is deeply saddened to see him go, but she keeps her composure when he leaves. She tells him she is tired of having him there and wants the house to herself now; she has many things to do. Brian knows his mother all too well and gives her a hug as he goes out the door.

Episode 5

Mrs. James readjusts to her new life. She is able to do most things, but accomplishing everyday tasks takes her longer. She finds the house quiet and lonely since Brian left, although her cats keep her company. Mrs. James avoids going to the Senior Center because she believes that everyone will talk about her. Brian calls her to ask how things are going. She tells him she is just fine and doesn't need anything ▼.

Episode 6

In the past several months, Mrs. James has lost her favorite cat and suffered a stroke. Her son came to help her recover and she liked having him with her. Now he is gone and she is experiencing yet another loss. Mrs. James is frustrated by some residual physical limitations and just wishes that Brian would come back. She watches TV but does not find this pastime enjoyable.

Episode 7
Mrs. James decides to go back to the Senior Center for the first time since her stroke. The only person she wants to see is Karen, the nurse at the Senior Center Nursing Clinic. Mrs. James is initially greeted by Jennifer, a student nurse, and Mrs. James announces that she is there to see Karen. She is glad no one is with Karen when she arrives. Karen measures her blood pressure at 120/78 mm Hg and her blood glucose at 122 mg/dL. Mrs. James enjoys visiting with her for 15 minutes before being interrupted by "a stupid old man" who wants to see Karen. Mrs. James wanders out to the main room and finds a group of ladies playing cards. They invite her to join them. Mrs. James tells them that she can only stay for a few minutes because she has other things to do, but she ends up staying for the entire afternoon. They suggest that she join them again the following week ▶.

Episode 8
Mrs. James decides not to join the ladies at the Senior Center for cards, but she goes for lunch twice this week. She wonders why she has not heard from Brian lately and decides to call him. They talk for a short while, and Mrs. James tells him about the ladies asking her to join them in card games. Brian encourages her to join them again sometime soon.

Episode 9
A nurse case manager by the name of Trish visits Mrs. James in her home to evaluate her progress since her discharge. Trish is impressed with the degree of independence Mrs. James has regained. She spends time explaining to Mrs. James the importance of exercise, diet, and medication. Although Mrs. James tells Trish she "already knows all that stuff," she does pay attention to what Trish has to say and finds the information helpful. If nothing else, Mrs. James begins to understand the complexity of diabetes and has a new appreciation for disease management.

Episode 10
Mrs. James sees Karen at the Senior Center again this week. She is annoyed when the student nurse, Jennifer Porter, is with Karen; Mrs. James doesn't know why that nosy student always wants to listen to what she has to say. Karen asks her about her medications and glucose measurements, but Norma just wants to visit. However, because she is self-managing her disease better, Mrs. James is able to recall her medications and her most recent glucose readings. She isn't sure when she should be going back to see her physicians, however. Karen checks her blood pressure and finds it to be 118/82 mm Hg; her glucose is 116 mg/dL.

Episode 11
Mrs. James sees the card-playing ladies at the Senior Center this week and is again invited to join them. She spends most of the afternoon playing cards and finds that she can beat them easily because they spend all of their time talking to one another instead of paying attention to the cards in their hands.

Episode 12
Mrs. James sees on the news that the city is holding a "Pet Adoption Bonanza" and all adoption fees are waived for the weekend. She convinces her neighbor to drive her to the shelter, and she finds a new kitten to adopt. Knowing that she might not be allowed to adopt a cat if the shelter knows she already has five cats, Mrs. James says she has only one other cat. When she gets home, she calls her son Brian and tells him about her new kitty ▼.

Episode 13
The Senior Center is promoting fitness by bringing in fitness guru Jack Blaine. Normally she would not attend, but Mrs. James thinks about the information she learned from Trish (the case manager nurse) and decides to attend to listen to what he has to say. When she gets there, she does not care much for Jack Blaine. In her opinion, his shorts are too tight and too short. "What is wrong with that man? Those shorts are awful," she says aloud to no one in particular. Mrs. James notices that nobody pays any attention to her comment. All the ladies seem to be in love with that Mr. Jack Blaine. Mrs. James leaves to go home to her cats.

Episode 14
Mrs. James is invited to spend a week at the home of her son Brian and his family. Brian has offered to drive to her home, board her cats in a kennel, and then drive her to his home several hours away. Mrs. James is reluctant to leave her home and her cats. However, because it has been years since she last visited with her grandchildren, she is anxious to see them. Mrs. James agrees to visit Brian and spends the rest of the week getting ready to go.

Episode 15
Mrs. James is out of town visiting her son Brian this week ▼.

JOHNSON HOUSEHOLD

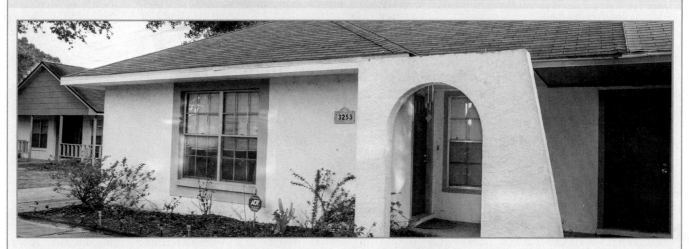

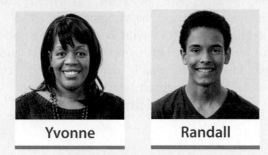

Yvonne   Randall

Housing	The Johnsons live in a small townhouse in Riverbank section, closer to Northwoods than to the river. The home is about 30 years old and they have a small yard and sidewalks in the area.
Parks and Recreation	There is a large recreation park nearby where Randall plays baseball. There is also a YMCA located in the area and several small parks.
Services	The high school Randall attends is located in the Riverbank area.

Key: ▶ = video clip   ▤ = medical record   ▽ = journal entry   📰 = news article

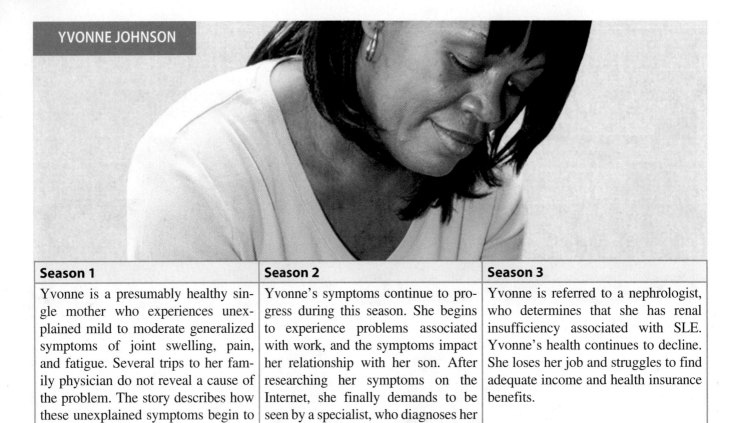

YVONNE JOHNSON

Season 1	Season 2	Season 3
Yvonne is a presumably healthy single mother who experiences unexplained mild to moderate generalized symptoms of joint swelling, pain, and fatigue. Several trips to her family physician do not reveal a cause of the problem. The story describes how these unexplained symptoms begin to affect her personal life.	Yvonne's symptoms continue to progress during this season. She begins to experience problems associated with work, and the symptoms impact her relationship with her son. After researching her symptoms on the Internet, she finally demands to be seen by a specialist, who diagnoses her with a connective tissue disorder.	Yvonne is referred to a nephrologist, who determines that she has renal insufficiency associated with SLE. Yvonne's health continues to decline. She loses her job and struggles to find adequate income and health insurance benefits.

Yvonne Johnson Season 1 Information

Episode 1

Yvonne Johnson is a 35-year-old African American female. She is a single parent to her 15-year-old son, Randall. Yvonne never married Randall's father and has always resented him because he left her for another woman when Randall was an infant. He lives in a nearby town and sees Randall several times a year. He sends Yvonne child support on a semi-regular basis.

Yvonne completed a Bachelor's degree in marketing 5 years ago but has been unable to break into the marketing field locally. Instead, she has been working full time as an administrative assistant for a large company. She is really not satisfied in her current job because she wants to be in the marketing field. In her opinion, she is underemployed. The positive aspects of her current job are excellent health insurance and other benefits and the proximity of work to her home. Although other opportunities are potentially available in other cities, she has lived in the Neighborhood most of her life and is not interested in leaving. Her parents and siblings live nearby, and she maintains a close relationship with them.

Over the past 4 years, Yvonne has noticed mild swelling in her hands and feet every morning. The symptoms began subtly not long after graduating from college and getting a job. She has always attributed the symptoms to her sedentary lifestyle and being somewhat overweight. More recently, she has been experiencing pain along with the swelling in her hands and feet.

Yvonne spends Saturday afternoon at her parents' home, helping her mother weed her garden and cut flowers for a bouquet. She shares with her mother that she has had pain in her hands for the past couple of months that she just can't seem to explain. Her mother tells her there is no reason that a healthy young woman should have pain and swelling in her hands and urges her to see a doctor about it. Yvonne decides her mother is probably right. The only healthcare provider she has seen in the past 10 years has been a nurse practitioner in a women's health office for her yearly pelvic exams. She makes an appointment with a family practice physician, Dr. Rowe, who is on her medical plan. She is unable to see Dr. Rowe for a few weeks.

Episode 2

Yvonne has been interested in a man at work (from a different department) for several months. After dropping hints of her availability and receiving no response, she was beginning to think he was not interested. However, he surprises Yvonne this week by asking her to accompany him to a community fundraiser event in a few weeks. She does not consider it a date but is hopeful the relationship will progress.

Episode 3

Yvonne has her appointment with Dr. Rowe, a family practice physician. She shares with Dr. Rowe that she has had pain in her hands for the past several months. When asked about other symptoms, she mentions the swelling in her hands and feet for the past 4 years. Dr. Rowe believes the pain is occupational in nature (typing) and suggests that she take ibuprofen. Dr. Rowe notices that Yvonne's blood pressure is slightly elevated (134/92 mm Hg), but attributes this elevation to her race and diet. He suggests that Yvonne try to lose a little weight and reduce her salt intake. Yvonne feels a little offended by the remark and she does not think her salt intake or weight have anything to do with her symptoms. However, she is polite and agrees to his suggestions ▶ ▼.

Episode 4

Yvonne has been exceptionally busy at work and has been frustrated with the lack of administrative support in the office. She feels that there are too many expectations of her and not enough time to complete all of the tasks she is assigned. Yvonne has hinted to her boss that perhaps another person should be hired, but her boss just ignores her.

Episode 5

Yvonne has had another exceptionally busy week at work and frequently feels tired. Her hands continue to hurt, and the swelling in her feet and hands also continues. At work, Yvonne has her annual evaluation. She is told by her boss that she has been doing excellent work, and the boss is still not willing to hire another office assistant. Yvonne's boss mentions administrative reorganization changes that are planned for next year and hints that she may be considered for a promotion. She is encouraged by the fact that her job situation has the potential to improve.

Over the weekend, Yvonne has a garage sale at her home, along with her sister and mother. She makes over $400 and is thrilled to get rid of so much stuff. After the garage sale, she feels very tired and elects not to go to her sister's house for dinner. Her sister criticizes her for feeling tired, pointing out that their mother has more energy than she does NEWS.

Episode 6

Yvonne attends a community fundraiser with Tim, a man from work whom she likes. She has a great time with him and thoroughly enjoys his company. She learns that he was married for 10 years and has been divorced for two. He mentions that he is not looking for a long-term relationship but enjoys friendships with women. Yvonne is not sure what to think about the comment but gets the hint to take it slowly ▼.

Episode 7

Yvonne has been trying to follow Dr. Rowe's advice for the past 3 months. Despite the fact that she has lost about 5 pounds, has avoided salty foods, and has been taking ibuprofen three times a day, she continues to have pain in her hands and swelling in her hands and feet. She also wonders if the symptoms are really associated with her work. She takes Randall for his annual sports physical examination and hopes to talk to Dr. Rowe while there. She learns that Dr. Rowe is out of the office, but is told that she is more than welcome to make an appointment. Yvonne considers this idea, but does not act on it ▼.

Episode 8

Yvonne thinks constantly about Tim, the man she has recently started to date. Although the relationship has not yet become romantic, she has seen him regularly and he occasionally is affectionate. Yvonne tells Randall she would like him to meet Tim. She knows he is not happy about the fact she is seeing someone, so she does not talk about it much. She is sure Randall would like him if he only gave Tim a chance.

Episode 9

Randall is trying out for the baseball team after school every day this week. Yvonne goes to work early so that she can leave in time to watch the tryouts. After practice, she takes Randall home and makes him dinner. She feels quite tired after a long day of work and all the running around after work.

Yvonne's relationship with Tim has finally become romantic. Yvonne was beginning to wonder if that would ever happen; he has been very slow to become sexually involved with her. She now considers the relationship serious and makes herself available to spend time with him as much as she can, while also attending to Randall ▼.

Episode 10

Yvonne decides it is about time for Randall to meet Tim. He comes over to the house for a few minutes to pick up Yvonne to go to a movie and is introduced to Randall. Randall does not say much and the interaction is very short. On the way to the movie, Tim comments to Yvonne that he senses Randall is not too happy about the situation.

Later that evening when Yvonne returns home, Randall tells his mother her boyfriend is a loser. Yvonne does not respond to the comment and figures it will just take Randall some time for him to get used to her having a boyfriend.

Episode 11

It has now been several months since Yvonne saw Dr. Rowe. She begins to notice that she has stiffness in her hands in the morning as well as continued hand pain and swelling in her hands and feet. She also does not feel rested when she wakes up and often needs to lie down when she gets home from work. She does not have the same energy on the weekends that she used to have. She continues to be unhappy in her current job and decides the symptoms are related to job dissatisfaction in her current position. She would quit, but thinks she might get the promotion at work if she just stays with it.

Episode 12

One afternoon this week, Yvonne goes to Randall's baseball game after work. Following the game, she is too tired to cook and stops for hamburgers on the way home. Randall tells her that it is okay with him to eat hamburgers and suggests they do this after every game ▽.

Episode 13

On Saturday, Yvonne watches Randall play in a baseball tournament all day. She wakes up on Sunday absolutely exhausted, and when she looks in the mirror, she notices a splotchy rash across her face. She also experiences increased pain in several of her joints, which really worries her. She cancels her plans to watch Randall's games and decides to rest all day on Sunday (despite protests from her son), expecting to feel better by Monday morning. However, instead she feels progressively worse. On Monday morning, she calls in sick and tries to get an appointment with Dr. Rowe. Dr. Rowe is unable to see her until the end of the week. Yvonne is advised to go to the Urgent Care Clinic or the Emergency Department (ED).

Yvonne's elects to go to the ED. Upon arrival, her blood pressure is 134/92 mm Hg. Yvonne tells the ED physician,

Dr. Gordon, about the red rash on her face, her excessive fatigue, and her other symptoms, including swelling and pain in her joints. She mentions that her finger joints and hip joints are hot and that the swelling in her lower legs has been present for 8 months. Dr. Gordon does not notice the rash on Yvonne's face because of her dark skin pigmentation. Based on her other symptoms, he suggests that Yvonne make an appointment with her primary care physician for a full workup to rule out a virus or arthritic condition. To keep her comfortable in the meantime, he gives Yvonne a 14-day prescription for prednisone (deltasone) in a decreasing dose. Yvonne gets the prescription filled that day and immediately begins to feel better ▷.

Episode 14

Yvonne finishes the prednisone (deltasone) prescription. She feels great! The swelling and pain are completely gone, and she has more energy than she has had in months. She feels so good that she decides she does not need to make an appointment with Dr. Rowe.

Tim comes over to her home twice this week. Randall says very little to Tim and leaves shortly after he arrives. Yvonne tries to talk with Randall about his rude behavior when Tim comes to their home. Randall becomes angry and yells at his mother. "I don't like him and I wish you would stop talking about him!" Yvonne wonders what she needs to do to help Randall accept Tim ▽.

Episode 15

Yvonne and Tim go on a weekend trip together when Randall visits his father for several days. She has fallen completely in love with him and, in her opinion, the relationship has become very serious, although she wishes he were more passionate sexually. She feels disappointed when Tim points out that Randall's resistance may make it more difficult for things to progress further. Not wanting to accept this, she does not tell Tim about the recent arguments she has had with Randall. Instead, she tells Tim that Randall really likes him but is just a moody teenager ▽.

Yvonne Johnson Season 2 Information

Episode 1

Yvonne has seen Dr. Rowe during the past year because of fatigue and pain and swelling in her hands and feet. Most recently, she was seen by a physician at the Emergency Department. He gave her a prescription for prednisone (deltasone), and this seems to have cured her. She has felt great ever since. Because she felt so good, she did not keep her appointment with Dr. Rowe, believing that

whatever it was that was bothering her has finally been resolved.

Work continues to be frustrating for Yvonne. Reorganization rumors are rampant, and many of her coworkers are concerned about their jobs. Her boyfriend Tim, who works for the same company, has decided to take a job elsewhere. He tells Yvonne he would rather find something else than get laid off. Yvonne remains hopeful that the reorganization will result in a promotion for her. For this reason, she has been putting extra effort into her work ▼.

Episode 2

Because Randall went out of town to see his father, Yvonne takes the opportunity to paint his bedroom, a project she has wanted to do for months. Tim helps her with the project and spends the night with her. It is the first time he has stayed overnight in her home since they started seeing each other. She hints to him they could save money by moving in together. He tells her, "I don't think that would work at all. Your son would not be happy about that! And there are some things about me that you don't understand." Yvonne feels disappointed and thinks that her son Randall seems to be holding back the relationship ▼.

Episode 3

Yvonne wakes up one morning this week feeling exhausted. When she gets out of bed and stands up, she experiences intense pain in her hips. Her hands are red, swollen, and painful. She also notices generalized swelling over her entire body. She realizes the symptoms are back and calls her family practice physician, Dr. Rowe, insisting that she be seen that day.

At Dr. Rowe's office, the medical technician measures Yvonne's blood pressure at 136/94 mm Hg. She tells Dr. Rowe about the current symptoms and their sudden appearance. She also tells Dr. Rowe about her previous visit to the ED. Dr. Rowe orders several diagnostic blood tests and sends her to the outpatient lab to have blood drawn. He asks Yvonne to return the following day. Yvonne has the blood drawn and spends the rest of the day in bed. She calls work and tells them she might not be in for several days. Although she knows there is nothing she can do about the situation, she worries about the impact of missing work again.

The following day, Yvonne returns to see Dr. Rowe. Dr. Rowe shares with Yvonne that some of her lab results are abnormal. Dr. Rowe tells Yvonne that many people have these abnormal results. They probably mean nothing, but there is a chance they could be related to a connective tissue disorder. Dr. Rowe gives Yvonne prescriptions for hydrochlorothiazide, 25 mg, to be taken once a day for blood pressure control, prednisone for a steroid "burst," and ibuprofen 800 mg to be taken three times a day for joint pain. He tells Yvonne to "watch things" for a while and see what happens. Yvonne wonders just what exactly she is supposed to watch. Between her feeling bad and Tim's job change, she does not see him at all for over a week ▶.

Episode 4

Yvonne begins feeling better almost immediately after taking the medications prescribed by Dr. Rowe. Within a few days, the pain and swelling are completely gone and she feels great! Because she missed several days of work last week when she was sick, Yvonne works late each day in an attempt to catch up. As a result, she is unable to spend much time at all with her boyfriend Tim. She has been worried about the number of sick days she has taken and the impact this may have on her performance evaluations ▼.

Episode 5

Yvonne is devastated when Tim meets her for coffee and tells her the relationship has run its course and he wants to "break it off." Yvonne is blindsided. She did not see this coming at all; she thought they had the perfect relationship! Crying, she asks him, "What did I do wrong? What can I do to make it right?" He tells her he really is not interested in a long-term relationship and it is clear she wants that. He also points out it would be very difficult to take the relationship further because of his own personal issues and because her son Randall is clearly not happy about the arrangement. Deep down, Yvonne knows Tim is right about Randall, and she feels angry about the fact that her son has ruined her opportunity. She is unable to see other issues in the relationship.

Episode 6

Yvonne continues to feel very sad about the fact that Tim "dumped her." On the bright side, she is feeling well physically and is completely pain free.

She turns her attention away from Tim, focuses on work, and prepares for a major presentation. She is hopeful that her presentation will be noticed by the company managers. One of her coworkers asks her if she plans to be sick again the week she gives her presentation, which makes Yvonne furious.

After work, she goes to the high school basketball game to watch Randall play ▼.

Episode 7

Yvonne has a discussion with Randall about getting a car. He wants a car of his own, but she can't afford to buy him a car and pay his car insurance. In addition, Yvonne is not so sure she wants him driving all over town anyway. She tells Randall that, if he wants a car, he can buy one for himself. Yvonne knows he won't be able to earn the money anytime soon ▼.

Episode 8

Yvonne is told a rumor in the office that ex-boyfriend Tim has a new girlfriend. Yvonne tells her co-workers that the story is ridiculous and that he would not already be seeing somebody else. Deep down, she feels very angry and wonders if he broke off their relationship for another woman.

Episode 9

Yvonne has a performance evaluation at work this week. She is told that she is capable of excellent work. The managers point out that every time she misses work, she tends to fall behind, and her coworkers end up having to do extra work to make up for her absence. They tell her she is still being considered for a promotion, but they would like to see these issues addressed. Yvonne tells them she thinks her illness is over, and that the medications she took seemed to have cured whatever was wrong with her. Yvonne decides she should be in each morning a bit early and stay a little later in the evenings to show that she is committed to the job.

On Friday night, Yvonne watches Randall play in a basketball game. After the game, Randall fails to come home by his midnight curfew. Yvonne is angry when he finally comes in at 1:30 a.m. He tells her it isn't his fault he's late, because he doesn't have a car to drive himself home ▶ ▽.

Episode 10

Yvonne's best friend calls and asks her if she would like to go to the beach with her next week over the 3-day weekend. Yvonne knows Randall is planning to visit his father and agrees to go. She decides she needs a bit of fun because she is still feeling down about being rejected by Tim ▽ [NEWS].

Episode 11

Yvonne and her friend go on a 3-day beach vacation. She has a great time but feels very tired by the time she gets home on Sunday afternoon. On Monday, she continues to feel tired at work. Initially, she thinks it is a case of "vacationitis," but then she notices the rash across her face again. Over the course of the next 2 days, the fatigue does not resolve, and she begins to experience joint pain and swelling again. Yvonne recognizes these symptoms and also notices that she has been forgetting details and "feeling foggy." She takes the rest of the week off from work to rest, but she does not improve.

Frustrated with the ongoing problems, Yvonne does an internet search for "fatigue and joint pain" and comes across websites that describe rheumatoid-type problems. She enters a rheumatology support bulletin board, posts her symptoms, and asks for advice. Many people respond to her posting, telling her that she should see a rheumatologist ▽.

Episode 12

This week, Yvonne continues to feel poorly. She misses 2 days of work but makes herself go to work the other days. She finds that trying to get to work and keep up with her projects is exhausting. She tries to go to work a little late and go home early to compensate for the exhaustion, but the schedule is just killing her. Yvonne also overhears some of her coworkers talking about her lack of productivity. Because of this criticism, she decides to make an appointment with Dr. Rowe again.

Randall tells Yvonne that he is getting a car from his father. She is angry with Randall's father for not talking with her about it first, but she is too tired to get into an argument with anybody. She tells Randall that car insurance is very expensive and that he will have to help pay for it ▽.

Episode 13

Yvonne sees Dr. Rowe this week. She tells Dr. Rowe what she learned by searching the internet and reminds her that the symptoms have been coming and going now for quite some time and getting worse. She tells Dr. Rowe that she was told by friends that she should see rheumatologist. Based on her symptoms and her lab values at her last visit, Dr. Rowe agrees.

Episode 14

Yvonne has missed several days of work during the past couple of weeks because she is so tired and feels poorly. When she does get to work, she has a hard time getting much done.

She is not thrilled that Randall has his own car now and makes it clear he will have to pay for part of the car insurance. She wishes Randall did not have to work on top of all his other activities, but she knows she really cannot afford his insurance right now. She is hopeful that, with a promotion at work, her income will improve.

Episode 15

It takes several weeks for Yvonne to see the rheumatologist. She has missed work about one-half of that time and is worried about the amount of time she has missed. At the rheumatologist's office, a detailed family history reveals that Yvonne's maternal aunt had rheumatoid arthritis and her grandmother had hypothyroidism. The rheumatologist repeats many of the same diagnostic tests previously ordered by Dr. Rowe. Yvonne tests positive for anti-DNA antibody, anti-Smith antibody, and antinuclear antibody (ANA). An initial diagnosis of undifferentiated connective tissue disease is made.

The rheumatologist tells Yvonne that this is a common initial diagnosis for people who have symptoms of autoimmune illness. The specific diagnosis will become clear over time, although it is likely that she has systemic lupus erythematosus (SLE). Because of the amount of protein in her urine, the rheumatologist also tells Yvonne she probably has renal insufficiency and refers her to a nephrologist. Yvonne is not sure exactly what all this information means, except that it has something to do with her kidneys. The rheumatologist gives her a prescription for hydroxychloroquine (Plaquenil), 400 mg two times a day, and tells her to return again next month ▽.

Yvonne Johnson Season 3 Information

Episode 1

Yvonne Johnson is a 36-year-old African American female. She is a single parent to her 16-year-old son Randall. She does not date at this point, primarily because Randall has not reacted well to her having relationships with men. Her parents and siblings live nearby, and she maintains a close relationship with them.

Yvonne has recently been diagnosed with an undifferentiated connective tissue disease and has been told it is most likely systemic lupus erythematosus (SLE). Yvonne is scheduled to see a nephrologist to evaluate her renal function. She is motivated to adhere to her recommended treatment regimen.

Yvonne continues to work as an administrative assistant, but she has a difficult time keeping up with the job demands. Because of her illness, she has missed a lot of work. Although she once believed she might get promoted, at this point she is just concentrating on keeping her job.

Recently Yvonne was told she might have renal insufficiency due to her lupus. This episode she reads about this on the internet and is very worried about her health status.

Episode 2

Yvonne has an appointment with the nephrologist this week. She is scheduled for outpatient urine and blood tests and a renal biopsy to rule out lupus nephritis. She has the biopsy at the Neighborhood Outpatient Surgery Center at the end of the week.

Yvonne misses 2 days of work this week to accommodate the appointments. Because she has missed so much work, she is reassigned to another position in the company, a position that is clearly a demotion. She finds many of the individuals who were once friendly and helpful to her now avoid her. Yvonne knows they don't understand how she feels.

Episode 3

Yvonne meets with the nephrologist again this week. She is told that the laboratory tests show protein in urine and an elevated creatinine level. These tests, along with the biopsy results, suggest she has progressive glomerulonephritis and renal insufficiency; they confirm a diagnosis of lupus nephritis. The nephrologist tells Yvonne that she has chronic kidney disease and is at risk for developing end-stage renal disease. To help preserve her renal function, the nephrologist prescribes a steroid burst of prednisone (deltasone) with

a tapering dose, cyclophosphamide (Cytoxan) and azathioprine (Imuran). Because her blood pressure is elevated despite taking hydrochlorothiazide, the physician adds metoprolol to her medication regimen. Yvonne tells the physician that she finds all of this information overwhelming and confusing. She is referred to the Neighborhood Patient Education Center for further patient teaching ▼.

Episode 4

Yvonne leaves work early for an appointment with a nurse educator at the Patient Education Center. At the center, Yvonne learns about her disease process, her medications, diet (low protein, low salt), and self-management strategies for lupus and renal insufficiency. She finds the session helpful and finally begins to understand the severity of her illness. Yvonne agrees to return for additional sessions with the nurse educator.

Episode 5

Yvonne is very concerned when she learns that Randall's best friend, Charles, ran over and almost killed a young boy who was riding his bike. Yvonne reminds Randall that he needs to be careful when driving ▼ [NEWS].

Episode 6

Yvonne finds that the new medications are helping somewhat, but she continues to experience joint pain and fatigue. She has great difficulty keeping up with her household and job responsibilities. Although she continues to go to work, she often feels poorly and misses work often. Yvonne has been unable to go to Randall's baseball games because of the need to avoid sun exposure. They have an argument, and she comes to understand that Randall is angry with her for being sick ▼.

Episode 7

Yvonne has a follow-up appointment with the nephrologist. Her urine output has decreased somewhat, and she is feeling puffy. Based on additional tests, she is told that her kidney disease has progressed, as evidenced by a further reduction of her creatinine clearance. Although her BUN and creatinine levels are borderline normal, she is told she is going to need dialysis treatment in the future. The goal at this point is to continue to preserve her kidney function for as long as possible. Yvonne is taught how to measure her urine output and instructed to reduce her daily fluid intake to 600 mL plus the measurable urine output from the day before. She is also told to measure her weight daily and report increases in weight over 4 pounds.

Yvonne notices Randall is out every night with his new girlfriend. She worries about the time they are alone and tries to talk with him about being careful with her and avoiding sexual contact, but this conversation results in another argument.

Episode 8

Yvonne is fired from her job this week with her employer citing poor quality of work as the reason for termination. She is devastated because she knows she needs the health insurance coverage not only for herself, but also for Randall. She signs up for COBRA coverage and is shocked at the cost of the monthly premiums. She realizes she will not be able to afford to pay the premium, particularly if she is out of work. She has prepaid her insurance until the end of the next month, so she is hopeful she can find another position before she has to pay for the COBRA coverage ▼.

Episode 9

Yvonne spends the entire week looking for work. She feels terrible and when she looks at herself in the mirror, she recognizes how tired she looks and is sure this is affecting her presentation to potential employers. She does not want to share with them what is wrong with her for fear that they will not be interested in hiring her. Yvonne feels fortunate that her mother and siblings are supportive of her situation and have promised to help her in any way they can ▼.

Episode 10

Yvonne is so tired this week that she is unable to look for a job. She sees her physician and is found to be Anemia and hypocalcemic. Her blood pressure remains within normal limits. She is given a subcutaneous injection of epoetin alfa (Epogen).

Episode 11

Yvonne scours the internet for job postings. She applies to anything that she might remotely be able to do, but it seems many other people are applying for the same positions. She knows that she will have to be persistent ▼.

Episode 12

Yvonne is feeling noticeably more energetic than in weeks past. A follow-up visit with her physician confirms that her RBC, hemoglobin, and hematocrit levels are elevated in response to the epoetin alfa (Epogen). Yvonne is able to get a temporary position. Although there are no benefits, she at least has some income for the time being. She realizes that she will not easily be able to get a permanent job. At the suggestion of a friend, she applies for Social Security disability. She is overwhelmed with the process ▼.

Episode 13

Yvonne talks at length with Randall's father about her inability to get full-time employment and to make ends meet. She asks him if he can help with additional child support so that she can better provide for Randall. He accuses Yvonne of wanting the money to pay for her medical bills and tells her that if he sends any additional money, it will be sent directly to Randall. He also suggests that Randall live with him to finish out his high school years ▶ ▼.

Episode 14

Yvonne receives notification that she has been turned down for the Social Security disability benefits because she has not had a documented disability long enough and she is currently employed by the temporary agency. Yvonne can't believe this news. She has to work to keep from losing her home, but if she works, she can't get disability. She does not understand how anybody gets disability benefits within such a system.

Episode 15

Yvonne has become excessively fatigued again and short of breath this week. She has experienced a 6-pound weight gain in the past 3 days and notices excessive swelling in her legs. Yvonne makes a call to her nephrologist, fearing the worst ▼.

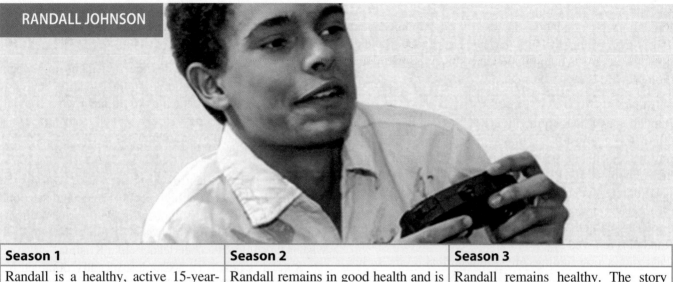

RANDALL JOHNSON

Season 1	Season 2	Season 3
Randall is a healthy, active 15-year-old. His story focuses on typical teen-related behaviors related to school, sports, and his social life. He is frustrated with mother, because he perceives her as being lazy.	Randall remains in good health and is active in school and sports. He hates the fact that his mother is always feeling sick, even though she looks fine. He gets a car during this season and must get a job to pay for car insurance and gas.	Randall remains healthy. The story focuses on typical adolescent behaviors and the impact of his mother's illness on his life.

Randall Johnson Season 1 Information

Episode 1

Randall is a healthy, athletic 15-year-old African American male. He lives with his mother Yvonne in a small but comfortable home. His father and stepmother live in a nearby town. Although he visits his father several times a year, he does not feel particularly close to him.

Randall is in his first year of high school. He is an excellent student, is very athletic, and has many friends. He loves social media and maintains a regular presence on Facebook. He is an avid sports fan and plans on playing basketball and baseball for the high school team. He is looking forward to taking driver education and getting his driver's license soon.

Randall spends hours reviewing the posts of his friends on Facebook. He posts several pictures of himself and his best friend, Charles. Randall and Charles regularly compare the number of "likes" to their postings. His mother is constantly telling him to be careful about what he puts on the site and is angry when she learns he has posted pictures of her. He does not understand what she is worried about ▾.

Episode 2

Randall spends most of the weekend hanging out with Charles. They go to the mall to meet some friends, play video games, and go to the golf course to hit balls on the driving range. He posts pictures of them hitting golf balls on Facebook. Randall does not know how to play golf, but he thinks he might like to learn.

Episode 3

Randall spends a 3-day weekend with his father. When he comes home, he tells his mother that it gets boring at his dad's house because he doesn't have any friends there. His father keeps trying to teach him some basics of woodworking in his workshop, but Randall is completely uninterested ▾.

Episode 4

Randall asks his mother to attend a parents' night for school athletics at school this week. He plans to go out for the baseball team and he is very excited for his mother to meet the coaches.

Episode 5

Randall helps his mother, aunt, and grandmother have a garage sale. He does not particularly like doing the work, but his mother promises to give him $25 for helping. He keeps himself entertained by taking pictures of people and some of the random items for sale and posting them to his Facebook page with sarcastic comments. He notices his mother is tired after the garage sale, but he figures she is just old and out of shape ▾.

Episode 6

Randall's mother mentions she went to a community event with a man from work and that he is very nice. Randall does not pay much attention to the comment, thinking his mother's life is pretty boring.

Episode 7

Randall sees a nurse practitioner at the Family Practice clinic for a physical examination. He hates having a physical exam, but he knows it is required for him to play high school sports. Randall mentions to the nurse that he would prefer his mother not to be in the room during the exam. The nurse practitioner asks Yvonne if she would mind staying in the waiting room during his examination; Randall is relieved that his mother agrees. All of his physical examination findings are within normal limits for his age ▶ ▽.

Episode 8

Randall's mother tells Randall she would like him to meet Tim. She wants to invite Tim over to dinner to given Randall an opportunity to talk to and get to know Tim. He is completely annoyed with her and can't stand the idea that his mother is even dating. Randall replies, "You are too old to date." Later he sees that the man his mother is spending time with has a Facebook page. He is not able to learn much about him other than the fact that he is a nerd ▶ ▽.

Episode 9

Randall and his best friend, Charles, try out for the baseball team this entire week. At the end of the week, he is thrilled to learn that he and Charles have earned starting positions on the Junior Varsity squad. After the announcement, Randall goes to Charles's house, where they have a celebration cookout for the other kids who made the team. He knows his mother has been tired a lot this week and assumes it is because she is spending time with her boyfriend, Tim ▽.

Episode 10

Randall has baseball practice every evening this week to get ready for the season opener. Following practice on three of the evenings, he goes to the gym with his friends to lift weights. He is so busy this week he does not bother to tell his mother about the open house at the high school.

One evening this week, Yvonne tells Randall she is going to a movie with Tim and that she would like him to meet Tim when he picks her up. When Tim arrives, he shakes Randall's hand and says, "Hello, Randall. It is good to meet you. Your mother has so many good things to say about you." Randall looks at Tim briefly, then looks at the floor and simply says, "Okay." Tim asks Randall a few more questions that he politely responds to and then they leave. Later that evening, when his mother returns home,

she tells Randall he was not very nice to Tim. Randall tells his mother that her boyfriend is a loser ▽.

Episode 11

Randall's baseball team loses the first game this week. Randall is very disappointed in the loss and feels that, if he had played better, his team would have won. Randall receives a "friend request" on Facebook from Tim. He is annoyed with the request and deletes it ▽.

Episode 12

Randall has an uneventful week at school. During the weekend, he goes to the high school dance and sees one of the cheerleaders, Kristina Martin, with Jared Williams (the quarterback of the high school football team). He wishes he could date cheerleaders like Kristina.

Randall's best friend, Charles, recently obtained his driver's license. Yvonne allows him to go out, but she worries about his safety because his friend is an inexperienced driver. Randall thinks that his mother is too protective and that he can take care of himself. The boys spend the evening cruising on one of the main streets in the Neighborhood with some of the other local high school kids. He gets home by 11:30 p.m ▽.

Episode 13

Randall plays in a 2-day baseball tournament over the weekend. His mother promises to watch all of the games. After going to all of the Saturday games, she says she is too tired to go to any of the Sunday games. Randall tells her that he really wants her to come and watch and is disappointed when she declines. At one of the games, he hits a home run and is angry that she is not there to see it. He imagines that she is tired because she is spending all her time with Tim ▽ [NEWS].

Episode 14

Randall is very annoyed because it seems like Tim is coming to their house a lot. He does not like to see his mother hugging and kissing him and hates to think about the other things they do when alone. Randall feels resentment toward Tim and hates the fact that his mother seems to prefer spending time with him. Randall copes with the situation by limiting his interactions with Tim and leaving the house when he comes over. Yvonne tries to talk with Randall about his rude behavior when Tim comes to their home. Randall becomes angry and yells at this mother. "I don't like him and wish you would stop talking about him!" ▶

Episode 15

Randall and his friends go out for pizza after a baseball game. While out with his friends, Randall learns that the parents of Jeremy (one of the guys at school) are out of town, and he is having a party. Randall knows the party would be a lot of fun but also knows his mother would be incredibly angry if he went. He tells his friends that he has other plans and goes home instead. Later in the week, Randall goes to his father's home. His mother tells him she will be spending the weekend with Tim. Randall is glad not to be home to see them together. He tells his father that his mom has a new boyfriend who is a real "dork head." ▾

Randall Johnson Season 2 Information

Episode 1

Randall is a healthy, athletic 16-year-old African American male. Randall is very close to his mother, but he does not like it when she dates men. He has been taking driver's education and will soon be getting his driver's license. He plays on the high school basketball and baseball teams.

Basketball season starts this week. Randall and his friends stay after school each afternoon for practice. He comes home just before dinner and posts pictures of himself at practice on Facebook with comments about making the team. Later in the evening, he completes his homework ▾.

Episode 2

Randall spends a 3-day weekend with his father. He tells his father about his mother's boyfriend and says that he really hates Tim. He also tells his father that he can't come to visit again for a while because his basketball games start next week and he'll be playing basketball every weekend. He suggests to his father that he come to see him play.

Episode 3

One morning this week, Randall is surprised by how ill his mother looks. She tells him she feels really bad and is going to stay home from work and see the doctor. She asks him to get a ride to and from school. She does not want to get out and drive any more than she must because she is feeling a lot of pain. Randall wonders why his mother is sick again ▾.

Episode 4

Randall and his best friend, Charles, go to the school dance with two of the girls from school. The girls spend all afternoon getting ready for the dance. In contrast, Randall and Charles hang out together until about an hour before they are scheduled to pick up the girls. Randall's mother takes their pictures. Randall is glad she is feeling better. The pictures get posted to Facebook ▾.

Episode 5

Yvonne tells Randall she is no longer going to go out with Tim. He is very glad to hear this news. He did not like Tim and really does not think his mother should be dating. He goes out and shoots baskets, relieved that their life can go back to normal now.

Episode 6

Randall gets his driver's license this week. He tells his mother he wants a car. Yvonne tells him they will have to talk about it, but in the meantime, he can borrow her car once in a while. Yvonne watches him play basketball over the weekend.

Episode 7

Randall continues to pester his mother about getting a car. He thinks he should be able to have one; most of his friends have been given a car by their parents. Yvonne tells Randall she can't afford to buy him a car or pay for the car insurance. If he wants a car, he'll have to get a job and buy one. Randall knows it will be nearly impossible to save enough money to buy a car any time soon ▶ ▾.

Episode 8

Randall is obsessed with getting a car. He talks about it constantly. He tells his mother everybody else has a car and it is not fair that he can't have one. At least his mother allows him to periodically drive her car. He posts car-related sites to Facebook with comments such as "my dream car" or "wishing to be driving this ride ▾."

Episode 9

Because his mother works late on Friday evening, Randall needs to catch a ride to his basketball game with Charles. After the game, he hangs out with his friends. He sends a text to his mother to let her know, but she does not answer. He does not come home until after 1:30 a.m. Yvonne is furious with him for coming home so late. Randall tells her he had no choice because he was with Charles and Charles was driving. He tells his mother that, if he had his own car, he could come home on time ▾.

Episode 10

Randall's basketball season has come to an end. They lose a game in the state basketball tournament in the opening round. He is disappointed that they don't win, but he does not dwell on it. He begins to think about tryouts for the track and field team ▾.

Episode 11

Randall spends a 3-day weekend with his father. He complains to his father about not having a car to drive. His father tells him that he will buy a car for him, and Randall can pay him back during the summer. Randall thinks this plan is awesome. He posts a photo of himself with the good news on Facebook: "getting hooked up with car - having a ride soon ▼."

Episode 12

Randall notices his mother is feeling bad again; she spends a lot of time just lying on the couch. Sometimes, she doesn't even make dinner, asking him to make himself a frozen pizza instead.

He tells his mother that he is going to get a car soon from his father, and she tells him he is going to have to help pay for the car insurance. Randall tells his mother that he is going to be on the track and field team, but he will get a part-time job to pay for the insurance ▶ ▼.

Episode 13

Randall gets a part-time job at a fast-food restaurant. His manager promises to be flexible with his work schedule to accommodate his track and field season. Randall is very pleased with the arrangement ▼.

Episode 14

Randall's father keeps his promise to buy a car for him. It is a late-model sedan, but he is thrilled to have it. He takes multiple pictures of himself and Charles with the car in a number of poses and posts them to Facebook. Later in the week, he meets with the insurance agent and is surprised at the cost of car insurance, but decides it's worth it to be able to have his own car. He figures out how many shifts a week he needs to work to pay for his portion of the insurance ▼.

Episode 15

Randall is adapting to his new schedule of school, track team practice, homework, and a few hours at work several evenings a week. He quickly finds that working at a fast-food restaurant is not a great job, but he's happy to make the money. He is aware that his mother has been going to the doctor a lot, but he does not ask her much about it ▼.

Randall Johnson Season 3 Information

Episode 1

Randall is a high school student and keeps a very busy schedule. He is an excellent student, plays on several high school sports teams, and most recently has started a part-time job at a fast-food restaurant to pay for a car and auto insurance. He has very little free time. He knows his mother has been sick, but he has not talked with her very much about it.

Randall has been increasingly worried about his mother. She has not been looking well and she is always so tired. He knows she has been going to the doctor a lot, but he does not specifically ask her what is wrong with her.

Episode 2

Tryouts for the baseball team are taking place this week. Randall literally goes from school to practice to work and does not get home until after 10:30 p.m. four nights this week. Although his mother tells him he can't maintain that schedule or his grades will suffer, Randall is confident he can keep up with everything. He wonders about the number of days his mother misses at work ▼.

Episode 3

Yvonne tells Randall that the doctor finally knows what is wrong with her, and she is going to have to take many medications and change her diet. Randall does not quite understand what is wrong with her, but he is aware she is always tired and looks swollen at times. He hopes the medications will make her better.

Episode 4

Randall makes the varsity baseball team this year and is thrilled. He shows his mother his schedule and tells her he hopes she can make it to his games this year. Randall's grades in school are beginning to be affected by his busy schedule. He does not share with his mother that he has C's in three of his classes, fearing that she will make him quit work. He is not willing to quit because having his own car to drive is more important to him than making A's in school. This week, Randall goes to the formal high school dance with Natalie, a girl he has had a crush on for several months. They have a great time, and she agrees to be his girlfriend. Randall posts all the good news to his Facebook page, including multiple pictures of himself with Natalie ▼.

Episode 5

Randall hears that his best friend, Charles, was speeding in his car when he accidentally hit a boy riding a bike. Charles is freaked out by the incident and calls Randall. Randall goes with Charles to the police department for questioning. Randall feels badly for Charles when his parents arrive. They are angry with him for wrecking the car, being careless, and almost killing a little boy. He knows Charles was probably texting when the accident happened and wonders if they will find out. Randall thinks it is pointless to yell at Charles about what happened; he already feels bad enough [NEWS].

Episode 6

Randall is angry with his mother and argues with her when she tells him she is going to miss another baseball game. He tells her that all she ever does is lie around, and he wishes she would quit being sick all the time. He posts his frustration with her on his Facebook page by placing a photo of a dog lying on a couch upside down with the message "Tired like a Dog - AGAIN."

Randall and Charles make a visit to Neighborhood Hospital to visit Marcus Young, the boy Charles injured with his car. Charles tells the boy how sorry he is for what happened. The boy's mom is very rude at first, but eventually she is nicer to them [▶] [▽].

Episode 7

Randall spends most of his spare time with his new girlfriend, Natalie. During the evenings that he is not working, Randall is at her house. His mother verbalizes concern about the time they spend together. Randall becomes angry with his mother and thinks that she does not want him to do anything but come home and watch her lying around on the couch [▽].

Episode 8

Randall finds his mother crying in the living room after coming home from a baseball game. She tells him she has been fired from her job because of her illness and is not sure what they are going to do. She tells Randall that they may have some tough times ahead. Randall does not think it's fair that they fired his mom just because she is sick. At the same time, he feels angry with her for letting it happen.

Episode 9

Randall's grandmother unexpectedly picks him up from school after baseball practice and tells him he is having dinner with her. He initially protests, telling his grandmother he has plans with Natalie, but his grandmother tells him to get on his cell phone and let Natalie know his plans have changed for the evening.

Randall's grandmother outlines what is going on with his mother in a way that he understands better. She points out to him that he is being very unfair in his assessment of his mother, who is doing the best she can. Randall's grandmother tells him to let her know if there is something he needs, and she will help him get it. She also suggests he talk to his father and let him know what's going on; maybe he can help out somewhat. Randall feels badly about some of the things he said to his mother in the previous weeks, but he still does not comprehend the seriousness of his mother's illness.

Episode 10

Randall helps his mother around the house this week. She is very appreciative of his efforts. He asks Natalie to come to his house on the evenings he is not at work. Randall retrieves his report card from the mailbox because he doesn't want his mother to see it. He knows it will just upset her, and he does not want her to worry about him anymore. He figures that, as long as he is passing, what she doesn't know won't hurt her [▽].

Episode 11

Randall and Natalie are together almost all the time unless he is at work or baseball. He notices that his mother does not even seem to mind that Natalie is there so much. It makes things much easier because Natalie helps him with homework and also helps him do things around the house. Randall thinks she is about the best girlfriend ever!

Episode 12

Randall had been thinking about attending college, but now he is starting to think that when he graduates, he will just get a job and work. He is fairly sure he is going to need to help his mother. He mentions this plan to his father, and his father insists that he needs to go to college. He tells Randall that his mother's problems are not his and that he needs to stay focused on his own priorities.

Episode 13

Randall's father suggests that he come to live with him since his mother is having such a tough time. Randall tells his mother and his father that there is no way he is going to move. He is not interested in changing schools, leaving his girlfriend, or leaving his mother. He tells his dad that he is paying for all of his car insurance at this point, and it may take longer to pay him back for the car than they had originally agreed.

Episode 14

Randall has become very close to his girlfriend Natalie's parents. They are aware his mother is sick and has lost her job, and they have been helping him by purchasing some of the things he needs. Most recently, Natalie's mother bought Randall some new jeans and shoes. He feels as if he has a second set of parents he can turn to for help. At some point, he wants his mother to meet them, but is not sure this is the best time for that.

Episode 15

Baseball season has come to an end. Yvonne did not see Randall play a single game, but at this point, he accepts this disappointment. He worries about his mother and elects not to go out for the track and field team so that he can help her more around the house and pick up additional shifts at work. He hopes to work enough hours to help his mother through the rough times that lie ahead [▽].

MARTIN & AMES HOUSEHOLD

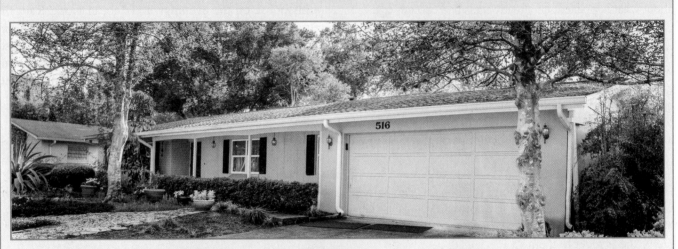

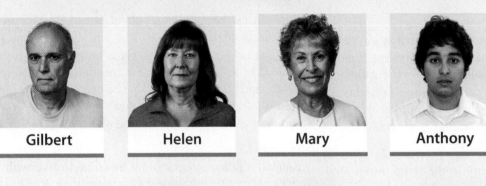

Gilbert **Helen** **Mary** **Anthony** **Kristina**

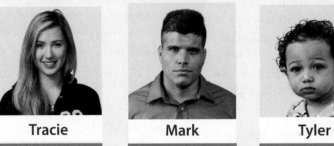

Tracie **Mark** **Tyler**

Housing	The Martins live in the Riverbank area. They have a mid-size one-story home. They are close to the river.
Parks and Recreation	There are parks in the area where Mark takes Tyler to play.
Services	The Neighborhood Hospital and clinics are across town from where the Martins live. Bus service does not extend into their area. The high school that Kristina and Anthony attend is close to their home.

Key: ▶ = video clip ▤ = medical record ▽ = journal entry [NEWS] = news article

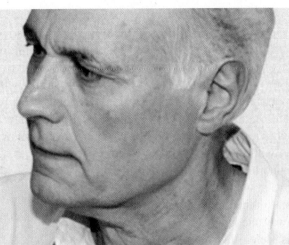

GILBERT MARTIN

Season 1	Season 2	Season 3
Gil is a healthy adult male with chronic back pain and hyperlipidemia. He tries to watch his diet and is compliant with medications. Gil is a very hard worker and wants to take care of everyone. He allows his mother to move into home after his father's death, which creates tension in the household and with his wife.	Gil has ongoing issues with chronic back pain. He allows his son, Mark, and grandson, Tyler, to move in (without consulting with Helen), until Mark can catch up on his bills. He does this not only for Mark, but also for the sake of his grandson. Gil is devastated when Anthony experiences psychotic episodes.	Gil continues to have ongoing issues with chronic back pain. The family home becomes chaotic with so many people in the home, Mark's devastating injury, and Anthony's mental illness.

Gilbert Martin Season 1 Information

Episode 1

Gilbert Martin is a 52-year-old Hispanic male who is married to Helen. They have been married for 18 years. Gil has a son (Mark) from a previous marriage, a stepdaughter Tracie (whom he has raised since she was 3), and two teenage children with Helen (Anthony and Kristina). He considers his marriage excellent, although he knows Helen does not get along with well with his mother, Mary, and oldest son, Mark. Because Gil's father recently passed away, he spends a lot of time helping his mother manage her home.

Gil works as a local delivery truck driver for a construction company. His job includes assisting with loading and unloading the truck. He has been in this position for over 20 years. Although he finds the pay to be competitive and he has health insurance, he gets no paid vacation. Gil speaks both English and Spanish - in fact his first language was Spanish. He often communicates with his mother in Spanish.

Gil considers himself to be in good health, with one exception - he has chronic back pain, which frequently makes him miserable. He usually manages the pain with over-the-counter analgesics. He has a prescription for oxycodone with acetaminophen, which he takes when the pain becomes severe, but he is unable to take the oxycodone on days he works. Gil also has a medical diagnosis of hyperlipidemia, for which he takes atorvastatin (Lipitor) 20 mg/day. He sees his physician once a year for cholesterol, triglycerides, and liver function tests. Gil has also been encouraged to eat a low-fat diet.

Gil spends the entire weekend at his mother's home, helping her pay bills and performing other various chores. She has been a widow for 6 months and does not seem to be managing her situation very well. She tells Gil that she is just too old to do these things alone and wishes that his father were still alive to take care of her. Gil feels responsible for his mother and knows that she must be very lonely.

Episode 2

Gil strains his back at work again this week while unloading his trailer. Because he is in severe pain, he goes to the Emergency Department, gets a narcotic pain medication and a prescription for cyclobenzaprine (Flexeril), a muscle relaxant. He is told to follow up with his primary care provider. He has to take several days off from work and is relieved that it is classified as a workmen's compensation injury, so that he gets paid despite being off work

While he is at his mother's house this week, Mary bakes Gil some cookies and takes the opportunity to let him know how much she appreciates his visit. She also shares with Gil how lonely she is. Feeling sorry for his mother, Gil suggests that maybe she could stay with them for a while. Mary immediately jumps at the opportunity to do so and tells Gil that she would love to move in with them. Gil had made the comment as a suggestion to think about and did not expect his mother to react the way she did.

When he gets home, Gil tells Helen that his mother wants to move in and that they should make room for her. He is disappointed in Helen's reaction but attributes her behavior to not feeling well and going through "the change." Gil makes arrangements for his mother to move in during the upcoming weeks and plans to help her sell her home ▶ ▼.

Episode 3

Gil tells Kristina and Tracie that they'll need to share a bedroom to make space for their grandmother. Gil spends several days helping his mother move. Mary moves to their home and brings with her more possessions than there is room in the house. He fills the garage with her boxes. Helen comments to Gil that there is now no room to park the cars. Gil experiences back pain for several days.

Episode 4

Gil continues to hear Kristina and Tracie argue about sharing a room. He does not want his mother to be aware of the issues they are having because he wants her to feel welcome. Gil talks to both of the girls and asks them to be more sensitive to their grandmother.

Episode 5

Gil is happy to see his mother involved in cooking meals. He knows that this makes her happy, and he wants her to feel welcome in their home. He also has always loved his mother's cooking and is happy to eat some of his favorite dishes (even though he knows that the meals are not optimal, considering his hyperlipidemia). When Helen complains to him about his mother sabotaging her diet, he suggests that she eat low-fat foods for breakfast and lunch, and limit what she eats at dinner.

Episode 6

Gil spends most of his evenings at his mother's home doing home repairs and getting it ready for sale. On Thursday evening, he strains his back while moving furniture. He is in a great deal of pain and considers going to the Emergency Department, but decides against it because he knows that he will have to wait for hours to be seen. Instead, he takes a sick day on Friday and spends the next 3 days lying down, using a heating pad, taking oxycodone with acetaminophen pain medication, and drinking a lot of beer to treat his back strain. He is aware that Helen is frustrated with his ongoing back pain, especially this time, because it was caused by his taking care of his mother. By Monday morning, he is able to go back to work, but he is still uncomfortable.

Episode 7

Gil is still suffering from back pain this week. Each day he goes to work and then comes home, takes pain medication, lies on the couch to watch TV, and drinks a few beers. Gil's mother, Mary, tells him that she wants to get a bone scan because her bone density screening, which was done at the health fair, was low. He makes an appointment for her to see Dr. Rowe, the family physician ▼.

Episode 8

Kristina tells Gil that Grandma is willing to let her use her car, but only if it is okay with him. He confirms this with Mary and decides that it wouldn't hurt to let Kristina drive that car. It would also get her to stop pestering him about buying her one. Helen is angry with Gil over this decision. Gil recognizes that she has been moody and again believes this is all related to her menopause.

Episode 9

Gil spends the evening lying down on the couch watching TV with a heating pad applied to his back. He is aware that Helen is very upset because Anthony and Kristina are late coming home from a school function. When Anthony arrives home, he sees Helen and Anthony arguing. He is concerned about the fact that Anthony came home without Kristina, and reminds Anthony that, no matter what, he must look out for his sister.

Episode 10

Gil and Helen attend the Neighborhood High School open house – an opportunity for parents to meet with teachers. Gil is pleased with Anthony's academic achievement as described by his teachers. One teacher pulls Gil aside and tells him that she has noticed that Anthony seems socially withdrawn. Gil responds to the comment, "He is a lot like I was at that age – pretty shy. I am sure that will change as he gets older."

Episode 11

Gil finally has his mother's house ready to put up for sale. He is hopeful that she will be able to get a good price for the home so that she will have her own spending money.

Episode 12

Gil and Helen ground Kristina for staying out past curfew after the high school dance. Gil backs Helen on this decision but wonders if Helen is being too tough on their daughter and blowing the situation out of proportion.

Episode 13

Gil strains his back at work again this week while unloading his trailer. Because he is in severe pain, he goes to the Emergency Department, gets a narcotic pain medication and a prescription for cyclobenzaprine (Flexeril), a muscle relaxant. He is told to follow up with his primary care provider. He has to take several days off from work and is relieved that it is classified as a workers' compensation injury, so that he gets paid despite being off work.

While resting at home, Gil and his mother have a short conversation in Spanish. When Mary gets up to leave, Helen criticizes Gil for "always speaking in Spanish" to his mother. He just does not understand why Helen is always mad at him ▼.

Episode 14

Gil notices foil in the windows of Anthony's room and wonders why it has been placed there. He asks Anthony about it and Anthony responds that it helps him sleep better. Gil tells him he can close the shades if the light bothers him, but Anthony insists that he likes the foil better. Although he does not find his son's answers logical, Gil decides that if it helps him sleep, he can keep the foil.

Episode 15

Gil manages to get Mary's house sold. He had hoped she would receive a nice sum of money to use for personal expenses. As it turns out, he is barely able to sell it for enough to pay off the mortgage and real estate broker fees.

Gilbert Martin Season 2 Information

Episode 1

Gilbert Martin is a 53-year-old Hispanic male who is married to Helen. His mother, Mary has recently moved in with Gil and his family.

Gil considers himself to be in good health, with one exception - he has chronic back pain, which frequently makes him miserable. He usually manages the pain with over-the-counter analgesics. He has a prescription for oxycodone with acetaminophen, which he takes when the pain becomes severe, but he is unable to take the oxycodone on days he works. He also has a prescription for cyclobenzaprine (Flexeril) 5 mg twice a day. Gil has a medical diagnosis of hyperlipidemia, for which he takes atorvastatin (Lipitor) 20 mg/day. He sees his physician once a year for cholesterol, triglycerides, and liver function tests. Gil has also been encouraged to eat a low-fat diet.

Gil's oldest son Mark (from a previous marriage) has fallen on hard times. He has been attempting to raise his 2-year-old son, Tyler, alone and has been experiencing significant financial difficulty. Gil wants to help his son and grandson out. Because Anthony has moved out of the house to go to school, Gil suggests that Mark and Tyler move in with them temporarily, to allow Mark to catch up on some of his bills. Gil cannot understand why Helen is so angry about this.

Episode 2

Gil is sympathetic to Helen's abdominal pain. He can tell that she is very uncomfortable and encourages her to go see the doctor about it. He overhears his mother telling Helen about goldenseal and recalls that his mother had her gallbladder removed when she was about 40.

Gil talks with Kristina about his concerns regarding her new boyfriend, Jared. He understands that she really likes him, but he is concerned about the obvious differences between high school and college-aged students. Gil tells Kristina that, if she is going to see Jared, he wants her word that she will not go into his dormitory room. Kristina assures her father that she won't do anything like that ▼.

Episode 3

Gil truly loves children and finds it enjoyable having a young child in his house again. While playing with Tyler, Gil takes the opportunity to look at Tyler's teeth (based on Mary's concerns); he, too, notices that Tyler's teeth appear to be in bad shape. When he mentions this to his son, he learns that Mark is aware of the problem but does not have the money to take Tyler to a dentist.

Gil hurts his back while doing some work around the house and ends up lying around for the next couple of days, taking pain pills and nursing a bottle of scotch.

Episode 4

Gil goes to the hospital to be with Helen for her surgery. He is amazed that they have taken her gallbladder out and that all she has to show for it are four Band-Aids on her abdomen. He feels sorry for her, as she keeps getting sick all evening, and he feels helpless for not being able to do anything for her. Kristina, Mark, Mary, and Tracie all come to the hospital that evening to visit.

Episode 5

Gil helps Helen as she continues to recover from her gallbladder surgery. She spends a good part of her time just resting. He asks the girls to help their grandmother take care of dinner, dishes, and general house chores. Gil's son Mark mentions a woman he recently met by the name of Shelly. He tells Gil she could be "the one." Gil is happy for his son, knowing he has been lonely since his falling out with Tyler's mother.

Episode 6

Gil receives a phone call from a woman named Louise, who introduces herself as a psychiatric mental health nurse practitioner. She informs Gil that Anthony was admitted to the hospital the day before, following an acute psychotic episode. Gil demands to know why he wasn't called earlier and asks multiple questions about his son's state of mind. Louise suggests that they make a visit to the hospital so that they can meet in person and see Anthony.

When Gil and Helen arrive at the hospital, both are anxious and afraid of what they might find. They learn that Anthony has been admitted to a locked acute care unit. Louise takes them into Anthony's room, where they find him hiding under the covers of his bed.

Gil and Helen talk with Louise for a time before participating in a team meeting. During the meeting, Gil asks what has happened to Anthony. The psychiatrist tells Gil and Helen that they are still gathering information, but it appears that Anthony had some type of psychotic break. Gil does not fully understand what "psychotic break" means, and the psychiatrist explains that Anthony had a break with reality. Helen and Gil find the meeting emotionally draining. Gil goes home and shares a 12-pack of beer with Mark.

Episode 7

Gil is very glad Anthony is coming back home. He is sure that the stress of going away to college contributed to his breakdown. Gil is confident that if Anthony lives at home in comfortable and familiar surroundings, the problem will go away. Gil talks to Mark and explains that it is very important for Anthony to feel comfortable at home. He asks Mark if he can let Anthony have his room back and is relieved that Mark agrees to do this ▼.

Episode 8

Helen tells Gil that Mark is not living up to his parental responsibilities with Tyler. She points out that he works, stays out late with his girlfriend, Shelly, sleeps in during the morning, and lets everybody else take care of Tyler. Gil admits that Mark is out a lot, but he also reminds Helen that helping him take care of Tyler is what families do. He agrees to talk with Mark about being more responsible, but he thinks that his wife is overly anxious and stressed out because of Anthony.

Episode 9

Gil hurts his back again this week while moving boxes in the garage. He is unable to complete the task and asks Mark to finish the project. Mark willingly does so, and Gil thinks that having Mark around the house is actually helpful. His mother, Mary, goes to the store and returns with pureed capsaicin. She applies it to his back and tells him this is a good treatment she learned from her grandmother. Gil finds the concoction causes some numbness to the area. That treatment in combination with a heating pad makes him feel pretty good.

Episode 10

Gil is aware that his wife is increasingly anxious. She tosses and turns in bed at night, keeping him awake. She has a hard time getting things done around the house. Gil suggests to Helen that she go see a counselor or someone to help her feel less anxious and settle down.

Gil is very concerned when Anthony decides to return to school. He tries to discourage Anthony from doing this, but it is clear to him that Anthony already has his mind made up.

Episode 11

Gil sees Anthony this week and is relieved that his son seems to be doing fine. He begins to think that he was wrong for discouraging him to return to school.

Episode 12

Mark tells Gil that his truck is finally paid off and he has caught up on all of his credit card debts. He tells Gil that things are getting serious between him and his girlfriend, Shelly. He asks Gil if he can stay a bit longer to save for a down payment on a house. Gil is proud of Mark's progress and does not consider his request to be unreasonable. He wishes that his wife could see the progress that Mark has made, instead of always being critical of him.

Episode 13

Gil gets another disturbing call from the hospital. Anthony has been arrested for indecent exposure and attempted assault on a police officer. He has been admitted to an inpatient psychiatric hospital again. Gil and Helen go to see their son and are confused about what might have happened NEWS.

Episode 14

Gil welcomes Anthony home and encourages him to do everything that he is asked to do in the therapy sessions. He assures Anthony that he has the support of his family, but says that he also needs to take measures to take care of himself.

Episode 15

Gil is notified by the insurance company that Anthony has almost reached his maximum coverage for psychiatric services. Gil is glad that Anthony has nearly completed his intensive outpatient program ▼.

Gilbert Martin Season 3 Information

Episode 1

Gilbert Martin is a 53-year-old Hispanic male who is married to Helen. They have been married for 19 years. Gil has a full house. His mother Mary, oldest son Mark, grandson Tyler, stepdaughter Tracie, and his two children with Helen (Anthony and Kristina) are all currently living in his home. Mark and Tyler will be moving soon into their own home.

Gil is especially concerned about his son, Anthony, who was recently diagnosed with schizophrenia. Gil is attempting to help Anthony adjust to living with this illness.

Gil and Helen have been very attentive to Anthony; they want to support him as much as possible. Gil is happy to see him working and making such good progress.

Episode 2

While the family is eating dinner together, Kristina tells everyone about the school dance she went to the previous evening and about her new boyfriend, Brian. Gil is glad to know that she has a new boyfriend because he was very leery about her last boyfriend, Jared. While Kristina is talking, Anthony has his eyes closed and then says, "Who cares about this? Just shut up." He then gets up and leaves the table. Gil is shocked by Anthony's behavior, but lets it go, knowing that he is still adjusting to his medications.

Episode 3

Gil takes his mother to the outpatient surgery center for the first of two cataract surgeries. He is glad that everything goes smoothly and hopes that his mother's vision improves.

Gil is happy to see Mark and Shelly looking for a home to buy. He likes Shelly and thinks she is good for Mark. To his mind, she has helped him settle down and will be a good mother for Tyler. Not only will he be glad to see Mark regain his independence, but he is also looking forward to having fewer people in the house.

Episode 4

Gil is devastated when he gets a phone call from the hospital, informing him that Mark has been involved in a serious car accident. He goes to the hospital immediately. When he arrives at the hospital, he is told by the Emergency Department charge nurse that Mark is in serious condition. Gil asks to see him but his request is denied. The charge nurse tells Gil that Mark is in the trauma room and he would just be in the way. He is told to take a seat in the waiting room.

Hours later, Gil is further devastated when he learns that Mark has a spinal cord injury and is paralyzed from the waist down. He is so distraught that, after meeting with the physicians, he goes home and gets drunk. Helen is angry with him for drinking because this is what caused Mark to be in the condition that he is in now ▼ NEWS.

Episode 5

Gil takes a week off from work to be with Mark. He attempts to be supportive, but he is aware of the difficulties that lie ahead for his son. Gil is not surprised by Mark's anger in response to fully understanding his injuries. Gil prides himself on being able to help family members in times of need, but he realizes that, in this particular case, he is completely helpless.

Episode 6

Gil continues to visit his son at the Rehabilitation Hospital. He can see that Mark is depressed. He knows that Mark is having difficulty finding anything to look forward to. Gil's mother reminds him of the need to pray for Anthony and Mark by going to the church. He was raised with such values, and his mother reinforces these in an important way for him. He goes with her to church and says the rosary NEWS.

Episode 7

Gil becomes angry when he learns that Anthony wants to stop taking his medications. Gil cannot understand why Anthony would even consider such a thing, especially in light of what happened the last time he stopped taking his medications. Perhaps it is because of the stress associated with Mark's injuries, but Gil tells Anthony that the family will be supportive of him - but only if he agrees to treatment. If Anthony does not undergo treatment, he will have to find someplace else to live.

A couple of hours later, Gil has to break Anthony's door down because it's locked and Anthony does not respond to his mother. Gil sees that his son has taken an overdose of medication and calls for an ambulance. Helen becomes upset, pale, and sweaty. She tells Gil that she has chest pain, and her neck feels like it is swelling shut. Gil really has his hands full and doesn't know if he should attend to Helen or to Anthony. Gil feels terrible and blames himself for Anthony's suicide attempt and Helen's near heart attack ▶ ▼.

Episode 8

Gil worries about his son Anthony, who is still hospitalized for inpatient psychiatric treatment. He has been told that Anthony no longer qualifies for outpatient treatment on the insurance plan. Gil is working with a social worker to get Anthony signed up for Medicaid coverage.

Episode 9

Gil is glad that Anthony is out of the hospital and wants to ensure his success with outpatient therapy. He tells Anthony that he is sorry for making him upset and just wants him to be better. Gil notices that, although Anthony talks with him, there is little emotion in his voice. Gil feels so sad about the conditions of both of his sons. He desperately wants to get drunk, but he knows this will only make things worse. He buries his feelings and tries just to focus on work.

Episode 10

Gil takes several days off from work at the end of the week to make the necessary arrangements for Mark's discharge home. He obtains a special bed and makes phone calls to arrange for a home health nurse to help with Mark's wound care. After Mark comes home, Gil hurts his back while trying to move him into bed. He must elicit Anthony's help to get Mark moved. Gil spends the next several days trying to rest his back before going back to work.

This week Tracie decides to move out of the house. Gil knows that this makes Helen very upset. Although he hates to see her go, he recognizes that the household has been in total chaos and understands her decision to leave.

Episode 11

Gil overhears Anthony yelling at his mother about not taking his medications. Gil and Anthony have another confrontation about Anthony's lack of compliance with his treatment. Anthony doesn't want to take the medications - he just can't take anymore! He says that he would rather live on the street. Anthony gathers a few things and storms out. Gil asks him where he will be, but Anthony does not answer. Gil notices that Anthony has left his medications in the bathroom ▶.

Episode 12

Gil learns that Anthony has been staying with Jason, a friend from high school. He attempts to call to find out how he is doing, but cannot reach him. Gil worries about both of his sons and his wife, and he wishes that he could make everything okay again. He does not know how to express what he is feeling. He feels the need to be "man of the house" and not show his emotions. Gil is glad that Kristina and Tracie have not had any problems.

Episode 13

Gil continues to feel very stressed out over all the recent events. He does not have any friends he has shared this with, and although he has talked to Father John at the church, he feels very lonely and powerless. Gil gets very drunk as a way to cope with the feelings he has.

Episode 14

Gil thinks about Anthony and Mark constantly. He is glad to see Tracie step up to take care of Tyler and he makes a point to spend time with Tyler each day. It is important to him to have a close relationship with his grandson, and he appreciates Tracie's efforts to bring Tyler over each day.

Gil also notices that Kristina has not been running around with her friends as much and is glad that she is home more. He is particularly glad that she has not been going out with Jared.

Episode 15

Gil learns that Anthony is staying in one of the homeless shelters in the downtown area. He is devastated to know that one of his children is on the streets, but he doesn't know what else to do. He knows that he cannot bring Anthony back into the house at this time, but he still worries constantly about him ▼.

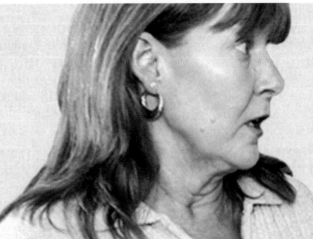

HELEN MARTIN

Season 1	Season 2	Season 3
Helen is Gil's wife. She is unhappy when Mary comes to live with them, finding her presence to be disruptive to the family. Helen is obese and has had cholelithiasis; she attempts to manage her condition through diet and weight loss.	In addition to the mounting chaos in her home, Helen has acute cholecystitis and eventually has a laparoscopic cholecystectomy. She has a great deal of post-op nausea. Helen is angry with Gil for allowing Mark and Tyler to move into the home. She is also very distraught about Anthony and his mental illness.	With Mark's injury, Anthony's mental illness, and her mother-in-law living in the home, Helen has anxiety attacks and is diagnosed with an anxiety disorder. She becomes further distraught when Tracie decides to move out of the house.

Helen Martin Season 1 Information

Episode 1

Helen Martin is a 48-year-old White female who is married to Gil. They have been married for 18 years. Helen has a daughter (Tracie) from a previous marriage, and she has two teenage children with Gil (Anthony and Kristina). She has been relatively happy in this marriage. Her primary frustration with Gil is that he always wants to take care of everybody and has a hard time saying no. She thinks he is generous to a fault. Helen has never gotten along well with Gil's adult son, Mark, or Gil's mother, Mary. For all the years they have been married, Mary has referred to Helen as a "gringa," which really annoys her. Helen often feels frustrated when Gil and his mother speak to each other in Spanish, because nobody else in the family can understand them.

Helen works as a teller at a bank. Although she finds her job monotonous, she appreciates the steady income. Helen is overweight and has tried to lose weight most of her adult life. She frequently diets and, in fact, has lost a great deal of weight in the past, but she just can't seem to keep it off. She blames menopause for her most recent weight gain.

Helen experiences indigestion following a few meals this week. She takes an antacid, believing the problem is just heartburn. She also experiences hot flashes.

Episode 2

Gil tells Helen that his mother wants to move in and that they should make room for her. Helen is furious with this decision for several reasons: Gil did not first consult with her, they don't have room for her, they cannot afford another person in the house, and Helen has never gotten along well with her mother-in-law.

Helen continues to have indigestion following meals; it does not occur following all meals, just sometimes. The discomfort is usually located in the upper right side of her abdomen, and sometimes it is quite painful. The pain can last for up to a couple of hours and then it subsides. Occasionally, she feels nauseous as well. To top it off, Helen experiences several episodes of hot flashes ▶

Episode 3

Helen is not happy about Mary moving into the house. Her two daughters are angry and fighting because they have to share a bedroom to accommodate their grandmother.

Helen thinks that this is very unfair to both the girls. Additionally, she overhears Gil and Mary talking to each other in Spanish. They know darn well that nobody else in the family speaks Spanish. She thinks that Mary does this intentionally so that she can talk to Gil in a way Helen can't understand.

Helen continues to experience pain and indigestion after meals. In fact, the symptoms have become more frequent. She decides to make an appointment to see her physician about the symptoms.

Episode 4

Helen has not slept well this week. She has had a hard time falling asleep because she worries about everything: the kids, money, problems at work, and recent problems on the national level that affect the country. Oftentimes, she gets up and paces about the house, trying to turn her mind off. About the time she falls asleep, she is awakened by Mary, who is watching TV in the den during the middle of the night. She asks Mary to keep the volume down so that she won't disturb the family. Helen also wakes at times because of hot flashes and night sweats.

Helen sees her family physician, Dr. Rowe, this week for indigestion. Based on Helen's symptoms, Dr. Rowe suspects that Helen has cholelithiasis and orders an ultrasound scan of the abdomen. The ultrasound confirms the presence of gallstones. The physician tells Helen that she has two options: (1) conservative therapy that would involve dietary modification (a low-fat diet and a reduced-calorie diet to promote weight loss); or (2) surgery to remove her gallbladder. Helen decides to try dietary modification. Dr. Rowe refers her to the Neighborhood Patient Education Center for more information. She is encouraged to use over-the-counter analgesics for pain ▼.

Episode 5

Helen goes to the Patient Education Center and receives dietary counseling from a nurse educator. She is taught about low-fat food options and is given sample menus and cooking techniques to minimize fat. Helen is very motivated to go on this diet to avoid the pain, and she looks forward to losing some weight.

Helen agrees to Mary's request to prepare dinner three times a week. Helen shares with Mary what she learned at the Patient Education Center, with an expectation that the meals Mary cooks will be prepared based on this dietary plan. She becomes angry when she finds that Mary essentially ignores her requests and is frustrated because the rest of the family members comment on how good dinner is when Grandma cooks. She believes that Mary is intentionally sabotaging her dietary efforts ▼.

Episode 6

Helen comes home one day after work this week and is unable to find anything because Mary has rearranged the entire kitchen. Helen feels angry and invaded. Mary defends her actions by claiming that Helen's kitchen was very disorganized and that she is just trying to help the entire family.

Episode 7

Helen becomes frustrated when she finds that Mary continues to rearrange things in the house and clean things that were already clean. Helen also notices that Mary is often unaware that the dishes she washes and puts away are still dirty, so Helen ends up rewashing dishes.

She has given up fighting with Mary over the dinner menu and has decided to take Gil's advice and limit fat intake at other meals, eating only small portions when Mary cooks.

Episode 8

Helen is angry when she learns that Mary and Gil have given Kristina permission to use the car. She does not feel that it is appropriate for Mary and Gil to make such decisions without her input. But, at this point, if she were to put a stop to it, she would end up looking like the "bad guy." Helen is so frustrated with this that she eats a large, fatty meal and ends up having 2 hours of indigestion, pain, and nausea as a result. She also has trouble sleeping that night. She blames Gil and Mary for the pain and loss of sleep.

Episode 9

Helen panics when Anthony fails to bring Kristina home after a school function. She tries to call Kristina's cell phone, but it is turned off. She becomes frantic and is sure that somebody has abducted Kristina. Helen gets in the car and drives to the school to see if she can find her daughter. On the way to school, she becomes increasingly anxious and begins to experience shortness of breath and tightness in her chest and throat. The closer she gets to the school, the worse the symptoms become. Helen's symptoms reach the point at which her heart is pounding in her chest and she feels like she is suffocating; she breaks out in a cold sweat. Helen pulls over to the side of the road and begins to cry. She tells herself to calm down and that everything surely will be all right. After a few minutes, Helen composes herself and continues driving to the school. When she gets to the school, she finds that the college fair is over and nearly everybody has left. When she gets back home, she finds Kristina there watching TV. Helen screams at her and wants to know where she was and why she didn't answer her phone. She tells Kristina that she almost had a heart attack and that her gallbladder acted up because of this situation ▶.

Episode 10

Helen goes to the Neighborhood High School open house with Gil to meet Kristina and Anthony's teachers. They are very complimentary about both of their children. One teacher who has taught both of them says they are really quite different from each other. Kristina is very outgoing and bubbly, and Anthony is very quiet and studious. Helen remarks that her daughter is quite the socialite.

Episode 11

Helen overhears Gil and Mary speaking to each other in Spanish again; for some reason this is really getting on her nerves. Why can't they speak so that others in the family can understand?

Episode 12

Helen is worried about Kristina when she fails to come home by 1 a.m. following a school dance. She attempts to text and call Kristina's cell phone, but it is turned off. She paces the house and alternately worries that Kristina has been in a wreck or that she is up to no good with her date. She feels a subtle tightness in her chest and slight shortness of breath, which she attributes to her gallbladder problems. When Kristina comes home, Helen grounds her for staying out an hour past her curfew and warns her that if she turns off her cell phone and can't be reached in the future, she may lose her cell phone privileges.

When Kristina protests, she reminds her who pays her phone bill each month. Helen feels frustrated because Tracie and Anthony never behaved in this way.

Episode 13

Helen overhears Gil and Mary speaking to each other in Spanish – AGAIN. When she mentions to Gil that she does not like it and it makes her feel left out, he tells her this is how they communicated with one another when he was growing up and it really is no big deal ▶.

Episode 14

Tracie tells her mother about the foil in Anthony's room and tells her the house looks awful with the foil, especially when the afternoon sun is shining on it. Helen agrees it does not look very good, but then again, she hates the pinkish color their next door neighbors used to paint their house, and the people who live across the street have weeds growing in their front yard. She hopes the neighbors complain so she can tell them what she thinks of their homes.

Episode 15

Helen begins to experience indigestion and pain again. She knows that she has not stuck with her low-fat diet very well. She is hopeful that the symptoms will subside with better eating habits.

Helen Martin Season 2 Information

Episode 1

Helen Martin is a 48-year-old White female who is married to Gil. They have been married for 18 years. She has been relatively happy in this marriage. Her primary frustration with Gil is that he always wants to take care of everybody and has a hard time saying no. Helen has never gotten along well with Gil's adult son, Mark, or Gil's mother Mary. Helen has had recent stress in her marriage because Gil's mother Mary is now living with them. Helen's son, Anthony, has recently left home to attend college nearby.

Helen has been experiencing ongoing abdominal pain due to gallstones. She has been trying to manage the problem through dietary modification, but this effort has not been successful.

Helen is furious with Gil for suggesting that Mark and Tyler move into their home. Helen and Mark have never gotten along very well, so she is very resentful that Gil gave Mark permission to live with them. Situations like these make Helen feel that Gil does not care what her opinion is. This makes her feel powerless. Helen thinks that Mark is a loser because he cannot seem to keep a job, and the party scene is more important to him than looking

for work or raising Tyler. She believes that Mark should have to figure out a solution to his own problems. Helen is also angry with Kristina for staying out late again. Helen grounds her, but she recognizes that this punishment has not been terribly effective with her in the past ▶.

Episode 2

Helen has an abrupt episode of intense abdominal pain and vomiting. She becomes sweaty and feels that her heart is racing. At first, she thinks that she is having a heart attack, but then she concludes the pain is probably being caused by her gallbladder. The pain lasts about an hour and then subsides. She has given up hope that conservative treatment will resolve anything. She has an appointment with Dr. Rowe the following day, who refers her to a surgeon. After meeting with the surgeon, Helen decides to go ahead with surgery to remove her gallbladder. She is scheduled to have the surgery in a couple of weeks.

Helen talks with Anthony this week. He tells her that he elected not to go to the football game. Helen wishes her son would interact more at school. She frequently feels anxious about his well-being.

Episode 3

Helen overhears Mary talking to Gil in Spanish. This makes her so angry. She assumes that Mary is talking about her or telling Gil things about the family that are not true. She really resents the fact that they have their own private communication that nobody else can understand. Later when she asks Gil what they were talking about, Gil tells Helen that Mary is concerned about Tyler's teeth.

Episode 4

Helen is anxious all week, worrying about her surgery - almost to the point of not being able to do basic tasks around the house. She goes to the hospital 2 days before the surgery for preoperative testing and blood work. On the day of surgery, she arrives at the hospital at about 6 a.m. She is in the surgical suite by 10 a.m. and has a laparoscopic cholecystectomy performed. The surgery goes smoothly, with no complications.

When Helen begins to wake up in the post-anesthesia care unit, she experiences a great deal of pain and nausea. She is given morphine and Ondansetron (Zofran) to treat her symptoms. She is transferred to the surgical unit when she is mostly awake and her vital signs are stable. She has no bleeding at the surgical site, her respiratory rate is 18, and her oxygen saturation is 97%.

Helen continues to have problems with pain and nausea throughout the afternoon and evening and has several episodes of emesis. On the surgical unit, she is given a 4-mg IV dose of ondansetron, which seems to do little for the nausea. She is also given 4 mg of morphine, which effectively eases her pain. She is unable to eat her dinner and has several more episodes of emesis during the evening. The pain and nausea make Helen increasingly anxious, to the point that she becomes tearful. Helen is then given a 4-mg IV dose of ondansetron, which helps her to relax and relieves her nausea. She finally falls asleep at about 3 a.m. Gil stays with her during this period, and although he can't help her, she appreciates his company.

The next morning, despite the fact that she has slept only a few hours, Helen feels much better. The nausea is gone, she has minimal pain, and she is able to eat. Her IV is discontinued, and she is discharged by mid-afternoon the day following her surgery.

Episode 5

Helen takes this week off from work to recover from her surgery. She spends a great deal of time with Tyler and actually finds the time quite enjoyable, although she would never admit this to anyone. She frequently feels anxious while at home about what might be going on at work. She does not leave her home often during her week off.

Episode 6

Gil informs Helen that Anthony has been admitted to the psychiatric unit at the hospital. Helen becomes very anxious and does not know what to think. She feels her heart racing and starts to cry. A while later, after having a chance to settle down, Helen goes with Gil to see Anthony. Upon arriving at the unit, Helen and Gil go into Anthony's room and find him hiding under the bedsheets. Helen approaches the bed and calls his name softly. Anthony peeks out from under the sheets and starts to cry uncontrollably. Helen cries also. Gil attempts to console Helen, but she continues to cry.

Louise, the psychiatric mental health nurse practitioner, asks Gil and Helen to accompany her to the day room. Helen wonders what she might have done to cause Anthony to act in this way. Louise obtains a family history from Helen and Gil. During this interview, it is revealed that Helen's maternal aunt spent many years at a psychiatric facility. She reports that her aunt was a bit "weird," but she can't give further details.

Helen and Gil later participate in a family meeting involving Louise, the psychiatrist, and Anthony. Both Helen and Gil find the meeting very difficult emotionally ▼.

Episode 7

Helen is glad that Anthony has moved back home. At the same time, she hates the commotion it has caused. Mark and Tyler are now sleeping in the family room, and the house feels very crowded and chaotic.

Episode 8

Helen is quite aware of Mark's late-night partying and talks with Gil about this. Although she does not come out and say it, she resents having to take care of Tyler. She is not interested in raising another child. She points out to Gil that the rest of the family (including herself) should not be responsible for taking care of Tyler just because Mark wants to party all the time. These recent changes in her household and going through menopause have placed quite a strain on Helen's marriage with Gil. These stressors make Helen feel anxious ▶ NEWS.

Episode 9

Helen continues to feel anxious about many things, including Anthony, Kristina, Mark, and Gil. Her symptoms have gotten so bad that just leaving the house makes her feel anxious, and she feels demoralized. Helen asks Tracie to accompany her to the grocery store.

Episode 10

Helen's anxiety escalates when Anthony returns to school. She is sure that he is in for further problems and is tearful when he goes back, despite her objections. At times Helen feels paralyzed by her anxiety. She is unable to work two days this week.

Episode 11

Helen is feeling a little better this week. Anthony is now back at school and seems to be doing fine. She is hopeful that his medications will continue to help him.

Episode 12

Helen notices Kristina has been looking thin and asks her about her weight. Kristina tells her Mom that she lost a few pounds, but it really has been no big deal and denies that there are any problems. Helen fails to notice that Kristina's report card came in the mail.

Episode 13

Helen is devastated when she learns that Anthony has been readmitted to the hospital. She is angry with him when she learns that he quit taking his medications. She feels her heart racing, and it is very hard for her to settle down. Gil again suggests that she go see a doctor. Helen is worried that she might have a heart problem and avoids making the appointment out of fear of having an anxiety attack at the physician's office [NEWS].

Episode 14

Helen is relieved when Anthony is discharged from the hospital and comes back home. She is determined to help him keep up with all of his medications. She worries that he will have another "episode." She tells Gil that Mark needs to move out and get his own place. Gil tells Helen that Mark is planning to move soon.

Episode 15

Helen's anxiety has reached the point at which she only goes out to go to work. She is fearful of having an anxiety attack in public. She has read that heart attacks in women have different signs than those in men, and she is convinced that she is at risk of having a heart attack. She asks Tracie to go with her nearly everywhere she goes. Tracie tells her mother that she needs to get checked out by a doctor.

Helen Martin Season 3 Information

Episode 1

Helen Martin is a 49-year-old White female who is married to Gil. They have been married for 19 years. Until lately, she has been relatively happy in this marriage. However, she has been feeling frustrated with Gil because he allowed his mother Mary and then his adult son, Mark, and Mark's son Tyler to move into their home. Helen has never gotten along well with Mark or Mary, so these changes have been difficult. The whole time Gil and Helen have been married, Mary has referred to Helen as a "gringa," which really annoys her. Helen also often feels frustrated when Gil and his mother speak to each other in Spanish, because nobody else in the family can understand them.

Recently, Helen had a cholecystectomy for treatment of gallbladder disease. More recently, she has been experiencing bouts of anxiety. Much of the anxiety has been due to her concern for Anthony and issues with her daughter Kristina. She has not formally seen a physician for the condition, although several of her family members have suggested she do so.

Helen is very attentive to Anthony. She pays close attention to his mood and behavior to be sure not to miss something. She makes sure that he takes his medications every day and helps him to get to work on time. She is glad that he has a job to go to every day and is hopeful that he is on the road to recovery.

Episode 2

Helen is glad to hear that Mark and Shelly are planning to buy a house. Mark has been living with them too long already, and Helen can't wait to see him leave. She is frustrated that Gil hasn't set more limits with Mark.

Helen is upset by Anthony's behavior at the dinner table when he tells Kristina to shut up. She wonders if the medication is causing him to act this way. Mary and Gil say some things to each other in Spanish, and that makes her even more upset [NEWS].

Episode 3

Helen becomes annoyed with Mary telling her that the family needs to be going to church together to pray for Mark and Anthony. According to Mary, if they don't pray at the church, the prayers may not be heard. She tells Mary that she is too stressed out and does not understand the Catholic way. Helen tells Mary that she will pray on her own.

Episode 4

Helen is upset when she learns of Mark's accident. She is angry with him for driving his truck drunk and is shocked to learn that his injuries have left him paralyzed. At the same time, she feels guilty about her resentment toward him. She wonders how he will ever be able to care for himself and how he will be able to raise Tyler. Helen is furious when Gil comes home from the hospital after seeing Mark and gets drunk [▼] [NEWS].

Episode 5

Helen and Gil spend a great deal of time at the hospital with Mark this week. Helen is worried about the long-term consequences of Mark's injuries. Although they have never been close, and despite the fact that he brought this on himself, Helen feels very badly for Mark. She wonders what lies ahead, not only for his life, but for Tyler's as well. This causes her to worry almost constantly.

Episode 6
Helen feels overwhelmed with trying to keep up with everything and the competing demands of her family. She often finds herself crying and unable to stop 🟦.

Episode 7
Helen is upset with Gil for yelling at Anthony. She hears him slam his door and decides that it is best to leave him alone for a while. After a couple of hours, Helen gently knocks on the door. Anthony does not respond, and she attempts to enter his room, but he has locked the door. She knocks louder, and he still does not answer. Gil finally forces the door open, and Helen sees Anthony lying on the floor, stuporous and incoherent. She sees a large (500-count), empty bottle of acetaminophen in the trash can. They call 9-1-1.

Finding Anthony on the floor causes Helen to have a severe anxiety attack. She begins to experience severe chest pain. When the paramedics arrive, they tell her that she needs to be seen in the Emergency Department (ED) as well. In the ED, Helen reports nausea, chest pain, shortness of breath, neck tightness, diaphoresis, and palpitations. She has a cardiac workup, which is negative. She sees a cardiologist in the ED, who orders Holter monitoring for one week to rule out a dysrhythmia. Helen is also given a prescription for 0.5 mg of lorazepam (Ativan) to take when she has anxiety ◤.

Episode 8
Helen sees the cardiologist this week, who determines that she has no evidence of cardiac disease. After taking a thorough history and learning about the recent events within Helen's family, the cardiologist refers her to a psychiatrist about a possible anxiety disorder. Helen is told that she cannot get in to see the psychiatrist for 3 months, so instead she agrees to make an appointment with a nurse practitioner at the Neighborhood Health Connections Clinic who specializes in mental health. Helen has been taking the lorazepam (Ativan) and finds that it helps her to feel better.

Episode 9
Helen sees Shawn Jacobs, the nurse practitioner, this week. Expecting to see a female nurse, Helen is very surprised by Shawn's appearance. Helen tells Shawn all about the issues she is experiencing in her family but embellishes the most about her son Anthony and how he almost gave her a heart attack a few weeks ago. She says that the lorazepam definitely helps, but that she also feels like she is "on a seesaw," up and down, feeling good, feeling anxious, then needing more medications. Helen agrees to start two new medications (Buspirone hydrochloride, 10 mg daily, and sertraline [Zoloft], 50 mg daily);

she also agrees to a lab test to check her thyroid. She is ready to agree to almost anything if it means getting better 🟦.

Episode 10
Mark is discharged from the Rehabilitation Hospital this week. It has been quite an ordeal getting ready for him to come home. Helen is glad to have the lorazepam to keep her anxiety under control. She feels very discouraged about the fact that she is now responsible for caring for a depressed paraplegic man and his son. The one positive thing, however, is that her mother-in-law, Mary, has made it clear that she is going to help take care of Mark. For the first time since she has moved into their home, Helen is glad to have Mary's help. Things get worse for Helen when Tracie announces that she has decided to move out of the house. Helen is so upset by this that she cries uncontrollably for hours. She feels overwhelmed and as though her life is spinning out of control. Tracie is the one solid person Helen knows she can count on.

Helen sees the nurse practitioner at Neighborhood Health Connections Clinic again this week. As she tells Shawn about her week, she loses her composure and sobs. Helen initially feels embarrassed, but she realizes that the nurse practitioner seems genuinely interested. Helen asks Shawn if he knows her son because she brought him to this same clinic earlier in the week. Shawn tells Helen that the clinic sees many patients and all cases are treated confidentially. His calm and nonjudgmental approach puts Helen at ease. Helen tells Shawn that she is still relying on the lorazepam to make it through the day. Shawn recommends an increase in her sertraline (Zoloft) and buspirone dosages. He suggests that she not take lorazepam unless she really needs it and asks her to come back in a week ▶.

Episode 11
Helen feels stressed from attempting to help care for Mark and is getting into regular arguments with Anthony about taking his medications. She does not know how much more she can take of all this. She is devastated when Anthony has an argument with Gil and storms out of the house.

Helen sees Shawn, the psychiatric mental health nurse practitioner, again this week and tells him about the latest events in her home and how upset she was that Anthony stormed out of the house. Despite all this, Helen reports feeling less anxious and believes the medications are helping her. The nurse practitioner provides Helen with information for caregiver resources and recommends family counseling. Helen would love to go, but she just does not think there is any way that she can afford the time or the expense.

Episode 12
Helen worries all week about Anthony and keeps hoping that he will come back home. Helen's friend, Martha, calls to tell her that Anthony is living with her son's friend, Jason.

She is relieved that Anthony is okay. Helen gets Jason's phone number and tries to call, but she is not able to reach Anthony. Helen also misses having Tracie and Tyler at the house. She wishes that Tracie and Anthony would both come home 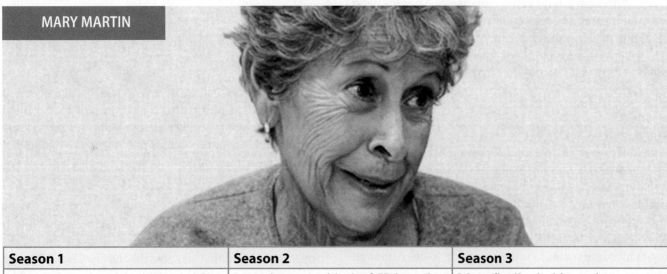.

Episode 13

Helen is pleased to see Tracie bring Tyler over to visit Mark every day. She can see how happy Tyler is with her and how good Tracie looks. Helen realizes that it is probably good for Tracie and Tyler to be out of the house, despite how much she misses them.

Helen makes another visit to the Neighborhood Health Connections Clinic this week to see Shawn Jacobs, the psychiatric mental health nurse practitioner. Helen tells Shawn that things are calmer this week and that Anthony is living at a friend's house but that he has not returned her calls. Helen asks if he has been coming to the clinic for his appointments and is not surprised to be told that

Shawn is unable to comment. Helen asks for a refill for lorazepam (Ativan) and is told that she should not need this anymore because her other medications are helping her. Helen hopes that Shawn is right!

Episode 14

Mark makes his first unassisted transfer from the bed to a wheelchair this week. Helen is glad to have something positive to think about. She wishes that she knew how Anthony was doing.

Episode 15

Helen is devastated to learn that her son Anthony has been at a homeless shelter. She pleads with Gil to go get him and bring him home, but Gil tells Helen that they cannot have that disruption in their home. Helen blames Gil for driving Anthony away. Helen makes an appointment to see Shawn at the Neighborhood Health Connections Clinic.

MARY MARTIN

Season 1	Season 2	Season 3
After being recently widowed, Mary moves in with Gil's family. She is a "busybody," and moving into the household disrupts the family. Mary is in good health, although she has cataracts and glaucoma, and is found to have osteoporosis.	Mary is very critical of Helen when Anthony has mental health problems, however, she is very supportive of Anthony. She continues to have problems with her vision.	Mary finally decides to have cataract surgery. Following surgery, she starts driving again. She attempts to help Anthony and takes care of Mark after his accident.

Mary Martin Season 1 Information

Episode 1

Mary Martin is a 75-year-old female who was recently widowed. She and her husband were married for 52 years when he died from cancer 6 months ago. She has a limited income, because her husband's pension terminated when he died. She receives $752 each month in Social Security benefits. Mary has not adjusted well to being alone. Her son, Gil, visits her frequently and helps her manage her home.

Mary does not see very well; otherwise, she is in excellent health. The only health-related problems she is aware of are cataract and glaucoma, for which she sees an ophthalmologist on a regular basis. The only prescription drug that she uses is Latanoprost (Xalatan) to manage her glaucoma (her dose is 1 drop in each eye once a day), and her only complaint about the eye drops is the cost. Although she has a car and driver's license, she does not drive very often due to problems with night vision. She prefers to get friends and family members to take her where she needs to go.

Mary is a devout Roman Catholic and is very active with parish activities. She feels frustrated because her son Gil and his family are not actively practicing Catholics. Mary's primary hobbies include cooking and quilting. She regularly goes to the Neighborhood Senior Center.

Mary is happy that Gil spent most of his time with her this past weekend. Not only does she enjoy his company, but she appreciates the fact that he takes care of things for her. Although it has been 6 months since her husband died, she has not become comfortable living alone. She tells Gil that she wishes his father were still alive to take care of her. To pass the time and combat loneliness, she spends a great deal of time at the Neighborhood Senior Center.

Episode 2

Mary bakes cookies for Gil this week and then calls him to invite him over for a treat. She wishes that he would spend more time with her because she feels so lonely. While Gil is visiting, she tells him that she is having a hard time managing her home. Gil tells her that perhaps she could stay with them for a while. This is exactly what Mary has been hoping for, and she immediately agrees that moving in with his family would be the best thing to do. Although she is not fond of Gil's wife, Helen, she loves her son and her grandchildren and knows that she will be much happier living with them. She quickly begins making plans to move. Mary goes to her quilting club and tells her friend Pam Allen and the other the ladies in the group that she is planning to move in with her son ▶.

Episode 3

Mary moves into Gil and Helen's home this week. She is unaware of the disruption that her moving in has created within the household. She has many possessions that she wants to bring with her to Gil's home, but space is somewhat limited. Several boxes of her possessions are placed in the garage, with the understanding that she will go through the boxes and determine what she wants to keep and what she wants to give away. Mary agrees to let Gil clean up her home in order to list it for sale ▼.

Episode 4

Mary is still in the process of fitting into the family. She has the house to herself during the daytime and feels a bit out of place, at times even wishing to be back in her home. At night she has trouble sleeping and frequently goes out to the den to watch television in the middle of the night.

Episode 5

Mary loves to cook and is actually very good at it. Mary tells Helen that she will make dinner for the family 3 nights a week. Helen agrees to this and asks Mary to try to keep the dinners low in fat because she is trying to stay on a diet. Mary knows what Gil's favorite foods are and also knows that Helen does not cook Mexican food as well as she can. Mary liked Gil's first wife much better than Helen and is not too concerned about cooking foods consistent with Helen's request. She is much more interested in preparing dinners that her son likes. She is very pleased that all of the family members (except Helen) comment on how good her dinners are. Mary also spends time this week at the Senior Center with her friends and goes out to get her hair and nails done ▼.

Episode 6

This week Mary decides that the kitchen cabinets need to be cleaned and reorganized; she proceeds to rearrange the entire kitchen to suit her needs. Mary thinks Helen is a lazy housekeeper and decides that it is a good thing that she is living with them to help them out and take care of her son, Gil.

Episode 7

Mary goes to the community health fair with her friend. While at the fair, she has a bone density screening performed and is told that she possibly has low bone density - a finding commonly associated with osteoporosis. The health fair nurse suggests that she contact her physician about getting a full bone scan so that her condition can be evaluated further. When Gil comes home from work that evening, she tells him that she needs to have a bone test done and would like him to arrange this for her 🔲NEWS.

Episode 8

Mary hears the argument between Kristina and her parents about the car. When Kristina asks Mary if she may drive her car, Mary decides it would be fine—but only if she promises to take care of the car and only if her father approves it.

Mary goes to the Senior Center for lunch and to play cards with her friends. She tells her friends that she must take care of her son because her daughter-in-law is lazy and does not cook properly. During lunch she notices her friend Beatrice eating two pieces of cake. Mary reminds Beatrice that she should not eat too much. Than Mary stops in the Senior Center Nursing Clinic and talks with Karen Williams and a student nurse by the name of Kayla Sharif. Mary tells them all about her bone density scan results and the recommendation to follow up with her physician. At the end of the week, Mary sees Dr. Rowe and tells him about the health fair. She asks Dr. Rowe about getting a bone test.

Episode 9

Mary has an appointment for the bone scan this week; following her scan, she asks Gil to take her to the beauty salon to have her hair and nails done. Later in the week, she observes Helen cleaning the house and determines that it is not being done correctly. She often follows behind Helen and repeats the cleaning so that the house is cleaned properly.

Episode 10

In a follow-up visit with Dr. Rowe, Mary is told that her bone scan shows evidence of decreased bone mineral density that is consistent with osteoporosis. She is told to increase her activity for weight-bearing exercise, increase her calcium intake to 1,500 mg per day, and take vitamin D supplements. She is given a prescription for alendronate (Fosamax). Dr. Rowe also tells Mary that new research points to a link between osteoporosis and celiac disease and suggests that she be screened. Mary agrees to the screening, and serologic autoantibody testing is performed.

Mary goes to the Neighborhood Senior Center this week and attends a leather craft class. During the class, she tells all the ladies about the medical tests, her new medication for osteoporosis, her new exercise regimen, and all the events happening at her home ▶.

Episode 11

Mary receives a phone call from the physician's office, informing her that her blood tests were negative for the presence of celiac disease. Mary still does not really understand what celiac disease is but is relieved to know that she doesn't have another condition to worry about. She walks around the block early every morning this week for weight-bearing exercise.

Episode 12

Mary has been living with Gil and his family for several months now and she finally decides to talk with him about her displeasure in their lack of involvement in the church. She tells Gil, "You and your children need to be more involved. That is how you were raised." She is disappointed by his lack of acknowledgement of her concerns and he simply says they have a different way.

Episode 13

Mary continues her walking routine. She also gets involved in some of the exercise classes offered at the Neighborhood Senior Center.

Episode 14

Mary has an appointment with her ophthalmologist this week, who notes that her cataract continue to worsen and recommends that she consider surgery. Mary does not admit that she is afraid to have surgery on her eyes. She tells the doctor that she might have the surgery at some point, but she is too busy to do it right now. The physician gives Mary a new prescription for her eyeglasses, which will help her vision at least for a little while. Mary is told to increase the amount of light and to use reading glasses or a magnifying glass for reading.

The physician also notes that Mary's intraocular pressure has increased since her last visit. She is asked how often she uses the latanoprost (Xalatan) eye drops. Mary admits to the ophthalmologist that she only uses the drops on Mondays, Wednesdays, Fridays, and Sundays, as opposed to every day. Mary explains that she does this because the drops are expensive and this regimen makes the drops last longer. The office nurse helps Mary find a prescription assistance program to help defray the cost of the eye drops.

A few days later, Mary is at the Senior Center and drops by the Nursing Clinic. She tells Jacob McCain about her appointment with the eye doctor and the eye drops and the cataract surgery. She tells Jacob that she finds all this information confusing and asks if he can help her understand the information. Jacob sits down with her and reviews information from a website.

Episode 15

Mary is angry that somebody hit her car in the school parking lot while Kristina was driving. She tells Kristina that she understands that the accident was not her fault, but she needs to take good care of the car. Mary is disappointed, but not really surprised, to learn that she only is getting $12,500 from the sale of her house.

While at the Neighborhood Senior Center this week, Mary hears that Mr. Jackson, the shuttle driver, is in the hospital with pneumonia. She makes a point of dropping by the hospital to visit Mr. Jackson so that she can fill him in on all the news from the center. This week, Mary is also saddened to hear that Pam Allen (one of the women from the quilting club and also from her church) recently had surgery for cancer. This brings back not-too-distant memories of her late husband's bout with cancer. Mary goes to the church to pray for Pam and her family.

Mary Martin   Season 2 Information

Episode 1

Mary Martin is Gil Martin's 75-year-old mother. About one year ago, Mary's husband of 52 years died from cancer. Because she was feeling so lonely, Mary jumped at the opportunity to move in with Gil's family. It is Mary's perception that Gil and his family need her because she can cook and clean for them. She has never felt that Gil's wife Helen was a good housekeeper.

Mary does not see very well; otherwise, she is in excellent health. She prefers to get friends and family members to take her places she needs to go.

She has always been fond of Mark and is glad that he is finally getting a chance to live with his father. She tells Helen that Gil has done the right thing by letting Mark and Tyler live with them. She tells Kristina that she should be happy to share a room with her sister. Mary says that, when she was growing up, she had to share a room with four of her sisters. Mary offers to babysit her great-grandchild, Tyler, whenever Mark needs help.

Episode 2

Mary notices that Tyler has no toys or books. She asks Kristina to drive her to her hair appointment and then to the discount store, where she buys Tyler toys, puzzles, and books.

Mary spends time with her friends at the Neighborhood Senior Center, telling them in detail all about her granddaughter, Kristina, dating a college boy, about the fact that Mark and Tyler have recently moved in with them, and how her daughter-in-law is so intolerant of other people's misfortunes. As she talks, she notices a small, white-haired woman walk by and scowl at her. She asks the ladies at the table who the woman is. Although a few ladies say that they have seen the woman before, nobody knows her name.

When Helen has her gallbladder attack this week, Mary tells her that she should just take goldenseal (*Hydrastis canadensis*) instead of having surgery. Mary swears this is the way her gallbladder problems were cured when she was 44 years old [NEWS].

Episode 3

Mary overhears Tracie commenting to Tyler about the condition of his teeth. With her bad eyesight, Mary really never noticed the condition of his teeth before. Later in the day, she is shocked at how bad they are—or at least what she can see. She mentions it to Mark and can tell by his response that he is aware of the problem. Mary talks to her son, Gil, about her concerns for Tyler's teeth and suggests that he talk with Mark about taking Tyler to a dentist ▶.

Episode 4

Mary takes over most of the household duties when Helen goes to the hospital for her surgery. She enjoys being in charge and making dinner for everyone. Mary has another visit with the ophthalmologist this week. She tells her doctor that her vision is foggy and that it has become hard to see clearly, even with the eyeglasses. The physician indicates that a stronger prescription of eyeglasses will help for now, but that she really needs to consider having the cataract surgery.

Episode 5

Mary hates the fact that Helen is home all this week and feels irritated when she complains about her pain. Mary prefers to have the house mostly to herself during the daytime when Helen is at work. Mary listens to the local news and wonders if they will ever get the forest fire put out.

Mary goes to her friend Pam Allen's home several times this week to help provide meals. She also recognizes that the Allens need help transporting their son, Gary, to work and other activities. Mary takes it upon herself to contact several women in the church and get them signed up to help ▼ [NEWS].

Episode 6

Mary is very saddened by the problems that Anthony has been experiencing. When it comes to light that mental health problems run in Helen's side of the family, Mary is quick to point out that it is obvious where Anthony's problems have come from. She gets a friend to pick her up to join in on the card games at the Neighborhood Senior Center. Mary tells everyone all the things happening in her household this week.

Episode 7

Mary is somewhat annoyed initially when Anthony moves back home, because Mark and Tyler take over the family room and this interferes with Mary's late-night TV watching. In the mornings, she encourages Mark to sleep in. She gladly takes care of Tyler because it makes her feel useful.

Mary talks Tracie into driving her to get her hair and nails done. On the way home, she asks Tracie to stop at the mall. At the mall, she buys Tracie some badly needed new shoes in appreciation for her time.

Episode 8

Mary overhears Helen sharing her concerns with Gil about Mark's late-night schedule. Mary tells Gil that he should not give Mark too hard a time for being out late. She points out to him that she likes taking care of Tyler, and it all seems to work out just fine.

Mary also is aware of how much Anthony is struggling. She tries to talk with Anthony to make him feel better, but can tell that he is just not interested. She thinks that he is lonely and just needs to have a girlfriend. She bakes him his favorite cookies to try to cheer him up.

Episode 9
Mary's son, Gil, hurts his back while moving boxes in the garage. She gets some pureed capsaicin and applies it to his back. She tells him that this is the best treatment for his back because it will numb the pain. It is a home remedy that she learned years ago.

Episode 10
Mary is hopeful that Anthony's return to school is successful. She believes that he has had a hard time in life because of Helen and believes that being away from her is what he really needs. Mary spends time at the Neighborhood Senior Center playing cards, although it is getting more difficult for her to play because of her vision.

Episode 11
Mary Martin goes to her quilting club and spends most of the time talking about all the problems with her eyes and the problems that Anthony is having. She also tells Pam Allen how glad everyone is to have her come back to the quilting club. Mary can see that Pam has lost weight and looks tired.

Episode 12
Mary decides that her eyesight has gotten bad enough that she should go back and see the ophthalmologist. She asks Tracie to help make an appointment for her because she has trouble seeing. She makes an appointment but cannot be seen for a couple of weeks.

Episode 13
Mary feels so sorry for Anthony and feels badly for her son, Gil. She wishes that Anthony did not inherit mental problems from his mother and wishes something could be done about it. Mary talks with Kristina about Anthony and tries to point out that he cannot help what is happening to him.

While playing cards at the Neighborhood Senior Center and attending her quilting group this week, Mary tells all of her friends about Anthony. She denies that he has mental health problems and does not believe that he needs the prescribed medications. She tells the ladies, "If he is crazy, it must be Helen's fault, because we don't have those kinds of problems on our side of the family [NEWS]."

Episode 14
Mary is very supportive of Anthony; she just thinks he is who he is. It is obvious to her that those people at the university don't understand him and are just mean. In her mind, Anthony would never hurt anyone. She wants everything to be okay for him. She tells Anthony over and over again that everything will work out and that he needs to let his father help him. She also encourages the whole family to go to church with her to pray for Anthony.

Mary does not feel a bit guilty about the fact that she has a bedroom to herself, while Mark and Tyler have to sleep in the family room. Instead, she finds the arrangement annoying because it interferes with her late-night television viewing.

Episode 15
Mary has an appointment with the ophthalmologist. He confirms that her vision has indeed become worse and tells her she really needs to have the cataract surgery. Mary has been very resistant to this but is now realizing that her loss of vision is affecting her quality of life. She talks with the doctor about the fear she has about eye surgery. The physician points out that, without the surgery, she will lose her sight – essentially, she has nothing to lose and everything to gain. Mary tells the physician that she will consider it.

Later in the week, Mary is at the Neighborhood Senior Center and speaks to Karen Williams, the nurse at the clinic there. Mary says that she is scared of cataract surgery because she heard people can go blind from it. Karen assures her it is a very common procedure that could potentially improve her vision and quality of life. Karen also says that three of the ladies who come to the Senior Center have had cataract surgery and suggests that Mary talk with them [NEWS].

Mary Martin Season 3 Information

Episode 1
Mary Martin is Gil Martin's 76-year-old mother. About 18 months ago, Mary's husband of 52 years died from cancer. Mary has been living with Gil and his family for about one year now.

Mary does not see particularly well. Otherwise, she is in excellent health; the only health-related problems she is aware of are osteoporosis, cataract, and glaucoma. She sees an ophthalmologist on a regular basis. The only prescription drugs and over-the-counter supplements that she uses include alendronate sodium (Fosamax) and calcium for osteoporosis, and latanoprost ophthalmic solution (Xalatan) to manage her glaucoma (her dose is 1 drop in each eye once a day). Her only complaint about the eye drops is the cost. Mary's vision has been getting increasingly poor; for this reason she has been considering cataract surgery.

Mary hears Tyler crying and investigates the problem. Even with her poor eyesight, she can see that the child is covered in hives and his lips are swollen. She asks Mark about this, and he tells her that he did not notice it. Mary tells Mark to take Tyler to a doctor immediately.

Mary returns to the ophthalmologist this week and tells him that she has decided to go ahead with the surgery. The ophthalmologist tells Mary that they will do surgery on one eye first and then wait 4 to 6 weeks before performing surgery on the other eye.

Episode 2

Mary is very interested in hearing Kristina talk about her school dance at the dinner table. Kristina shows her a picture of Brian and she agrees that he is very handsome. While Kristina is talking about the dance, Anthony tells her to shut up because nobody cares about her stupid dance. He then gets up and leaves the table. Mary tells Gil in Spanish that she is really worried about that boy and wonders if the medications are making him act this way. Responding back to her in Spanish, Gil tells her to leave him be – he is just needing some space.

Episode 3

This week Mary has her first cataract surgery. The day before surgery, she asks Kristina to take her to the church so that she can pray to the Virgin Mary for her health. She also sees Father John and asks him for a blessing.

Gil takes Mary to the Neighborhood Outpatient Surgery Center for the cataract surgery on her right eye. She is instructed to put ketorolac tromethamine ophthalmic solution (0.4%) and gatifloxacin ophthalmic solution (0.3%) in her eyes 4 times a day for 2 days following the procedure. She stays awake during the procedure. Anesthetic eye drops are used, so she does not feel anything at all. After the surgery, she is sent home with a bandage and eye shield over her eye. She is told to wear it until she returns to the office in the morning for a postoperative check. Mary does not experience any pain or problems that afternoon or evening.

The following morning, she is examined by the ophthalmologist, who tells her that everything looks great. Mary is amazed at how bright and brilliant colors are; she notices immediately that the "foggy" sensation is gone. Mary is instructed to use the eye drops that were given to her preoperatively, along with prednisolone ophthalmic solution (Pred Forte) (1.0%) eye drops 4 times a day for a week; the following week, she is told to use the ketorolac and prednisolone eye drops twice a day for another week.

Episode 4

Mary gets a phone call from Gil and is told about Mark's accident. She is devastated! She cannot believe that Mark will never walk again. She refuses to believe that Mark was responsible and is sure that somebody else must have caused the accident and left the scene. Mary tells Gil that the people who had the party should be sued for getting Mark drunk [NEWS].

Episode 5

Mary goes with Gil and Helen every day to see Mark at the hospital. She takes prayer cards and brings him a statue of the Virgin Mary to help him heal. At home, she prays the rosary for him with the hopes of a full recovery. She asks Father John to include Mark in his prayer intentions at Sunday mass.

Episode 6

Mary tells Gil and Helen that the whole family needs to be going to church together to pray for Mark and Anthony. She stresses that if they don't say their prayers at the church, the prayers may not be heard. She is glad when Gil goes with her and is not surprised that Helen does not, since Helen did not have a Catholic upbringing.

Episode 7

Mary is very upset about Anthony's suicide attempt. She worries about Anthony and wishes that there was something she could do for him. She blames Helen for upsetting him to the point of wanting to kill himself. She is very concerned for her son, Gil, considering the toll all this stress must be having on him. In her opinion, Anthony has a special gift of sensitivity that others don't appreciate and he has been unfairly labeled as having a mental illness. Mary tells Anthony that she believes that God is trying to communicate with the family through him [▼].

Episode 8

Gil takes Mary in for her second cataract surgery – this one on the left eye. She experiences the same exact course of events as with the previous surgery and has no problems with her postoperative recovery. Mary is so pleased with the outcome of her surgery that her only regret is that she did not do it sooner.

Episode 9

Because Mary feels her vision is greatly improved, she decides to start driving again. She tells Kristina that she wants to have her car back. Kristina does not think this is fair and tells Mary that she needs the car for school and cheerleading. Mary is also somewhat angry to see that Kristina has not done a good job caring for the car. It is full of trash, and there are many stains on the seats and carpet.

Mary learns that Pam Allen (a church parishioner and friend from the quilting club) died this week. She signs up to take food to the family. She bakes a chicken casserole and takes it to the Allen's home. She talks briefly with Clifford Allen. The conversation with Clifford causes Mary to reflect on her husband's death from cancer. Mary feels very sad for the rest of the week [NEWS].

Episode 10

When Mark is discharged home, Mary decides to make him her new project. She wants to take care of him and is willing to do whatever it takes to help him recover. She tells Mark that she will make him whatever he wants to eat, recognizing that he has been eating poorly since the accident. It makes Mary very sad to see Mark's condition. She cannot bear the thought of her precious grandson confined to a bed and wheelchair.

Mary watches with great interest when the home health nurse comes to see Mark. She asks the nurse many questions so that she can take good care of him. Being Mark's primary caregiver makes Mary feel very useful, but the amount of care he requires is overwhelming.

Episode 11

In addition to having great concern for Mark, Mary is deeply concerned about Anthony. She does not directly criticize her son, Gil, but she blames Helen for driving Anthony away and out of the house. She believes that he would be okay if everybody could just be more patient with him. She goes to the church to pray for her troubled family. She sees Father John and talks with him. He assures her that they will say a prayer for Mark and Anthony at Sunday's mass.

Episode 12

Helen and Mary bicker back and forth about all the issues in the family and why Anthony has left. When Kristina walks in and grabs her keys, Helen asks her where she is going. Kristina simply says, "Away from this crazy house!" Mary tells Helen that she needs to keep Kristina home more and accuses her of driving Kristina away too ▶.

Episode 13

Every day, Mary talks to Mark about the people at church who are praying for him and explains that the Virgin Mary and Jesus are there to help him get better. She does everything she can think of to get him to eat and is disappointed when he doesn't. She has been meticulous about taking care of his wounds and is pleased at the progress that she can see 〔NEWS〕.

Episode 14

Mary is delighted when Mark transfers himself out of bed and into a wheelchair without assistance for the first time. She recognizes that this is a major milestone and is hopeful that it will encourage him to become more independent.

Episode 15

Mary is concerned about her grandson Anthony being on the streets. She makes a point of driving by the parks and through the downtown areas every day, hoping to see Anthony. She knows that he is out there somewhere and wants to find him so that she can bring him home. Mary is embarrassed by the fact that her grandson is homeless and does not mention it to her friends at the Neighborhood Senior Center. It is, in her opinion, completely unacceptable for one of her family members to be homeless.

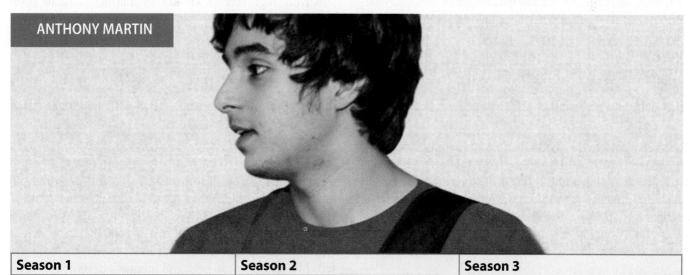

ANTHONY MARTIN

Season 1	Season 2	Season 3
Anthony is Helen and Gil's son. He is in his final year of high school, is a loner, and does not participate in many activities. He begins to display some odd behavior during this season, but it goes unnoticed by his parents.	Anthony moves out of house and into college housing. He has a psychotic episode requiring hospitalization and is diagnosed with schizophrenia. He tries to go back to school, but has a second episode and drops out of school. He moves back home.	Anthony is in outpatient treatment, but is not compliant with his medications. He has a suicide attempt, another hospitalization, and more outpatient treatment. Eventually he leaves home after constant fighting with his parents and becomes homeless.

Anthony Martin Season 1 Information

Episode 1

Anthony is the 17-year-old son of Helen and Gil Martin. He lives with his parents and two siblings, Tracie and Kristina. He gets along with his family but still feels somewhat isolated. His parents are not aware that he feels this way and perceive him to be a quiet, serious child. He tends not to interact with family members very much and prefers to isolate himself in his bedroom.

Anthony is in his senior year of high school. Although he is an excellent student (has a 3.9 GPA), he does not participate in any school-related activities, with the exception of science fairs. He has few friends and rarely socializes, because he is more comfortable being alone. Many of the kids at the high school consider him to be weird, but he is never teased or bullied. For the most part, he just blends in with the other kids. His typical routine involves going to school, coming home, and then working part-time; three nights a week, Anthony bags groceries at the local grocery store. He gets along well with his coworkers. In fact, the cashiers (who tend to be middle-aged women) like it when he works, because they perceive him to be very polite and shy.

Anthony is in excellent health and, with the exception of dental exams, has not needed health-related care since entering high school.

Anthony is somewhat annoyed with his sister, Kristina, because she was named captain of the cheerleading squad this week and has been talking about it nonstop. He doesn't understand how she can't see that cheerleading is a trivial and worthless activity. When Kristina asks Anthony if he would like to see some of her cheers, he tells her, "When I get bored enough, I'll let you know." He wonders why she wants to talk to him about cheerleading.

Episode 2

Anthony goes to the football game at the high school this week with his friend Jason. Jason is Anthony's lab partner in a chemistry class and is one of Anthony's only friends. Jason comments to Anthony about how "hot" his sister Kristina is as they observe her on the field doing cheers. He tells Jason, "Don't make me sick – it is bad enough living with her. I don't want to hear you talk about her."

Episode 3

There is a lot of commotion at the house this week. Anthony's grandmother has moved in, and the girls are fighting because they now have to share a bedroom to make room for their grandmother. Anthony is relieved that he won't have to share his space. He hears his mother yelling at his father about the situation. Anthony likes his grandmother and does not think that her moving in is that big a deal.

Anthony works a few shifts at the grocery story this week. While working, his mind wanders and thinks it is weird that his grandmother gave birth to his father [NEWS].

Episode 4

Anthony's bedroom is next to the den. In the middle of the night, he wakes up to the sound of the television coming through his heating vent. He goes into the den and finds his grandmother watching a movie. Mary tells him that she has had trouble sleeping at night ever since his grandfather died. Anthony wonders why his grandmother sits in the room next to his during the middle of the night [▼] [NEWS].

Episode 5

Anthony likes his grandmother's dinners. The food is quite good, although he wonders if she does something to his food because he previously heard her mention folk remedies from Mexico. He picks through the food to make sure that she has not put something weird in his food.

Anthony does not understand why his mother has to argue so much with his grandmother. Although he finds his job boring, he is relieved to go to work so that he doesn't have to listen to the arguing. On the nights that he is home, he mostly stays in his room and listens to classical music with his headphones on.

Episode 6

Anthony starts thinking about his options after he graduates from high school. He knows that he wants to get a degree in mathematics, but he does not know for sure what kind of a job he might get with a degree like that – maybe he should get a graduate degree in physics. He also is interested in astronomy and space exploration and thinks it would be interesting to be a scientist in one of those areas. While at work, he daydreams about space exploration and aliens [NEWS].

Episode 7

Anthony starts exploring college opportunities. Because of the limited financial help that his parents can offer, he knows that he will need to get an academic scholarship or settle for attending the local college, which he would like to avoid. His mother has verbalized that she thinks he should stay at home and go to the local college like Tracie. Tracie tells him that if he can get a full scholarship somewhere, he should take it and get away. Anthony submits applications to several colleges and scholarship programs [▶] [▼].

Episode 8

Anthony enters an exhibit in the school science fair, hoping to win one of the top three exhibit awards and the opportunity to show in the state science fair. If he were to place at the state science fair, he would win an academic scholarship to one of the large universities in the state. He does not tell his parents about the science fair because he would rather go alone. He is disappointed that he does not win one of the three top awards and suspects that it is because the judges plotted against him.

Episode 9

Anthony attends a college fair night at the high school. His sister, Kristina, wants to go along with him. He is mostly annoyed with this, but he agrees to take her. Anthony visits most of the booths and picks up a few more applications. He does not see Kristina at all after they get there. When he is ready to go, he looks for her everywhere. After searching for 30 minutes, he just goes home. When he gets home at 9 p.m., Helen and Gil are angry with him for not bringing Kristina home.

Anthony goes to his room, angry that his parents blame him for Kristina's actions. After Kristina comes home, Mary tells Anthony not to worry about it. She points out that his mother got hysterical over nothing. Anthony is indifferent to his grandmother's attempts to make him feel better ▶.

Episode 10

Anthony goes to the high school open house with his parents. He starts to make the rounds with his mother and father to meet some of his teachers, but then gets bored with the talk and tells his Dad that he will just meet him in the lobby when he is done. On the way home, Anthony does not ask about or comment on any of the teachers that his parents met.

Episode 11

Anthony receives acceptance letters to several colleges. Although he has been offered scholarships from the large university in the state, he knows that they will not total enough for him to be able to attend. A small college about 45 minutes away from home has offered him

a scholarship that would not only pay for his tuition and books but also pay for him to live on campus. As much as he wants to go to the big university, he decides that this is his best option and commits to the small college. His grandmother, Mary, comments that he will feel more comfortable at the small college anyway.

Episode 12

A girl at school asks Anthony to the formal school dance. Anthony is not interested in girls and does not want to go to the high school dance. He tells the girl that he has other plans and cannot go. He sees his sister getting all excited about the dance and wonders what her problem is.

Episode 13

Anthony overhears Kristina and Tracie arguing over earrings. He thinks to himself about how earrings could be made to have secret global positioning devices implanted within them to study movement of humans – similar to devices used in studying migratory patterns among birds or whales.

Episode 14

Anthony takes his grandmother to the eye doctor this week so that his parents don't have to take off from work. While waiting for her, he reads a magazine article about the damaging effects of sun to the skin. Anthony begins to think about radiation from space and becomes very concerned. He does not share his concerns with anyone, but when he gets home, he places foil over the windows in his bedroom to block radiation from entering.

Episode 15

Anthony is very upset with Tracie when he finds out that she took the foil off the windows in his room. She tells him that it makes the house look really wacky to have foil in the windows. He tells her that it is important to him and he likes it. He replaces the foil the next day ✉.

Anthony Martin Season 2 Information

Episode 1

Anthony is the 18-year-old son of Helen and Gil Martin. He recently graduated from high school and was accepted into a college nearby with an academic scholarship that pays for his tuition and dormitory. He just moved into the dormitory and has a roommate named Jeff. He gets along fine with Jeff, although they are really not friends. Anthony is taking a full, typical freshman curriculum and hopes to earn a degree in mathematics. Because he tends to be a loner, he does not feel particularly close to many individuals. He prefers not to interact much with the college kids.

This Saturday, there is a large party on campus that is sponsored by the student life center and dormitory. His new roommate, Jeff, and several other guys invite Anthony to join them. They tell him that he needs to loosen up a bit and have some fun. He declines, explaining that he has homework to do. Anthony leaves the dormitory and goes to the library so that nobody will bother him.

Episode 2

The biggest football game of the year is held at the college this week. Recognizing that he is not socializing much, Anthony's roommate, Jeff, suggests that he go to the game with the guys. Anthony tells Jeff that he doesn't like large crowds and prefers to stay at the dormitory. That afternoon, Anthony has the dormitory practically to himself. He likes the fact that it is quiet, but he wonders what people who are still in the building are doing.

Episode 3

When Anthony goes to class, he looks at his instructor and also several of the students and thinks they are staring at him. He wonders why they are looking at him and whether they share secrets about him. He wonders if they are talking about him after class.

Episode 4

Many of the students in Anthony's political science class have decided that Anthony is "spaced out" and keep their distance from him. Several times he has verbalized his opinions about government conspiracy theories involving mind control, radiation poisoning, and aliens that listen to conversations on earth. He also has begun to dress in mismatched or poorly kept clothes. Anthony suspects that his roommate, Jeff, has been spying on him. In addition, he wonders if his parents have implanted a radio transmitter in his head and are reading his thoughts ▽.

Episode 5

Anthony tells Jeff that he has been receiving secret messages from the television, newspaper, and radio about a government conspiracy occurring on campus. Jeff thinks his roommate is "wacko" and puts in a request for a change in roommates. However, he is told that the earliest possible time that his request could be honored would be at the semester break.

Episode 6

Anthony's roommate, Jeff, comes home from classes and finds Anthony hiding under a table. Jeff attempts to coax him out, but Anthony refuses to move. Anthony talks in gibberish (using Neologisms) and accuses Jeff of plotting to get him expelled from college. Jeff sees that Anthony has a knife, so he immediately leaves the room and summons the residence hall director, who promptly calls the campus police.

Anthony refuses to come out from under the table when the campus police arrive; he becomes agitated and shouts at them. He accuses them of reading his mind and plotting his death. The police observe that he is tightly holding a knife and that his jaw muscles are tightening. Police call for backup and do a "take down." Anthony is combative the entire time – flailing and kicking. He is placed in handcuffs and is transported by police to the Neighborhood Hospital Emergency Department. There he is evaluated, sedated, and then admitted to the inpatient psychiatric unit with an initial diagnosis of acute

psychosis. Anthony spends the rest of the week on the inpatient unit 🗒.

The following day, Louise, a psychiatric mental health nurse practitioner, obtains Anthony's permission to call his parents and speak to them about his condition. Louise informs Anthony that morning that his parents will be in to see him later. Anthony does not react at all to this news.

When his parents arrive to see him, Anthony is hiding under the sheets in his bed because he is afraid. He begins to cry when he sees his mother. Later in the morning, Anthony participates in a meeting involving Louise, Dr. Jacobe (a psychiatrist), and his parents. During the meeting, Anthony becomes very agitated, gets up, and leaves the room.

Episode 7

Anthony stays at the inpatient psychiatric unit for 5 days. He is started on Olanzapine 5 mg once a day; by discharge, his dose is increased to 10 mg per day. He participates in patient education sessions for his medication and attends group psychotherapy. He is discharged home with an outpatient psychiatric appointment the following day. The insurance company authorizes Anthony to participate in intensive outpatient treatment ▽.

Episode 8

Anthony continues to live at home and attends outpatient therapy sessions with Dr. Jacobe. The sessions are effective, as evidenced by his increased attention to hygiene, ability to carry on conversations, reduced agitation, and lack of hallucinations. He also has been very hungry and has put on a little weight. Anthony has come to trust Dr. Jacobe – he believes that Dr. Jacobe is the only person who understands him. He continues to take the olanzapine and is now up to a dose of 15 mg daily. Anthony is anxious to return to school, but he is strongly advised to take a semester break before going back to school. He is somewhat overwhelmed by the constant commotion at home and spends most of his time in his room 🗒.

Episode 9

Anthony's brother, Mark, suggests that they go to a shooting range. He used to go shooting frequently with his father, and sometimes Anthony would also come. However, it has been a number of years since Anthony has been at the range. After they leave the range, they pick up a pizza and take it home to eat. Overall, Anthony enjoys the afternoon, but he does not say much to Mark during the day, nor does he say much about it when they get home.

Episode 10

Despite the fact that he has missed nearly a month of school, Anthony wants to return to college. He speaks to an academic counselor, who informs him that the date to withdraw from classes has passed. She encourages him to talk with his instructors. She also tells him that in some cases they can do an administrative withdrawal. Anthony informs his parents that he is going to go back to school. He is confident that he can catch up and is sure that his instructors will work with him. Gil, Helen, and Mary all attempt to dissuade him, as does Dr. Jacobe, the psychiatrist. Against everyone's advice, Anthony goes back to school.

Episode 11

Anthony does not like the way the medication makes him feel and decides to take a lower dose than was prescribed. Without telling anyone, Anthony cuts back on the amount of medication he is taking.

Episode 12

This week, voices from the television begin to tell Anthony that medications are poisonous. Anthony stops taking his medication.

Episode 13

While walking to a late morning class, two girls spot Anthony lying naked in the grass near the center of the main campus. They are frightened by this and call the campus police. When the campus police confront Anthony, he accuses them of trying to kill him, and he becomes combative. A large crowd gathers to watch the naked student battling with the officers. The police transport Anthony to the Emergency Department. Anthony is delusional and accuses the nurses of inserting electrodes into his head. He is placed in seclusion and sedated. He eventually calms down and becomes compliant. Anthony is admitted to the inpatient psychiatric facility.

Later the same day, Anthony refuses to take the medication given to him by a nurse because he thinks it is poisonous. He is argumentative at first, but he quickly becomes combative and hits the nurse in the head with his fist. Security is called to assist and, against his wishes, Anthony is sedated with 10 mg of haloperidol (Haldol) and 1 mg of lorazepam (Ativan) and placed in seclusion. Eventually, he calms down. However, even after calming down, he continues to refuse medications. It becomes necessary for Dr. Jacobe, the psychiatrist, to file for the appointment of a conservator to make decisions on Anthony's behalf regarding medications 📑 ✉️.

Episode 14

Anthony spends most of the week in the inpatient psychiatric unit. He is started back on olanzapine 10 mg PO and gradually makes progress. He is discharged home with a referral for 10 days of intensive outpatient therapy.

Episode 15

Anthony continues to go to his daily intensive outpatient therapy sessions with Dr. Jacobe. He makes a great deal of progress. When he is notified by the university that he has failed all of his classes, he tells Dr. Jacobe that he is ashamed, feels like a failure, and will never try to go back.

Anthony Martin Season 3 Information

Episode 1

Anthony is the 18-year-old son of Helen and Gil Martin. He had been enrolled at the local college, but had **Psychotic episodes** and subsequently was diagnosed with **schizophrenia**. He was hospitalized and then completed intensive outpatient treatment. Currently, Anthony is taking **olanzapine** 10 mg PO to treat his condition and sees a psychiatrist once a week.

Because of his mental health disorder, Anthony fell behind and failed all of his classes. He has made a decision not to return to college. He has moved back home and now lives with his parents and three siblings (Mark, Tracie, and Kristina), his nephew, Tyler, and his grandmother, Mary.

Anthony returns to his previous job as a courtesy clerk (bagger) at the local grocery store - the same store where Gary Allen works. Although he interacts very little with his coworkers and customers, Anthony is able to comply with the job description. Anthony's boss would like to see him be more cheerful and friendly toward the customers, but he is aware of Anthony's condition and has been told that a change in demeanor may come with time.

Episode 2

While at the dinner table, Anthony's sister Kristina is sharing stupid details about her recent high school dance. Anthony tries to ignore her voice but he can't, and it really irritates him. He finally loses his temper and says to her, "Nobody cares about your stupid dance. Just shut up!" He then gets up, leaves the table, and walks out of the room. He goes back to his room and lies down, trying to calm himself. He soon falls asleep ▶️.

Episode 3

Helen makes certain that Anthony takes his medication every day. Despite being on the medication, he becomes suspicious that his supervisor and Gary Allen are talking about him. He reports his suspicions to Dr. Jacobe during an outpatient visit. Dr. Jacobe compliments Anthony for recognizing this symptom and suggests that it may be necessary to change his medication ✉️.

Episode 4

Despite all of the commotion in the house, Helen makes sure that Anthony gets to his weekly appointment with Dr. Jacobe. He tells Dr. Jacobe that he knows that Gary Allen is spying on him and reporting his activities to the boss. Dr. Jacobe changes Anthony's medication to Quetiapine (Seroquel XR). Helen is instructed to give Anthony 50 mg at bedtime the first day; 100 mg at bedtime for the next 3 days, and then 300 mg at bedtime thereafter.

Episode 5

This week Dr. Jacobe asks Anthony about his symptoms. Anthony admits that he no longer believes that his coworkers are talking about him, but he reports feeling very tired and sedated. The psychiatrist assures him that over time these symptoms will subside.

Episode 6

Anthony continues to feel sedated and has difficulty thinking clearly. He is no longer hallucinating, but he doesn't like the way the medication makes him feel.

Episode 7

Anthony tells his father about the way the medication makes him feel and that he doesn't like taking it. Gil becomes uncharacteristically angry with Anthony and tells him that he *will* take his medications or he will have to move out of the house. Anthony becomes very upset, runs to his room, and slams the door. He feels that nobody understands and decides that it's time to just end it all. He picks up a large bottle of acetaminophen and takes all of the pills remaining in it, as well as all of his prescription medication. Later, his mother finds him on the floor in a stupor. She calls 9-1-1. An ambulance takes Anthony to the Emergency Department. He is later admitted to the ICU for treatment of a drug overdose.

Episode 8

Anthony returns to inpatient psychiatric treatment and remains in the hospital for 1 week. He has insurance coverage for inpatient treatment, but he no longer qualifies for outpatient treatment on his insurance plan. The social worker tries to find an outpatient program for Anthony and helps him apply for Medicaid. Anthony remains in the hospital for 8 days. Now his diagnosis is major depression with psychotic features. He is placed on Citalopram (Celexa) 20 mg daily. His antipsychotic medication is changed to Risperidone (Risperdal) 1 mg twice a day. The Risperdal is very expensive.

Episode 9

Anthony is discharged home this week and referred to the Neighborhood Health Connections Clinic for follow-up. He can't afford the intensive outpatient treatment anymore, so he is assigned to the mental health clinic and receives an appointment for the following week. He also applies to a medication assistance program to help offset the costs of his medications while waiting for Medicaid approval. During the week, Helen helps Anthony take his medication. He remains calm.

Episode 10

Helen and Gil take Anthony to his first appointment at the mental health clinic this week. Anthony sees Shawn Jacobs, who introduces himself as a nurse practitioner who specializes in mental health. Anthony feels angry and is not really interested in talking to this guy. The one person he grew to trust was Dr. Jacobe, but he has been told that he won't be seeing him anymore. He wonders why he can't just go back to Dr. Jacobe. Anthony knows that it has to do with an insurance issue, but Anthony wonders why Dr. Jacobe won't see him anyway. When asked by the nurse practitioner for permission to talk with his parents to gain a better understanding of his condition, Anthony loudly yells, "NO!" When asked if he would consider injections as opposed to oral medications, he says that he will think about it. For now, he agrees to take his medication consistently.

Episode 11

Anthony begins to argue with his mother when she confronts him about not taking his medication. Helen expresses intense frustration and is highly anxious about Anthony. Gil is well aware of the effect this is having on Helen and suggests to Anthony that he move out of the house. Anthony becomes upset, gets up, and storms out. He goes to his friend Jason's apartment and asks if he can stay there for a while. His friend agrees to let him stay but has no idea about the problems that Anthony has been having. Anthony stops taking his medication.

Episode 12

Anthony is still staying at his friend Jason's apartment. He has not been going to work, and he has not been taking his medication. Not wanting to talk to his parents, he does not return any of their calls.

Episode 13

Anthony begins to exhibit odd behavior again. His friend Jason has always known that Anthony is a bit different. He wonders what is going on with him – if he is just in a bad mood or what the deal is. Jason knows that he has not been getting along with his parents and wonders if that is the issue.

Episode 14

Anthony's behavior has gone from what his roommate Jason considers "odd" to "bizarre." Jason wonders why Anthony does not have a job and why he never leaves the apartment. He is not sure what Anthony is doing with his time. Jason tells Anthony that if he is going to stay with him much longer, he will need to help him pay rent.

Episode 15

Anthony has a major argument with Jason about Anthony's weird behavior and his failure to help Jason pay rent. Jason tells him to move out. Having nowhere to go, Anthony sleeps in a local park. Not only is he not taking any medication, but now Anthony is also out on the street 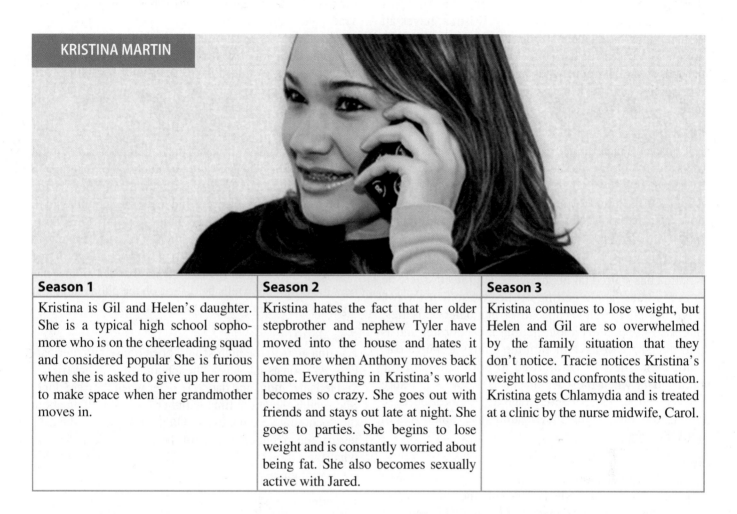.

| KRISTINA MARTIN | | |

Season 1	Season 2	Season 3
Kristina is Gil and Helen's daughter. She is a typical high school sophomore who is on the cheerleading squad and considered popular She is furious when she is asked to give up her room to make space when her grandmother moves in.	Kristina hates the fact that her older stepbrother and nephew Tyler have moved into the house and hates it even more when Anthony moves back home. Everything in Kristina's world becomes so crazy. She goes out with friends and stays out late at night. She goes to parties. She begins to lose weight and is constantly worried about being fat. She also becomes sexually active with Jared.	Kristina continues to lose weight, but Helen and Gil are so overwhelmed by the family situation that they don't notice. Tracie notices Kristina's weight loss and confronts the situation. Kristina gets Chlamydia and is treated at a clinic by the nurse midwife, Carol.

Kristina Martin Season 1 Information

Episode 1

Kristina is the 16-year-old daughter of Helen and Gil Martin. She lives with her parents, brother Anthony, and step-sister Tracie. She gets along with her siblings, but considers her step-sister Tracie to be way too serious and her brother Anthony to be a bit strange.

Kristina is a fairly typical sophomore who attends the local high school. She is on the junior varsity cheerleading squad at school and has a very busy schedule. Although she has always been close to her family, she feels closest to her circle of friends, and she is considered popular among the kids at school. Kristina is an average student who usually puts friends and school activities well ahead of school-related work. She is an avid user of the social media site Facebook and posts to her personal page on the site several times a day. She is in excellent health and has not needed health-related care outside of annual physicals to participate on the cheerleading squad.

Kristina is named captain of the junior varsity cheerleading squad this week. She is thrilled because she knows that as captain she is expected to work out with the varsity squad and serve as their first backup. She and her friends on the squad spend time after school making posters for pep rally week.

Episode 2

Kristina has cheerleading activities associated with the high school football game and is thrilled to be cheering at a varsity game - something very rare for a sophomore. Her brother Anthony is at the game with his creepy friend Jason, who seems to be staring at her. Kristina posts pictures of herself cheering at the varsity game on her Facebook page 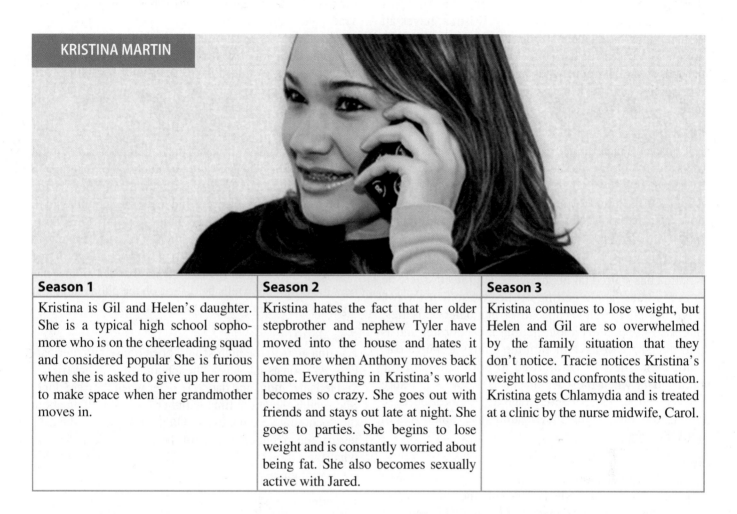.

Episode 3

Kristina is furious when she is told to give up her bedroom to make space for her grandmother. She does not think it is fair and asks why her grandmother can't just sleep on the pull-out bed in the den. Kristina moves all of her things into Tracie's room and finds that there is not enough space for her stuff. She removes everything on half of the bedroom walls and hangs up her posters instead. She and Tracie have a fight about what should be hung up in the room.

Episode 4

Kristina and Tracie argue frequently about having to sharing a room. Gil talks to the girls about being more sensitive to their grandmother. Kristina is annoyed with the whole situation and comments that none of her friends have to share rooms. Her frustrations are evident from her postings on her Facebook page.

Episode 5

Kristina has started taking driver education classes. She is very excited about getting her license so that she can drive herself to school and all of her other activities. She asks her parents about getting a car for her and is told that she will have to earn the money to buy a car. Until then, she will be allowed to borrow one of the family cars when they are not in use. She is not sure how she will ever earn enough money for a car because she is too busy with cheerleading and other school activities.

Episode 6

Kristina tells her mother that she is going to her friend Roslyn's house for a sleepover with the cheerleading squad. The girls go to the mall until closing time, and then hang out at the pizza place near the high school until it closes. Then they stand around in the parking lot, talking to some of the guys from the high school until 2 a.m., when they are told by the police to go home. Kristina has a blast and thinks that it's dumb that the cops had to run them off. After all, they weren't doing anything wrong. She posts pictures of herself with the guys on her Facebook page.

Episode 7

Kristina overhears Anthony talking with Tracie about college to get her opinion about best options. She hopes that Anthony plans to move out of the house when he goes to college (unlike her sister), so that she can have a room to herself.

Episode 8

Kristina completes her driver education classes. Kristina posts pictures of herself with her driving certificate on Facebook. She has a fight with her parents because she wants to start driving herself to school so that she doesn't have to get rides to cheerleading and other activities. In her opinion, she should be given a car to drive. Helen tells her that she has to earn money for her own car - just like Tracie and Anthony have done.

Kristina asks her grandmother if she can use her car, since she does not drive it very much anyway. Her grandmother agrees to this, if it is okay with her father. Gil decides it would be okay and gives permission - as long as she takes good care of the car.

Episode 9

Kristina goes with Anthony to the high school career night and college fair. She goes with the intention of meeting up with her friends and hanging out with them. They decide that the college fair is boring and leave the school to go to a fast-food restaurant. When Kristina returns to the school, she realizes that Anthony has already left, and she has to get a ride home with her friends. She does not get home until 10 p.m. and is surprised to learn that her mother has become frantic. She tells her friend on the phone later that night, "My mother needs to take a chill pill."

Episode 10

Kristina goes to the high school open house with her parents. As soon as she gets to the school, she sees her friends and tells her mom and dad to text her when they are done. She spends the entire time with her friends, talking about the upcoming sporting event. On the way home, she asks her parents about every one of the teachers they met and what they thought about him or her. She then adds her own commentary.

Episode 11

After cheerleading practice, Jared Williams, a senior and the quarterback of the football team, comes up to Kristina and asks her to the upcoming school dance. Kristina is so happy because he is considered one of the hottest guys in the school. She knows that the dance will be the most important night of her life, and she needs to look fabulous. Both her mother and grandmother give her money to go shopping. She spends hours at the mall this week with her friends looking for the perfect dress. Kristina finds a beautiful, low-cut, strapless dress similar to one she saw in a celebrity magazine. She buys the dress a bit small and vows to diet so that she can fit into it.

Episode 12

Kristina has practically starved herself during the past couple of weeks so that she can fit into the dress she bought for the high school dance. She spends all afternoon getting ready with her girlfriends. They do each other's hair, makeup, and nails. She is happy that she is able to fit into the dress, and her friends keep remarking on how skinny and beautiful she looks. Kristina has a curfew of 12:30 a.m., but doesn't come home until after 2 a.m. She is grounded for the following week. She is told not to go anywhere except school and home, and she is not allowed to drive. Her parents also tell her that if they are unable to reach her by cell phone in the future, she may lose cell phone privileges. Despite being grounded and not driving for a week, Kristina decides it was well worth it. She calls her friends to let them know all about the date and how stupid her parents are for grounding her.

Episode 13
Kristina takes a pair of Tracie's earrings from her dresser because she thinks that they will look good with her outfit. She doesn't bother to ask Tracie because she figures that Tracie would just say no. Kristina predicts correctly that Tracie will be angry with her. She tells Tracie that she is just selfish for not sharing.

Episode 14
Kristina has another date with Jared and has a great time. They go to a local sporting event and then to a party afterwards. She thinks he is very sweet and wonderful and she likes that he touches her a lot. She feels so lucky to be dating him because he is a senior and the most popular boy in the school and she is only a sophomore. She posts on her Facebook page pictures of her and Jared. Several senior girls post mean messages about Kristina being a little snot and that sophomore girls should not date senior guys. Kristina knows that they are just jealous because she is thin, cute, and a cheerleader ▾.

Episode 15
This week at school, Kristina runs into another car in the parking lot. Although she does not damage the other car, Kristina gets a dent in her grandmother's car. She tells her parents that she is not sure what happened to the car, but somebody must have hit it in the parking lot.

Kristina Martin Season 2 Information

Episode 1
Kristina is the 16-year-old daughter of Helen and Gil Martin. She lives with her parents, grandmother, step-sister Tracie, step-brother Mark, and his son Tyler. Her brother, Anthony, recently moved out of the house to attend college. Kristina was looking forward to moving into Anthony's room when he moved to college. She becomes angry when she learns that Mark and Tyler are moving into the room instead. Kristina has always gotten along with Mark, although he has never lived with them before, but Kristina wishes that she could have her own room again.

Kristina has recently completed her driver education class and has a provisional driver's license.

Kristina gets a call from Jared Williams (the guy she went to the school dance with several months ago), inviting her to go with him to an on-campus party at the college. Jared recently graduated from high school and is now playing on the football team at the local college. In fact, he lives in the same dormitory as Kristina's brother Anthony. Kristina is excited about going on a date with Jared and hanging out with college kids. She ends up getting drunk that evening. Jared takes her back to his dormitory room and has unprotected sex with her. She has never had sex before and she wonders if anyone will know what she and Jared have done. She also wonders if Anthony will find out. Jared drops her off at home at 2 a.m. Kristina is grounded for a week for being out past her 12:30 a.m. curfew ▾.

Episode 2
Kristina's parents are not happy that she is seeing Jared, and suggest that she date the guys at high school instead. Since she has had sex with Jared, there is no way she is going to stop seeing him now. She likes the idea of going out with an older guy because it makes her feel older.

Mary asks Kristina to take her to the store to buy toys for Tyler. On the way over to the store, she talks to Kristina about the need to be careful when dating college-aged boys. Kristina thinks her parents and grandmother are just old-fashioned.

Episode 3
Kristina has not been doing well in school lately because she has been busy socializing instead. She receives a letter from the academic advising office informing her that she is close to being placed on probation and will not be allowed to continue on the cheerleading squad if her grades don't improve. Kristina is disappointed that Jared does not call her to hang out with him after the college football game this week. She ends up spending time with her friends instead ▾.

Episode 4
Kristina spends two evenings this week alone with Jared in his dormitory room. She is glad that she has not seen her brother because she doesn't want him to tell her parents that she is on campus with Jared and alone in his dorm room. She posts regularly to her Facebook page

about her and Jared so everyone knows they are together. One of Kristina's friends tells her that Jared is also going out with some girls at the college. Kristina dismisses this, believing that her friend is just jealous that she is dating an older guy. She decides to lose 5 pounds because she thinks her butt looks big in the mirror.

Kristina is relieved that her mother's surgery went well. She goes to the hospital with Tracie, Mark, Helen, and her dad the evening following her mother's surgery. She watches her mother get sick and thinks it is gross. She hopes that she never has to have surgery ▾.

Episode 5

Gil has asked Kristina and her sister to help Mary with all the chores around the house while their mother recovers from her surgery. Kristina has never taken much of an interest in cooking before this, but she loves working with her grandmother to prepare dinner. She learns a lot in just a week. She posts pictures of the food that she and her grandmother prepare on Facebook ▾.

Episode 6

Kristina is aware that her brother is in a psychiatric hospital and recognizes how upset her mother and father are over the situation. Kristina doesn't really understand very much about Anthony's problems, but she is concerned for him. She does not tell any of her friends about Anthony because she finds the whole thing embarrassing. Kristina has lost the 5 pounds she set out to lose and is very happy with the way she looks. She likes the compliments from the girls at school about how skinny she is ▾.

Episode 7

Kristina finds her home increasingly chaotic with Anthony moving back home and Mark and Tyler living in the family room. She continues to see Jared and has been hitting the college party scene frequently. Her parents are so distracted with Anthony that they don't pay attention to the fact that she is with Jared as often as she is. She has had sex with Jared on several occasions now and is worried about getting pregnant. She asked Jared about using condoms, but he told her he doesn't like the way they feel. Kristina goes to the Neighborhood Community Health Department to get birth control information after learning from her friends that she can get birth control pills there. Carol Ramsey, the nurse at the clinic, talks with her about protecting herself from sexually transmitted infections and pregnancy. Kristina is really only interested in getting birth control pills.

Episode 8

Kristina is taking birth control pills, but she has heard from her friends that birth control pills cause weight gain. She is worried about getting fat while taking them, so she decides that she needs to lose more weight to prevent that from happening.

Episode 9

Kristina goes to see Jared at the college and they have a good time, but she can tell he is a bit distracted. She does not see or hear from him for several days after this. She becomes worried when he doesn't answer his cell phone or respond to her text messages. She drops by to see him, but he is not in his dorm room. He finally sends her a text that just says, "*Sorry, been busy. Talk soon.*"

Episode 10

Kristina gets a text from Jared telling her that he is breaking up with her. He does not offer an explanation. Kristina is crushed! She wonders what she did wrong. Her calls and texts go unanswered. She does not dwell on it too long, though, and turns her attention to her cheerleading and high school friends. Her Facebook page posts reflect her feelings, "I'm so over you," and, "You weren't that good ▾."

Episode 11

Kristina is glad that Anthony has gone back to school because Mark and Tyler have moved back into his bedroom. She has been asked out by Ray, one of the guys on the basketball team at the high school. Ray wants to get Kristina drunk because he has heard that she "puts out." They go to a party, and Kristina gets drunk and has sex with Ray. She is glad that she is still on the birth control pills ▾.

Episode 12

Several of the kids at school talk about Kristina after Ray tells many of the guys about the party. Kristina is angry about the rumors and decides that, if she weren't so fat, people wouldn't talk about her. She vows to lose another 5 pounds.

Episode 13

Kristina is mortified by the fact that her brother was seen running around naked at the college and got arrested. The kids at the high school hear about the incident and are talking about it. Kristina feels angry with her brother for ruining her reputation. She gets a call from her old boyfriend Jared, who tells her that everybody at the dorm thinks Anthony is a psycho. He tells her that he misses her and asks her to come by and see him. She goes to see Jared and is hopeful that they are back "on" as a couple.

Episode 14

Kristina feels sorry for Anthony when he comes back home. She is amazed at how different he looks compared to last year, when he was in high school. Kristina also feels sorry for her mother. She can see that her mom is constantly nervous and upset. Kristina hates not having any control over all the craziness in her home and wishes that there was something she could do to make it stop. She is also upset that Jared is ignoring her again. She wonders if the only reason he sees her is for sex.

Episode 15

Tracie suggests to Kristina that they take Tyler to the mall together and do some shopping. Kristina wants a new dress for an upcoming school dance so she agrees to go. Kristina has been asked to the dance by Brian, one of the "stud" football players on the varsity team who recently broke up with his girlfriend. She accepts his

invitation, knowing that everyone will be talking about it. She hopes that Jared hears about it and it makes him jealous.

While at the mall, Kristina tries on a few dresses and shows them to Tracie. Kristina becomes very defensive when Tracie tells her that she looks like she has lost a lot of weight. Kristina tells her, "No I have not – and you must just be jealous of me to say that." Secretly, she is glad to know that she looks thin.

Kristina Martin Season 3 Information

Episode 1

Kristina is the 17-year-old daughter of Helen and Gil Martin. She lives with her parents and grandmother, her three siblings, Tracie, Anthony, and Mark, and her nephew Tyler. She gets along with her siblings but she considers her sister Tracie way too serious and is embarrassed by her brother Anthony for being crazy.

Kristina is a fairly typical high school junior. She is on the varsity cheerleading squad at school and has a very busy schedule. Kristina has recently become sexually active.

Kristina sees Jared every couple of weeks; she would like to see him more, but there are other guys at high school that are "hot," and she is going to have fun. She has decided that she is definitely going to move into a dorm when she goes to college because it is so cool.

Episode 2

Kristina attends the school dance this week with Brian. She likes Brian because she knows that he is a high-profile date, considering his social status at the school. He is also very attractive. However, if she had the choice, she would rather be with Jared. After the school dance, Kristina and Brian go to the "after party" hosted by the parents of one of the cheerleaders. Kristina gets very drunk at the party, and ends up having sex with Brian in one of the back bedrooms ▼.

Episode 3

Pictures of Kristina and Brian making out at the party are posted on Facebook from the party the previous week and she hopes that Jared sees the photos. She is angered when Brian's ex-girlfriend writes a post under the picture that reads, *"Pathetic that someone enjoys being with leftovers."* Kristina posts a reply: *"Pathetic is a jealous ex who did not have a date."*

Kristina has managed to get her grades back up so that she is no longer at risk for probation from cheerleading. She is glad about this because, in her mind, cheerleading is the most important thing that she does ▼.

Episode 4

Kristina is freaked out when she learns about Mark's accident. She is so worried for him. She goes with her parents and grandmother to see him at the hospital every day. She posts several things about her brother's injuries on Facebook.

Kristina spends all of her spare time with her new boyfriend, Brian, and he provides her comfort during this time of stress. His parents work late, so she goes to his house several times after school and has sex with Brian. She likes how hot he is and also posts several pictures of herself with Brian. She loves how many "likes" she gets ▼ NEWS.

Episode 5

Kristina gets a text from Jared telling her that they need to talk. She is sure that he is jealous and wants to talk with her about her new boyfriend and wanting to get back together. When she calls him, he tells her that he got Chlamydia from her and that she needs to be tested. Kristina has heard of Chlamydia but is not too sure what it is.

Kristina goes to the community health department and tests positive. She learns from Carol Ramsey, the nurse midwife, that Chlamydia is a sexually transmitted infection. She is given azithromycin (Zithromax) and is told to abstain from sex for one week. The nurse talks with Kristina about safe sex practices and encourages her to inform all of her sex partners. Kristina knows that she has not had sex with anyone else except Brian and Ray and is sure she did not get anything from them. She also knows that she has not been with Jared since being with Brian. Kristina asks the nurse if this means that Jared cheated on her. She also begs Carol not to tell her parents.

Episode 6

Kristina is embarrassed and humiliated when she has to talk to Brian and Ray about needing to get tested for Chlamydia. When she talks to Ray, he is shocked and just says "okay."

When she talks to Brian, he is furious and breaks up with her, calling her many very unpleasant names.

Kristina finds out that Jared had been having sex regularly with multiple girls at the college while he was having sex with her. She figures that this is how she got infected with Chlamydia. She is angry with him for getting her infected and causing her breakup with Brian. In some ways, Kristina does not want anything to do with Jared, but at the same time, she really wants to be his girlfriend. She is embarrassed to talk to anybody about what has happened and is afraid that her parents will find out. She hopes that Brian won't tell anyone.

Episode 7

Kristina is feeling very stressed out about what is happening with her family. When Anthony tries to kill himself, she can't understand it, and she doesn't know how to respond. In many ways, she feels almost invisible. She loses more weight to make herself feel attractive. In the past 6 months, Kristina has lost 20 pounds. She is 5'2" and now weighs 90 pounds.

Episode 8

In Kristina's opinion, her entire world is terrible. Her old boyfriend cheated on her and gave her Chlamydia, her mother suffers from anxiety, one brother is paralyzed, and her other brother is crazy. Kristina has become exceedingly thin, to the point where her friends constantly talk to her about her weight. Her parents have not commented on her weight, and she wonders if they even notice. When her sister, Tracie, asks her how she is doing and what is wrong, Kristina shares with her all that is troubling her. She takes comfort in her older sister's concern and is relieved to have somebody to talk with. Although Tracie encourages her to talk with their mother about these issues, Kristina elects not to do so because she perceives that her mother is nearly at a breaking point. She does not want to talk with her father because she does not want to disappoint him ▶.

Episode 9

Kristina sees Brian's Facebook postings and is relieved that he has not posted anything negative about her. All of his posts focus on basketball and other sports topics. Nobody has mentioned to her that there are rumors about her having Chlamydia, so she is pretty sure that the information won't get out. She sends Brian a few text messages but they go unanswered ▼.

Episode 10

Mark comes home from the hospital this week. Kristina no longer looks at his presence in her home as an inconvenience; rather, she is happy to have him there. She helps her mother and grandmother take care of him. Kristina is sad to see Tracie leave this week to move in with John. The pleasure of having a bedroom to herself is minimized by the loss she feels.

Episode 11

Anthony leaves the house after a fight with her parents. Kristina is upset and calls Tracie to tell her what happened. Tracie invites Kristina to spend the night at her apartment with John and Tyler; Kristina chooses to do this rather than go out with her friends. Tracie comments to Kristina that she is looking better, but she notices that Kristina gets dizzy when she stands.

Episode 12

Kristina's mother is constantly talking about Anthony and Mark, and quibbling with Mary. Kristina sends Tracie a text with the message:

"Mom driving me crazy~!"

She soon gets a text back from Tracie:

"B home in hour, come by 2 talk"

Kristina goes to Tracie's apartment and talks with her about what is going on with her mom and Anthony. She tells Tracie, "Even Grandma is really getting on my nerves. She says that she feels sorry for Mark having to be stuck there all the time."

Episode 13

Jared sends Kristina a text message, asking her to come see him and telling her that he wants to get back together with her. When Kristina reads the message, she calls her sister Tracie and asks her what to do.

Episode 14

The situation at home has brought Kristina and Tracie much closer. Kristina thinks Tracie is the most reliable person she can talk to. She spends an increased amount of time with her. She secretly wishes that she could move in with Tracie and John, but knows that would be asking too much.

Episode 15

The kids at school are talking about Anthony. Kristina is angry with many of them, including some of her "friends" on the cheerleading squad. Having them ask her questions about what has happened to him makes her feel embarrassed, and she doesn't really want to talk about it. For the first time in her entire life, she finds herself wishing that she weren't the center of attention among her peers ▼.

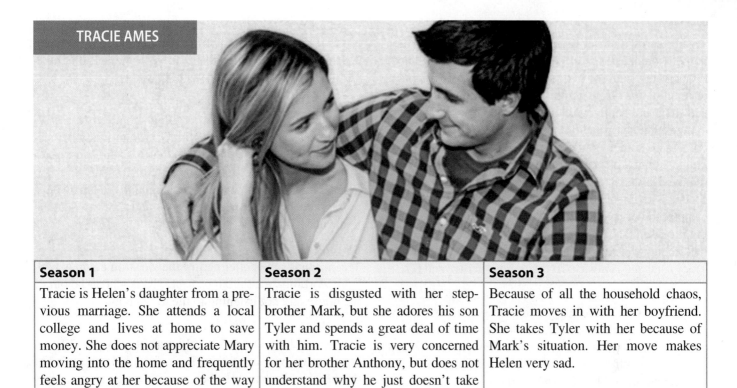

TRACIE AMES

Season 1	Season 2	Season 3
Tracie is Helen's daughter from a previous marriage. She attends a local college and lives at home to save money. She does not appreciate Mary moving into the home and frequently feels angry at her because of the way Mary treats her mother.	Tracie is disgusted with her step-brother Mark, but she adores his son Tyler and spends a great deal of time with him. Tracie is very concerned for her brother Anthony, but does not understand why he just doesn't take his medications.	Because of all the household chaos, Tracie moves in with her boyfriend. She takes Tyler with her because of Mark's situation. Her move makes Helen very sad.

Tracie Ames Season 1 Information

Episode 1

Tracie Ames is a 20-year-old college student. She is Helen's Martin's daughter and Gil's stepdaughter. Tracie was 3 years old when her mother married Gil, so he essentially has raised her as his own daughter. Although Tracie has had a very positive ongoing relationship with her biological father Rick, she has always lived with her mother and is very close to Helen.

Tracie attends the local college and is working on a degree in English. She hopes to be either a high school or college English teacher when she completes her degree, with a long-range goal of being a writer. She is a very serious young woman and is very goal driven. She has been on the Dean's list every semester since beginning school. Tracie has earned scholarships, which help her with tuition, and she lives at home to save money. She would love to live on campus or in an apartment, but to do so would require her to get a full-time job, and she is concerned that this would affect her success in school. Tracie has a part-time student employment position as a writer/editor. She has been in a monogamous relationship with her boyfriend John for one year. He attends the same college and lives in an apartment near campus. Tracie has a Facebook page, but she rarely posts on it. She finds that most posted information is irrelevant and she generally thinks people post too much personal information on the site.

Tracie is in excellent health; she has no medical conditions requiring ongoing care. She watches her weight, exercises regularly, and does not smoke or use illicit drugs or alcohol. She goes for annual examinations each year. The only prescription medication she takes is an oral contraceptive. She does not use any over-the-counter medications on a regular basis.

This episode Tracie attends a political rally on the college campus with her boyfriend, John. She has never aligned herself specifically with one political party, but she is fascinated with the process and the behavior of individuals at such rallies. Specifically, she thinks that many people are foolish in their behavior and she recognizes the many double standards that are presented ◢.

Episode 2

Tracie sees Kristina's postings on her Facebook page with pictures of herself as cheerleader at a varsity football game. Tracie smiles to think how one's perspective about what is really important can change so much in just a few short years. Tracie finds the whole cheerleader thing trivial now, compared to some of the world's social issues.

Episode 3

Tracie learns that her grandmother is moving into their home. To make room for her, she is told that she will need to share her bedroom with Kristina. Tracie feels that it was unfair for Gil to do this without asking her mother, and she is not happy with the situation. However, she recognizes that her grandmother may need some assistance.

Tracie comes home from class and finds that everything she hung up on two walls of her bedroom has been removed by Kristina and replaced with posters of rock groups and celebrities. To make matters worse, Kristina has placed her possessions all over the room and is burning incense. Tracie suggests to Kristina that they need to talk about what it means to share a room; Kristina tells Tracie that she is always trying to boss her around ▽.

Episode 4

Kristina drives Tracie crazy and Tracie can't stand having to share a room with her. Gil talks to her and Kristina about being more sensitive to their grandmother. Tracie thinks to herself, "You are not my father, and she is not my grandmother," but she says nothing.

Episode 5

Tracie is trying to study for a test that will be given the following morning. Her sister is playing rock music in the bedroom and talking on the phone with friends, so she moves to the den. She then hears her mother arguing with her grandmother, Mary, about the way dinner was prepared. She later hears her mother arguing with Gil about Mary intentionally ignoring her diet. All this commotion is distracting, so Tracie goes to John's apartment to study for the evening ▽.

Episode 6

Tracie continues to be annoyed with Kristina. She finds her to be very immature and self-centered. She seems to think the world revolves around her cheerleading, friends, and driving. She is not sure if Kristina is getting worse, or if these behaviors are just more noticeable now that they are sharing a bedroom. Tracie finds that it is very difficult to study and do her part-time editing job at home, so she spends an increasing amount of time at John's apartment. Mary tells Tracie that she should spend more time at home. Helen agrees, but won't say so, as she does not want to support Mary. Tracie has dinner with her father, Rick, and tells him about all of the changes that have been occurring at her home. Rick suggests that she move out, but does not offer to help her financially with alternative living arrangements.

Episode 7

Anthony sits down to talk with Tracie about colleges, asking her opinion about the pros and cons of the college she attends. Tracie listens as Anthony tells her that he wants to get away to the big university; she replies that she goes to the local college and lives at home because it is cheap. As she listens to Anthony, she thinks to herself that he is getting stranger the older he gets ▷.

Episode 8

Tracie overhears her parents arguing about Kristina driving Mary's car and is angry with Gil for allowing her sister to do so. She does not think that it's fair and knows that Kristina will not take good care of the car. She also is beginning to see that Mary is manipulative. Tracie does not appreciate the things Mary says and the way that she treats her mother ▽.

Episode 9

Tracie spends the better part of the week on campus with John working on a school project. She is glad to be out of the house and not listening to the arguments.

Episode 10

Tracie and John are on school break at college. They go out of town with her father, Rick, for a long weekend at the beach. She has only been to the ocean a few times in her life and is thrilled to go. She is happy to get away from some of the commotion that constantly happens in their household.

Episode 11

Tracie and John are still on school break from college. They decide to take an overnight camping trip. Tracie is amazed at how many skills John has. She never went camping as a child and wishes that she had more experience with these sorts of things ▽.

Episode 12

Tracie and her mother spend an afternoon together shopping and having lunch. It has been a long time since the two of them shared some time like this. Tracie tells her mom that she misses spending time like that with her. Tracie learns from her mother that she is going through menopause and that she has not been feeling like herself lately.

Episode 13

Tracie sees Kristina wearing her earrings and asks her where she got them. Kristina tells Tracie that she borrowed them and forgot to ask, but didn't think Tracie would mind. Tracie tells Kristina that she is not to touch any of her stuff, and Kristina tells Tracie that she is selfish for not sharing.

Episode 14

Tracie pulls up in front of their house and sees a bright reflection from the sun in the windows of Anthony's room. She goes into his room and sees that foil has been placed in the windows. She wonders what it is for and tells her mother that it looks awful.

Episode 15

Tracie is embarrassed by the way their house looks with foil in the windows. She makes a command decision and goes into Anthony's room when he is away and removes the foil from his windows. When he comes home, he is frantic and wants to know who removed the foil.

Tracie tells him that she took it down because it makes the house look ridiculous. She is surprised at his reaction. She finds his behavior really odd and she does not understand his reasoning for wanting foil to be on the windows. The next day she notices that the foil is back. She decides that she will let Gil or her mother deal with it.

Tracie Ames Season 2 Information

Episode 1

Tracie Ames is a 20-year-old college student. Tracie attends the local college and is working on a degree in English. She has been in a monogamous relationship with her boyfriend John for 18 months.

This episode Gil's 27-year-old son Mark moves into the house with his 2-year-old son Tyler. Tracie is not sure that she agrees with Gil for letting Mark move in with them, but she also recognizes that he has fallen on some tough times. Mainly, she feels sorry for Tyler and is glad that the family might be able to make a difference in her nephew's life.

Episode 2

Tyler quickly becomes attached to Tracie, and she does not mind one bit. She is glad to see him take an interest in books and puzzles, and she is happy to read to him in the evenings ▼.

Episode 3

Tracie continues going to school in the daytime and spending time with Tyler in the evening. She notices that Tyler's teeth look bad and wonders why Mark hasn't done anything about them.

Episode 4

Tracie is glad her mother's surgery went well. She is hopeful that her mother's ongoing abdominal pain will be a thing of the past.

Episode 5

Gil asks Tracie to help more around the house with meals and general cleaning while her mother recovers from surgery. Tracie is glad to help, but as it turns out, her sister, Kristina, and Mary seem to be in a good routine for making meals. She contributes by cleaning up the dishes and helping with the shopping.

Episode 6

Anthony is hospitalized this week because of his strange behavior, and Tracie is very concerned about him. She is also very concerned about her mother. She recognizes that her mother has been increasingly anxious about everything happening in the family, but this situation with Anthony has been especially difficult for her ▼.

Episode 7

Tracie wonders just how much more chaotic her family could possibly get. With Anthony back home, as well as her grandmother, Mark, and Tyler, the house is quite full. She finds herself spending an increasing amount of time with her boyfriend, John, even though her mother doesn't approve.

Episode 8

Tracie sees a notice in the paper about a dental screening. She mentions this to Mark and is not surprised when Mark doesn't seem to think taking Tyler to the screening is a priority. Tracie gets Mark's permission to take Tyler herself.

At the screening, Tracie is told that Tyler has "bad teeth" and must be seen by a dentist. Tracie explains that her brother cannot afford a dentist. She is given a referral to community health services and is told that dental care is offered there on a sliding-scale payment plan. When asked, Tracie explains that Tyler is given a bottle at night and a sippy cup during the day. Tracie is told that these habits are a huge contributing factor to his poor dental condition and that the family needs to put water in his bottle at night ▼ [NEWS].

Episode 9

Tracie talks with her other family members about the need to stop giving Tyler milk or juice in his bottle at night. They make attempts to do this but give in when he screams.

Episode 10

Tracie is glad that Mark takes Tyler to the dentist. She suspects that Tyler might need to have teeth pulled and can't bear the thought that he might blame her. She is anxious when he comes home and can tell that he has been through an ordeal.

Tracie is glad that Anthony made it back to school. She is hopeful that he can put the bad experience behind him and succeed. She thinks he is much too serious and hopes that he can make friends and just have some fun. She is concerned about her mother's obvious problems coping with the situation and wishes that she could relax a bit.

Episode 11

Tracie knows that Kristina has been out late and has been drinking because she can smell it on her breath when she comes in at night. She talks to Kristina and suggests she "cool it." Kristina tells Tracie to mind her own business ▶.

Episode 12

Tracie learns that Mark is going to stay a little longer at the house to save up for his own home. She is almost relieved that he is not moving yet, because Tracie loves Tyler and hates the thought of him moving away from her.

Episode 13

Anthony is readmitted to the hospital this week because he stopped taking his medication and his delusions returned. Tracie feels badly for Anthony, but also angry with him for not taking his medication. She does not understand why he would just quit taking it. This relapse is obviously his fault. She is very concerned about her mother's reaction ◪ [NEWS].

Episode 14

Tracie is glad to see her brother back at home, but feels the commotion of the household is back up a notch. No wonder her mother is so anxious!

Episode 15

Tracie agrees to watch Tyler for an afternoon and she convinces her sister Kristina to go with her and Tyler to the mall. Tracie is shopping for a pair of jeans while Kristina is looking for a dress for an upcoming school dance. Kristina tries on a few dresses and shows them to Tracie. Tracie is struck not only by how beautiful her sister is, but also by how exceedingly thin she is. Tracie tells Kristina that she looks like she has lost a lot of weight. Kristina denies the weight loss and tells Tracie that she is obviously just jealous ◪.

Tracie Ames Season 3 Information

Episode 1

Tracie Ames is a 21-year-old college student. Tracie attends the local college and is working on a degree in English. She lives at home to save money, but she has been considering other options due to the large number of people who live in the home. Tracie has been in a monogamous relationship with her boyfriend John for two years. He attends the same college and lives in an apartment near campus.

Tracie knows that if she is to move out of the home, she needs to find full-time employment for the last year of school. She has been working part-time on campus as a writing editor and has been offered a full-time position with benefits at a small publishing company located in town. The company owner would like to keep Tracie on staff once she finishes her degree, so Tracie is told that she will be flexible with her hours, allowing her to continue taking her classes. Tracie decides to take the position and see whether she can manage working full-time and going to school ◪.

Episode 2

Tracie and John discuss living together. Now that she is working full-time, she has decided this is perhaps her best option. The one thing that makes her reluctant to move is her attachment to Tyler.

Tracie tells her mother that she is thinking of moving in with John because the house is so crowded. Helen responds that Mark is planning to buy a house with his girlfriend, Shelly, so there will be more room in the house again soon. Tracie senses that her mother does not want her to move.

Episode 3

Tracie is excited for Mark and Shelly to buy a house together, but she is not excited for Tyler to go with them, because she is sure that Shelly does not love Tyler the way she does. She hopes that Mark and Shelly buy a home close by so that she can still see Tyler regularly.

Episode 4

Tracie is in disbelief when she learns that Mark had a serious automobile accident and has permanent injuries. She is further devastated over the impact it will have on the entire family. She wonders just how much more chaos her family can take. Tracie and Mary team up to keep the house organized and functional, while Helen and Gil try to manage the problems with Anthony and Mark.

Episode 5

Tyler has been throwing temper tantrums all week. Tracie recognizes that he is used to a certain level of attention; he is now not getting it because everyone has been so focused on Mark and Anthony. She decides to make specific time each day to read to him and play, even though her heart is heavy with grief ◪.

Episode 6

Tracie takes Tyler to see Mark at the Rehabilitation Hospital. Mark begins to cry when he sees Tyler and tells Tracie that he is depending on her, since there is no way he can ever be a good dad for his son. Tracie cries along with him and vows to make sure that Tyler is always cared for ◪.

Episode 7

Anthony attempts to commit suicide this week. Tracie is very worried about her mother and Gil. She finds them blaming themselves and each other 🟦.

Episode 8

It is obvious to Tracie that Kristina has been losing weight. She can also tell, when Kristina comes in late at night smelling of alcohol, that she has been partying. It is also obvious to her that Helen and Gil seem only to be going through the motions, as they deal with so many issues within the family. Although they have never been particularly close, Tracie talks to Kristina about her concerns, not from the perspective of a bossy older sister, but rather out of concern for her health and well-being. To Tracie's surprise, Kristina opens up and shares with her all the problems she has been experiencing, including being sexually active with Jared and getting Chlamydia. Tracie listens to her sister as she cries about all that has been troubling her. She also says that she feels lost in the family because others have bigger problems than she does. Tracie encourages Kristina to talk with their mother and to try to stop losing weight.

Tracie talks with her boyfriend, John, about living together and wants to know if he would agree to letting Tyler live with them as well. Tracie is very happy that John agrees to the idea. In fact, John says he looks forward to spending time with them.

Episode 9

Tracie visits Mark at the Rehabilitation Hospital this week. She shares with Mark her interest in moving out of the house and in with John, and requests his permission to take Tyler with her, promising to bring him over to the house regularly to visit. Mark tearfully agrees to this. He also tells Tracie that Tyler is due for more shots at the community health clinic. Tracie agrees to take him for his shots.

Kristina continues to confide in Tracie and share with her the things that are bothering her. Tracie is happy to finally feel close to her sister, who has always been very self-centered. She realizes that she has the potential to have a positive influence on Kristina and hopes that moving out of the house will not be a deterrent to this ▶.

Episode 10

Tracie tells her mother and Gil that she and Tyler are moving to John's house to provide more room for Mark when he comes back home. She is not surprised by her mom's protests, but she did not expect Helen to break down and cry. Gil tells Tracie that she should do what she thinks is best. As long as Mark agrees to Tyler living with her, he will support the decision. Tracie feels sorry for her mother, but at the same time she recognizes the need to get herself and Tyler away from the constant chaos ✉.

Episode 11

Tracie and Tyler have settled into their new home with John. Tracie is very happy to have Tyler with her and makes every attempt to be a good parent to him.

Tracie gets a call from Kristina and learns that Anthony has had another fight with Gil and her mother and has left the house. She knows that her mother is devastated, and Tracie feels a bit guilty about leaving when she did. At the same time, she is enjoying her time with John and thinks that Tyler is adjusting well to his new living arrangement. Tracie invites Kristina to spend the night if she wants to get away from the house.

Episode 12

Tracie gets a text from Kristina with the message, "*Mom driving me crazy~*!"

Tracie texts her back, "*B home in hour, come by 2 talk.*" Kristina shows up at Tracie's apartment and talks with her about what is going on with Anthony. She says that she feels sorry for Mark having to be stuck there all the time.

Episode 13

Tracie takes Tyler to see his father every evening. She can see how depressed Mark is and feels badly for him. She is glad that Mark is so positive about Tyler's living with her because she knows deep down that it's the best thing for him ✉.

Episode 14

Kristina has been spending a great deal of time with Tracie. Tracie is glad to be able to provide some level of sanity for Kristina, but she also feels a bit stressed out because of her limited free time. She considers asking Kristina to help her by watching Tyler so that she can study.

Episode 15

Tracie finds that going to school, taking care of Tyler, and working is becoming very taxing. Living in an apartment is more expensive than she imagined. She is glad that she is able to rely on her sister, Kristina, and John to help her with Tyler. She goes to the financial aid and scholarship office at the college to see about possible financial assistance to help her get through this time.

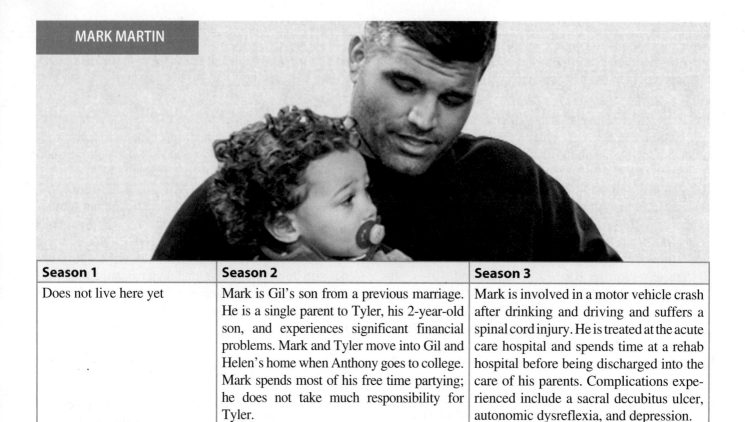

MARK MARTIN

Season 1	Season 2	Season 3
Does not live here yet	Mark is Gil's son from a previous marriage. He is a single parent to Tyler, his 2-year-old son, and experiences significant financial problems. Mark and Tyler move into Gil and Helen's home when Anthony goes to college. Mark spends most of his free time partying; he does not take much responsibility for Tyler.	Mark is involved in a motor vehicle crash after drinking and driving and suffers a spinal cord injury. He is treated at the acute care hospital and spends time at a rehab hospital before being discharged into the care of his parents. Complications experienced include a sacral decubitus ulcer, autonomic dysreflexia, and depression.

Mark Martin Season 1 Information

Does not live here yet.

Mark Martin Season 2 Information

Episode 1

Mark Martin is Gil's 27-year-old son. Mark is a single parent to his 2-year-old son Tyler. Mark has held a variety of odd jobs while attempting to support himself and Tyler, but he has fallen deeply into debt. He has reached the credit limit on all of his credit cards and is struggling to make his car payment, apartment rent, and child care payments. At Gil's suggestion, Mark has moved into his father's house so he can get caught up on bills. Currently, Mark is working as a security officer for a private security company. His employment provides minimal health insurance for him and Tyler and does not include dental coverage. Mark hopes to start taking classes at the local college and work toward a degree, but he is not sure what he wants to do with his life. Mark gets along very well with Gil, Anthony, and Kristina, but he has never felt close to Helen or Tracie. His father married Helen when

he was 10 years old. Even at that time, Mark could tell Helen resented him. Although Mark always lived with his mother, he spent a lot of time with his father's family. Mark is a regular user of the social media site Facebook and posts to his personal page on the site a couple times a week.

This episode Mark and Tyler settle into Gil and Helen's home. Mark realizes that the house is pretty full and promises Helen that he will stay only as long as he has to. He apologizes to Kristina for ruining her plans to move into Anthony's room and thanks her for being so flexible. During the evening, Mark goes to work and leaves Tyler at the house, assuming that nobody will mind taking care of him. He appreciates the fact that his grandmother is also willing to help, but he is not sure she can see well enough to care for Tyler adequately. Mark posts his relocation news to his Facebook page ◥.

Episode 2

Mark makes a change to the evening shift so that he can take care of Tyler during the daytime, and his family members can take care of him in the evening while he works. Mark quickly realizes that, between the savings in rent and child care, he can pay off most of his bills within 6 months. This motivates Mark to get along with his family members as well as he can.

Episode 3

Mary mentions to Mark that Tyler's teeth seem to be in bad shape. Mark does not pay much attention to his grandmother. He knows that she can't see very well and that she has a tendency to meddle in other people's business. He tells Mary that he already knows about the teeth and it's under control. In truth, Mark has never paid any attention to Tyler's teeth. When Gil asks Mark about Tyler's teeth, Mark tells his dad that he is aware of the problem but has been short on cash and is not able to afford to take him to the dentist. He also tells Gil that he is not too worried about it, because they are just his baby teeth and they'll fall out eventually anyway. Mark posts pictures of him with Tyler on Facebook page with the message, "Kid has bad teeth - who knows a good cheap dentist?" ▼

Episode 4

After getting off the evening shift, Mark goes to a party he heard about on Facebook. He meets up with some of his friends, but the majority of people there he does not know. While at the party he meets a woman by the name of Shelly. He has been reluctant to get seriously involved with another woman since his ex-wife left his life in such a mess, but Shelly seems a lot different. He hopes to continue to see her ▼.

Episode 5

Mark finds that working the evening shift is great. He can work and then go out and party with friends after work. He often does not come home until 2 or 3 a.m. In the mornings, he gets up to take care of Tyler, but he ends up taking a nap most mornings or early afternoons while other family members watch him. Mark's love life has really picked up as well. He has been seeing Shelly almost every day since they met ▼.

Episode 6

Gil tells Mark about the serious situation with his brother, Anthony. Mark always considered Anthony to be weird, but he is really surprised that he flipped out and was admitted to a psychiatric hospital. He can't imagine his brother being violent at all.

Episode 7

When Mark is told by Gil that Anthony is moving back home, Mark gladly moves out of Anthony's room and takes over the family room. Mark finds that he likes this better anyway, because the family room has more space for him and Tyler. Mark has been partying so much this week that he has stopped getting up in the mornings to care for Tyler. He sleeps until noon nearly every day, knowing that his grandmother is caring for Tyler ▼.

Episode 8

Tracie tells Mark about a free dental screening and suggests that he take Tyler to it. Mark tells her that he has plans with his girlfriend on that day, but he gives her permission to take him. Later that day, Tracie tells Mark that Tyler's teeth are in bad shape and he needs to have dental care immediately. Tracie has already made the appointment for Tyler and tells Mark he needs to take him to the appointment. Mark agrees to take care of it.

Gil talks to Mark about coming in so late each night and not taking more responsibility for Tyler. Mark comes home immediately after work for a couple of nights, but then he is back to his party scene with his girlfriend, Shelly. On some nights, he spends the night with Shelly, comes in at about 6 a.m., and then crashes on the couch in the family room. Mark updates his status on Facebook to: "In a relationship ▼."

Episode 9

Mark knows that Anthony has been very down about his psychiatric problems and decides to help him cheer up. On a day off, he takes Anthony out to the shooting range. Gil used to take Mark and Anthony to the shooting range periodically when they were younger, but it has been years since they did this. Mark can see that Anthony still has incredible accuracy. After they leave the range, they pick up a pizza and take it home to eat. The entire time they are together, Mark tries to engage Anthony in conversation and finds it a real challenge. He wonders if Anthony doesn't say much because of the medications. In any event, Mark knows that Anthony is really a messed-up kid ▼.

Episode 10

Mark moves back into Anthony's bedroom this week. Although he liked the extra room he had in the family room, he hated not having any privacy. Tracie reminds Mark to take Tyler to the community health center for the dental clinic. Mark is not thrilled about taking Tyler because of the cost, but he is relieved when he learns that the clinic provides services on a sliding-scale payment plan and is willing to help him out with the costs. While taking a history, the nurse asks Mark about Tyler's immunizations. Mark knows he has had "some," but can't remember which ones, and he does not have Tyler's shot records. The staff at the clinic stress to Mark the importance of having his child immunized. Mark is also told by the staff to replace the juice with water in Tyler's sippy cup ▼.

Episode 11

Mark continues to party and spend time with his girlfriend Shelly most nights after work. He knows that between his grandmother, Helen, and Tracie, Tyler is well cared for. Mark posts pictures of himself with Shelly on his Facebook page ▼.

Episode 12

Mark gets his truck paid off this week and has finally been able to pay off most of his credit card debt. He tells his Dad that he would like to stay a little longer to save for a down payment on a house. He is feeling good about getting himself out of debt and celebrates by taking his girlfriend, Shelly, away on a weekend vacation out of town ▼.

Episode 13

Mark and Shelly take Tyler to the park. He is disappointed that Tyler does not want anything to do with his girlfriend. He knows that Tyler loves Tracie, but he wants him to love Shelly, too.

Episode 14

Mark and Tyler have to move back into the family room when Anthony gets discharged from the hospital. Mark is hopeful that he and Tyler can move out soon. He is thinking about asking Shelly to marry him.

Mark takes Tyler back to the dental clinic for more dental work. The nurses at the clinic also give Tyler immunizations and ask Mark to bring Tyler back in 2 months.

Episode 15

Mark realizes that he needs to figure out a better plan for employment – especially if he decides to get married. He looks into some of the classes at the local college and is not sure how he can manage taking classes, taking care of Tyler, and working. He feels a little discouraged and wonders how he can possibly advance out of his security officer job. At the same time, Mark enjoys the guys that he works with. He parties with them three times this week.

Mark Martin Season 3 Information

Episode 1

Mark Martin is Gil's 27-year-old son. Mark is a single parent to his 2 1/2 year-old son Tyler. Mark has been living with Gil and Helen for the past several months because he had fallen deeply into debt and needed help caring for his son. Mark has been steadily working the evening shift as a security officer for a security company. He has recently been able to pay off his truck and credit card debt and is currently saving for a down payment on a house. He has a girlfriend, Shelly, whom he hopes to marry in the near future. Mark talks about taking classes at the local college and working toward a degree, but he is not sure what kind of a career he wants to pursue.

Mark is healthy, although he is a smoker and consumes alcohol on a regular basis. Mark parties after work and often does not come home until the early morning hours.

Early in the week, Mark is at home watching a movie. Tyler keeps interrupting him, so Mark gives him some shelled peanuts to eat to keep him quiet. A few minutes later, Tyler is crying. Because Mark is busy watching a movie, he fails to notice the hives on his son. Mary points out the problem to Mark and tells him to take Tyler to the Emergency Department at Neighborhood Hospital.

Episode 2

Mark thinks he has saved up enough money for a down payment on a house. He talks with a real estate agent, Rachel Reyes, who agrees to help him find a small home

that he can afford. Mark takes Tyler back to the community health clinic for another set of immunization. He is told to return in 2 months.

Episode 3

Mark and Shelly go out to look at several homes this week with Rachel Reyes, the realtor. Mark and Shelly see several homes they like, but Mark is unsure about being able to make the house payments. Mark and Shelly have decided to get married at the end of next year, but they plan on living together once he has a house. Mark changes his status on Facebook to: "Engaged." ▼

Episode 4

Mark and several friends from work go to a party 20 miles north of town in the afternoon. He stays there all afternoon and into the evening, and continues to party into the early morning hours. Mark is drunk when he leaves the party at 3:15 a.m. On the way home, while driving on a rural road, Mark crosses the center line in his truck, sees an oncoming car, swerves to avoid the vehicle, and rolls his truck four times. Mark is not wearing his seatbelt and is ejected. The driver of the oncoming car sees the accident and calls 9-1-1 for help.

It takes the volunteer emergency medical technicians (EMTs) 20 minutes to arrive at the scene. Mark is highly intoxicated but awake. His arms are flailing, and he can answer questions. He is strapped to a backboard and transported to the Emergency Department (ED) at

Neighborhood Hospital, where it is a very busy night. The EMTs tell the ED nurse that Mark is in stable condition.

The ED nurse completes an assessment and realizes quickly that Mark does not have movement or sensation in his lower extremities. She informs Dr. Gordon of the situation and asks him to examine Mark immediately. After an extensive workup and evaluation, Dr. Gordon diagnoses Mark with a spinal cord injury. A neurosurgeon is called to consult on his case. He is told his has a fractured vertebra in his back, requiring surgery to stabilize the bones in his back, and is sent to the OR shortly thereafter.

After surgery, Mark is admitted to the Neurosurgical Intensive Care Unit. Upon admission to the unit, a large red area is noted on his sacrum. As he gains an awareness of his surroundings and his circumstances, Mark is told he has fractured vertebrae in his back, and that he severed his spinal cord. When Mark asks if he will regain feeling and movement in his legs, he is told that, no, the injury will leave him with paraplegia.

Episode 5

Mark is devastated as the reality of his injuries sinks in. He is very angry. Shelly spends a great deal of time at the hospital, and he wonders why she even bothers. He knows that they will never buy the house they had dreamed about, and that it is unlikely she will want to marry him now. He is scheduled for surgery this week to stabilize the spinal fracture. The skin over the reddened sacral area remains intact. Several people come by to see Mark, but he is not interested in visiting with anybody.

Episode 6

This week, Mark is transferred to a Rehabilitation Hospital. The day he arrives, the nurse notices a discolored area over his sacrum. By the following day, the discolored area has opened up, revealing a large decubitus ulcer. A large amount of purulent drainage comes from it, and a wound care specialist is called in to consult.

The nurses also recognized that Mark is very depressed and unmotivated. He lacks interest in turning or doing any of the rehabilitation exercises. Following a mental health consultation by Shawn Jacobs, a nurse practitioner with psychiatric and mental health expertise, Mark is started on duloxetine (Cymbalta) for depression.

Episode 7

Mark remains at the Rehabilitation Hospital. Shelly has been spending less and less time with him. When she comes to see him, she says very little. Mark asks her why she even bothers coming if she won't talk to him. Shelly asks Mark, "What am I supposed to say?" and this triggers a fight. Shelly leaves in tears. Mark has a visit from Shawn Jacobs, the psychiatric mental health nurse practitioner. Mark tells Shawn that he is still feeling very depressed. Mark mentions the fight he had with Shelly and that he is furious. Mark is surprised that Shawn does not try to sugar-coat the incident and has a no-nonsense approach. Mark kind of likes that about him but is too angry to talk very much.

Episode 8

Mark is very depressed. Shelly was in a few days ago and told Mark that she has to get on with her life. She cannot spend all her time looking at him sitting in a chair. Mark became angry with her and told her never to come back. She threw her engagement ring at Mark and told him she was done. Since then he has not been motivated to do anything, and he has had frequent angry outbursts with the nursing staff. When they attempt to point out the benefits of exercise and therapy, he comments that there is no point.

Shawn Jacobs, the psychiatric mental health nurse practitioner, makes a visit to see Mark. Mark tells him that his life is essentially over. Shawn acknowledges that he has experienced yet another painful loss. He encourages Mark to talk about how he is feeling with friends and family members as he feels up to it. When his father, grandmother, and occasional friends come by to visit, Mark does little to interact.

Episode 9

Mark is still at the Rehabilitation Hospital and is still not engaged in his care. One afternoon, there is a delay in performing his catheterization. While checking on Mark, the nurse notes that Mark is flushed and has tachycardia. His blood pressure starts to rise. The nurse recognizes the signs of autonomic dysreflexia and knows this is a potential emergency. An in-and-out catheterization is immediately performed on Mark—850 mL of urine is returned with the catheterization.

Mark's sister, Tracie, visits Mark and shares with him her plans to move out of the house. She asks Mark if she can take Tyler with her. When asked why, Tracie tells Mark about the constant commotion in the home and says she wants to shield Tyler from the drama. For the first time since the accident, Mark breaks down and sobs in Tracie's arms. He feels so sad about his situation and at the same time is relieved to know that Tracie would do this for Tyler. He knows that his father and grandmother mean well, but he agrees with Tracie's assessment. He knows that things will get crazier once he goes home. He thanks her for taking care of his son and only wishes there was a way he could repay her. He tells Tracie she is truly a living angel.

Episode 10

Mark is discharged from the Rehabilitation Hospital to Gil and Helen's home. He has been transferred to a new medical group and will continue outpatient rehabilitation for the next several weeks. Mark's new medical group has a preferred psychiatrist who will begin following Mark for depression. Gil and Helen have had to make many modifications to their home to accommodate him. Mark's grandmother, Mary, lets him know that she is going to take care of him and get him well. Mark appreciates her interest in him, but he recognizes that she obviously does not understand how he is feeling. She is more interested in seeing him get well than he is.

Episode 11
Mark can hear his father and Helen arguing with Anthony about not wanting to take his medication. Mark feels very angry with Anthony and wishes that he would just shut up and take the damn medication. The home care nurse comes to see Mark three times this week for wound care. She reminds Mark about the need to change positions, turn, and eat. Mark has had a poor appetite, partly because he hates having to be dependent for toileting. He hopes to be able to get out of bed and to a real bathroom soon. He continues to work on upper body strengthening and transfers with a physical therapist in the outpatient rehabilitation clinic.

Episode 12
Mark's mood is improving. He is becoming increasingly engaged in his care and is starting to see value in life again. He is pleased with the progress that he has made with his psychiatrist and now openly talks about the accident. He finally has quit blaming others and accepts his role in the situation. Mark is becoming increasingly close to Tracie and John. They come over regularly and Mark can see that Tyler is very happy with them. Mark is even happier that Tyler still calls him Daddy ▼.

Episode 13
Mark is happy to see his son nearly every evening. He can see that Tyler is well cared for and that he loves Tracie. He finds himself wishing that he had been a better parent to Tyler and that he could do many things over again. He has so many regrets. If only he had a second chance! ▼

Episode 14
Mark's decubitus ulcer is nearly healed. This week, he is finally able to transfer himself from the bed to a wheelchair without assistance. He is elated and takes even greater interest in building his upper body muscle strength to facilitate transfers. He can see that his grandmother and parents want to help, but he finally is beginning to acknowledge that he needs to make more of an effort himself.

Episode 15
Mark hears that his brother is sleeping in the park. He feels angry with his brother for wasting his life. He wishes that he could trade places with him.

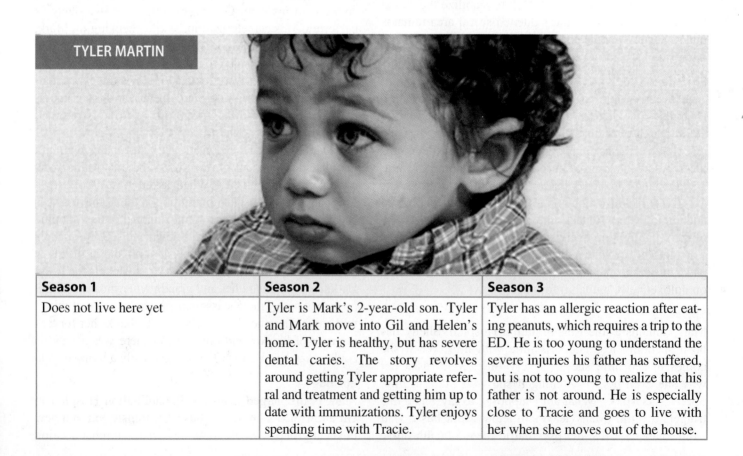

TYLER MARTIN

Season 1	Season 2	Season 3
Does not live here yet	Tyler is Mark's 2-year-old son. Tyler and Mark move into Gil and Helen's home. Tyler is healthy, but has severe dental caries. The story revolves around getting Tyler appropriate referral and treatment and getting him up to date with immunizations. Tyler enjoys spending time with Tracie.	Tyler has an allergic reaction after eating peanuts, which requires a trip to the ED. He is too young to understand the severe injuries his father has suffered, but is not too young to realize that his father is not around. He is especially close to Tracie and goes to live with her when she moves out of the house.

Tyler Martin Season 1 Information

Does not live here yet.

Tyler Martin Season 2 Information

Episode 1

Tyler Martin is Mark's 2-year-old son and Gil's grandson. Tyler has really only known his father, because his mother began abusing drugs shortly after he was born, and he has not seen her since he was 6 months old. Tyler has been going to various babysitters since he was 1 month old. He and his father have recently moved to his grandparents' home. Tyler loves living there because of all the attention he gets. He also no longer has to go to day care.

Tyler has generally been in good health, although Mark has not consistently taken him for routine infant/child care. He is of normal weight and generally has a good appetite. Tyler still loves his bottle, and each night he is given a bottle of milk or juice to help him go to sleep.

Mark gives Tyler a sippy cup of juice and puts him in front of the TV. Tracie sits down next to Tyler on the couch; Tyler crawls into her lap and falls asleep.

Episode 2

Tyler is enthralled with the toys and books that his great-grandmother has bought him. He immediately sits down on the floor to play with the blocks, with a sippy cup of juice within arm's reach. In the evenings, Tyler sees Tracie studying at the table. He runs to his room to get his new books and holds them up to her to read.

Episode 3

Tyler has quickly become very comfortable at Gil and Helen's home. During the daytime, he spends time with his daddy. In the evenings, he loves the attention from Gil, Helen, Mary, and especially Tracie. He sits in Tracie's lap at every opportunity. Tracie tells Tyler that his teeth look bad and asks him if his daddy has ever taken him to a dentist. Tyler does not know what any of this means.

Episode 4

Tyler's daddy brings a lady to the house to meet him. He tells Tyler that the lady's name is Shelly and she is his girlfriend. Tyler does not quite know what that means, but he is not interested in talking to the lady. He buries his head against Mark's chest so that he does not have to look at her.

Episode 5

During the daytime, while Tracie is at school, Tyler follows his grandmother around almost constantly. She is not usually at home during the day, and he is happy to spend time with her. Tyler likes the fact that Helen plays with him.

Episode 6

Tyler wants some lunch. Nobody is at home except for his daddy, who is asleep in the bedroom. Tyler pushes a chair to the counter and climbs up on the counter. He is able to open the cabinet and find an open package of cookies. Tyler sits on the counter and eats. Eventually his daddy comes in and scolds him for getting up on the counter.

Episode 7

Tyler and his daddy move their stuff into the family room. They sleep on a pull-out bed instead of a regular bed. Tyler sometimes wakes up at night. His daddy is not at home, but he sees his great-grandmother watching TV. She refills his bottle and tells him to go back to sleep.

Episode 8

Tyler goes to the dental screening clinic with Tracie. At the clinic, a man looks at his teeth and says that they are in bad shape. Tyler wonders how his teeth have been "bad." He is given a toy and a toothbrush, and the assistant shows Tracie how to brush Tyler's teeth.

Episode 9

Tyler is frustrated when Tracie takes his sippy cup full of juice away and gives him water instead. He screams at night for his bottle and does not stop crying until somebody gives him a bottle with juice or milk.

Episode 10

Tyler has a follow-up dental appointment at the community health center. A history is taken, and his height and weight are measured and plotted for 27 months. His length is 91 cm (60th percentile) and weight is 13.2 kg (55th percentile), which are plotted on a growth chart. The dentist finds that two of Tyler's teeth are rotted at the gum line and that he has cavities in five teeth. The two rotted teeth are extracted, which is a frightening experience for Tyler. When they get home, he immediately runs to Tracie to hold him.

Episode 11

Tyler hates the fact that his sippy cup has water in it. He screams at the top of his lungs and throws the sippy cup across the room. Mary gets him some juice and puts it in the cup to keep him from crying.

Episode 12

Mark tells Tyler that he and Shelly are going to be away for a few days for a trip. He cries and says, "I want to go, too." When Mark tells Tyler he has to stay, Tyler has a temper tantrum. After they leave the house, Tracie picks up Tyler and suggests that they read a book together. Tyler soon forgets his daddy has left.

Episode 13

Tyler goes to the park with his daddy and Shelly. He wants Tracie to go to the park, too, but she is not at home. He does not want Shelly to hold him. When she tries to hold him, he cries and kicks his feet until she puts him down.

Episode 14

Tyler has another terrifying experience at the dentist because he receives very painful shots and has five teeth filled. Because his immunization status is unknown, he is given HBV, DTaP, Hib, IPV, and PCV immunizations during this visit.

Episode 15

Tyler goes to the large shopping mall with Tracie and Kristina. He rides in a stroller while they shop for some clothes. Later they take him to the food court and he helps Tracie eat a soft pretzel. He gets cheese all over his face. Tracie and Kristina laugh hysterically and take his picture with their phones.

Tyler Martin Season 3 Information

Episode 1

Tyler Martin is Mark's $2^1/_2$-year-old son and Gil's grandson. Tyler and his father have been living at his grandparents' home for the past several months. Tyler has become attached to his aunt, Tracie, as a mother figure. He prefers Tracie to all other family members.

Tyler has generally been in good health, although he had bottle mouth (multiple dental caries and rotting teeth), which required extraction of some of his teeth and fillings in others. Tyler also has been behind on his immunizations, and his father has been taking him to the community health center to get caught up on these.

Tyler is bored and wants his daddy to play with him. Instead, Mark gives Tyler a handful of shelled peanuts to eat. Shortly after eating the peanuts, Tyler begins to cry. His mouth feels funny, and he is itchy all over. He runs back to his father crying, but Mark fails to look at him and just tells him to be quiet. After his great-grandmother discovers the problem, Mark takes Tyler to the Neighborhood Hospital Emergency Department, where he is seen and treated by Dr. Gordon for an allergic reaction.

Episode 2

Tyler has become a very stubborn toddler. He gets angry if he does not get his way. He gets even angrier when his father yells at him or tells him to be quiet. When he throws a tantrum, Tracie or Helen puts him in the back bedroom and closes the door. He is told he can come out when he calms himself.

Episode 3

Tyler goes with his father and Shelly to look at homes. Tyler is not interested in this activity and gets very cranky when he is taken in and out of his car seat at each house. He wants to be home. Mark and Shelly get frustrated with Tyler.

Episode 4

Tyler is told by Tracie that his daddy is sick and at the hospital. He is unable to understand the severity of his father's injuries. Tracie elects not to try to take Tyler to see his dad until he is in a little less critical state.

Episode 5

Tyler wants somebody to play with him but nobody – not even Tracie – is doing anything with him other than feeding him, bathing him, and putting him to bed. Tyler gets very cranky and throws several temper tantrums this week.

Episode 6

Tyler is happy to see his daddy, but he does not understand why he is in the hospital and why Tracie and Daddy are so sad. Tyler sits on top of his dad on the bed and plays with a stuffed animal; he also shows his dad the book that Mary bought for him.

Episode 7

Tracie has purchased some play dough at the supermarket. She sits down with Tyler at the kitchen table and plays. She makes shapes out of various colors and asks Tyler to match the colors. She sees that he is actually quite good at this skill.

Episode 8

Tyler has a new activity book that Tracie has given to him. The activity book is a book about the body, and Tyler learns how different body parts work. He is able to look at the pictures and point to the body part and state the name; then he shows Tracie the location on her and then himself.

Episode 9

Tracie takes Tyler back to the community health clinic for his second round of HBV, DTaP, Hib, IPV, and PCV immunization. His height and weight are plotted on a growth chart at 33 months. His length is 95 cm (60th percentile) and weight is 14.4 kg (60th percentile).

Episode 10

Tyler has a new place to live. He moves with Tracie to John's apartment. Tyler sees several toys, books, and markers. He immediately sits down and scribbles. Tracie tells Tyler that this is his new home.

Episode 11

Tyler has adjusted to the change in his living environment without any difficulty and considers John's apartment his home. Tracie and John have quickly established a consistent routine for him, and he thrives on this routine. He sees his father, grandmother, and grandfather every day. His favorite stuffed animal is always nearby.

Episode 12

Tyler loves Tracie and John, but he is always very excited to see Daddy. Tracie spends the afternoon making sugar cookies and helps Tyler decorate a special one for Daddy. He puts frosting on the cookie and adds sprinkles to the top. He is very proud to give it to Daddy when he sees him that evening.

Episode 13

Tyler sees his daddy every afternoon or evening at his grandmother's house. He wonders why his father always lies in bed. He can tell his daddy is sad because he doesn't say very much and doesn't want to play.

Episode 14

When he goes to see his father, Tyler actually spends most of his time interacting with his great-grandmother, Mary, or his grandfather, Gil. He especially likes to spend time with his grandfather. Gil takes him to the park to play on the playground equipment, plays ball with him in the yard at their home, and lets Tyler sit on a tall stool to watch as he works in his workshop.

Episode 15

Tyler sees his daddy move from the bed to the wheelchair. He climbs up into his father's lap and laughs with delight as Mark navigates about the house in the wheelchair.

OCAMPO HOUSEHOLD

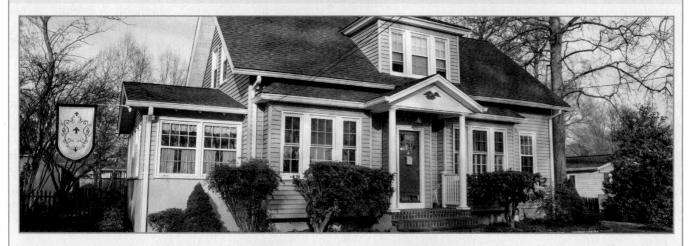

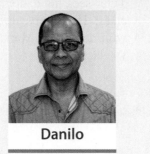

Danilo

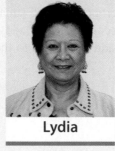

Lydia

Housing	The Ocampos live in a two-story home in Northwoods. Their home is about 20 years old. They have a large yard with a garden and trees.
Parks and Recreation	There is a small park located nearby within the housing development where Danilo takes Lydia for picnics.
Services	There is a golf course nearby where the Ocampos used to play golf. There is also a shopping plaza near the area where they can shop. The Neighborhood Hospital is located several miles away in the downtown area.

Key: ▶ = video clip   ▤ = medical record   ▽ = journal entry   [NEWS] = news article

DANILO OCAMPO

Season 1	Season 2	Season 3
Dr. Ocampo has class II heart failure and is a full-time caregiver to his wife Lydia. This story depicts the day-to-day life of disease management and the caregiver role. Danilo does not want any outside help. He maintains a very consistent schedule for Lydia, and they get along quite well. When Lydia falls and breaks her hip, he spends all of his time at the hospital at her bedside because he is not confident she will get good care without him.	Danilo reluctantly agrees to Lydia's transfer to a rehabilitation hospital. Danilo's perception is that Lydia is receiving poor care at the facility. Eventually she is discharged home. He initially has the help of a niece, but after she leaves, he is unable to care for Lydia. He tires easily and is fatigued. He develops acute exacerbation of heart failure, has a myocardial infarction, and dies.	

Danilo Ocampo Season 1 Information

Episode 1

Dr. Danilo Ocampo is a 74-year-old retired pathologist. He lives in his home with Lydia, his wife of 51 years. Their only child, a son, was killed at age 22 in an automobile accident. Danilo was born and raised in the Philippines and came to the United States when he was 23. He is the last living member of his immediate family. He has a 77-year-old sister-in-law, several nieces and nephews who live in the Philippines, and one grand-niece who attends college in the United States; no relatives live nearby.

Dr. Ocampo's health has been declining for the past few years. He has a medical history that includes hypertension, myocardial infarction, angina, and class II heart failure. Because of these cardiovascular disorders, he takes multiple medications. He has a good understanding of the pharmaceutical properties of the medications. At times, he is not sure he gets good health care because of all the medications he takes. He often does not believe

they are helpful because he experiences many side effects and has required multiple admissions to the hospital. He usually feels better after a few days in the hospital, but he typically checks himself out of the hospital before his physicians are ready to discharge him.

Although at one time in their lives they were very active socially and involved with their church, at this point they rarely go out. A deep-seated cultural value is that appearance is important. With Lydia's dementia, Danilo fears her behavior or appearance may be seen as unacceptable, and he wants to avoid such shame.

Dr. Danilo Ocampo is a full-time caregiver for his wife Lydia who has Alzheimer. He maintains a very consistent schedule for Lydia, and they get along quite well. He has been resistant to outside help, believing he can care for her better than anyone else.

This episode Danilo takes Lydia with him to the store to pick up a prescription refill and other household items they need. While walking through the store, he notices that Lydia is wearing two different shoes, despite the fact that he set her clothes out for her this morning. He hopes nobody will notice! Danilo and Lydia have always followed the tradition of dressing well, particularly in public, so mismatched shoes are an embarrassment. He looks through some craft supplies to find projects for Lydia to work on at home.

Episode 2

One of Danilo's favorite hobbies that he is able to maintain while caring for Lydia is gardening. He has always kept a meticulous lawn and flower garden. While outside weeding, Danilo experiences angina pain. He immediately sits down, takes out a nitroglycerin tablet, and places it under his tongue to dissolve, noting a slight burning sensation. Within a few minutes the chest pain subsides, and he goes in the house to rest ▼.

Episode 3

Danilo has a typical week at home and is feeling pretty good. On one day this week, he goes to the bank, grocery store, and home super center for some basic items. He rarely leaves Lydia for more than 1 hour at a time when running errands. While out, he calls her to be sure she is fine. When he comes home, he finds she has removed her shirt and is sitting on the couch watching TV. The vacuum cleaner, which was in the closet when he left, is a few feet away. He asks her why she is not wearing a shirt. She laughs and says, "I don't know!" She also does not know why the vacuum cleaner is out ▼.

Episode 4

Danilo encourages Lydia to do some things in the kitchen. He recognizes that her Alzheimer's disease is causing continued mental decline and hopes his efforts will keep her as functional as possible. He also recognizes that she is past the point at which she could live by herself and decides he probably needs to meet with an attorney to discuss care for Lydia, should he precede her in death. He has never formalized any such documents in the past ▼ [NEWS].

Episode 5

This week, while out grocery shopping, Danilo hands Lydia the list of things they need to buy and he asks her to help by reading the list and crossing off the items they place in the basket. Danilo does this purposefully to help Lydia with cognitive skills and to assess changes in her cognitive function. While waiting in the checkout line, one of the neighbors from down the street stops to say hello. Danilo can tell Lydia does not recognize him and he quickly covers for her by saying to Lydia "Lydia, do you remember me telling you about their trip?" Danilo then gathers their things and tells him goodbye. He hopes Lydia's dementia is not outwardly noticeable ▶.

Episode 6

Dr. Ocampo has an appointment with his attorney, Mr. Wolf, to discuss planning for Lydia in the event of his death. He is encouraged to write a living will and durable power of attorney. He also discusses in general terms how best to manage her health care. He is encouraged to explore life care communities, board and care homes, and assisted living facilities. Although he does not make any immediate decisions, he knows he needs to get serious about doing something for Lydia ▼.

Episode 7

Danilo gets out Lydia's knitting supplies and suggests she make something. Lydia struggles to think about something to make. He tells Lydia their niece, Kristina, has a birthday coming up and perhaps she could make her a scarf. Lydia has knitted for years, and Danilo tries to give her projects to work on that she can easily do. She spends all day working on the scarf. She proudly shows him the scarf when finished. He asks her who the scarf is for, and Lydia becomes frustrated when she cannot remember. Danilo gently reminds her that the scarf is for their niece Kristina. He helps her wrap the scarf and gets it ready to mail ▼.

Episode 8

Because the weather is beautiful, Danilo goes through the drive-through of a fast-food restaurant to pick up some chicken and then takes Lydia to a park for a picnic. Lydia does not say much, but he enjoys spending a quiet afternoon with her out of the house.

Episode 9

Danilo gets up early in the morning and takes a shower while Lydia is sleeping. When he is finished he returns to the bedroom and notices Lydia is no longer in bed. He walks through the kitchen, dining room, the guest bedrooms, and bathrooms. Lydia is nowhere to be found. He goes to the living room and notices the front door is open and suddenly realizes she may have gone outside. He looks in the yard and still does not see her. Down the street he spots her walking in the middle of the road, still wearing her red robe and pink slippers. He rushes down the street to get her, hoping none of the neighbors will see her. In the midst of all this, he experiences angina pain. He has to ignore the pain until he gets Lydia safely back inside the house. Danilo immediately places a nitroglycerin tablet under his tongue and gets no pain relief after five minutes. He takes a second nitroglycerin pill and is relieved when the pain begins to subside.

Episode 10

Danilo wakes up in the middle of the night to the screams of his wife. He finds her on the floor in the bathroom and recognizes from the position of her leg that she has broken her hip. He calls for an ambulance to take her to the emergency department. The day of her surgery, Danilo spends the entire day at the hospital. He is concerned that nobody will know how to best care for his wife. She is confused, and he can see that she is scared. He tries to calm her as best he can. Eventually, late that evening, he goes home exhausted and not feeling well himself.

The next morning, Danilo arrives at the hospital at about 10 a.m. He finds Lydia in restraints, yelling for help. Her breakfast tray is untouched. Danilo is frantic and calls for the nurse. Lydia's primary nurse is Bobby. Danilo complains to him about the current condition of his wife and the poor care she is receiving. Bobby tries to explain that there had been an emergency on the floor that morning and that the restraints were necessary to keep Lydia safe. Danilo removes the restraints, cleans Lydia up, and feeds her breakfast. A nursing technician comes by the room. She tells Danilo she had not fed Lydia or bathed her yet today because she knew Danilo would come to the hospital this morning, and she figured he would prefer to feed and bathe his wife. Danilo feels angry and decides he cannot trust the hospital staff to care for Lydia.

Episode 11

Danilo has had a frustrating and exhausting week. Lydia remains in the hospital with complications stemming from her surgery. He becomes very anxious about Lydia's care and has ongoing arguments with the nursing and medical staff. He asks many individuals the same questions about her condition, care, and plans for discharge, but he gets different answers from everyone. He feels he must be at the hospital during meal times, or Lydia will not eat. It is Danilo's perception that her complications have resulted from inappropriate care and that he needs to get her out of the hospital and back home if she is to survive.

Danilo spends as much time at the hospital as he can. As a result, he quits attending to his own self-care. He has become increasingly short of breath and is very fatigued. He notices his legs have become edematous. Danilo goes to the drugstore to use the "self-serve" blood pressure machine and finds his blood pressure is elevated (152/106 mm Hg). Still, he resists the idea of seeing his physician or going to the emergency department, for fear of being admitted. Instead, he increases his dose of Furosemide (Lasix) and lisinopril by one-half tablet each per day and tries to get a bit more rest ▼.

Episode 12

Danilo continues to be short of breath and fatigued, but the swelling in his legs has lessened. He also checks his blood pressure at a drugstore and finds that it has dropped to 142/98 mm Hg, which he finds acceptable. He reduces his medication doses to normal levels. While he is at

the hospital, Zainah Kattan, the staff nurse assigned to Lydia's care, and a student nurse ask him how he is feeling. He tells them the focus of their care should be Lydia, not him. He later feels bad for being short-tempered with the nurses.

A discharge planning meeting is held a few days later to discuss arrangements for Lydia to be transferred to a rehabilitation hospital as soon as a bed is available. Danilo argues with the discharge coordinator and nurse, Bobby Schofield, about taking her home so that he can take care of her properly. He is especially concerned about her decline in cognitive function since being hospitalized. He is quite sure this will improve if he can just get her home.

Danilo becomes annoyed when the student nurse, Jennifer Porter (who happens to be in the meeting), speaks up and tells the discharge coordinator that Danilo has been looking very tired. The discharge coordinator reinforces to him that the care she will receive at the rehabilitation hospital will be excellent, will facilitate her recovery, and will allow him needed rest. Knowing he is unlikely to win this battle, Danilo reluctantly agrees. Deep down he knows he has pushed his limits in the past few weeks ▶.

Episode 13

A bed finally becomes available at the rehabilitation hospital, and Lydia is transferred there. Danilo notices she has become more confused again. Because of the experiences at the other hospital, Danilo is not trusting of the care Lydia will receive. He spends most of his time at the rehabilitation hospital and talks with the staff frequently about Lydia's needs and care.

Because of the amount of time Danilo has spent at the hospital, Danilo has had very little time to keep the house in order. He feels ashamed when he thinks about how poorly the house looks. Reluctantly, Danilo hires a housekeeper to come to the house twice a week. His mood improves when he comes home to a clean home.

Episode 14

Danilo is unhappy with the lack of progress he has seen during the week Lydia has been at the rehabilitation hospital. She is still confused. The hospital staff gets her out of bed frequently, and she yells and cries. He wishes they would leave her alone so she could rest and wonders if they remember that she is an old woman with a broken hip.

Danilo continues to go back and forth between the hospital and his home. He feels exhausted and frequently is short of breath from trying to take care of his wife at the hospital. Although the housekeeper is helpful, he still has things to take care of at home. He does not take his medications consistently, has a hard time sleeping, and gets little rest. Danilo experiences several episodes of angina, which he manages successfully with nitroglycerin.

He goes to the physician's office without an appointment and is seen by a nurse practitioner. He makes it clear that he will not agree to being admitted, but he feels as though he'd better check in, given his ongoing symptoms. The nurse practitioner auscultates his heart and lungs, noting fine crackles in the lower bases bilaterally; no extra heart sounds are noted. She also observes pitting 3+ edema in the lower extremities. The nurse practitioner tells Danilo he really should be admitted and tries to talk him into an overnight stay to help reduce his symptoms. When he refuses, the nurse practitioner makes several suggestions that would offer social support, such as Meals on Wheels to help minimize the stress of keeping up his home. After checking his potassium level (3.9 mEq/L), she increases his Furosemide (Lasix) and lisinopril to the maximum dose levels and asks Danilo to come back to see her the following week.

Episode 15

Danilo continues to feel tired and frequently experiences angina. He believes if he could take Lydia home he would feel better because he wouldn't have to do all of the running around that he does. He also believes he can take better care of her than the people at the rehabilitation hospital and continues to argue with the nursing and medical staff about the care she receives. The discharge coordinator meets with him and tries to help him understand the progress that Lydia is making. Danilo does not believe that she is progressing all that much.

Danilo Ocampo Season 2 Information

Episode 1

Dr. Ocampo's wife has dementia, and she recently has suffered a hip fracture. She spent several weeks at Neighborhood Hospital and more recently was admitted to the rehabilitation hospital. Danilo has been very distressed about the care Lydia has received and her increased level of confusion. It is his opinion that she has not been well cared for, and he wants to bring her home to take care of her himself.

Throughout Lydia's hospital and rehabilitation experiences, Danilo has kept the family back in the Philippines informed about Lydia's condition. Lydia's sister tells Danilo they could come to the Philippines so that more family members would be available to help him care for Lydia. Danilo knows that relocating her to the Philippines would not be in Lydia's best interest. As an alternative, Lydia's sister suggests that her granddaughter, Kristina, come to stay with them for a few months. Danilo welcomes the offer of help from a family member. Danilo speaks with the medical staff about discharging Lydia and tells them that his niece is coming to stay with them to help care for Lydia. They agree to a discharge next week.

Episode 2

Danilo's grand-niece, Kristina, has arrived to stay with them. She is the granddaughter of Lydia's sister. Kristina is a college student and is between semesters. Danilo is very happy to bring Lydia home and feels sure that she will improve once she is back home.

Episode 3

Danilo is happy to have Kristina at their home to help him. She not only has been caring for Lydia, but she has also been taking care of many things around the home. Danilo is feeling more rested than he has for the past couple months. He continues to employ the housekeeper so that Kristina can have more time to spend with Lydia.

Episode 4

Danilo talks with Lydia's sister (Kristina's grandmother) by phone to give the family an update about Lydia's condition. Danilo tells her that Lydia is doing much better now that she is home and since she is being taken care of by Kristina. Lydia's sister tells Danilo more members of the family will plan to come to the United States to take care of Lydia, but Danilo says they are doing fine right now, and maybe in the upcoming months their help might be needed.

Episode 5

Danilo continues to feel good. He has energy, and the swelling in his legs has subsided. He is aware that Kristina's school break is coming to an end. She offers to take a semester off from school to stay with them longer. Although he likes having Kristina around to help, he knows she feels a sense of obligation because they are considered the elders. Danilo knows that Kristina needs to continue her education and he believes that he can take care of Lydia independently. He encourages her to go back home.

Episode 6

Danilo is somewhat surprised at how much work it takes to care for Lydia. Since Kristina left, Danilo has not been able to sleep very well because Lydia is often awake at night. He also finds that keeping up with the laundry, shopping, and preparing meals is tiring. He did not appreciate just how much Kristina was helping until she left. Despite this, Danilo is sure they will manage just fine ▾.

Episode 7

Danilo is very concerned about the need to keep Lydia looking as good as possible. Personal appearance is a deeply embedded value among Filipinos, and Lydia would feel a great deal of shame if she were aware of how she looks. He wonders how Kristina was able to keep her hair looking so good. Danilo takes her to a hair salon to get her hair done right. Danilo continues to have several episodes of angina that he treats with nitroglycerin tablets ▾.

Episode 8

Danilo has not kept up with management of his own health. For example, he has not consistently taken his medications and is not getting adequate rest. During the middle of the night this week, Lydia attempted to leave the house. Because of situations such as this, Danilo is unable to sleep well. He attributes his poor sleeping patterns to caring for Lydia, but he also is not sleeping well because of orthopnea. He experiences shortness of breath frequently while awake and has noticed an increase in edema in his legs over the past couple of weeks.

Episode 9

Danilo has been feeling progressively more fatigued. He is unable to sleep more than a few hours at a time. Twice this week he has had episodes of angina, which he promptly treats with nitroglycerin. He knows he should make an appointment with his cardiologist, but he becomes concerned that, if he is admitted to the hospital, Lydia could be sent away from their home for care. He decides to self-manage by increasing his dose of furosemide (Lasix). He feels better the following day. He is well aware his condition is not optimal and is now considering arranging for a home health assistant to come to the home each day to help with Lydia's personal care [NEWS].

Episode 10

Danilo ran out of his lisinopril medication last week. Although he called in for a refill, he has been too tired to drive to the drugstore to pick up his prescription. He is feeling increasingly fatigued and short of breath. The leg edema has increased significantly over the past couple of days, and he again self-medicates with furosemide (Lasix). Following a sleepless night, Danilo continues to feel even more fatigued. He is too tired to help Lydia with anything. He begins to cough and experiences slight pressure in his chest. This is relieved, but the sensation soon returns. Within a few hours, he is coughing up blood-tinged, frothy sputum and realizes he is in trouble. Danilo calls 9-1-1.

Paramedics respond to the Ocampo home about 15 minutes after the call. By this point, Danilo is extremely anxious and somewhat confused. The paramedics note his vital signs (respiratory rate 36 breaths/minute; heart rate 132 beats/minute; blood pressure 100/60 mm Hg; oxygen saturation 85%). They immediately placed him on oxygen and a cardiac monitor. They note that he is in sinus tachycardia. An intravenous line is started, and 4 mg of morphine sulfate and 80 mg of furosemide (Lasix) are administered.

The paramedics transport Danilo to the emergency department (ED). In the ED, Dr. Gordon quickly makes a diagnosis of acute heart failure and myocardial infarction. Danilo's condition further deteriorates shortly after arriving in the ED. He goes into ventricular fibrillation and, despite exceptional emergency care and resuscitative efforts, Dr. Danilo Ocampo dies ☰ ▶ [NEWS].

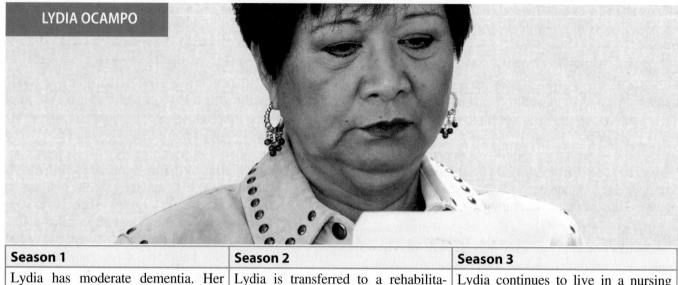

LYDIA OCAMPO

Season 1	Season 2	Season 3
Lydia has moderate dementia. Her husband cares for her in the home, and she rarely goes out in public. The consistent routine at home that Danilo provides helps Lydia function at an optimal level. Lydia falls and breaks her hip in episode 10 and is admitted to the hospital for an ORIF. Confusion escalates at the hospital. Issues managing her post-op pain, nausea, infection, and anemia also present.	Lydia is transferred to a rehabilitation hospital for continued care. She receives appropriate care, yet she continues to be more confused than she was prior to her fall. A niece comes to help with her care when she is discharged home. After Danilo dies, she is placed in a nursing home.	Lydia continues to live in a nursing home. She has no visitors. She gradually declines, due to lack of mobility and poor nutrition. She becomes confined to bed, does not eat, becomes incontinent, and develops a decubitus ulcer. Lydia eventually dies.

Lydia Ocampo Season 1 Information

Episode 1

Lydia Ocampo is a 69-year-old female who has been married to Danilo for 51 years. Their only child, Emilio, was killed at age 22 in an automobile accident. His death devastated Lydia, but over time she adjusted adequately and coped with the loss. Lydia was born and raised in the Philippines and came to the United States with Danilo when she was 18. Lydia has one 77-year-old sister who is still alive, but all of her other 8 brothers and sisters have passed away. She has several nieces and nephews still living in the Philippines whom they have not seen in years and one grand-niece who is attending college in the United States. She and Danilo have no relatives nearby.

Lydia's overall physical health is good, and her only known condition is Alzheimer's disease. She has had dementia for several years. Her husband is her caregiver, and she benefits from the consistent routine that he provides. Lydia rarely socializes and spends most of her time at home. She is fully ambulatory and feeds, dresses, and toilets herself. She is often confused and is easily distracted.

This episode Danilo places Lydia's clothes on the bed so she can get dressed to go to the store with him. She puts on one shoe and then goes to the closet to find another shoe. She ends up wearing mismatched shoes - a brown slip-on shoe and a blue sandal. While walking in the store with Danilo, he asks her about the shoes and she is surprised to see that they don't match.

Episode 2

Lydia is out in the yard with Danilo, helping him pull weeds. She loves being outside and listening to the birds sing. She cannot remember which plants are weeds and which plants should not be pulled, so she asks him over and over if she can pull a plant out.

Episode 3

Danilo leaves Lydia at home for about an hour while he runs errands. He assures her that he will only be gone for a little while. While he is out, Danilo calls Lydia and tells her that he will be home soon. Although Lydia had forgotten he had left the house, she tells him she is doing just fine. She gets out the vacuum cleaner to do some cleaning and unsuccessfully tries to turn it on, not realizing it is not plugged in. Frustrated, she just leaves it and sits down to watch TV. For no particular reason she removes her shirt. When Danilo comes home, he helps her put her shirt back on and puts the vacuum cleaner in the closet.

Episode 4

Lydia helps Danilo make dinner. She is still able to do many routine things in the kitchen herself, but with assistance. Unassisted, Lydia may do such things as place food to be baked in the refrigerator instead of in the oven, leave burners on, or put food items in the dishwasher. With verbal cues, she is better able to stay on track. While in the kitchen preparing dinner, Lydia is getting ready to heat soup on the stove and places a plastic container on the burners. Danilo reminds her to use a saucepan instead of a plastic bowl. She comments on how silly she is. After dinner is over, Lydia begins to empty the dishwasher (before it has run) and starts putting dirty dishes away in the cupboards. She gets stuck when she can't remember where plates go. Danilo stops her and tells her the dishwasher has not yet cleaned the dishes ▶.

Episode 5

Lydia goes to the grocery store with Danilo. She is charged with reading the grocery list. Lydia proudly locates many of the items and places them in the basket. She gets somewhat agitated when she can't locate canned green beans. She picks up several cans of vegetables without being able to differentiate green beans specifically.

While in the checkout line, a man starts talking to Danilo. She does not recognize him, but thinks that she should. After they leave Danilo reminds her that the man is their neighbor. She does not remember that he is a neighbor, but she recognized him.

Episode 6

Lydia goes into the den to watch television. Several of her favorite television shows come on in the middle of the day, yet she cannot remember the names of any of them. She becomes frustrated because she can't figure out how to turn on the television. Danilo turns on the television; noting her frustration, he tells her that he finds the remote controls confusing, too ▽.

Episode 7

One of the things Lydia has done for years is knit. Danilo keeps her well supplied with yarn so that she can keep busy with projects. She spends all day knitting a scarf for her niece as a birthday gift. She proudly shows it to Danilo when she is finished. He asks her who the scarf is for, and Lydia becomes frustrated when she cannot remember. Danilo gently reminds her that the scarf is for their niece Kristina. He helps her wrap the scarf and get it ready for mailing.

Episode 8

Lydia goes with Danilo for a picnic. She enjoys being outside and watching the animals. She sees a playground and thinks about her son, Emilio. She wonders aloud if he has come home from school yet. Danilo reminds her that he died many years ago. She then remembers he died and feels sad, but she still wants to go home to be sure that he is not home alone.

Episode 9

Shortly after waking up in the morning, Lydia wonders where her son, Emilio, is. She looks in the house and then determines he must be outside. She opens the front door and walks out into the street, calling his name. A short while later, Danilo is at her side and tells her she needs to go home. She protests, telling him they must find Emilio. He reminds her again that he died a long time ago.

Episode 10

During the middle of the night, Lydia gets out of bed to urinate. While rushing to the bathroom, she experiences urinary leakage. Her foot slips on the floor, causing her to fall on the ceramic tile floor, hitting the toilet and edge of the tub on the way down. She screams in pain, awakening Danilo. An ambulance takes her to the emergency department, where she is diagnosed with a left hip fracture. She is sent to the operating room for an open reduction internal fixation (ORIF) of the left hip. She is admitted to the medical-surgical floor following surgery.

When Lydia wakes up, she finds a dramatic change in her surroundings and is extremely confused. She does not know where she is or what is happening to her. She is in a strange room, in a strange bed. There are strange sounds and smells all around her. She is in pain. She feels nauseous and vomits several times. She has uncomfortable tubes in her arms. She attempts to resolve this by pulling them away from her body, but they are quickly replaced. A large object is placed between her legs, making it difficult for her to change positions and get comfortable. Strangers come into her room and do things to her regularly. She tries to fight them off to protect herself. She yells frequently for somebody to help her and speaks in Tagalog, her native language. She tries to get out of bed to escape the situation, only to be scolded. Although she is fairly calm when Danilo is with her, she is often restrained when he is not present. When Lydia is tied up, she becomes terrified and cries for help. She refuses to eat unless Danilo feeds her, because she is afraid that the strangers are trying to poison her 🗏 ▶.

Episode 11

Lydia remains at the hospital because she has developed an infection in her incision and needs intravenous antibiotics and dressing changes. She is pale, and her hemoglobin and hematocrit have dropped to 7 g/dL and 30%, respectively; thus, she requires a transfusion of 2 units of packed red blood cells for anemia. Her oral intake has been inadequate, but she has been well hydrated by the intravenous fluids. She has been incontinent ever since the Foley catheter was removed. Attempts at physical therapy have been unproductive. The physical therapists are successful at transferring her from the bed to a chair, but this requires nearly full assistance.

She continues to be more confused than she was when at home but is calmer than she was immediately after surgery. However, the nursing staff often finds her to be uncooperative. Danilo is with her much of the time, and she finds his presence and the sound of his voice comforting.

Episode 12

Lydia remains at Neighborhood Hospital. She is still confused, but she is beginning to recognize some of the nurses and is becoming familiar with the routine on the floor. She no longer has an IV, but she still is getting wet-to-damp dressing changes to the incisional wound. The wound is no longer infected and is beginning to heal. Lydia's hemoglobin and hematocrit levels are still low (10 g/dL and 36%), but within an acceptable range. She still has not progressed with physical therapy, but she is more cooperative when they come to work with her than she was last week. Her nutritional intake improves, particularly when Danilo is present to feed her. She remains incontinent.

Episode 13

Some strangers come into Lydia's room, place her on a hard cart, and put her in the back of a van. She is sure she is being kidnapped. She yells and tells the intruders to leave her alone. She is wheeled into another building and placed in another room and a different bed. Her confusion increases for several days after her transfer to the rehabilitation hospital.

Episode 14

Lydia remains in the rehabilitation hospital, where she is receiving excellent care from the nursing staff. She is placed on a very consistent routine, which has resulted in improvements in her nutritional intake. She is also beginning to make progress with physical therapy by getting out of bed regularly and using the toilet. Although she is still more confused than she had been at home, her level of confusion has decreased dramatically.

Episode 15

Lydia continues to progress well at the rehabilitation hospital.

Lydia Ocampo Season 2 Information

Episode 1

Lydia has Alzheimer's disease and, until recently, she experienced relatively good health. A few months ago, she fell and broke her hip. She spent several weeks at Neighborhood Hospital. Her recovery was slow due to a number of postoperative complications that included anemia, nutritional deficits, a wound infection, and a high level of confusion. In recent weeks, she was admitted to a rehabilitation hospital, where she is making progress, both nutritionally and from a mobility standpoint. At this time, she remains confused. She needs assistance ambulating, bathing, toileting, and getting dressed. Her appetite has improved, but she requires verbal cues and encouragement to eat.

Danilo comes to see her every day. Danilo tells Lydia she needs to work on getting out of the rehabilitation hospital. He tells her Kristina will be coming. Lydia lights up, recalling the name of her great niece [NEWS].

Episode 2

Lydia is discharged home. She recognizes her surroundings but remains confused and requires full care. A girl is in the home caring for her, but she does not remember who she is. She asks the girl if she knows her son Emilio. Kristina tells Lydia over and over again she is her niece.

Episode 3

Under Kristina's care, Lydia makes great progress in her recovery. Kristina tells Lydia about what is happening with family members. Lydia is delighted to hear about the family, although she is still somewhat confused. Sometimes she seems to know who Kristina is, and some days Lydia asks her 4 or 5 times who she is and what she is doing. Lydia is beginning to eat well. She likes the food prepared by Kristina. She is also gradually becoming more independent, although she still requires help with mobility.

Episode 4

Kristina has done a superb job getting Lydia in a consistent routine and sensing when Lydia is getting overly tired. She has quickly learned that Lydia is sharpest when she is well rested. Kristina also recognizes that some of

Lydia's long-term memory is intact, so she spends time with Lydia talking about past events.

Episode 5

Although Lydia continues to require assistance with ambulation, she is using a walker and is eating independently now. Kristina has enjoyed caring for Lydia and has been pleased with her progress. She leaves this week to go back to school. Lydia does not understand why she left, but she misses her. She believes Kristina may have been her sister.

Episode 6

Lydia is missing the ongoing activity and stimulation she received with her niece. Danilo gets her out of bed, but she ends up sitting in a chair and sleeping off and on most of the day. She gets up to go to the bathroom with his help and she sits in the kitchen with him while he prepares their meals. She feels frustrated and agitated when she tries to tell Danilo something and can't remember what she wants to say or can't remember how to do something. The housecleaner who comes to the home twice a week has to reintroduce herself to Lydia each time she is there 🟥NEWS.

Episode 7

Each morning, Danilo puts out Lydia's clothes. He encourages her to dress herself as much as possible and then helps her finish. She also does as much of her own personal hygiene as she can and sometimes does not recognize when she forgets steps in a process – such as putting toothpaste on a toothbrush. Danilo repeats instructions over and over to Lydia so she can complete as many tasks as possible. Sometimes it takes nearly two hours for Lydia to get bathed and dressed.

Episode 8

During one night this week, Lydia gets out of bed, walks through the house completely naked, and attempts to go out the front door. Danilo hears her trying to open the door and directs her back to bed. Fearing that she might do this again, Danilo sleeps very little the rest of the night. The next day, Lydia thinks she hears her son, Emilio, and attempts to go out the front door to find him ▶.

Episode 9

Lydia has not slept at night for a week now. Her confusion has increased to the point that she is unaware of the time of day – although she is aware she is at home. She attempts to get up out of bed, and Danilo either puts her back in bed or helps her up and sits with her until she is ready to sleep. She frequently calls Danilo "Emilio." Danilo patiently reminds her that Emilio died a long time ago.

Episode 10

This past week, Lydia has only been out of bed to use the restroom. Danilo has been too tired to help her, and she has not independently made the effort to get up. She also has not eaten very much. When paramedics respond to the 9-1-1 call, they find Lydia curled up in bed. She asks them who they are and begins to yell when they put her on a cold, hard cart. She is sure the men are going to kill her. At the emergency department, the nurse tells Lydia her husband has died and attempts to elicit information regarding next of kin. Lydia is unable to answer the questions.

Because there is no medical need for hospital admission, Lydia remains in the emergency department for 30 hours while the hospital social workers work with local authorities to get her an emergency placement into a nursing home.

Episode 11

Lydia remains at the nursing home. She is persistently confused and alternates between being passive and uncooperative. During the past few weeks, a case manager has been working on Lydia's case. She is able to locate paperwork in the home and in a safety deposit box. She also finds the name of Danilo's attorney, Mr. Frank Wolf, and contacts him. The case worker attempts to contact Lydia's 77-year-old sister in the Philippines to inform her of Danilo's death and Lydia's situation. She first dials a phone number left in the files, but the person who answers the phone does not speak good English. The case worker is unsure who the person is or if the person understands the conversation. A letter is prepared and mailed to the sister.

Episode 12

In the several weeks she has been in the nursing home, Lydia has become progressively dependent on her caregivers and accuses them of being her kidnappers.

Danilo's attorney, Mr. Wolf, is contacted this week by the case manager. Although Danilo never made any decisions regarding care for Lydia, he did give Mr. Wolf power of attorney in the event he or Lydia was unable to make decisions independently. Because of the discussion he had with Danilo in the months preceding his death, Mr. Wolf elects to keep Lydia in the nursing home facility and proceeds with trust-related activities.

Episode 13

Lydia remains in the nursing home. She has lost her sense of time and does not know where she has been or how she ended up here. She does not trust any of the nursing personnel and is uncooperative about basic hygiene and eating.

Episode 14

Lydia remains in the nursing home. She is placed in a wheelchair and is taken to the dining hall for each meal. After her meal, she either sits in a wheelchair in the hall or lies in bed in her room. Lydia has become progressively less responsive, and her nutritional status has gradually declined.

Episode 15

Lydia remains in the nursing home. She sleeps a good part of the day while sitting in a wheelchair. At night, she often cries out for help and does not understand why nobody will help her. She is sometimes incontinent and the nursing staff places her in diapers. She finds the diapers hot and uncomfortable and often pulls them off. Some of the nursing aides scold her for misbehaving.

Lydia Ocampo Season 3 Information

Episode 1

Lydia is a 70-year-old widow who currently lives at a nursing home. She has Alzheimer's disease, and her health has steadily declined in the past year. She has been in the nursing home for several months now and has become completely dependent. Her attorney, Mr. Wolf, has Power of attorney over Lydia and is overseeing her care. He has proceeded with the process of selling the family home. The money will be placed in a trust to care for Lydia until she dies.

In this episode Lydia's grand-niece contacts the social worker involved in Lydia's case. Her grandmother (Lydia's sister) received the letter from the social worker informing her of the situation but had to find somebody to translate the letter. She then asked Kristina to contact the social worker to learn more about the situation. After learning that Lydia is in a nursing home, Kristina calls the nursing home to get information about her care, but she is told they cannot provide information about Lydia. Frustrated, Kristina contacts the social worker again who refers her to Mr. Wolf. After speaking with the social worker, Kristina talks with her grandmother again who urges Kristina to travel to the Neighborhood and bring Lydia home to the Philippines.

Episode 2

Lydia remains in the nursing home. She has become fairly unresponsive to her caregivers. She sleeps often and only gets up out of bed when the nursing assistants get her up. She has developed a decubitus ulcer over her sacrum.

Episode 3

An estate sale was held at Danilo and Lydia's home last week. The home was listed for sale and is purchased by a middle-aged couple who are in the process of relocating to the community. Proceeds from the sale of the home have been placed in a trust for Lydia's ongoing medical care.

Episode 4

Lydia's grand-niece, Kristina, has a few days' break from her college courses and pulls enough money together to travel to the Neighborhood. She goes to the nursing home where Lydia is and is shocked to see her condition. Lydia does not recognize Kristina and interacts very little with her. Kristina sees her in diapers and can see she has a decubitus ulcer. Kristina feels like all of this is her fault. She feels a great deal of shame for leaving her great aunt and uncle and returning to school. She feels that if she had stayed to take care of Lydia, none of this would have happened.

Kristina tells the manager of the nursing home that she would like to make arrangements to take Lydia home with her to the Philippines. She is told the manager cannot legally release Lydia, because Mr. Wolf has the legal authority over her care. Kristina makes an appointment to see him.

Episode 5

Kristina is able to get an appointment with Mr. Wolf. She tells Mr. Wolf she wants to take Lydia out of the nursing home and take her to the Philippines. Mr. Wolf questions the logic of this request, given Lydia's condition. Mr. Wolf also questions the circumstances of care for Lydia in the Philippines. He tells Kristina that he has a legal duty and obligation to carry out the wishes of Danilo and that there was no mention of Kristina or of Lydia's going to the Philippines. Kristina asks if she can just take Lydia home to care for her in the United States, but she acknowledges her apartment is not set up for this. Since the Ocampo's home has been sold, she has no local accommodations to care for her great-aunt, either.

Episode 6

Lydia sleeps most of time. She does not get out of bed very often. When she is placed in a wheelchair, she often falls asleep. She is not interested in eating or communicating. She talks very infrequently and has become completely dependent for all aspects of her care. Despite efforts to turn her, Lydia's ulcer has increased in size. A wound care nurse comes to see her for ulcer management.

Episode 7

Lydia's grand-niece, Kristina, has convinced Mr. Wolf, the attorney, to provide travel funds from the estate that allow her to travel back and forth from school to visit Lydia and to help care for her in the nursing home. Mr. Wolf also gives permission to the nursing home to allow Kristina access to her medical condition and care. This seems to be the best option. Kristina no longer feels guilty for abandoning her great-aunt, and she is able to communicate with her grandmother in the Philippines about what is happening with Lydia. Kristina arranges to spend every other weekend with Lydia. Lydia sleeps most of the time while she is there, but Kristina makes good use of her time by studying.

Episode 8

Lydia has very poor nutritional intake, and the decubitus ulcer has not responded well to treatment. She is completely incontinent of urine and stool and now does not get out of bed at all. Despite attempts to feed her, she eats very little. Mr. Wolf, Lydia's attorney, is informed of her declining condition, and a do-not-resuscitate order is obtained. Mr. Wolf contacts Kristina and lets her know of Lydia's deteriorating condition.

Episode 9

Kristina is with Lydia all weekend. Lydia is awake periodically but does not communicate or respond at all to Kristina's presence. Kristina talks with her mother (who lives in the Philippines) via web communication on her smart phone and shares Lydia's condition this way so that the family can better understand the situation.

Episode 10

A nursing assistant taking morning vital signs walks into Lydia's room and finds that Lydia has died during the night. The nursing staff contact Kristina, letting her know that Lydia has died. Mr. Wolf is also contacted, and he prepares a letter notifying Lydia's sister of her passing.

REYES HOUSEHOLD

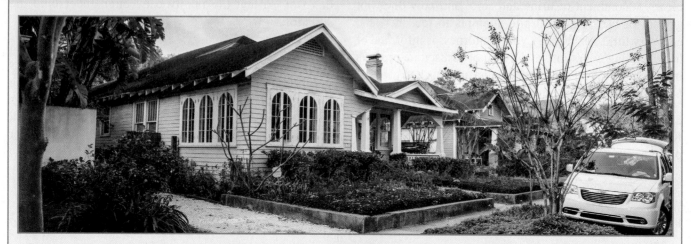

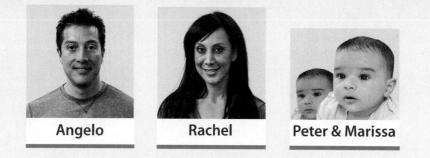

Angelo   **Rachel**   **Peter & Marissa**

Housing	The Reyes family lives in a one-story home in Northwoods district. Their home is about 5 years old.
Parks and Recreation	There is a fitness center nearby where Angelo works out regularly. There is a golf course located in the Northwoods area, as well as walking trails near the lake.
Services	There is an upscale shopping plaza located near the Reyes home. The Neighborhood women's center is also close to their home.

Key: ▶ = video clip   ☰ = medical record   ▽ = journal entry   [NEWS] = news article

ANGELO REYES

Season 1	Season 2	Season 3
Angelo is a healthy male with well-controlled type 1 diabetes mellitus. He and his wife go through infertility workups. The story also addresses his daily management of DM. He has an episode of vitreous hemorrhage with the threat of retinal detachment and undergoes an outpatient vitrectomy procedure.	The story follows his experiences associated with his wife having a high-risk pregnancy. In addition, Angelo gets the flu and develops ketoacidosis. He is treated in the ED and does not require hospitalization.	Angelo is supportive of his wife during her difficult pregnancy, but is frustrated that she won't slow down at the advice of her physician. His babies are born during this season, and the story depicts the stress associated with being a parent of infants in the NICU.

Angelo Reyes Season 1 Information

Episode 1

Angelo Reyes is a 40-year-old Hispanic architect who has been married to Rachel for the past 3 years. He has had type 1 diabetes mellitus since the age of 13. Despite recent advances in diabetic management, he has followed the same treatment plan for a number of years and has been resistant to change because he has had excellent glycemic control. He attributes his successful disease management to a very structured lifestyle. His daily routine is as follows:

- Wakes up at 5:30 a.m. and checks his blood sugar. If within a normal range, he gives himself an insulin injection (22 units Regular/12 units NPH), takes a shower, and gets dressed. He eats a bowl of cereal and a banana each morning for breakfast and leaves the house about 6:30 a.m., arriving at work by 7 a.m.
- At 10 a.m., he eats a snack (usually an apple or raisins).
- At noon, he checks his blood sugar; if it is within normal range, he eats a sandwich and fruit.
- Between 12:30 and 1 p.m., he walks at a park close to his office.
- At 2:30 p.m., he eats another snack (such as a granola bar or soda).

- Leaves the office at 5:30.
- Arrives home by 6 p.m., checks his blood sugar, and administers his evening dose of insulin (16 units Regular/8 units NPH).
- Eats dinner at 6:30 p.m
- Three nights a week, Angelo goes to the gym at 7:30 p.m. to work out. On these evenings, he may slightly decrease the dose of insulin to compensate for the exercise.
- Checks his blood sugar at 9:30 p.m., has a snack of peanut butter and crackers, and goes to bed immediately after the evening news at 10:30.

Since getting married, Angelo's wife has been very anxious to get pregnant and start a family, but they have been unsuccessful. Rachel has extensively researched infertility on the internet and has, in Angelo's opinion, become obsessed with getting pregnant. Although he would like to have a child, he has not been enthusiastic about infertility workups, partially because of the huge expense involved. However, after 3 years without a pregnancy, he agrees to begin the process because he knows how important it is to Rachel ▶ ▽.

Episode 2

Rachel has an initial workup with her gynecologist today. She comes home after the appointment and tells Angelo that he needs to have an examination by an urologist, because (in her words) he may be "the problem." Rachel has the name of an urologist and asks Angelo to make an appointment to get checked ▶.

Episode 3

Angelo calls to make an appointment with the urologist. He is embarrassed when he talks about the reason for the appointment. He tells the scheduler he has been advised to be evaluated as part of an infertility workup. Angelo finds it stressful simply to make the appointment and does not look forward to the process.

Episode 4

Angelo has an appointment with the urologist and needs to take off from work during the morning to go. He does not tell his coworkers why he is gone that morning because he finds the process a major invasion of his privacy. He dreads going to the examination. Because the appointment is at 9:30 a.m., Angelo takes his morning snack with him and ends up eating a box of raisins on the exam table while waiting for the physician to come into the examination room.

The urologist takes a history and learns that Angelo has had type 1 diabetes mellitus (DM) since age 13. Further, it is revealed that Angelo has a positive family history for type 1 DM (his uncle). Angelo's medical history reveals no past exposure to chemicals, no past trauma to his genitalia, no history of sexually transmitted infections, and no history of impotence. A physical examination reveals no abnormalities of his reproductive organs or testes. The urologist gives Angelo lab requisitions for a blood test to assess hormonal levels and a semen analysis. He is instructed to obtain a semen sample within the next couple of weeks, following 48-72 hours of abstinence from ejaculation. Angelo is very embarrassed about this entire process and leaves the physician's office feeling humiliated.

Episode 5

Angelo is notified by the urologist that all of his lab results are normal. He feels relieved that the "problem" does not lie with him. Rachel expresses surprise that his results are normal. Angelo has an A1c test done this week; his level is 7.0% ◣.

Episode 6

Rachel has her first appointment with the infertility specialist this week, and she shares with Angelo every detail about the visit, including all the tests and the general game plan. Angelo wonders just how much this is all going to cost and hopes that, if they are successful, there will be money left over to raise the baby.

Episode 7

Rachel reviews with Angelo the various tests they need to have in the upcoming weeks as part of the infertility workup. She asks him to be sure he arranges time off from work. He can see that this process is not only likely to cost a lot, but also will require flexibility with his work schedule. He elects not to tell anyone in the office about the process they are beginning.

Episode 8

This is the week Rachel has her postcoital exam. Angelo is very embarrassed about the idea that he has to leave work to have sex with his wife, knowing she is going to be examined shortly thereafter. He goes along with this because he knows how important it is to Rachel, but he finds the process very embarrassing. On the day of the test, he fakes having stomach cramps at work so he can have an excuse to go home.

Angelo finds that having sex on demand for a test is not at all enjoyable and is in fact stressful. Additionally, he has to eat lunch earlier than normal and is unable to take his lunchtime walk. Because he is not planning to go back to work, Rachel asks Angelo to go with her to the appointment. He feels embarrassed, knowing the physician is examining his wife right after they had sex. At 2 p.m. Angelo eats his mid-afternoon granola bar snack while in the waiting room and wonders if eating lunch too early will cause problems for him later that day. At 6 p.m. that same evening, Angelo's glucose levels are much higher than normal, and he adjusts his insulin dose. He decides to skip working out at the gym that evening ◣.

Episode 9

Angelo thinks his wife is acting very moody this week. She learns her hormonal levels are the probable cause of the infertility and that she needs to have a hysterosalpingogram. This creates a great deal of tension between the two of them, and Angelo finds the situation very stressful. Angelo also notices that his glucose levels are running consistently higher this week. He has a hard time making the necessary adjustments with his diet and insulin to get it under control.

Episode 10

Angelo has been giving a great deal of thought to the stress he has been experiencing related to the infertility workups. He is quite sure Rachel has also been under a great deal of stress. He mentions to Rachel that the process for infertility seems to be more involved than he imagined and wonders if they should stop pursuing it. Rachel becomes very upset with him for making such comments and points out that she was willing to do an adoption but that he was unwilling to do that, too. As much as Angelo hates to admit it, he realizes he has not been completely fair to Rachel and vows to be more positive ◣.

Episode 11

Rachel tells Angelo about her experience getting the hysterosalpingogram, and he is glad he was not there when she "lost it." He thinks she is taking this whole pregnancy thing a bit too far, but he says nothing.

Episode 12

While at work one morning this week, Angelo notices a "glob" appear in the visual field of his left eye. He calls his ophthalmologist immediately and is told to come into the office.

At the ophthalmologist's office, Angelo describes the vision in his left eye as "patchy" – he sees multiple dark reddish-black spots. Although he is generally still able to see, he can't focus on small details easily. Reading, for example, is difficult. The physician tells Angelo that he is having another vitreous hemorrhage, but this time, he is at risk for retinal detachment. He is advised to have a vitrectomy and is scheduled for the procedure the following day as an outpatient at the hospital. Because he will undergo general anesthesia for the procedure, he may not eat or drink anything after midnight. The procedure is scheduled for 8 a.m.

The next morning, Angelo gets up at 6 a.m. and checks his blood sugar; because it is 124 mg/dL and he is not able to have breakfast before the procedure, he decides to administer one-half of his normal morning dose of insulin. Angelo arrives at the hospital at 7 a.m. and is taken to the outpatient surgery department to prepare for the procedure. At 8:30 a.m., Angelo is still waiting to go to surgery. Rachel asks the nurses about the delay and is told they are waiting for the doctor, but it shouldn't be much longer. At 9 a.m., Angelo is still waiting in the preoperative holding area and begins to get anxious about the effect of the delay on his blood sugar. At his request, the nurse checks his blood glucose level, and it is 108 mg/dL.

By 9:20 a.m., Angelo is in surgery, and the vitrectomy procedure is performed without any complications. By 12:15 p.m., Angelo is ready for discharge. He is given prescriptions for moxifloxacin hydrochloride ophthalmic solution (Vigamox) and prednisolone ophthalmic solution (Pred Forte) and told to avoid strenuous activity for the next couple of days. He is scheduled to see his ophthalmologist the following week.

Episode 13

Angelo elects to take a week off from work following his surgery. He sees the ophthalmologist, who tells Angelo that the surgery was a success and there was no evidence of retinal detachment. Angelo is relieved.

He goes with Rachel for her Biopsy and is glad everything goes smoothly. She is not feeling well after the procedure, so he spends the afternoon with her. He worries a little bit about the amount of work he has missed lately due to his eye surgery and all of Rachel's tests ▼.

Episode 14

Angelo's vision is gradually improving, and he goes back to work this week.

Episode 15

Angelo goes on a vacation with Rachel this week - a Caribbean cruise they booked last year. Had he known he was going to have eye surgery or the infertility tests, Angelo would not have planned the trip. Because a large deposit for the trip was made, he agrees they should still take the trip. He also realizes that if they have a baby there will be few opportunities for a trip like this. Despite his initial reservations, he has a wonderful time on the trip ▼.

Angelo Reyes Season 2 Information

Episode 1

Following her latest visit with the infertility specialist, Rachel tells Angelo she is going to start taking a drug that will help her get pregnant by stimulating ovulation. She tells Angelo that they will have to have sex on specific days for this to work. Angelo does not like the idea of a "sex-on-demand" routine.

Episode 2

Rachel has her ovulation cycle confirmed and is taking her first course of therapy. Rachel wants to have sex twice a day for several days to improve their chances of getting pregnant. He finds this to be a real challenge.

Episode 3

Angelo feels bad for his wife when she has her menstrual period. He has come to believe that having a baby is just not in the cards for them. Although this disappoints him, he can envision a long and happy life without children. He wishes there was something he could do to relieve his wife of the ongoing disappointment that she experiences; he wishes that she could be more accepting of the situation ▼.

Episode 4

Angelo has the A1c test done this week, and his level is 6.7%. He is pleased that he continues to have excellent glycemic control.

Episode 5

Angelo has a terrible time at the company picnic because of the smoky air conditions caused by the nearby forest fires. He is surprised that the picnic was not cancelled. One of his coworkers has Asthma and did not come because of the poor air conditions.

Episode 6

Angelo is shocked and very excited about the news that Rachel is finally pregnant. At the same time, he remains cautious, because he knows things might not work out. Angelo also quickly realizes that a 2-week vacation he secretly planned will fall around Rachel's due date, so it will have to be cancelled. He is glad he did not tell Rachel about it, or she would have felt badly.

Episode 7

Rachel asks Angelo to go with her for her first prenatal visit. He hates to miss work, but he wants to support her in every way that he can. He is excited to see the baby on the ultrasound, but then is shocked when the technician points out the presence of two babies. Twins! Angelo does not know what to think or say.

Episode 8

The flu has been going around the office for the past few weeks. Angelo thinks he has been spared until he wakes up in the morning on Monday feeling achy and tired. Still, he does not feel all that bad, so he decides to go to work. Throughout the day, he feels progressively worse. He leaves work in the mid-afternoon so that he can go home to lie down. Because he is not particularly hungry at dinner, he eats a small meal and accordingly gives himself a reduced dose of insulin.

By late in the evening, Angelo is vomiting and beginning to run a fever. He continues to vomit well into the next day (Tuesday). His entire body aches, and he feels so tired that it's an effort to get out of bed. He sleeps off and on the entire day, only getting up to go to the bathroom to vomit and urinate. Despite not eating, his glucose level is elevated, but he is reluctant to give himself insulin, fearing his glucose levels will plummet. By Wednesday morning, the vomiting subsides. Angelo believes he is on the road to recovery, but he remains very nauseated. He begins urinating frequently but is also drinking a large volume of fluids because he is exceedingly thirsty. Angelo knows he has some catching up to do because of the amount of fluids lost the previous day. He continues to sleep off and on.

When Rachel comes home, she takes Angelo to the Neighborhood Hospital emergency department (ED). By this time, Angelo is in no position to protest. He is treated by Dr. Gordon for acute diabetic ketoacidosis and dehydration. He is treated with fluids and insulin, and then sent home after spending 7 $\frac{1}{2}$ hours in the ED.

Episode 9

Angelo has a follow-up visit with the internal medicine physician who manages his diabetes. They discuss the recent events that led to the diabetic ketoacidosis. Over the past year, the physician has suggested changing Angelo's insulin and dosing, but Angelo has been resistant to changing because of the excellent control he was experiencing. The physician could not argue that point. However, given the recent events, the physician asks if Angelo would consider changing insulin and dosing. Angelo agrees to try the new approach. His new insulin and dosing are: glargine (Lantus) 17 units subcutaneously at bedtime and lispro (Humalog) +/- 14 units subcutaneously at each meal based on blood glucose, anticipated dietary intake, and activity level.

Episode 10

Angelo feels very sorry for Rachel and how bad she is feeling with nausea and fatigue. He wishes he could provide comfort but he feels completely inadequate. He takes care of all the household chores so that she can rest.

Episode 11

Angelo is happy to see that Rachel is back to her usual self. He is pleased that the pregnancy is progressing well and starts to think about how they might arrange the spare bedroom into a nursery.

Angelo has been using his new insulin and dosing schedule for several weeks now and has been pleased with the results. He will know more when he has his next A1c test.

Episode 12

This week is Rachel's birthday. Angelo buys her a diamond bracelet to honor her motherhood. The bracelet is expensive, but he figures this may be one of the last opportunities he has to buy his wife a nice gift. After the babies are born, assuming Rachel stays at home to care for them, they will have to make adjustments to their budget.

Episode 13

Angelo has been busier than usual at work this past week. He has a new project that is very time consuming. To accommodate the need to increase his work hours and yet maintain his schedule, two evenings a week (after coming home and taking his insulin and eating dinner), he goes back to the office from 6:30–9:30 p.m. He is still able to have his evening snack and be in bed by 10:30 p.m. He also decides to go to his office for a few hours over the weekend. He does not like to go back to the office, but he recognizes the need to stay on his regimen.

Episode 14

This week Angelo clears out the spare bedroom to begin preparing a nursery for the babies. Although he thinks it is a little early to do so, Rachel wants to get things ready.

Rachel has selected a "bunny" theme for the nursery. They go shopping for nursery furniture and Rachel picks out many of the accessories ▽.

Episode 15

Rachel talks with Angelo about taking childbirth education classes in the evening next month at the Neighborhood Patient Education Center. He has heard all about such classes from his friends who have become fathers. He is interested in going, but he is not so sure about the process. He is somewhat concerned that the classes will interfere with his evening dinner, insulin, and exercise regimen. He hates the thought of having to make changes when he has established a routine that works so well for him.

Angelo Reyes Season 3 Information

Episode 1

Angelo has been going with Rachel to childbirth classes during the past couple of weeks. He has been able to adjust his schedule so that it does not interfere with his diabetes management too much. He finds the classes very informative, and they make him feel much more a part of the pregnancy. He is excited when Rachel tells him they are going to have a boy and a girl.

Angelo meets with his physician to discuss his diabetes management since changing insulin. His A1c test level is 6.6%, so Angelo considers the new insulin management effective. He has a conversation with the physician about the possibility of getting an insulin pump. He worries that, after the babies are born, he won't be able to stay on the strict schedule he has been following for all these years. After talking with the physician, he decides not to rush into anything and instead will think about it for a while ▽.

Episode 2

Rachel tells Angelo about the babies being in a breech position and that Dr. Tito told her to "slow down." Rachel tells Angelo that Dr. Tito obviously does not know about the real estate business. Angelo reminds Rachel that Dr. Tito does know the pregnancy business. He encourages Rachel to reduce her workload and cut back to part-time until the babies are born. Angelo senses that this is not what Rachel wants to hear.

Episode 3

Angelo suggests to Rachel that she cut back her work to half days - go in at 10 a.m. and leave the office by 2 or 3 p.m. Rachel tells him it just is not possible to do what she needs to take care of with a schedule like that. Instead, she insists she can work in two breaks during the day and has a comfortable couch in her office so she can recline. Angelo is concerned that Rachel is not taking the physician's recommendation very seriously ▽.

Episode 4

Angelo gets a phone call from Rachel. She tells him that Dr. Tito wants to put her in the hospital because of some swelling and a headache, but she doesn't have time for this. Angelo becomes angry with Rachel for putting her career before her well-being and potentially the well-being of the babies. He tells her that refusing hospitalization is not an option, and she needs to do exactly what Dr. Tito suggests.

Episode 5

Angelo can see that Rachel continues to look swollen, especially around her face. When she tells him her headaches have returned, he insists she call Dr. Tito immediately. He leaves work to take her to Dr. Tito's office. Shortly thereafter, he is on his way to the hospital with her, worried that Rachel and the babies are in danger.

Angelo is told that Rachel will have a cesarean section later in the evening. Angelo immediately begins to plan how he will manage his diabetes around the change in his schedule for the day. He is nervous all day as they wait for her surgery, because he knows the babies will be premature and is worried about their survival. He finds the hospital chapel and spends time praying for Rachel and his unborn children. He has never felt such a sense of fear and desperation in his entire life, but he knows he needs to be strong for Rachel.

Angelo is present during the delivery of his children. He is thrilled and scared at the same time. They are so tiny! They are taken to the Neonatal Intensive Care Unit shortly after birth. Angelo stays with Rachel as they complete the procedure, relieved that she is safe ▽ [NEWS].

Episode 6

Angelo is relieved that the babies seem to be doing better. The first few days were very difficult for him, because he felt as though he had no control over the situation. He also felt somewhat helpless in providing emotional comfort to Rachel. He goes with Rachel after work each evening to spend time with the babies ▽.

Episode 7

Angelo continues to go to the hospital each evening after work to see the babies. He can see the gradual improvement in their conditions and is amazed to see how quickly they are growing.

Episode 8

Angelo and Rachel visit their babies at the hospital each day. While at home, Rachel mentions her interest in exploring nursing school in the future. She tells Angelo she can see how fulfilling a career being a nurse could be – especially in comparison to her realtor job. Angelo listens in support. He tells her there will be plenty of time to consider such options in the future, but for now they will have their hands full once the twins are home 🗞.

Episode 9

Angelo is excited to know that the babies are coming home next week. Angelo's mother calls and tells him she wants to visit at their home when the babies leave the hospital. Angelo is reluctant to allow her to come because she is a heavy smoker. He tells her she will be able to see them when they are a little older and agrees to let her see them every day online ▼.

Episode 10

The babies are home at last. Angelo is more than willing to help Rachel, but he is just not sure how to help. He cannot believe the amount of work that goes into taking care of two tiny babies.

Angelo convinces his mother to delay her visit until the babies get a little bigger, and when they will be at a lower risk for an Infection. Angelo's mother is offended at his request, reminding Angelo that she raised him and his brother and did not seem to make her children sick ▼.

Episode 11

Angelo and Rachel continue to adjust to life with two tiny babies. Angelo feels tired from the frequent nighttime feedings and at times wishes he could just get a good night's sleep. He often feels guilty leaving the house to go to work because Rachel is alone at home caring for the babies ▼.

Episode 12

Rachel's mother is visiting this week. Angelo gets along well with his mother-in-law. Although she is very helpful with the babies, having her in their home is a disruption to their routine. Rachel, on the other hand, really seems to be enjoying her mother's help ▼.

Episode 13

Angelo has an A1c test this week and is pleased to learn that his results are 6.5%. He is a bit surprised that the results are that good, because his routine has been altered with the babies being home and having Rachel's mother visiting. Angelo talks with Rachel about the length of her mother's visit and suggests it is time for her to go.

Episode 14

After several weeks, Rachel's mother finally leaves and Angelo and Rachel have the house and the babies to themselves. Angelo was ready for her to leave long ago but she did not seem to pick up on any of his hints that she had been there long enough.

Episode 15

Angelo encourages Rachel to stay at home, rather than go back to work. He admits that finances will be tight, but he feels it is the only answer. He is completely against putting Peter and Marissa in day care due to the risk of their getting sick, and he really does not want anybody else coming into their home to care for the babies.

RACHEL REYES

Season 1	Season 2	Season 3
Rachel is trying to pregnant. She begins infertility work-ups and becomes obsessed with getting pregnant. The story describes the stress associated with this process, not only for Rachel, but also for her husband.	Rachel completes her infertility work-ups and begins taking Clomid. She finally becomes pregnant (with twins). This story follows her pregnancy. She represents a high-risk pregnancy.	As the pregnancy progresses, Rachel develops preeclampsia. She is told to slow down her work activities After developing HELLP syndrome, Rachel is taken for an emergency cesarean section, and her infants are delivered prematurely. She feels a great deal of regret, but is relieved when she is able to take them home.

Rachel Reyes Season 1 Information

Episode 1

Rachel is a healthy, happily married 38-year-old Hispanic woman. She and her husband Angelo have been married for 3 years and have been attempting to conceive a child ever since. Rachel and Angelo have both been heavily focused on their careers all of their adult lives. Rachel works as a realtor in a large real estate company. She is physically active, tries to eat a healthy diet, only drinks alcohol occasionally, and does not use any tobacco products.

Rachel has been very anxious to get pregnant and start a family. She stopped taking oral contraceptives shortly after getting married. After one year of failing to conceive, Rachel began searching the Internet for sites related to pregnancy and infertility. Rachel's research made her very aware of the huge expense associated with infertility workups and treatment, as well as the lack of insurance coverage for this expense. She and Angelo have been hopeful that she would get pregnant without intervention. Although she considers adoption a potential alternative, Angelo is against this idea, citing that he is not interested in raising someone else's child.

Acutely aware that her biological clock is ticking, Rachel has become increasingly obsessed with having a child. She spends many hours researching the process for infertility options on the internet. She finally convinces Angelo that they should consult infertility specialists to help them conceive. She makes an appointment with her women's health physician for an initial infertility workup ▼.

Episode 2

Rachel has her first appointment with her gynecologist to discuss her concerns regarding her inability to get pregnant. During this workup, a medical history is taken, which includes age at menarche and a description of menstrual cycles. Rachel shares with the gynecologist the notebook documenting her temperatures and dates of intercourse for the past year. The physician notes the lack of a biphasic temperature curve, suggesting inadequate hormonal function and ovulation. Rachel's history also includes evidence of rubella immunity. The doctor performs an examination, which includes a pelvic exam, Pap smear, and a culture for gonorrhea and chlamydia. The gynecologist refers Rachel to an infertility specialist and suggests that her husband be examined by an urologist. Despite the information about her temperature pattern suggesting hormonal dysfunction or a problem with ovulation, Rachel is quite sure the problem lies with Angelo because he has type 1 diabetes mellitus ▼.

Episode 3
Rachel sells two homes this week and is thrilled! She suggests to Angelo they apply the funds from the home sales to the infertility workups.

Episode 4
Angelo sees the urologist this week. Rachel wants to know everything that happened at the visit and what he learned. She is disappointed to learn that Angelo has no answers for her, and she will have to wait for the Semen analysis test to be completed before she knows more. Rachel learns from her gynecologist that the Pap smear a few weeks ago was normal, and the culture was negative.

Episode 5
Angelo tells Rachel he got his lab results back and his semen analysis is normal. She was convinced that her diabetes was the problem and thought for sure the infertility problem was with him. She has an appointment with the infertility specialist soon, and she remains hopeful the problem will be easily addressed.

Episode 6
Rachel has her first appointment with the infertility specialist. During this initial visit, a thorough history is obtained. Rachel shares with the physician the ovulation charts she has maintained and the results of Angelo's semen analysis. The physician outlines the general plan for the infertility workup and explains that the process is not only expensive, but long and drawn out, which can be very frustrating. The diagnostic process could take several months and require time away from work to complete the exams. The following blood tests will be run at one time: thyroid and androgen levels; daily blood samples for follicle-stimulating hormone (FSH), luteinizing hormone (LH), and progesterone; and prolactin levels for 1 month to evaluate hormonal production and regulation. The physician suggests that Rachel begin these tests within a couple days of starting with her next menstrual cycle. Other planned tests include a postcoital exam, hysterosalpingogram, endometrial biopsy, and laparoscopy. Rachel assures the physician that she and Angelo want to proceed.

Episode 7
Rachel blocks out time in her calendar for all the diagnostic tests she needs to have. She is glad she has not used any of her sick leave time and also has annual leave time

built up. However, she can see that scheduling all the tests could make her job challenging ▼.

Episode 8
Rachel has scheduled a postcoital exam this week because she is expected to ovulate within the next few days. The test will assess the quality of the cervical mucus and characteristics of the sperm. Rachel and Angelo were instructed to abstain from intercourse for several days prior to the exam. Because the sample of cervical mucus must be obtained within a few hours of intercourse, Angelo needs to come home during the middle of the work day to accommodate Rachel's 1 p.m. appointment ▼.

Episode 9
Rachel has a follow-up visit with the infertility specialist to discuss the lab results. Her thyroid and androgen levels are within normal range. Her follicle-stimulating hormone (FSH) level failed to rise early in the cycle, the luteinizing hormone (LH) level failed to rise midcycle, and the progesterone level failed to rise at end of the cycle. The prolactin level is normal. The results of the postcoital exam show that the sperm are mobile, and the cervical mucus is thicker than expected. The physician tells Rachel that these results point to a probable imbalance in hormonal regulation as the cause of the infertility. She wants to complete the other diagnostic tests, however, to rule out other coexisting problems.

Episode 10
Rachel becomes angry when Angelo begins to question if they are doing the right thing with the infertility workups. He tells Rachel the process has been very stressful for him and maybe it is not worth it. Rachel can't believe he is even saying this. She tells him that she wants a baby and he could have avoided all this if he would have gone along with an adoption. She tells him at this point she is not willing to stop the process ▼.

Episode 11
Rachel is scheduled for a hysterosalpingogram to visualize her uterus and fallopian tubes. This test needs to be done within one week following menses. Rachel had wanted to do this test last month, but she was out of town at a realtor continuing education program. Rachel's test is scheduled for 9 a.m. She plans on taking the early part of the morning off from work, with the intention of being in the office by late morning.

On the day of the test, there are scheduling problems at the radiology office because one of the technicians called in sick. Rachel is furious at the suggestion that her appointment be rescheduled for the following month. She yells at the receptionist, telling her that she MUST have this test today. The receptionist tells Rachel that, if she is willing to wait, they could probably work her in, but it would likely be in the afternoon. Rachel agrees to wait. She calls work and tells them she is not sure when she will be in, but that she will come as soon as she can. Rachel's test is finally done at 3 p.m.; following the test, Rachel just goes home ▾.

Episode 12

Angelo has a problem with his eye, requiring outpatient surgery. Rachel takes a day off from work to take him to his procedure and then take care of him at home afterward. Angelo is scheduled to have his procedure at 8 a.m. At 8:30 a.m., he is still in the pre-op holding area. Rachel asks the nurses what they are waiting for and is told they are just waiting for the doctor to arrive. At 9 a.m., they are still waiting in pre-op holding, and Rachel can see that Angelo is getting a bit anxious about his blood sugar. She goes to the nurses' desk and begins yelling at the staff, telling them that her husband is a diabetic and can't lie there all day without eating. The nurses attempt to apologize, but Rachel isn't interested in hearing their excuses. When the operating room technician comes to take Angelo into surgery, Rachel lets her know the delay in the surgery is unacceptable. The technician is annoyed with Rachel and could not care less about what she thinks.

Later in the day, after they are home from the hospital, Rachel gets a phone call from her physician, informing her that the results of her hysterosalpingogram are normal ▾.

Episode 13

Rachel has an endometrial biopsy performed to evaluate the quality of her uterine lining. Rachel experiences pain and cramping during and after the procedure, so she takes the rest of the day off from work.

Episode 14

Rachel receives a follow-up report from the endometrial biopsy that the results are normal. This week, she has her laparoscopy procedure, which she hopes will be the last diagnostic test. The laparoscopy shows no evidence of endometriosis ▾.

Episode 15

Rachel and Angelo take a much-needed vacation together. They had booked a Caribbean cruise last year before starting the infertility workups. Had they not put down a large deposit when they booked the trip, Rachel is not sure they would be taking the trip. However, she finds it is exactly what they need!▾

Rachel Reyes Season 2 Information

Episode 1

This week, Rachel has another appointment with her infertility specialist. The physician reviews the tests performed and the results, and explains the next steps to take. The decision is made to start Rachel on a prescription of clomiphene citrate (Clomid). She will need to take the drug for 5 days starting on the fifth day of her cycle. She is told that, because this drug stimulates ovarian activity, there is an increased risk of multiple pregnancies. Rachel has already read about Clomid and is anxious to get started. The physician tells her that, with luck, she might become pregnant in the next few months. Rachel purchases several home ovulation test kits on the way home from her appointment so that she can plan intercourse to coincide with ovulation cycles ▶.

Episode 2

Rachel is anxious to begin the medication to help her get pregnant. On the 5th day of her cycle, she starts her course of clomiphene citrate (Clomid) 50 mg a day for 5 days. With her ovulation test kit, Rachel confirms ovulation. She and Angelo have sex as often as possible for the next several days ▾.

Episode 3

Rachel has been performing a home pregnancy test every day to see if she has become pregnant. When she starts her period this week, Rachel is devastated and misses work. She attributes the failure to get pregnant this month to working too many hours.

Episode 4

Rachel continues to feel sad that she did not get pregnant. She wants the medication to work, but she is also aware that, if she does not get pregnant after 4 cycles, it is not likely to work. She thinks about getting pregnant nearly all the time and worries about what to do next if the medication is not successful ▾.

Episode 5

Rachel determines she is ovulating again. She and Angelo have sex at least twice a day and she starts her second attempt to get pregnant using clomiphene citrate (Clomid). With this cycle, her dose has been increased to 100 mg a day for 5 days.

Rachel and Angelo go to a picnic with Angelo's architectural firm this week. However, the nearby forest fire causes the air conditions to be very bad, so they leave early. Almost everyone at the picnic is feeling the effects of the air. Rachel has a mild cough after being out in the smoky air all day. She worries that inhaling the smoky air might negatively impact her ability to get pregnant ▽.

Episode 6
This week, Rachel tests positive for pregnancy with one of her home tests. She runs the test a second time to be sure it is positive. She is so excited that she calls Angelo at work to tell him the news and also calls the physician's office. She is asked to come in the following day to confirm the pregnancy. The following morning, Rachel runs another home pregnancy test as soon as she wakes up to be sure she is still pregnant. At the infertility specialist's office, Rachel's pregnancy is confirmed with yet another pregnancy test. She is referred to Dr. Gayle Tito at Neighborhood Women's Health Services for prenatal care, because of her expertise in working with older pregnant women. It is suggested that Rachel schedule a prenatal visit within a few weeks ▽.

Episode 7
Rachel has her first prenatal visit with Dr. Tito. She asks Angelo to go with her for moral support. During the visit, a comprehensive history and examination are completed. While getting an Ultrasound, Rachel is shocked when she is told that it appears as though they will have twins. She knew that was a possibility, but she really did not believe it would happen ▤ ▽.

Episode 8
Angelo stays home sick with the flu for a couple of days. On Wednesday, Rachel has a home showing that lasts until late afternoon. When she finally gets home at 6 p.m., she is shocked at how Angelo looks. He is lethargic, flushed, and breathing very fast. Rachel knows he is in trouble and that she needs to take him to the Neighborhood Hospital Emergency Department.

Rachel spends the entire evening into the early hours the following morning with Angelo while he is treated for Ketoacidosis. It scares her to think about what might have happened if she had not come home when she did. It also makes her realize how fragile Angelo is when he becomes ill ▽.

Episode 9
Rachel has begun to adjust to the idea of having twins. She knows that she is not the first person in the world to have the experience, but she worries that it will be difficult. She has been feeling very tired and nauseated. She knew to expect this, but she did not realize just how nauseated and fatigued one might get with a pregnancy. She suspects that having twins and keeping up her busy

schedule are both contributing to her symptoms. She is at 10 weeks and has another prenatal visit with Dr. Tito this week ▤ ▷.

Episode 10
Rachel pushes through a long and busy week at work. Between the fatigue and the nausea, she feels miserable. She begins to wonder if she will be able to manage both pregnancy and work ▽.

Episode 11
At long last, the nausea that Rachel has been experiencing has begun to subside. She has her 14-week prenatal visit and is pleased that her pregnancy seems to be progressing well ▤ ▽.

Episode 12
Rachel celebrates her 39th birthday this week. Angelo gives her a beautiful bracelet. She loves the bracelet Angelo bought for her, but she worries about how much he might have spent on it. Rachel enjoys a very busy and successful month as a realtor. She has been able to sell five homes - an all-time record for her. She is pleased that her client base and number of referrals are growing. At the same time, she is beginning to realize that much of the work that has gone into her business will be for nothing after she has the babies. She is thrilled about being pregnant, but also aware of what she will lose ▽.

Episode 13
Rachel regularly feels her babies move. She finds the sensation strange, yet pleasant. She does not have any nausea at this point, but she has been experiencing Constipation and continues to feel tired. Rachel has her 18-week prenatal visit ▤.

Episode 14
Rachel goes shopping with Angelo to select furniture for the nursery. She also selects bedding and decorative items and is excited to put the nursery together ▽.

Episode 15
It has been a very busy week for Rachel. She picks up two new clients and is working hard to arrange to show them homes. She has been frustrated with one client to whom she has now shown more than 40 homes in the past 3 weeks; he still cannot seem to make up his mind. At this point, she is not sure she will ever find him something he is willing to buy. Fortunately, Rachel has more energy than she had in past weeks.

Rachel sees Dr. Tito again this week for her 22-week prenatal visit. She talks with Angelo about getting signed up for childbirth education classes at the Neighborhood Patient Education Center ▤ ▽.

Rachel Reyes Season 3 Information

Episode 1

Rachel's pregnancy continues to progress, and she continues to maintain a busy work schedule. Overall she has been feeling well, except that she has noticed swelling in her hands and feet at the end of the day and has been having intermittent contractions. She and Angelo have been going to childbirth classes, and Rachel has decided that she will breastfeed her infants, although she isn't sure how one does this with twins. She sees Dr. Tito this week for her 28-week prenatal visit. An ultrasound shows that the babies are growing - and that she is going to have a boy and a girl ▤ ▽.

Episode 2

Dr. Tito has asked Rachel to come in every 2 weeks for prenatal visits at this point in her pregnancy. During this visit, Rachel shares with Dr. Tito that the swelling in her hands and feet has increased. She also tells Dr. Tito that the babies are very active, and she admits to occasional uterine contractions. During the examination, Dr. Tito determines that Rachel's babies are in a breech position.

Dr. Tito talks with Rachel about her work schedule and learns that she has been as busy as ever because her real estate business has grown. She tells Rachel that she really should reduce her work schedule, or at least slow down and find time during the day for rest. Rachel wonders how she will be able to cut back her hours at this point without giving her clients to other realtors ▤ ▶.

Episode 3

Rachel has done little to cut back on her work schedule. She has built in two 45-minute periods during the day when she lies down on a couch in her real estate office. However, she finds this to be a huge inconvenience. While lying down, she spends her time catching up on email or answering phone messages ▽.

Episode 4

Rachel has her 32-week appointment with Dr. Tito this week. She reports that the swelling in her hands and feet has not improved (despite resting like the doctor advised), her face feels puffy, and that she has had a headache for the past couple of days. She also admits to continued intermittent contractions. Dr. Tito, concerned about the symptoms, the observed edema, the elevated blood pressure, and the protein in urine, strongly recommends that Rachel be admitted to the hospital to rule out preeclampsia. Rachel tells Dr. Tito that she has a couple of closings later in the day, but perhaps she could be admitted the following day. After Rachel talks with Angelo, she agrees to the admission.

Rachel stays in the hospital for 48 hours. During this brief hospitalization, the headaches go away, and the edema decreases. Rachel's liver enzymes are found to be elevated, she has protein in her urine, and she continues to have edema in her feet. She is given steroids (betamethasone 12 mg intramuscularly once a day for 2 days) to help the babies' lungs develop, in case they are born prematurely. Rachel is told that the babies are still in a breech position and that she must rest to avoid serious complications. She arranges to begin her maternity leave immediately, deciding that selling homes is not worth the risk of having further problems with this pregnancy ▤.

Episode 5

Rachel is now at 33 weeks gestation. The headaches and facial puffiness that Rachel experienced last week have returned. She takes a couple of Tylenol tablets, but they are not effective. Rachel is evaluated by Dr. Tito, who immediately admits her to the hospital. Upon admission, a few blood tests are run. Her blood pressure is in the 160/100 mm Hg range. After the test results come back, she is told her liver enzymes are worsening and the fibrinogen and platelet count have dropped. Dr. Tito explains that Rachel has developed HELLP syndrome (*h*emolysis, *e*levated *l*iver enzyme levels and a *l*ow *p*latelet count) and needs to have a cesarean section delivery in the early evening. She is told she may not eat or drink anything until after the surgery. Rachel is glad she saw a video about this in the prenatal class so that she has an idea of what to expect.

A magnesium sulfate drip is started, causing Rachel to feel hot and panicky. She is assured by the nurse that these symptoms will subside after the initial bolus is in. A neonatal nurse practitioner visits Rachel and Angelo to inform them about what to expect after delivery. They are told the babies will be in the neonatal intensive care unit (NICU), and the couple will be allowed to visit them and ask questions. The nurse encourages breastfeeding the babies and discusses the use of a breast pump.

Rachel cries off and on all day, blaming herself for putting the babies in this position. If they do not survive, she will never forgive herself, and she is sure Angelo would never forgive her either. In the early evening, Dr. Tito successfully delivers both infants by cesarean section. Rachel sees her babies, briefly noting that they both have black hair, before they are taken to the NICU. She asks if they are healthy, but is only told that they will be evaluated immediately. Rachel is glad Angelo is with her ▤ ▽.

Episode 6

When Rachel is discharged from the hospital, she feels cheated because she cannot bring the babies home. She goes to the hospital every day in the morning and at night to see them, and Angelo accompanies her every evening. She is using the breast pump every 3 hours. She is happy that she is producing breast milk for her babies and is thrilled when she is allowed to hold them for the first time.

Rachel has a postpartum checkup with Dr. Tito this week. Although she generally feels well, she reports feeling easily fatigued. Her blood pressure is now 128/82 mm Hg, and her incision is healing well. She is reminded not to lift heavy objects or drive for several weeks. Contraception is discussed with Rachel, but she doesn't think she will need it because she needed Clomid to get pregnant ◩.

Episode 7

Rachel is pleased that Peter and Marissa are doing so well. She continues to make trips to the hospital every day, spending as much time as she can with them. With the help of a lactation consultant, she begins to breastfeed the babies. She comes to know the nurses and other medical personal very well and has developed an interest in the work they do. She asks them many questions about their roles and the procedures they do. She is amazed at how many types of healthcare providers are involved with Peter and Marissa's care, including physician, nurse, pharmacist, occupational therapist, respiratory therapist, and social worker. With all these various providers, she is impressed by how well these health professionals work together as a team for the benefit of the babies and parents on the unit ◩ [NEWS].

Episode 8

Peter and Marissa continue to progress. Rachel is told by the nurses that they should be able to go home in a few weeks. Rachel considers her job as a realtor. Although she has always enjoyed it and has been successful at it, she begins to think about the possibility of going to nursing school in the future. As she watches the nurses interact with parents and care for the infants, she perceives this to be a much more fulfilling career than selling homes. She talks to Angelo about her interest in nursing as a career ▶ [NEWS].

Episode 9

Peter and Marissa remain at the hospital but have made steady progress. Rachel is told by the nurses that she can expect to take them home next week ◩.

Episode 10

Rachel and Angelo are finally able to bring Peter and Marissa home. Rachel is instructed to feed them every 2-4 hours, alternating between breast and bottle feedings, until they are breastfeeding well. Rachel and Angelo quickly learn about the fatigue associated with caring for infants. With twins, it seems at times to be overwhelming. They are told to keep the infants home as much as possible, to keep them away from smoking, to keep them away from anyone who is sick, and to practice good hand hygiene. They are given information about car safety seats as well. Two days after the babies' discharge, Rachel takes them to see Carolyn Marquette, the pediatric nurse practitioner at Neighborhood Pediatrics for a follow-up visit ▶ ◩.

Episode 11

Rachel has another follow-up visit with Dr. Tito this week. Her blood pressure is now 122/72 mm Hg, and her incision has completely healed. A Pap smear is done, and she is told she does not have to return for another visit for a year, unless problems arise. She admits to Dr. Tito that she feels pretty tired; now that the babies are home, she is not getting much sleep.

Episode 12

Rachel takes the babies to see Carolyn Marquette, the pediatric nurse practitioner at Neighborhood Pediatrics, for another appointment. She is pleased to learn that the babies continue to gain weight. Her mother comes from out of town to spend the week at their home to help. Rachel is glad to have the help because she feels so tired. At the same time, she feels the need to watch her mother constantly to be sure she washes her hands before touching the babies.

Episode 13

Rachel and her mother take the babies to Neighborhood Pediatrics for their 2-month immunizations this week. Carolyn Marquette, the pediatric nurse practitioner, tells Rachel about the need to give the babies palivizumab (Synagis), a prophylactic medication to prevent respiratory syncytial virus (RSV), the following month. They will need to have this immunization every month for up to three doses. This medication, she is told, is very expensive and will cost as much as $1,000 for each dose for each baby, dose. Rachel is advised to check with her insurance company to ensure coverage.

Angelo talks with Rachel about the length of her mother's visit and asks if she will be leaving soon. Rachel has loved having her mother stay with them but can tell her husband is ready for her to go ▶ ◩.

Episode 14

Rachel's mother tells Rachel she really needs to get back home and hopes she does not mind if she leaves. Rachel lets her mother know how much she appreciates her help, but assures her that she can manage the babies with Angelo's help. Although Rachel is more than ready for her mother to leave, she is sad to see her mother go ▼.

Episode 15

Rachel's maternity leave is up at the end of next week. Her boss at the real estate office has left a message on her phone, telling her they are all looking forward to her return to work. Deep down, Rachel believes that she should give up her career to care for her babies. Although she loves her career, she feels strongly that Peter and Marissa are now her top priority. She explores the possibility of not going back to work and adjusting to one income.

Rachel and Angelo get a letter from the insurance company, denying coverage for the Synagis immunizations; they are told they will have to cover this expense on their own. Rachel makes a call to the nurse practitioner to inquire about this situation ▼.

PETER & MARISSA

Season 1	Season 2	Season 3
Not born yet	Not born yet	Peter and Marissa are born prematurely, due to their mother's preeclampsia. There are initial problems with thermoregulation, glucose regulation, and respiratory status. Infant care for healthy premature newborns is emphasized in this story.

Peter & Marissa Reyes Season 1 and 2 Information

Not born yet.

Peter & Marissa Reyes Season 3 Information

Not born yet.

Episode 5

Peter and Marissa Reyes come into the world this week at 6:52 p.m. on Thursday at 33 weeks' gestation. At birth, Peter and Marissa have Apgar scores of 6 and 7 at 1 minute, respectively; at 5 minutes, their scores are 7 and 7. They are briefly introduced to their mother and father before being taken to the NICU for evaluation and stabilization.

In the NICU, they are dried off, weighed, placed under a warmer, and examined by the neonatal nurse practitioner, who notes that the findings are consistent with 33 weeks' gestation. Because the infants become slightly dusky during the exam, blow-by oxygen is administered, and their color pinks up. Over the next 15 minutes, however, Peter begins to exhibit grunting and nasal flaring, and his oxygen saturation level drops to 84%. Respiratory therapy is called, and the technician initiates continuous positive airway pressure (CPAP). Blood gases and chest x-ray reveal that Peter is developing respiratory distress syndrome. The neonatal nurse practitioner intubates him and administers surfactant down the endotracheal (ET) tube, followed by bagging. Additional surfactant is administered for a few minutes, and the ET tube is removed. Oxygen is administered at $1/4$ liter by nasal cannula, and his symptoms resolve. Peter's oxygen saturation improves to 92%. Marissa's oxygen saturation remains stable at 94% on nasal cannula oxygen. Both of their body temperatures remain stable.

In addition to temperature and respiratory support, Peter and Marissa require nutrition and fluid support. Screening glucose levels are drawn; Marissa's glucose is 55 mg/dL, whereas Peter's is only 24 mg/dL. A bolus of D10W intravenous solution is administered to Peter, followed by a continuous infusion. An hour later, Peter's glucose is 44 mg/dL. Both infants are supported on peripheral parenteral nutrition (D12.5% with 2% amino acids) for several days.

The infants begin to exhibit yellowing of the face when they are 36 hours old, prompting a bilirubin assessment. Marissa and Peter's bilirubin levels are 6.0 mg/dL and 6.8 mg/dL, respectively. The following morning, their bilirubin levels climb to 12 mg/dL and 13 mg/dL, respectively, requiring phototherapy. Their eyes are covered and, wearing only a diaper, they are placed in an isolette for 3 days. Over that time, their bilirubin levels slowly decrease.

Episode 6

Peter and Marissa remain at the hospital. At the beginning of the week, their weights are 1,550 and 1,600 grams, respectively. They remain on peripheral parental nutrition (PPN) for several days and then graduate to feedings fortified with breast milk through a feeding tube. Both babies' average intake is about 150 mL/kg/day. They also both have an ultrasound to rule out intraventricular hemorrhage; the findings are negative.

Episode 7

Peter and Marissa gain weight steadily this week. Peter now weighs 1,625 grams, and Marissa weighs 1,700 grams. They have improved with their feedings and are now taking approximately 250 mL/day.

Episode 8

Peter and Marissa continue to gain weight and grow. So far they have avoided many complications common to prematurity. Their mother and father have been a regular presence in the hospital unit where they have been since their birth.

Episode 9

Peter and Marissa continue to do well in the hospital. Peter's weight is up to 1,800 grams, and Marissa's weight is 1,900 grams.

Episode 10

Peter and Marissa come home from the hospital this week. They are seen 2 days after discharge by the pediatric nurse practitioner. Their weights are 2 kg and 2.1 kg, respectively.

Episode 11

Peter and Marissa spend most of their time sleeping. They awaken every few hours for feeding – often at the same time.

Episode 12

Peter and Marissa remain healthy and both are making good progress in weight and doing well with breastfeeding.

Episode 13

Peter and Marissa are now 2 months old. During an office visit, Peter weighs in at 2.8 kg, and Marissa weighs 3.0 kg. They receive their immunizations (HBV, DTaP, Hib, IPV, and PCV).

Episode 14

Peter and Marissa listen with interest to the sounds they hear when their mother plays music in the home. They smile in response to the silly faces made by their mother and father.

Episode 15

Peter and Marisa have become fascinated with their hands. They notice that each of their fingers is separate and attached to their hands – and there are two of them that can be brought together. They use their hands to touch and explore various things within reach.

RILEY HOUSEHOLD

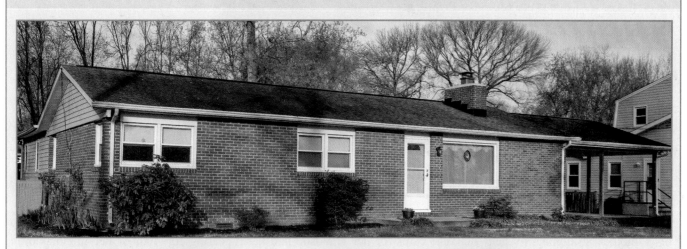

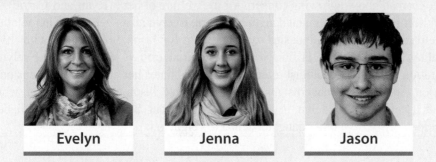

| **Evelyn** | **Jenna** | **Jason** |

Housing The Rileys live in a small single story home in the Southend. They live close to the manufacturing area.

Parks and Recreation There are only a few parks in the area, and some of them are in disrepair.

Services There is bus service to the area and a grocery store within walking distance.

Key: ▶ = video clip   ☰ = medical record   ▽ = journal entry   [NEWS] = news article

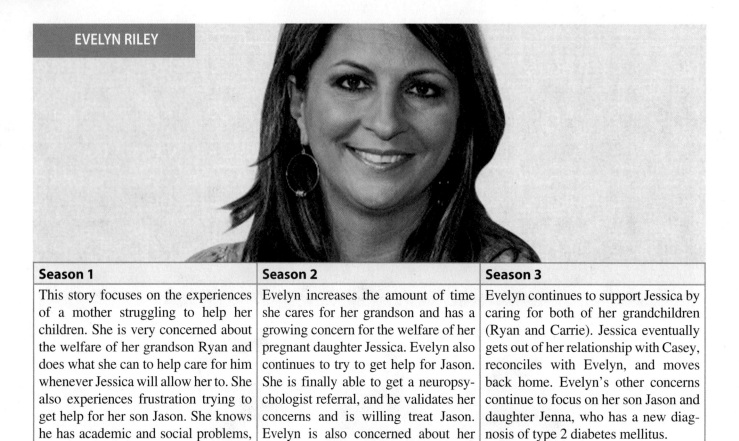

Season 1	Season 2	Season 3
This story focuses on the experiences of a mother struggling to help her children. She is very concerned about the welfare of her grandson Ryan and does what she can to help care for him whenever Jessica will allow her to. She also experiences frustration trying to get help for her son Jason. She knows he has academic and social problems, but can't seem to get help.	Evelyn increases the amount of time she cares for her grandson and has a growing concern for the welfare of her pregnant daughter Jessica. Evelyn also continues to try to get help for Jason. She is finally able to get a neuropsychologist referral, and he validates her concerns and is willing treat Jason. Evelyn is also concerned about her other daughter Jenna's weight gain.	Evelyn continues to support Jessica by caring for both of her grandchildren (Ryan and Carrie). Jessica eventually gets out of her relationship with Casey, reconciles with Evelyn, and moves back home. Evelyn's other concerns continue to focus on her son Jason and daughter Jenna, who has a new diagnosis of type 2 diabetes mellitus.

Evelyn Riley Season 1 Information

Episode 1

Evelyn is a 38-year-old single mother in good health. Her ex-husband left Evelyn and her children about 10 years ago. She has never remarried and is not currently involved in a romantic relationship. Although she receives a small amount of child support from her ex-husband on a regular basis, he has had very little contact with her or the children in the past 10 years; in fact, he has not seen his children for over 8 years. Evelyn considers herself religious and is very involved with the Neighborhood Christian Church. She enjoys interactions with members of the church community and finds prayer to be an effective coping strategy for her somewhat challenging life circumstances. Evelyn works out of her home as a medical transcriptionist. She supplements her income by working at a retail store at the mall in the evenings a few nights each week.

Evelyn has three children. Her oldest, Jessica Riley, is 17 and a new mother. Evelyn's relationship with Jessica was good until Jessica became an adolescent. Since that time, it has been very strained, especially after Jessica became pregnant. Jessica moved out of the house when she was 6 months pregnant to an apartment a short distance away. At this point, Evelyn tries to help her daughter by taking care of her baby, Ryan, when Jessica goes to school and sometimes in the evening. Evelyn's other children, Jenna (13) and Jason (11), live in the home with her. Evelyn has been frustrated by the ongoing school and social problems that Jason has been experiencing. For the past year, she has been attempting to get an appropriate referral to help him, but she feels she has been going in circles within the system.

Evelyn teaches Bible school classes each Sunday for an hour before the regular church service. Her daughter Jenna is in the class she teaches (7th and 8th grade students). At the same time Jason attends a class for 5th and 6th grade students taught by another teacher. By teaching the Bible classes each week, Evelyn partially fulfills a lifelong desire to be a teacher ▼.

Episode 2

Evelyn is asked by Jessica to babysit Ryan for a few hours in the evening so that she can go to her friend's house for a party. Evelyn begins to become concerned when Jessica fails to pick up the baby by midnight. Jessica finally calls about 1:30 a.m. and tells her mother that she will just pick up Ryan in the morning. Evelyn is angry with Jessica because of her lack of responsibility.

Jason is involved in another fight at school this week. Evelyn is asked to come in for a counseling session with the teacher, principal, and counselor. The counselor suggests that Jason's behavioral issues are related to poor or inconsistent discipline in the home. Evelyn says she disagrees and believes that he has some sort of learning problem. She requests that Jason be tested ▼.

Episode 3

Evelyn goes with Jessica to take Ryan for his 2-month well-baby check-up. Jessica tells her mother that her new boyfriend Casey is going to move in with her, so Evelyn will only need to watch Ryan during the daytime. Evelyn expresses concern and says she's happy to continue caring for Ryan. Jessica tells her mother that she can raise her own baby ▼.

Episode 4

Jason comes home with a note from his teacher that he failed to complete his volcano project and that Evelyn needs to ensure that he completes his homework. Evelyn was not aware that Jason even had a volcano project – this was the first she had heard of it. Evelyn also gets a phone call from the school nurse, Violet Brinkworth, telling her that Jason's vision is only 20/100 in both eyes. The nurse suggests that she take Jason for an eye examination.

Episode 5

Evelyn takes Jason to an optometrist this week who determines that he needs glasses. Evelyn hopes that the glasses will help Jason do better in school. Despite her optimism, she knows deep down that Jason has some kind of learning problem and wishes she could get him some help. Evelyn makes sure Jason gets his homework completed each night this week, but it is a major task ▼ [NEWS].

Episode 6

Jessica drops Ryan off to be cared for by Evelyn while she runs a few errands. Evelyn is concerned about her grandson Ryan. She gives him a bath, changes his clothes, plays with him, and then rocks him to sleep after feeding him. When Jessica picks him up several hours later, Evelyn voices several concerns, including that Ryan does not seem to be gaining much weight and that he often looks dirty - today he had dried milk on his neck and his clothes were not clean. Evelyn also questions whether living with Casey is in Jessica and Ryan's best interest. Jessica gets

very defensive and angry, accusing her mother of disliking Casey and trying to make her feel dumb. Jessica says that, if she continues to criticize her, she won't let her take care of the baby anymore. Evelyn decides it is best to back off, because she wants to continue taking care of Ryan ▼.

Episode 7

Jenna tells Evelyn she is having a period. When Evelyn starts to tell Jenna that everything is okay and it is normal for women as they mature, Jenna puts her hand up and says, "Yeah I know, I learned about this stuff in school. I just need some tampons." When Evelyn comes home from the store with tampons and feminine napkins, Jenna tells her that she just wants the tampons. None of her friends use napkins. Evelyn warns her not to flush the tampons down the toilet or the plumbing will get stopped up. The following day, Jason informs her that the toilet is overflowing onto the floor. When Evelyn asks Jenna about this, she denies flushing tampons and suggests that Jason just uses too much toilet paper. Evelyn is unable to clear the blocked toilet and has to call a plumber ▼.

Episode 8

Evelyn arranges a party for Jason and several of his classmates in an attempt to help him make friends. Only a few kids show up at the party, and Evelyn notices that few interact directly with Jason. She continues to feel frustrated with Jason over the ongoing homework battles. She notices that his complaints of headaches have stopped, but the problems with schoolwork remain. The assistant scoutmaster, Pat Richman, tells her that Jason had a "meltdown" at the Boy Scout meeting this week ▼ [NEWS].

Episode 9

Evelyn's church holds an annual youth group pancake breakfast fundraising event. She spends several hours at the church in support of the event and has a chance to talk with Pastor Jeff about her son Jason's problems at school. Evelyn is interested to know if Pastor Jeff has any suggestions for helping Jason. Pastor Jeff suggests that Jason would benefit from having an adult male role model to interact with more and offers to spend a few hours a week with Jason by having him help at the church. Evelyn likes the suggestion and they agree on a time that works for both of their schedules.

Episode 10

Ryan is 6 months old this week. Evelyn gets Jessica's permission to take Ryan to his well-baby check-up and to get immunizations. The pediatrician tells Evelyn that Ryan is falling a bit behind on his weight and to feed him more. Evelyn again tries to talk to Jessica about Ryan's care, but Jessica tells her mother to shut up and mind her own business.

Evelyn receives a phone call from the principal's office at Jason's school because Jason was involved in another fight. She feels at her wit's end with her son; she just can't seem to control him at times. She talks with the school counselor again about getting a referral to a neuropsychologist. The counselor continues to suggest that the problems seem to be the result of inadequate discipline but agrees that a medical problem might explain some things. Evelyn is advised to start with her family physician. Evelyn schedules an appointment with Dr. Rowe to see if she can help with Jason's situation ▶ ✉.

Episode 11

Evelyn learns this week that Jessica is pregnant again and has quit school. Evelyn tells Jessica that the last thing she needs right now is another baby. She has another fight with Jessica about the fact that she is going nowhere in life and needs to get her act together.

Evelyn takes Jason to Dr. Rowe, the family physician, to see if she can offer any help with Jason's ongoing problems. Dr. Rowe's initial response to Evelyn as she discusses the problems is one of skepticism. He tells Evelyn that most 11-year-old boys are hard to control. Dr. Rowe says Jason will outgrow the problems but she needs to discipline him more. Evelyn is furious with the accusation and frustrated by the lack of response she is experiencing. She specifically requests a referral to a neuropsychologist, but Dr. Rowe does not feel that it is indicated at this time ✉.

Episode 12

This week, Jason's Boy Scout leader tells Evelyn that Jason is no longer welcome to participate in the troop because he bit one of the other scouts during a meeting. Evelyn calls Pastor Jeff to let him know of the situation, hoping that when he spends some time with Jason this week, he might be able to determine what happened ▶.

Episode 13

Pastor Jeff talks with Evelyn after Bible class to inform her that Jason got into a fight with two boys in his class. Jason's teacher does not want him in his class anymore. When Evelyn protests, Pastor Jeff reminds Evelyn that all the Bible class teachers are volunteers and he can't afford to lose a volunteer over this. Also, Pastor Jeff explains that volunteer teachers are not trained to deal with behavioral issues and he can't expect them to be responsible for these kinds of issues. As a compromise, Pastor Jeff suggests Jason attend Evelyn's class in the hopes that he will get along better with older students ✉.

Episode 14

Evelyn, Jenna, and Jason go out of town to visit Evelyn's mother and are gone all week. While they are gone, Evelyn's grandson, Ryan, is hospitalized. Evelyn does not find out about Ryan's illness until they return. She is angry that Jessica did not call her about the situation immediately.

Episode 15

Jessica tells her mother that she has found a new preschool for Ryan to attend during the daytime, and she wonders if Evelyn can babysit Ryan in the evenings. Despite the fact that this would cut into her hours working at the mall, Evelyn agrees, knowing it will be in Ryan's best interest.

Evelyn Riley Season 2 Information

Episode 1

Evelyn is a 39-year-old single mother in good health. She has three children. Her oldest, Jessica Riley (18), is the mother of a 10-month-old son and is expecting another baby. Jessica lives in a one-bedroom apartment with her son, Ryan, and boyfriend Casey. Evelyn does not like Casey and fears for her daughter's and grandson's safety. She helps Jessica as much as possible by taking care of Ryan when Jessica works in the evenings. Evelyn's other children, Jenna and Jason, live in the home with her. Evelyn has been frustrated by the ongoing school and social problems that Jason has been experiencing. For the past year, she has been attempting to get an appropriate referral to help him, but she feels she has been going in circles within the system. This episode Evelyn agrees to serve as a chaperone for an overnight Bible camp. She is a bit concerned knowing that several of the boys Jason has ongoing problems with will be attending. She does not want him get into any more fights. She notices that when he interacts with older kids and adults, he seems to do just fine. Evelyn wonders if the real issue for Jason is excessive bullying at school. She takes the opportunity at the spiritual retreat to pray about this situation – and for Jessica, too. Evelyn takes Ryan to his 12-month well-child exam for Jessica and reports to Jessica on his progress.

Episode 2

Evelyn spends most of her day catching up with medical transcription work. She works 3 evenings at the mall and takes care of Ryan two evenings this week. She feels exhausted!

Episode 3

Evelyn receives a call from the school, informing her that Jason has been involved in another fight. The school administrators request that she come to the school immediately for a meeting. At the meeting, the principal and counselor suggest that they might need to expel Jason because of his ongoing behavioral issues. Evelyn becomes very angry and recaps the effort she has made, pointing out that she has been attempting to get help for her son for the past couple of years but has met resistance every step of the way - both from the school and in the community. Evelyn suggests that, before the school decides to expel her son, perhaps they should pay attention to the needs of the students and actually try to facilitate a solution to the problem.

The school counselor looks back over Jason's file, considers what Evelyn has said, and admits that perhaps they have not been as helpful as they could have been. The counselor vows to help Evelyn with a referral to a neuropsychologist ▼.

Episode 4

Evelyn notices that Jenna has been gaining weight and suggests to her that they go out for walks or to the gym. Jenna tells her mother she is too tired and wants to just hang out. Evelyn hopes that Jenna passes this "teenage laziness phase" soon. She tells Jenna that she will only buy two bags of chips a week at the store, so she needs to make them last. She also decides to start making Jenna her lunches to ensure that she eats healthy foods at school [NEWS].

Episode 5

Evelyn feels a bit overwhelmed with work and trying to help Jason, Jessica, and Jenna work through their own issues. Despite this, she agrees to teach another year of Bible classes at the church. Jason has done well in her Bible study class, so she figures it is one way for him to have a positive experience. It also keeps her in good graces with Pastor Jeff, who continues to mentor her son [NEWS].

Episode 6

Evelyn takes Jason to his first appointment with the neuropsychologist. Jason meets with the psychologist independently first and then with Evelyn. The psychologist asks for Evelyn's permission to obtain copies of Jason's school records, which would provide a history from the school system's perspective about his behavioral issues. The neuropsychologist also obtains permission from Evelyn and Jason to talk with his current and former teachers ▼.

Episode 7

Evelyn invites Jessica to the house for a family get-together. She is relieved when Jessica and Ryan arrive at the house without Casey.

Episode 8

Jessica asks Evelyn if she can watch Ryan each night this week, explaining that she needs to get more hours in to pay some bills, because Casey is out of work again. Evelyn agrees to do this and arranges for Jenna to watch Ryan while she works her shifts at the mall. Although she is angry that Jessica must work more hours, she is glad that Casey is not taking care of Ryan.

Evelyn takes Jason for his second visit to the neuropsychologist, who interviews Evelyn regarding Jason's behavior at home. Evelyn tells him that Jason is impulsive, can't attend to homework for more than 15 minutes at a time, has a hard time getting organized, and frequently forgets books and homework. The psychologist shares with Evelyn what he learned from the school records. She is angry to hear that there is repeated documentation of references to her child as obstinate and mean-spirited. One entry even implies that the school might consider investigating his home situation ▶.

Episode 9

Evelyn gets a call from the front office at school informing her that Jason needs a clean pair of pants because he sat in some glue. When she arrives, it is obvious to her that Jason has been crying. He tells her about what some boys had done, and that they had gotten in trouble and not him! The office staff confirms his story and tells Evelyn everything is fine. Evelyn is happy that for once, the school did not blame Jason for a behavioral situation. Perhaps there is hope! ▼

Episode 10

This week Evelyn takes Jason to another appointment with the neuropsychologist. After meeting with Jason, the psychologist shares with Evelyn that he has contacted Jason's previous and current teachers. He tells Evelyn that he is impressed by the consistency of the descriptions from the past three teachers. They all state that Jason is unable to attend to tasks, is easily distracted, can only attend to a task for 5-10 minutes, does best in very structured situations (especially if they remove distractions and provide frequent prompts), and seems to do best in a consistent routine. These symptoms suggest Attention deficit hyperactivity disorder (or ADHD).

Evelyn agrees with this analysis, because it is consistent with what she sees at home. She is relieved that somebody finally believes her and that there really is a problem other than a lack of discipline. The psychologist suggests medication and environmental modifications in the classroom. He also suggests family counseling - primarily to benefit Evelyn, because it is hard to be a single mother of a child with ADHD. Evelyn agrees to talk with the school to see what kinds of modifications can be made available for her son. She is not so sure about having Jason take medication, because she has heard many negative things about medications used to treat ADHD ▶ ▼ [NEWS].

Episode 11

Evelyn takes her grandson, Ryan, to the pediatrician's office because of poor eating, fever, and congestion. She does not want to take the chance of Ryan becoming severely ill again.

This week, Evelyn tells the principal about the ADHD diagnosis made by the neuropsychologist and the need for classroom accommodations. The principal and counselor are relieved to hear that there may be a way to help Jason. They request additional testing in the district office.

Episode 12

Evelyn takes Jason down to the school district offices for additional testing. She is so glad to finally be getting the cooperation she felt she should have had two years ago.

Evelyn, Jenna, and Jason take care of Ryan several nights this week because Jessica is very tired after work. She is glad for their help, even though Jenna keeps running off to the computer.

Episode 13

Evelyn gets a phone call from Jessica, who is crying. Jessica tells her mother that she is going to the hospital in an ambulance and needs her to pick up Ryan from her apartment. Evelyn later learns that Casey has been arrested and is suspected of injuring Jessica. She is relieved when she learns that Jessica's baby is born healthy. Evelyn hopes Jessica will get away from Casey now ◼.

Episode 14

Evelyn is thrilled to see and hold her new granddaughter, Carrie, but she is disappointed when Jessica tells her that she and Casey have worked things out. She wants to shake sense into her daughter, but at the same time feels helpless. She worries about the safety of her daughter and her two grandchildren and is glad Social Service is following up on the situation ◼.

Evelyn attends a meeting with the school nurse, counselor, principal, teacher, and neuropsychologist to set forth an individualized educational plan (IEP) for Jason. In this plan, recommendations are made by the professionals and the school system to structure the classroom and assignments. The purpose of the IEP is to establish specific goals for Jason during the academic year. Because he has poor reading skills, one goal that everyone agrees to is for Jason to read at his grade level. Another goal is to improve his social skills and to become more accepted by his peers. Finally, it is suggested that he focus on self-management skills, such as remembering to bring home and turn in homework. The neuropsychologist suggests that Jason's desk be placed in the classroom away from the window and that he be given two sets of textbooks - one for home and one for school. Furthermore, additional hands-on activities to increase Jason's academic engagement are recommended, as is a quiet environment for testing. It is also again suggested that Jason start taking a medication such as amphetamine and dextroamphetamine (Adderall), which the psychologist strongly believes is necessary for Jason to make progress.

Episode 15

Based on the results and recommendations from the neuropsychologist, Dr. Rowe agrees to start Jason on a prescription of amphetamine and dextroamphetamine (Adderall) to manage his symptoms. Evelyn has ambivalent feelings about this. Although she knows that her son needs help, she wonders if drug therapy is the right answer. Dr. Rowe tells Evelyn she will need to see Jason at weekly intervals to adjust the dose until the optimal response is obtained ◼ [NEWS].

Evelyn Riley Season 3 Information

Episode 1

Evelyn is a 39-year-old single mother in good health. Her ex-husband left Evelyn and her children about 11 years ago. She has never remarried and is not currently involved in a romantic relationship. Although she receives a small amount of child support from her ex-husband on a regular basis, he has had very little contact with her or the children. Evelyn considers herself religious and is very involved with the Neighborhood Christian Church. She enjoys interactions with members of the church community and finds prayer to be an effective coping strategy for her somewhat challenging life circumstances. Evelyn works out of her home as a medical transcriptionist. She

supplements her income by working at a retail store at the mall in the evenings a few nights each week.

Evelyn has three children. Her oldest, Jessica Riley (18), is the mother of an 18-month-old son, Ryan, and a 6-week-old daughter, Carrie. Evelyn's relationship with Jessica is strained. Jessica lives in a one-bedroom apartment with her two children and boyfriend Casey. Because of his abusiveness, Evelyn does not like Casey and fears for her daughter's and grandchildren's safety. Evelyn's other children, Jenna and Jason, live in the home with her. After several frustrating years, Evelyn has recently been able to get Jason help with his ongoing school and social problems. He has recently started taking amphetamine and dextroamphetamine (Adderall) and receiving special accommodations at school to facilitate his learning. Evelyn has noticed that Jenna has gained weight. Knowing it is a sensitive topic, Evelyn gently attempts to suggest that she watch her weight.

While talking with Jessica on the phone this week, Evelyn is suddenly cut off. When she calls back a few minutes later, Casey answers the phone and tells her that Jessica suddenly had to go the bathroom. Evelyn thinks this is odd. A few days later, Evelyn sees a bruise on Jessica's face. Jessica explains that she ran into a door, and answers "no" when asked if Casey hit her. Evelyn does not believe Jessica's explanation.

Evelyn helps care for her grandchildren when Jessica is working.

Episode 2

Evelyn receives a phone call from the school nurse, Violet Brinkworth, about Jenna. The nurse tells Evelyn that she is concerned about Jenna's weight gain and suggests that she have a medical evaluation to determine if there is a condition that might explain it. Evelyn confirms with the nurse that she has noticed the weight gain and is concerned, but it never occurred to her to take her to see a physician.

Evelyn also thinks it is odd that Jason has run out of his amphetamine and dextroamphetamine (Adderall) at home but assumes she was given too few at the pharmacy. Evelyn calls Dr. Rowe's office to ask for a refill for Jason. Evelyn is questioned about the need for a refill and asked if it is possible her children are taking the extra doses. Evelyn replies "No, why would they do that?" She is told to keep track of the doses because it is not uncommon for teens to take the drug when it is not prescribed for them. Later in the day, she Jason about the missing doses and he says he does not know. Evelyn takes Jenna to see Dr. Rowe, as suggested by the school nurse. She is glad that Dr. Rowe listens to her when she shares her concerns - unlike her previous experiences when trying to get help for Jason. Evelyn is surprised at the number of lab tests ordered and is worried. She has problems sleeping because of all of her concerns. She prays that everything will work out ▶ [NEWS].

Episode 3

Evelyn takes Jenna to see Dr. Rowe, as suggested by the school nurse. She is glad that Dr. Rowe listens to her when she shares her concerns – unlike her previous experiences when trying to get help for Jason. Evelyn is surprised at the number of lab tests ordered and is worried. She has problems sleeping because of all of her concerns. She prays that everything will work out [NEWS].

Episode 4

This week when giving Jason his morning dose of amphetamine and dextroamphetamine (Adderall), Evelyn believes some pills are missing so she counts them out. Sure enough, five are missing. She asks both Jenna and Jason if they know anything about this and both say they don't. She decides to hide the medication and she is going to count the pills every day.

The special teachers at school recommend some educational video games for Jason. They know he loves to play video games, and evidence suggests that they can be an effective learning tool with the right programs. Although he initially shows a lack of interest, Evelyn observes Jason playing the new video games during the evening.

Episode 5

This is an overwhelming week for Evelyn. She learns that her daughter Jenna has diabetes, Jason is an emotional wreck after being involved in another fight at school, and she notices bruises on Jessica's face again. She wonders about the effect that all of this stress is having on her own sanity and which of the problems should concern her most. How can she manage it all? Evelyn is relieved to know that Carrie and Ryan have not been harmed. She tells Jessica that she knows Casey is beating her and pleads with her to get away from him. Evelyn sleeps very poorly all week because of all her worries ▶ ✉.

Episode 6

Evelyn takes Jenna to an appointment with Dr. Yin, the pediatric endocrinologist. Dr. Yin talks with Evelyn and Jenna about diabetes and outlines the major components of treatment. She writes a prescription for Jenna and asks them both to work with Marjorie, the certified diabetic educator (CDE). She talks with Evelyn privately about typical psychosocial issues and adherence issues associated with teens who have type 2 diabetes.

Evelyn announces to both Jenna and Jason that there will be changes in the foods they eat and explains that the changes will benefit all of them ✉.

Episode 7

Evelyn is again very disturbed by the obvious beatings her daughter is enduring. She pleads with Jessica to get away from Casey – or, if nothing else, to let her keep the children so they are not near him. Evelyn does not understand why Jessica won't talk with her about the trouble she is in.

Evelyn and Jenna have additional meetings with Violet Brinkworth and with Marjorie, the diabetic nurse educator, this week. Evelyn had heard of diabetes, but she had not realized the complexity and seriousness of the disease.

Jason invites a classmate to spend the night this weekend. It has been many years since Jason has had a friend to their home for a sleepover. Evelyn is pleased to see that her son has a friend [NEWS].

Episode 8

Evelyn is out running errands when Jenna calls her to say she is going to the Neighborhood Mall with friends. Later in the day, Jenna calls her and asks her to pick her up. When Evelyn arrives at the mall, she is surprised by how dressed up Jenna is. On the way home, Jenna tells Evelyn she got separated from her friends and could not find them. Evelyn asks why she was so dressed up. Jenna tells her mother she just wanted to look pretty.

Her oldest daughter, Jessica, calls Evelyn excited to share her good news: Casey proposed to her and they are going to get married. Evelyn wants to scream, but she tells her daughter she is happy for her.

Episode 9

At 4 a.m., Evelyn gets a phone call from her oldest daughter. Jessica tells her mother that she left Casey, but she is hiding because she is afraid he will come looking for her and her children. Jessica does not reveal her location, but she asks her mother to call her employers to let them know she will be gone for a few weeks.

Evelyn feels so helpless, knowing the trouble her daughter is in, yet she is thankful that Jessica and the grandchildren are away from Casey. She wonders how many more problems she will have to deal with. Evelyn sees Casey driving by her home several times this week and worries what he might do.

Evelyn does not tell Jenna and Jason about Jessica. She figures they have enough on their minds, and she does not need to burden them with Jessica's problems [mail].

Episode 10

Casey knocks on the front door and asks Evelyn if she would help him find Jessica and the kids. He tells Evelyn that they have had some problems, but he is ready to work things out. Evelyn is glad she doesn't know where Jessica is. She does not share any information with Casey, but she worries that he will find Jessica and the children.

This week, Evelyn meets with staff members from Jason's school and learns that he is doing better since he began taking the medication and following the educational plan. Evelyn is pleased with this news [mail] [NEWS].

Episode 11

Evelyn is relieved to learn that Casey has been arrested and is in jail, but is very upset that he killed two people from her church in an automobile accident. She is relieved that Jessica is able to come out of hiding and return to her apartment. Evelyn worries, however, that Casey will find a way to post bail and harm Jessica [NEWS].

Episode 12

Evelyn talks Jessica into attending church with Jenna and Jason. Jessica had attended regularly until she moved out. Evelyn suggests that it might be helpful to reconnect with some of her friends from the church and to pray for the two victims killed by Casey. After church, Evelyn takes Jessica, Ryan, Carrie, Jason, and Jenna out for brunch. It is an expense she can barely afford, but Evelyn believes it is very important for Jessica to feel more connected with her family [NEWS].

Episode 13

Evelyn feels a sense of relief when she thinks about each of her three children's recent challenges. Jessica and her children are currently out of harm's way. Jason is making progress at school and finally has a friend his own age. Jenna finally seems to have embraced her diabetes treatment. Jenna shows Evelyn her glucose numbers each day and they have been consistently within normal range. She knows Jenna has been unhappy about the treatment plan, but she is very glad she is following it [mail].

Episode 14

Over the past few weeks, Jessica has spent a great deal of time at home with Evelyn. Evelyn talks with Jessica about the need to let go of past anger and move forward. For the first time in several years, Evelyn feels as if she and Jessica really understand each other. Evelyn suggests that Jessica and the kids move back home until she can get back on her own two feet. When Jessica agrees to this, Evelyn is overjoyed.

Episode 15

Evelyn, Jason, and Jenna help Jessica and her kids move back home this week. Evelyn knows the transition may be hard at first, but she is relieved to know that her daughter and grandchildren are safe.

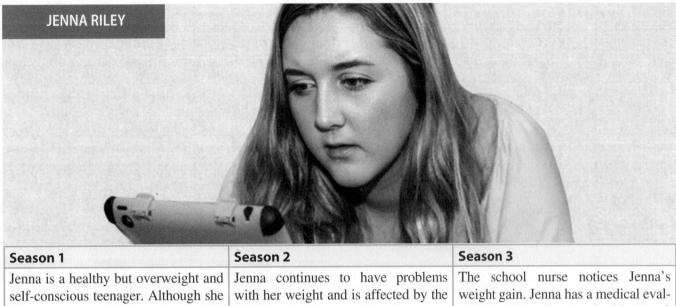

JENNA RILEY

Season 1	Season 2	Season 3
Jenna is a healthy but overweight and self-conscious teenager. Although she has many friends, she experiences rejection by them at times. She excels in academics. This story focuses on her experiences related to being an overweight 13-year-old.	Jenna continues to have problems with her weight and is affected by the problems her sister and brother experience. She reacts to stress by eating, causing her to continue to gain weight. Her mother has quit buying junk food, but Jenna gets the food she craves at school.	The school nurse notices Jenna's weight gain. Jenna has a medical evaluation and is diagnosed with type 2 DM. The rest of the story in this season depicts issues related to diabetic management of an adolescent.

Jenna Riley Season 1 Information

Episode 1

Jenna is a healthy but overweight 13-year-old girl who lives with her mother, Evelyn, and brother, Jason. Her older sister, Jessica, lives a short distance away in her own apartment with her infant son, Ryan. Jenna misses having her older sister around and looks up to Jessica. Jenna has had minimal contact with her father and does not really even know him.

Because her mother works a few evenings each week, Jenna is responsible for her younger brother Jason. She gets along okay with her brother, but she thinks he is weird. She is a good student in the seventh grade at the local middle school. She has many friends and spends a great deal of time on the phone or in computer chat rooms talking with friends in the evening. Jenna is self-conscious about her weight. She knows she should try to lose weight, but she doesn't really know how and doesn't have much discipline when it comes to resisting snacks. She finds it very hard not to join in with her friends when they eat.

Jenna goes to Bible school class each Sunday. Her mother is the teacher for her class this year, and she is not too thrilled about this. She loves her mother but does not like the fact that she is her teacher for these sessions. Jenna does not feel as though she can be "herself" and also worries that her mother will do something to embarrass her in front of her friends ▼.

Episode 2

Jessica's baby spends time at the house several times in the evening this week. Jenna likes it when Ryan is there and fantasizes about the day she will have a baby of her own. She hears her mother wondering out loud when her sister is going to pick up Ryan and take him home.

Episode 3

Jenna goes on an outing with the youth group at her church to an amusement park located in a city 3 hours away. She boards a bus at 7:30 a.m. and does not arrive back until 11:30 p.m. Jenna and her friends take photos of themselves at the amusement park. Jenna posts these to her Facebook page. She specifically brags about riding the "Widowmaker" roller coaster six times in one day. Jenna is careful only to post pictures of herself from the shoulders up so it is not so evident how heavy she is ▼.

Episode 4

Jenna attends a slumber party at her friend's house. They stay up all night, eat popcorn and pizza, and drink soda while watching movies. The girls also practice applying makeup, painting their fingernails and toenails, and doing each other's hair. One of the girls asks Jenna about a dark streak across the back of her neck near her hair line; Jenna looks in the mirror and sees the streak but doesn't know what it is. She unsuccessfully tries to wash it off. Because it does not hurt and is hidden by her hair, she doesn't think much more about it. The following day, Jenna sleeps the entire afternoon and does none of her chores ▼.

Episode 5

Jenna's brother comes home with new glasses this week. Jenna is quick to tell him the glasses make him look weirder than he already did.

Episode 6

Jenna is aware that her mother and sister are fighting about Jessica's boyfriend and about the baby. She finds this upsetting and eats half a package of cookies after school. Jenna's mother becomes angry when she learns this and tells Jenna that she needs to start watching what she eats.

Episode 7

Jenna has her first menstrual period. She recognizes what it is because of classes she had at school and because of things her friends told her. She is actually relieved to have her first period because all of her friends had periods and she wondered if something was wrong with her.

Evelyn buys Jessica some tampons and feminine napkins and tells Jenna not to flush these down the toilet. Jenna does not want Jason to see her tampons in the trash and figures they are small enough to flush. The following day, the toilet is stopped up and overflows onto the floor. Jenna denies flushing tampons and suggests that Jason just uses too much toilet paper ▼.

Episode 8

Jenna is teased at school by several of the boys in her class about being a "piggy." This hurts Jenna's feelings tremendously. Jenna and her friends make a pact not to talk to the boys until they apologize. Jenna eats three pieces of cake at Jason's party.

Episode 9

Jenna's youth group holds an annual pancake breakfast fundraising event. She gets to the church very early to help set up the tables and chairs and then spends time in the kitchen helping to serve the pancakes. She loves pancakes and has three plates over the course of the morning. She posts to her Facebook page so that everyone can see she is involved with volunteer work with her church ▼.

Episode 10

Jenna gets her report card at school this week and is pleased that she has all A's again. She likes the fact that people consider her smart. Jenna is aware that her brother has been in a fight at school again. She does not understand why he fights all the time and why he just can't sit down and do his homework the way she does. She is angry at him for making their mother upset. Jenna also knows that her mother is very worried about Ryan and Jessica. Jenna spends most evenings this week on Facebook while eating chips and drinking soda.

Episode 11

Jenna knows that Jessica is pregnant, but she still does not have a good understanding of how that all happens. Her mother is so wrapped up in that situation and with Jason that Jenna feels almost invisible. She has gained several pounds over the past few months, but she does not feel she has any control over her eating. She sometimes hates the way she looks and feels.

Episode 12

Jenna goes to a slumber party with several girls. The girls talk about their boyfriends at school. Jenna does not have a boyfriend, and she suspects the reason is that she is fat. Although she remains friends with the girls, she begins to feel like an outsider because of her weight. She wonders why she can't be skinny like her sister, Jessica.

Jenna's brother was kicked out of Boy Scouts this week. She wonders why he can't control himself.

Episode 13

There is an announcement at school that tryouts for the school Spirit Squad will be held in a couple of weeks. Jenna's friends talk about the tryouts and ask Jenna if she plans to try out. The girls on the Spirit Squad tend to be the popular girls at school. Jenna would love to be on the squad, thinking it could help her to become popular. However, she is becoming increasingly self-conscious about her weight and worries that people might laugh at her. She tells her friends that her mother doesn't have enough money for the uniforms and other expenses associated with Spirit Squad, because all their money goes to help her pregnant sister. She posts this information on her Facebook page in order to gain sympathy. Jenna likes getting this type of attention.

Jenna is unhappy when her mother informs her that Jason will be attending Bible class with her starting next week. It is bad enough that her mother teaches the class, but now her brother has to be there, too. Jenna hates being embarrassed by her family! ▼

Episode 14

Jenna goes out of town with her mother and Jason to visit her grandmother. Jenna loves to spend time with her grandmother, but she knows she has been sick lately with thyroid problems.

Episode 15

Jenna learns that all of her friends have made the Spirit Squad. She wishes she had tried out, but she did not want to face the possible embarrassment of not making the squad because of her weight. She is sure that her friends feel sorry for her because of what she posted on her Facebook page. However, she is told by some of her friends she was just "having a pity party."Sometimes Jenna feels really tired in the middle of the afternoon. One day she goes to the school nurse's office and ends up taking a nap there ▼.

Jenna Riley Season 2 Information

Episode 1

Jenna is a healthy but overweight 13-year-old girl who lives with her mother Evelyn and brother Jason. Her older sister, Jessica, lives a short distance away in her own apartment with her son, Ryan, and boyfriend, Casey. Jenna misses having her older sister around and looks up to Jessica.

Because her mother works a few evenings each week, Jenna is responsible for her younger brother Jason. She also often watches her nephew Ryan when he spends time in their home. Jenna is self-conscious about her weight. She knows she should try to lose weight, but she doesn't really know how and doesn't have much discipline when it comes to resisting snacks; she always feels hungry! She finds it very hard to not join in with her friends when they eat. Jenna goes to an overnight Bible camp with her youth group. Her mother is a chaperone but fortunately she does not directly supervise her activities. She has a lot of fun with the girls in her group and posts several of the activities to her Facebook page ▼.

Episode 2

Jenna had planned to hang out with her friends after school this week, but they now have Spirit Squad practice. Because Jenna is not on Spirit Squad, she feels hurt and left out. Jenna goes home and eats cookies. She hides the box of remaining cookies under her bed.

Later this week she cares for Ryan. While caring for him she doesn't think about the Spirit Squad once.

Episode 3

Jenna wakes up one morning this week with a huge pimple. She has been noticing little pimples lately, but she thinks this one can be seen from a mile away. Her mother does not even comment on the pimple. Jenna realizes her mother has been very distracted between worrying about Jason and Jessica.

Jenna frequently stays after school to watch her friends at Spirit Squad practice. One day after school this week, the Spirit Squad girls are making posters for the assembly. When Jenna offered to help, she is told that only Spirit Squad members could make the posters.

She watches Ryan one evening again this week.

Episode 4

Jenna is irritated with her mother for commenting on her weight and is further annoyed when she suggests they go out for a walk or to the gym. Jenna feels very tired in the afternoon and evening - too tired to get into an exercise routine.

Jenna becomes further annoyed when she is unable to find her favorite chips or cookies in the kitchen after school. Using her allowance, she buys candy from the store and hides it in her room so that her mother won't know she has it ▶ [NEWS].

Episode 5

Jenna is asked to babysit for a family from her church. She has watched her nephew, Ryan, before, but she has never had a real job or been paid to do this. She loves making money and tells her mother she wants to babysit more in the future ▼ [NEWS].

Episode 6

Jenna recognizes that her clothes are fitting tightly. She asks her mom if they could go shopping sometime soon, but she does not explain why. She is relieved when her mother does not comment about her weight gain. Jenna has more pimples on her face and is beginning to really hate the way she looks.

Episode 7

Jenna helps her mother make a cake for their family get-together. She secretly eats four pieces of cake over the course of the day and is glad that her mother doesn't notice. She feels very tired and spends the entire evening lying on the couch and watching TV [NEWS].

Episode 8

Jenna takes care of her nephew, Ryan, twice this week while Evelyn works at the mall. Jenna and Jason absolutely love taking care of Ryan. They find many games to play with him during the evenings.

Jenna hates the fact that she has more pimples. She washes her face three times a day, but the pimples continue to develop ✉.

Episode 9

Jenna has not been included in any activities with her friends on the Spirit Squad for quite some time now. She posts on her Facebook page indirect insults to them such as, "The truth comes out who your REAL friends are." She sees their posts that are directed at her that read, "Don't you HATE people who throw themselves pity parties?" She notices she has only 137 friends and they each have over 400 friends ✉.

Episode 10

Jenna hates the fact that there is (in her opinion) nothing good to eat at their house anymore and hates the lunches her mother makes for her. She usually trades most of her lunch away to other kids for foods that she likes. She constantly wants to drink soda pop and often drinks five cans in a day. She frequently needs to get up in the middle of the night to urinate. Jenna thinks this is causing her to be even more tired, and she vows to quit drinking sodas after 9 p.m.

Jenna spends an increasing amount of time on Facebook. She wants to prove to the mean girls on the Spirit Squad (who used to be her friends) that she is popular. She sets a goal of having over 500 friends. She sends out friend requests to many people she does not know, but look interesting. She also accepts friend requests from anybody, whether she knows them or not ✉ [NEWS].

Episode 11

Jenna is pleased with the number of friends she now has – she is up to 316 friends. She does not have as many friends as some of the girls on Spirit Squad, but she has many more than she did. She does not actually know many of her new Facebook "friends" – many of these are people that she sent friend requests to.

Episode 12

Jenna has a new Facebook friend by the name of Tom. He sent her a friend request and she accepted. Since then he has been sending her private messages telling her she is very pretty. Jenna loves the attention. He tells her he lives in a nearby city. She tells Tom all about her school and tells him she is a cheerleader ✉.

Episode 13

Jenna's sister has her baby this week. Jenna loves holding the new baby. She also found out that Casey hit Jessica and had to go to jail. Jenna wonders why her sister has such a jerky boyfriend. Jenna and Tom (her new friend on Facebook) send private messages back and forth several times a day. She tells him all about what has been going on. She begins to think of him as her boyfriend ✉.

Episode 14

Jenna is disappointed that no boy asks her to the roller skating party. All of her friends on the Spirit Squad were asked by boys from school. Jenna decides to go to the party anyway. Her friends on the Spirit Squad practically ignore her at the party, so Jenna spends time with some of the other girls. Jenna takes comfort in the fact that she regularly communicates with Tom on Facebook and knows that if he lived in the same city he would ask her out.

Jenna wants to lose weight but doesn't know how. Even though her mom has tried to force her to change her eating habits, Jenna can't stay away from soda and can't stop eating junk foods at school. She also feels too tired after school to exercise ✉ [NEWS].

Episode 15

Jenna brags on Facebook about her secret boyfriend. One of the girls from the Spirit Squad posts, "Your boyfriend must be an imaginary friend because nobody would want to date a fat girl like you." At Tom's request, Jenna has not revealed his identity. She figures he is just shy and guys don't like to post things about girls on Facebook anyway. She also realizes he has not actually asked her to be his girlfriend, but based on the things he writes, she is sure he thinks of her in this way ✉ [NEWS].

Jenna Riley Season 3 Information

Episode 1

Jenna is a healthy but overweight 14-year-old girl who lives with her mother Evelyn and brother Jason. Her older sister, Jessica, lives a short distance away in her own apartment with her boyfriend, Casey, and her children, Ryan and Carrie.

Jenna has recently gained a lot of weight. She is very self-conscious about her weight and believes her friends avoid her because she is fat. She knows she should try to lose weight, but she doesn't really know how and does not have much discipline when it comes to resisting snacks; she always feels hungry! She frequently hides the foods that she eats so that her mother will not make comments about what she is eating.

Jenna has been babysitting several days a week - either for free for her nephew and niece or for pay for two families at church. She does not mind taking care of her nieces and nephews, but she hates to turn down paid babysitting jobs because she has to take care of Jessica's kids. She knows Jessica does not have any money, but at the same time she does not think it is always fair. She posts comments on her Facebook page about having to babysit - AGAIN.

Jenna tells her friends at school that her dopey brother is taking medication for his ADHD problem. She is asked by one friend if he is taking Adderall. Jenna is not sure. Her friend tells Jenna that Adderall is the best thing for losing weight and she should try it. Jenna goes home and checks. Sure enough, Jason is taking Adderall. Jenna takes some pills - thinking there are so many in there nobody would ever notice. She takes one and loves the way it makes her feel. If it could help her lose weight, it would be great! ◥

Episode 2

During a gym class activity, Jenna goes to the school nurse, Violet Brinkworth, complaining of a twisted ankle. After examining the ankle, Violet talks with Jenna about other things that might be bothering her. Jenna tells the nurse that nobody wanted her on their team because she is too slow and that one of the boys told her she had a body like a penguin.

As the nurse talks with her more, Jenna shares that she has gained a lot of weight and is not happy about the fact that she is so heavy. She does not understand why she cannot be skinny like her sister. The nurse notices a dark pigmentation on the back of Jenna's neck and suggests to her that perhaps she might need to see a doctor to determine why she is gaining so much weight. Violet gets Jenna's permission to contact her mother about this matter.

At home, Jenna's mother surprises her when she asks if she knows why Jason is missing some pills. Jenna denies knowing anything about it. She decides she needs to take pills less often ▣.

Episode 3

Jenna continues to be rejected by her former friends on the Spirit Squad. She tries to join them at lunch, but she is frequently told that the table is already full. She goes to the practices to watch, but the girls ignore her presence. She is no longer invited to join them in any activities. She is sure they don't want to hang around with her anymore because she is fat.

She has an appointment with Dr. Rowe, the family physician, this week. Dr. Rowe takes a history and completes a physical exam. During the family history, Jenna is surprised to hear her mother report that obesity and diabetes run in her father's side of the family. Both her father and paternal grandmother have the disease.

Jenna's blood pressure is 120/78 mm Hg, and her body mass index (BMI) is 24.8, which places her at the 90% percentile for girls aged 14. A capillary blood glucose test done in the office is 158, and a urine dipstick shows a trace of glucose. Dr. Rowe also notices acanthosis nigricans on the back of Jenna's neck.

Based on the history and clinical findings, Dr. Rowe recognizes the need to test Jenna for diabetes. He orders an outpatient Thyroid-stimulating hormone blood test and a fasting blood glucose test to be performed on two different days. A follow-up appointment is scheduled for 2 weeks later. In the meantime, Jenna is encouraged to try to lose some weight by changing her dietary patterns and by exercising.

Episode 4

Jenna goes to the outpatient lab for blood tests on two different days this week. She hates the fact that she is unable to have breakfast until after her blood is drawn. After getting to school on both mornings, Jenna eats some doughnuts purchased from the snack machine. Jenna's mother announces to Jason and Jenna that 5 pills are missing from Jason's medication bottle and demands an explanation. Jenna denies knowing anything about it and wonders what the big deal is. A few days later when she tries to take a dose, the container is gone. Her mother seems to be on to her and has hidden the medication.

Jenna spends most of her time after school on Facebook. She posts many details about her medical workup and writes, "It sucks to be stuck by needles." Also, her communication with Tom has intensified. In several messages, he tells her that he has fallen in love with her and wants to meet her in person. He asks Jenna where she lives. Jenna wants to meet Tom, but she is afraid that he won't love her when he realizes how fat she is ◥.

Episode 5

Jenna returns to Dr. Rowe's office this week for a follow-up visit. Dr. Rowe tells Jenna and Evelyn that, based on the history, lab results, and other clinical findings, Jenna has type 2 diabetes. He recommends that a pediatric endocrinologist manage Jenna's diabetes and he provides her mother with a referral. Jenna has heard of diabetes before but doesn't know much about it. Although she doesn't think it is too big a deal, she enjoys posting many details of the experience on her Facebook page.

Tom, Jenna's Facebook boyfriend, continues to ask her to meet him. Jenna finally admits to Tom that she is a little overweight. Tom tells Jenna that it doesn't matter - that he loves her and wants to meet her. He also admits to Jenna he is really 20, not 18 like he originally told her. Jenna is pleased with the fact that Tom still loves her but wonders if she should be dating a 20-year-old guy.

Jenna finally tells her friends at school about Tom. They warn her not to tell him anything else and suggest that she stop communicating with him. Jenna thinks her friends are just jealous ▶ ▼.

Episode 6

It is report card time and, once again, Jenna has made straight A's. The recent teasing from her peers has been difficult, but she feels very proud to see her name near the top of the honor roll list.

Jenna has an appointment with Dr. Rena Yin, a pediatric endocrinologist, this week. Another history, work-up, and blood tests are completed. Dr. Yin elects to start Jenna on Metformin (Glucophage), 500 mg twice daily, to be taken with meals.

Jenna and Evelyn also meet with Marjorie, a nurse who is a certified diabetic educator (CDE), to begin the process of learning about diabetes self-management. Marjorie outlines the four major components of self-management: nutrition therapy, an increase in physical activity, self-monitoring of blood glucose, and drug therapy. Jenna immediately likes Marjorie because she doesn't make her feel uncomfortable about the fact that she is fat. She seems to accept her just the way she is.

Tom continues to suggest that he meet Jenna in person. He tells her he would like to drive to her city and take her on a real date. Jenna has been told not to completely trust everything people say online, but she is sure Tom is honest. Instead of agreeing to meet him, she gives him her cell phone number so they can talk ▶ ▼.

Episode 7

Jenna continues to meet with Marjorie, the CDE. The primary focus of initial education efforts is self-monitoring of blood glucose. Marjorie teaches Jenna how to perform a finger stick and measure her glucose level. She is instructed to do this twice a day for a few weeks to see how the new medication is working. Jenna hates poking her finger.

Over the course of meeting with Marjorie, Jenna opens up to her and tells her about the teasing at school and about her boyfriend Tom, whom she met on Facebook. Concerned about what Jenna might be telling this man, Marjorie talks with Jenna further about the situation and points out that it could be a very dangerous situation for her. Jenna tells Marjorie that Tom is not that way. Marjorie shares a brochure on Internet safety for teens and asks her to read it so they can discuss it on their next visit. She also suggests that Jenna talk with her mother about this.

Jenna talks and texts with Tom on the phone regularly. She tells Tom about what Marjorie said and he tells her that there are a lot of bad people out there – "Good thing I am not one of them!" He asks Jenna when he can meet her.

Episode 8

Jenna finally agrees to meet Tom in a public place at Neighborhood Mall. Feeling a bit nervous, Jenna asks Wendy, one of her friends, to go with her. Jenna puts on her best outfit and uses extra makeup. The girls get a ride to the mall from Wendy's mother and they agree to be picked up in 3 hours. Shortly after arriving at the mall, Wendy sees some other friends and tells Jenna she will be right back. Jenna waits at the appointed place when a man approaches her. He tells her he is Tom and hands her a flower. He tells her she is even more beautiful in person that he imagined and asks her if she is alone. She tells him her friends are at the mall with her. Jenna is surprised to see that in person Tom looks much older than 20. They spend nearly two hours together at the food court. After having some lunch, he suggests they leave the mall together – promising to take her home. Jenna tells Tom she has a ride and that her friend Wendy is probably waiting for her. While Jenna is sending a text to Wendy, asking her to come by the food court, Tom gets up and tells Jenna he is going to the restroom and will be right back. Jenna never gets a response from Wendy, and Tom does not come back and does not answer his phone. Jenna ends up calling her mother to pick her up from the mall.

Episode 9

Jenna does not hear back from Tom. He "unfriends" her on Facebook and later his account disappears. She texts him a few times but he doesn't answer. She wonders what she did wrong and why he suddenly disappeared. Although she feels disappointed, she does not dwell on it very long.

Jenna has completed most of the initial diabetic education. She feels like she learned a lot, but does not perceive her disease to be really all that bad. Marjorie suggests to Jenna that she attend diabetes camp to be held in a few months. Jenna likes the idea of going to a camp with other girls who have the same problem.

Although she adheres to the finger pricks and medication regimen, Jenna does not stick to her diet or attempt to increase her activity. The new diet leads to many fights with her mother. There are so many limitations on what she can eat that she often feels left out among her friends at school. She posts detailed information about her diabetes on Facebook in order to gain attention and sympathy. She posts a picture of herself with the message "Sticking my finger with a needle. Diabetes sucks ▼."

Episode 10

Jenna has no interest in following a diet. She finds herself thinking about food all the time and ends up eating compulsively at school. Jenna quickly figures out that, if she doesn't stick to her diet, the elevated glucose level is stored in the memory of the glucose monitor. She tries to erase the higher numbers so that Marjorie and her mother will not see them, but she is afraid she might break the meter and get into trouble. Instead, she figures out she can use her friend's blood to register good blood glucose measurements on the monitor 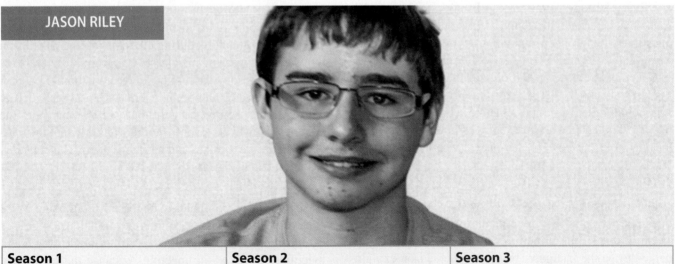.

Episode 11
Jenna learns that Casey is in jail and sees his picture and story on the local evening news. She hopes none of her friends recognize him as the man who is with her sister. Jenna also learns that he has been beating up Jessica, and Jessica has been trying to get away from him. Jenna is afraid of Casey and hopes she never sees him again.

Jenna continues to eat whatever she pleases at school. She frequently feels very tired and grouchy. Jenna has noticed that if her blood glucose levels are high, she can lose weight more easily. She does not understand how this works, but she likes the idea of losing weight. She continues to use her friend's blood for the glucose measurements.

Episode 12
Jenna's sister Jessica goes to church and then brunch with them this week. Because her mother is with her, she is forced to order food from the menu that is on her diet plan. She wishes she could eat the chocolate chip pancakes that Jason eats. Feeling sorry for herself, Jenna takes a picture of her meal and posts to Facebook with the message "Forced to eat healthy because of my diabetes."

Episode 13
Darren, one of Jenna's friends, figures out how to alter the memory on the blood glucose device. Jenna tells him what numbers to program into the monitor and figures out that this frees her from having to follow a diet (except when at home). She is quite sure that nobody will ever know the difference.

Episode 14
It has been a couple of months since Jenna began a treatment plan for diabetes management. She has a follow-up visit with Dr. Yin (the pediatric endocrinologist) and Marjorie, the CDE. She proudly shows her record of blood glucose levels from her blood glucose monitor, which reflects excellent glycemic control. She claims to have been following the diet, exercising, and taking her medication. She also tells them she has lost some weight - maybe 7 pounds. Dr. Yin and Marjorie note that she has lost 4 pounds since her last visit and that her Hb A1c level is 10.2%. Dr. Yin and Marjorie recognize the need for additional education with Jenna and confront her about the measurements recorded on the glucometer.

Episode 15
Jenna is excited about the fact that Jessica is moving back home with them. She has missed her older sister and loves her children. Despite some of her recent disappointments with the diabetes and excessive weight gain, Jenna takes comfort in the close relationships she experiences within her family.

JASON RILEY

Season 1	Season 2	Season 3
Jason has a history of academic and behavioral problems at school. His mother has been trying to get help for him for some time, but with no luck. It is determined that he needs glasses, but these don't resolve the problems at school.	Jason's problems at school continue. He gets into fights frequently and does poor academically. He is finally referred to a neuropsychologist, who diagnoses Jason with ADHD. Jason starts taking Ritalin, and an IEP is developed at school.	After adjusting to new medication and the IEP, Jason slowing begins to make academic progress, and his social skills improve. He begins to make a couple of friends.

Jason Riley Season 1 Information

Episode 1

Jason is an active, healthy 11-year-old boy. He is currently in fifth grade at the public grade school near his home. He lives with his mother, Evelyn, and his 13-year-old sister Jenna. He has never had much contact with his father. Jason's home life has been somewhat stressful the past year or so because of ongoing fights between his mother and oldest sister Jessica that resulted in Jessica moving out of the house. Jason gets along well with his mother, but he has typical sibling conflicts with Jenna.

Jason has had problems in school for the past 3 years. Teachers report that he has difficulty staying on task and won't follow directions. Although he made some progress last year with his fourth-grade teacher, his grades have been consistently poor. His mother tries to help him with homework after school or in the evenings, but these sessions frequently turn into battlegrounds. It takes Jason hours to complete fairly simple assignments, resulting in a great deal of frustration for him and his mother. The fact that he frequently comes home from school with headaches further aggravates the situation. In addition to problems with academics, Jason has problems with social interactions. His teachers at school find him to be disruptive in the classroom. During the past year, he has frequently been sent to the principal's office for misbehaving. He is often teased at school. Most of his time at home is spent playing video and computer games and watching TV.

Every Sunday Jason goes to Bible school class. His mother is a teacher for Jenna's class and so there is no question whether they are going to attend each week. Jason hates attending Bible school because he does not like any of the boys in the class. Many of them are in his class at school, too. He gets teased pretty regularly at school and it just continues at Bible school. He also does not like his teacher because he does nothing to stop the teasing from the boys in the class. He is pretty sure the teacher does not like him.

Episode 2

Jason gets in a fight at school this week when a classmate does not give him the green paint during an art activity. Jason is sent to the principal's office because he is perceived to be the instigator by the teacher. Jason explains to the principal that he wanted the green paint, but nobody would give it to him, so he punched his classmate to get it. He tells his mother he had a headache all day at school.

Episode 3

Jason comes home from school with a headache twice this week. His mother suggests that he join the Boy Scout troop associated with his school, hoping he'll get interested in something besides video games and make some friends. Jason is not thrilled about the idea, but he agrees to try it.

Episode 4

Violet Brinkworth, the school nurse, performs vision screening tests at Jason's school this week. Violet tells Jason he may need glasses. He attends his first Boy Scout meeting and finds that some of the boys in the troop are the same ones who often tease him at school. Still, he likes the Scoutmasters and decides to go again next week. Jason fails to complete a volcano project at school, and his teacher sends a note home to inform his mother. His mother grounds him for a week, which he thinks is "just dumb."

Episode 5

Jason's mother takes him to the optometrist's office this week to get fitted for glasses. Jason hates the fact that he has to wear glasses, but the eye doctor says they might help his headaches go away. The following day Jason is teased at school for wearing glasses, and Jenna tells him he looks like a nerd. Jason has already earned his first badge in his Boy Scout troop and takes interest in finding out how to advance to the next rank. He does not care much for the other boys in the troop, but he really likes the leaders, especially Mr. Richman.

Episode 6

Jason hates wearing his new glasses because the kids at school tease him when he wears them. To avoid further teasing, he puts them in his backpack when he gets to school. Unfortunately, during class his teacher asks Jason why he is not wearing his glasses – in front of several kids in the class. Jason tells him he left them at home. Later in the afternoon he intentionally breaks his glasses before getting home, hoping he will not have to wear them the next day. However, Jason's mother runs down to the optical shop before it closes and has them fixed. The next day, Jason reluctantly wears the glasses.

Episode 7

At school, Jason continues to be teased about being weird and for wearing glasses. Sometimes he takes his glasses off when he gets to school. He is still going to Boy Scout meetings. He likes the meetings because the leaders do not tolerate teasing among the boys. His favorite Boy Scout leader is Pat Richman. He is looking forward to going on a hike over the weekend with his troop.

Episode 8

Jason has a party at his house this week. Only some of the kids he invited come to the party. He also has a bad meeting at Boy Scouts this week. He got confused listening to directions while working on a badge and became disruptive. When he is disciplined by the head Scoutmaster, he becomes angry and has a temper tantrum. The assistant scoutmaster, Pat Richman, helps him to settle down and talks with his mother briefly after the meeting [NEWS].

Episode 9
Jason and his mother and sister attend a pancake breakfast fundraising event at the church. After a few hours, Jason is bored and gets permission from his mother to walk home. He is happy to have the house to himself and sits down to play video games. When his mother arrives home, she tells Jason that he will be spending a few hours a week with Pastor Jeff, helping him at the church. Jason likes Pastor Jeff but does not like the idea that he has to spend more time at the church. He thinks he goes there enough already.

Later in the week, Jason reports to the church to help Pastor Jeff. He is asked to help organize the hymnals for next Sunday's mass and to fold bulletins. Jason does not like the work, but he thinks Pastor Jeff is cool.

Episode 10
Report cards come out this week. Jason has a C, two D's, and an F. On the playground at recess, he gets into a fight with another boy who teases him for being dumb. Jason is unable to concentrate long enough to complete his homework assignments that evening, leading to another fight with his mother. She tells him he can't watch TV for two days. This makes him angry, and he gets on his bike and rides away, despite Evelyn's demand that he stay home. He goes to the nearby park, finds a stick, and hits the playground equipment.

One of the kids that Jason invited to his party several weeks ago is having a birthday party. All of the kids at school are talking about it, but Jason does not get invited. He does not understand why he doesn't get an invitation. He feels hurt, but he is too embarrassed to ask his friend about it [▶].

Episode 11
Jason is taken to a doctor's appointment to get some help with all the problems he is experiencing. He finds the discussion between his mother and Dr. Rowe very embarrassing. He also knows that Mom is really mad at Jessica, but he does not know why.

While working for Pastor Jeff at the church this week, Jason is asked to unpack a shipment of supplies and place them in the storeroom. He tells Pastor Jeff about the mean boys in Scouts and at school.

Episode 12
This week, Jason becomes angry at the Boy Scout meeting during a game. In his frustration, he bites one of the other scouts. The Scoutmaster takes Jason home and tells his mother that he can no longer come to the meetings. Jenna teases her brother about being so dumb that he can't even be a Boy Scout. His mother sends him to his room, where he spends the rest of the evening. He feels like such a failure. He wishes he could just kill the boys in the Scout troop.

Episode 13
Jason has a fight with two boys during Bible class. The boys are the same ones he was in a fight with in the Boy Scout troop. They were making fun of him for getting kicked out of Scouts. Jason is told by Pastor Jeff that he will now be attending the Bible class taught by his mother. Jason points out that is the 7th and 8th grade class, and Pastor Jeff tells him he is getting special permission to go to class with the older kids.

Episode 14
Jason goes to his grandmother's house this week with his mother and sister Jenna. He enjoys being away from school, but he is miserable that he does not have a computer or video game to play while there. His sister annoys him, and they frequently argue. He spends most of his time watching TV until his mother tells him to go out and play. He goes outside and throws rocks at cars from behind a hedge.

Episode 15
Jason has been attending Bible class with his mother and sister for a few weeks now. He does not have any friends in the class– in fact they pretty much ignore him — but nobody is teasing him. Jason figures he is not getting teased because his mother and sister are there. At the church, Jason helps clean music stands for the choir and he helps to fold, stack, and store folding chairs that were used for a function the previous day.

Jason Riley Season 2 Information

Episode 1
Jason is an active, healthy 12-year-old boy. He is currently in fifth grade at the public grade school near his home. He lives with his mother, Evelyn, and his 14-year-old sister, Jenna. Jason has ongoing problems in school with academics and with social interactions. During the past year, he has often been sent to the principal's office for misbehaving. He was kicked out of Boy Scouts and his Bible study class. He is frequently teased at school. Most of his time at home is spent playing video and computer games and watching TV. He has been working a few hours each week at the church with Pastor Jeff.

This episode Jason attends an overnight Bible camp with his church. He isolates himself from most of the kids when he can and entertains himself by playing games on his phone. He also offers to help the adults. He finds he enjoys the company of adults more than of people his own age.

Episode 2

Jason is the target of teasing at school in gym class. His mother suggests that he resolve problems by talking to his teachers instead of getting into fights. He tells the gym teacher about the teasing in the locker room, but he doesn't think the teacher listens or even cares. The boys in the class call him a "girly-boy" and make fun of him for telling the teacher. After school, Jason tries to share this experience with his mother, but she is busy taking care of his nephew Ryan. This makes him angry, and he runs into his room and tears up one of his school books.

Episode 3

Jason is bullied again by some of the boys in school this week. He tells the boys if they tease him again he will bring a knife to school and stab them. The boys report Jason's threats of stabbing them to the teachers. Because of his ongoing problems and his verbal threat, the school administrators threaten to expel him.

While at the church helping Pastor Jeff, Jason tells him about the trouble he got into at school. Pastor Jeff asks Jason if he really would consider taking a knife to school and Jason tells him no, but he wanted to scare the mean boys. Pastor Jeff reinforces to Jason that he needs to find other ways to address such conflict.

Episode 4

Jason does his best to ignore the ongoing teasing at school and resists the temptation to get into a fight. He is forced to do group work and can't seem to sit still. He hates the kids in his group and is disruptive. When redirected by the teacher, he thinks he is being picked on. It has reached the point at which he really hates going to school. He wishes he could go to a different school where the kids are nice.

Episode 5

Pastor Jeff gives Jason some money for helping him at the church over the past several months. Jason uses the money to buy a new video game he has been wanting. Once he gets the game, he plays non-stop for hours at a time over the next several days.

Episode 6

Jason's mother takes him to the neuropsychologist for an evaluation this week. The psychologist talks with Jason in an attempt to get to know him. He asks Jason what he likes to do, what he finds fun, and what school is like for him. Jason tells him that he doesn't like school because the other kids are dumb and they pick on him. Jason also shares that the teachers do not like him. He tells the doctor that he has a "job" at the church and that he likes Pastor Jeff. Jason undergoes psychometric testing ▶.

Episode 7

Jason enjoys the family get-together that his mother has planned. He likes it when his oldest sister Jessica is at home and they are all together. Jason also is glad to see his mother happy for a change.

Episode 8

Jason has another visit with the psychologist this week. He talks more with Jason about school and what his life is like in his home. Jason tells the psychologist about Jessica and her baby, and the fact that she is going to have another baby. He also tells the psychologist about mean kids at school and that he gets blamed for everything. He tells him that he wishes some of the other kids at school were dead. He admits that he has a hard time remembering what he needs to do for school once he gets home.

Episode 9

Two boys in Jason's class at school pour a bottle of glue on Jason's chair and he sits in it. He is so angry he turns over his chair, screaming that he hates everyone. This time the teacher recognizes what happened and disciplines the other two boys. She then sends Jason to the office to call his mother so she can bring him a different pair of pants to wear for the rest of the day. For the first time that Jason can remember, he is not being blamed for a problem.

Episode 10

The psychologist tells Jason that he believes the reason he has trouble at school is because of a problem known as Attention deficit hyperactivity disorder (or ADHD). He asks Jason if he would be willing to take some medication and maybe make some changes at school to help him feel better. Jason agrees to try the medications and changes at school, but he is sure the kids will still tease him.

Episode 11

Jason's mother has a meeting with the principal and counselor. He is embarrassed by the fact that they are talking about him. He wonders if they will make fun of him. After school he goes to the church to talk with Pastor Jeff about the meeting at school. Pastor Jeff tells him it sounds like positive progress, and he does not think the principal and counselor will make fun of him. It sounds like they want to help.

Episode 12

Jason takes tests this week at the school district offices. He is told that the tests will help his teachers help him learn better.

Episode 13

Jason's sister, Jessica, has her baby this week. He knows that his mother has been very upset and that she does not like Jessica's boyfriend. He overhears his mother tell a friend that Casey was arrested. Jason wonders what it is like to go to jail and is excited to see the new baby.

Episode 14

The neuropsychologist meets with Jason and Evelyn again this week to discuss positive reinforcement and time management strategies. Specifically, he suggests that Jason spend more time interacting with others and less time playing video games at home, unless the video games are educational. He also talks to Jason about taking the medication.

Episode 15

Based on the reports from the school counselor and neuropsychologist, Dr. Rowe (the family practice physician) agrees to write a prescription for amphetamine and dextroamphetamine (Adderall) for Jason. Dr. Rowe starts Jason off on 5 mg twice a day (first dose when he wakes up and the second dose around lunch time). Dr. Rowe also mentions the dose will be adjusted to response. Jason is asked to return weekly until the optimal response is obtained.

Jason Riley Season 3 Information

Episode 1

Jason is an active, healthy 12-year-old boy. He lives with his mother, Evelyn, and his 14-year-old sister, Jenna. He has never had much contact with his father. Jason's home life has been somewhat stressful during the past year or so because of fighting between his mother and his oldest sister Jessica, and the fact that Jessica just had another baby.

Jason has had problems in school (both academically and socially) for the past several years. Recently, he was diagnosed with Attention deficit hyperactivity disorder (or ADHD) and began taking medication for it. At school, an individualized educational plan and special accommodations have been developed. He continues to work a few hours each week at the church with Pastor Jeff. The church staff members have really come to enjoy Jason, and he feels like it is one place that he fits in.

Jason takes amphetamine and dextroamphetamine (Adderall) before school every morning and again at lunch time, requiring a trip to the nurse's office. Jason feels a bit nervous and less hungry ever since he started to take the medication. He does not want any of the kids to know he takes medication. Likewise, he doesn't want the other kids to know he has a "special plan," because he is afraid of being teased. At home, Jason is not happy about having limits placed on playing video games. He is not interested in reading books or doing other activities and feels angry about the changes expected of him.

Episode 2

Jason has been taking the new medication (amphetamine and dextroamphetamine [Adderall]) for several weeks. Evelyn asks Jason if he knows why he is almost out of medicine and Jason indicates he does not know. He just takes his medication when she gives it to him.

Episode 3

Jason has been taking amphetamine and dextroamphetamine (Adderall) for a month now and his dose has been stabilized to 10 mg twice a day. He feels less agitated and has a calmer presence. He has not been in any fights for several weeks and has been able to understand the teacher's instructions in class. Despite this, he gets teased for going to a resource room and for being dumb and weird. The fact that he has no friends makes him feel sad and angry. No matter how hard he tries, nobody likes him. But at least the school work doesn't seem as hard as before. Jason does not like the restrictions placed on video games at home. Sometimes, he plays them late at night after his mother goes to bed, but then he is very tired during school the following day.

Episode 4

Pastor Jeff talks with Jason at length about his feelings. Jason wishes Pastor Jeff were his father. He believes Pastor Jeff is the only person in the world who truly understands him. When he goes to the church to work, everyone is nice to him, and it is the one place where he feels wanted. Jason thinks about maybe being a pastor someday when he grows up.

At home, Jason misses playing his video games. However, based on the recommendations from his special teachers at school, he is given other computer games to play that are educationally oriented. He does not enjoy these as much as playing combat games, but he finds them more enjoyable than watching television or reading.

Episode 5

Jason has a fight at school this week. One of the boys sees him in the nurse's office when he goes to get his lunchtime medication and tells all the other kids that Jason takes pills because he is crazy. The kids start calling him "Crazy Jazy." Jason tries to ignore the teasing, but he finally punches one of the boys in the stomach and tells him, "I'm going to kill you." He is sent to the principal's office, and his mother is called when he is unable to settle down. He feels out of control and screams, yells, and shouts obscenities at the top of his voice. The school principal tells Evelyn to keep him home from school for the rest of the week.

Episode 6

Report cards are distributed this week. Jason is disappointed because he got all C's and a D. He is surprised (and relieved) that his mother signs the report card and does not even comment on the grades. Jason has a better week at school. The boys who teased him previously keep their distance and make no comments to him. A new student at the school named Brian talks with Jason about a video game they both have.

Jason learns that his sister Jenna has diabetes. His mother announces that there are going to be big changes in the way the whole family eats. She will not have any junk food in the house, and everybody is going to eat breakfast every morning. Jason hates having his sister's problems affect the food he has to eat.

Episode 7

Jason's new friend, Brian, spends the night this weekend. They spend most of their time playing video games - his mother has allowed them to play whatever game they want. Jason is very happy to have a new friend ▼.

Episode 8

Pastor Jeff listens with great interest as Jason tells him about his new friend, Brian. Pastor Jeff knows Brian and his family; they recently moved to the Neighborhood. Brian's father told Pastor Jeff that Brian has Asperger syndrome and had difficulty making friends. He finds it ironic that Jason and Brian found each other within a matter of a few weeks.

Episode 9

Jason has gradually been doing better in school. He has been keeping up with assignments and is better able to follow instructions. He has not been involved in any fights recently. Jason and Brian have another friend named Mike, and Jason is very happy to have two friends at school. Jason is somewhat aware of Jessica's problems with Casey and overhears his mother mentioning to Jenna that Jessica is hiding from him. He

does not fully understand where she might hide and pictures Jessica and her kids hiding in a closet or under a bed ▼.

Episode 10

A meeting is held this week with Jason, his mother, his teacher, the principal, and the school counselor. Jason is thrilled when his teacher shares with everyone the progress that he has made over the past month. Jason can tell that his mother is happy with the news, but she does not seem as excited as he thought she might be. He feels a bit disappointed with her response.

Episode 11

Jason learns that Casey killed somebody in a car accident and is in jail. He wonders why Casey did that and why he is so mean to his sister, Jessica. The following day, Jason tells Pastor Jeff about Casey. Pastor Jeff tells Jason that the people who were killed were church members and they will be having services at the church the following day. Jason feels very bad about the situation.

Episode 12

Jason is glad to see his sister Jessica. On their way to church, Jason tells Jessica that Pastor Jeff said the people Casey killed belonged to the church. Jessica does not reply to the comment, and his mother says they are aware of this, and he should not discuss it further.

Episode 13

Brian invites Jason and Mike to go on a fishing and camping trip over the weekend. Jason is thrilled to catch his first fish. Brian's father teaches the boys how to clean fish with a knife. Jason has never seen the inside of a fish before. They later cook fish over the campfire for supper. While sitting around the campfire, the boys talk about video games and Jason talks about Pastor Jeff ▼.

Episode 14

Jason tells Pastor Jeff about his camping trip with his two friends, Mike and Brian. Recognizing the importance of building on these friendships, Pastor Jeff tells Jason he would like to meet Mike. Pastor Jeff contacts Mike's father to get permission for his son to join them for pizza. Jason thinks Pastor Jeff is the best.

Episode 15

Jason is glad that his oldest sister is moving back home. Although he is not too interested in the baby, Jason loves to play with his nephew, Ryan. Ryan breaks Jason's head set, but instead of becoming angry, Jason remains calm ▼.

RILEY & HOLMES HOUSEHOLD

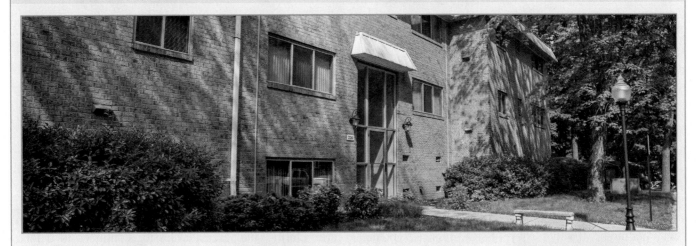

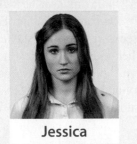

Jessica

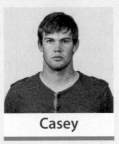

Casey

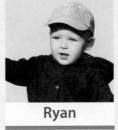

Ryan

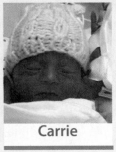

Carrie

Housing	Jessica lives in a small 2 bedroom apartment in the Southend district. She lives close to the downtown area. She is several blocks from her mother.
Parks and Recreation	There are only a few parks in the area and some of them are in disrepair.
Services	There is bus service to the area and the restaurant where Jessica works is close by. Neighborhood Hospital and Women's Health Services are located on the other side of the downtown area from the Riley/Holmes apartment.

Key: ▶ = video clip   ☰ = medical record   ▼ = journal entry   NEWS = news article

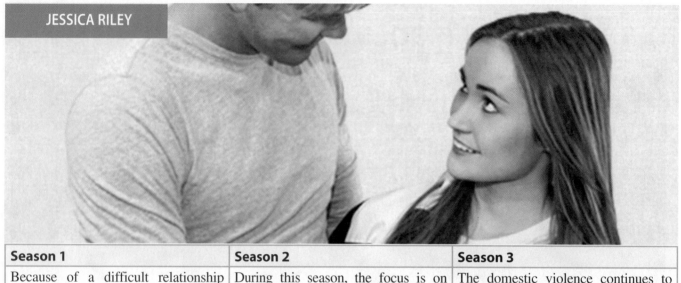

JESSICA RILEY

Season 1	Season 2	Season 3
Because of a difficult relationship with her mother, Evelyn Riley, Jessica recently moved into her own apartment with her infant son. She is trying to go to school, work, and take care of her baby. She is struggling financially. Early on in this season, she meets Casey. He moves in with her and she gets pregnant again.	During this season, the focus is on Jessica's prenatal care. During the pregnancy, she becomes the victim of domestic violence. Near term (38 weeks), she is kicked in the abdomen by Casey, causing her to go into labor. She delivers a healthy infant daughter.	The domestic violence continues to escalate. Jessica continues to defend Casey, believing that he will eventually become a good father. Eventually she seeks refuge in a shelter. Jessica and her kids move back home with Evelyn, and she plans to go back to school and finish a degree so that she can support herself.

Jessica Riley Season 1 Information

Episode 1

Jessica Riley is a 17-year-old single mother of a 1-month-old infant, Ryan. Ryan's father ended his relationship with Jessica when she was 4 months pregnant. She has not seen or heard from him since that time, but she has been told by friends that he left the state. Her relationship with her mother, Evelyn, has been strained for the past several years and worsened when she became pregnant. Because she was constantly fighting with her mother, Jessica moved out of her mother's home into a small, one-bedroom apartment when she was 6 months pregnant.

Jessica grew up in a single-parent home. Her father left the family when she was 7. She is the oldest child and has two younger siblings, Jenna and Jason. She recently completed her GED and is now trying to go to school part-time for an associate's degree in cosmetology at the local community college. She also works nearly full-time as a waitress at a restaurant, but because she has been supporting herself and her baby, she struggles financially. Her mother, Evelyn, helps by watching her baby a few hours each day. Additionally, Jessica receives government assistance in the form of WIC coupons and Medicaid. Jessica does not exercise and eats mostly fast food. She smokes about one-half of a pack of cigarettes a day and drinks alcohol socially when she parties.

Jessica often feels overwhelmed while trying to care for her infant, work, and go to school. Ryan experiences colic almost every night, spits up frequently, and cries constantly. She is so tired of listening to Ryan cry! Jessica has made several visits to the Emergency Department (ED) during the past couple of weeks, but the doctors (in her opinion) don't do anything. She had tried to breastfeed her baby, but concluded that she did not have enough milk, so she switched to formula. She believes this may be causing Ryan's colic. Jessica is not getting enough sleep; she feels nervous and exhausted. She misses being able to go out with her friends whenever she feels like it ▼ [NEWS].

Episode 2

Jessica's friend Amy invites her to a party at her home. Jessica believes she deserves a break from Ryan and asks her mother to watch him for a few hours. Jessica is thrilled to go out! At the party, she meets a guy named Casey, and they spend the rest of the evening together. Jessica calls her mother and tells her she will just pick Ryan up in the morning. Casey goes with Jessica back to her apartment and spends the night with her ▽.

Episode 3

Jessica and her mother, Evelyn, take Ryan for his 2-month well-baby visit at the pediatrician's office. Jessica met the pediatrician at the hospital when Ryan was born. She tells the pediatrician about her ongoing problems with Ryan's colic and that she has a hard time getting enough sleep. The pediatrician assures her that this stage will pass and praises her for the weight Ryan has gained since birth.

Jessica has been with Casey almost constantly since meeting him at the party a few weeks ago, and they decide to live together. Casey moves in with Jessica and Ryan and agrees to watch the baby in the evenings so that Jessica can work more hours. Jessica is thrilled to have someone to take care of her and Ryan. She tells her mother that she only needs Evelyn to watch Ryan during the daytime. Evelyn expresses concern about the live-in boyfriend and offers to keep Ryan, but Jessica tells her mother that she can raise her own baby ▽.

Episode 4

Jessica works every evening this week. She is so happy that Casey has moved in with her. She likes the idea of Ryan being able to stay home as opposed to being dragged out the door to her mother's house or to a daycare center. When she is with Casey, he is so good to Ryan. She is glad he seems to love her son. However, one evening when returning home from work, she asks Casey how the baby is and he replies, "The kid cries too much! ▽"

Episode 5

Jessica is working many extra evenings and likes the fact that she is starting to have a little more money to spend. In her opinion, having Casey live with her to care for Ryan is a perfect situation. However, she sometimes wonders if Ryan is being fed when Casey takes care of him. One time she finds a nearly full bottle of milk with him in the crib, and he always needs his diaper changed when she comes home. Casey sometimes yells at Jessica when she returns home about her "damn baby that won't quit crying" and says she has turned Ryan into a spoiled brat - the reason he cries so much is because he just wants attention. Although she has some concerns, she doesn't say anything for fear that Casey might leave her. She loves and needs Casey ▽.

Episode 6

Jessica asks her mother to take care of Ryan for a few hours so she can run errands. When she comes back several hours later, she has another fight with her mother. Evelyn voices her concerns about Ryan not gaining enough weight and says that he looks dirty - he has dried milk on his neck, and his clothes are stained. She also questions whether living with Casey is in Jessica's or Ryan's best interest. Jessica gets very defensive and angry, accusing her mother of not liking Casey and trying to make her feel dumb. Jessica tells her mother that, if she continues to criticize her, she won't let her take care of the baby anymore.

Jessica is concerned when Casey informs her he was fired from his job this week. He tells her not to worry - that he can get another job fast ▽.

Episode 7

Jessica has her 18th birthday this week. She and Casey celebrate by going out for pizza. Jessica hopes that Casey gets another job soon. She is picking up as many hours as she can to pay the bills. Ryan is due for his 4-month well-baby check-up and immunizations. Because she has a test at school, Jessica cancels the appointment ▽.

Episode 8

Casey is still out of work and Jessica gives him money to buy beer and food. She does not mind one bit because he is so much fun. Jessica has been introduced to all of Casey's friends and they often come to the apartment to party. This is very convenient, in Jessica's opinion, because she does not have to get a babysitter. During such parties, she often props Ryan in an infant seat on the floor next to the couch so she can keep an eye on him.

Episode 9

Jessica is relieved that Casey has a job again, but unfortunately he won't get paid until next week. She has to work several extra shifts to have enough money for the rent, which is due at the end of the week. She is feeling very tired from working extra shifts. It is hard enough making ends meet just for Ryan and herself, but having Casey also live with her without an income creates a significant financial strain. She is sure that now that he has a job, things will get much easier and they will have plenty of money ▽.

Episode 10

Jessica experiences nausea and fatigue 4 days this week. She also notices breast tenderness. She recalls that these symptoms are similar to how she felt shortly after she became pregnant with Ryan. Although she thinks it is possible that she is pregnant, she is pretty sure she is not because she just had a baby, and her menstrual cycles have been irregular. She cannot recall when her last period was, but she decides just to wait and see when she gets her next period.

Jessica allows her mother to take Ryan for his 6-month check-up and immunizations this week. After the visit, Evelyn reports that, according to the pediatrician, Ryan is falling a bit behind on his weight and needs to be fed more. Evelyn again voices her concerns about Ryan's care. Jessica tells her mother to shut up and mind her own business.

Episode 11

Jessica continues to be nauseated and has a hard time keeping anything down. While at work, she becomes dizzy and faints. Her coworkers urge Jessica to go to a doctor to get checked out. She goes to the Neighborhood Hospital Emergency Department and, following a workup, is told that she is pregnant. Jessica is instructed to follow up with her healthcare provider for prenatal care. Jessica quits going to school because she recognizes that, with another baby on the way, she will need to work more hours to make ends meet ▶ ▽.

Episode 12

Jessica goes for her first prenatal visit at the same women's healthcare practice where she went when she was pregnant with Ryan. On this visit, Jessica meets Carol Ramsey, a nurse midwife, and immediately likes her. An ultrasound scan shows her pregnancy to be about 16 weeks' gestation.

Jessica is advised to decrease or stop smoking, avoid alcohol, eat a nutritious diet, and take prenatal vitamins. She is instructed to go to the outpatient lab within a couple of days for a multiple marker screen (mms). Later in the week, Jessica goes with Casey to a party where she is introduced to Amanda Hardin - Casey's friend Robert's new girlfriend. Jessica thinks Amanda is really cool and hopes they can become friends ▶ ▽ [NEWS].

Episode 13

Over the past few weeks, Jessica notices that Casey has become increasingly possessive. He frequently questions her about men she works with at the restaurant and discourages her from hanging out with her friends. One afternoon this week, Jessica receives a phone call from Rick, a male colleague from work asking her to cover a shift for him. Casey immediately questions her about Rick in an accusatory manner. He pushes her backward onto the couch ▶.

Episode 14

Ryan has had a cold all week. Because Evelyn is out of town, Jessica's friend Megan agrees to babysit during the day while Jessica is at work. When she picks up Ryan, Megan tells Jessica that he did not eat anything, and she thinks he has a fever. Jessica knows he has been sick all week and observes that Ryan is sleeping. She is glad he is finally not crying. When she drops off Ryan at home on her way back to work for the evening shift, she asks Casey to keep an eye on him because he might have a fever.

When Jessica gets home from work later in the evening, she finds Casey asleep on the couch. She picks up Ryan and feels how hot he is. He is also limp, like a rag doll. Jessica notices that he is making funny noises when he breathes. She is frightened and immediately takes him to the Neighborhood Hospital Emergency Department, where Ryan is admitted with dehydration and bronchiolitis. While at the hospital, he is also diagnosed with Respiratory syncytial virus (RSV) and Failure to thrive.

Episode 15

A few days after Ryan is discharged from the hospital, a social worker makes a home visit, meeting with Jessica alone while Casey is at work. A detailed history is taken, and issues regarding child care, feeding practices, and Casey come to light. Based on the visit, the social worker advises Jessica to take Ryan to Kangaroo Junction Preschool, a special school for children at risk for domestic abuse or neglect, during the daytime and to Jessica's mother's house in the evenings. Specifically, the social worker recommends that Casey not care for Ryan. Fearing Casey's reaction to the situation, Jessica tells Casey that the lady from the hospital made her aware of a free daycare service for kids, and that her mother wants to watch the baby more often during the evenings. She is relieved that Casey does not question her further on this.

Jessica also goes for her 20-week prenatal visit. When Carol Ramsey, the nurse midwife, asks her how things are going, Jessica admits to fatigue, but confirms that she is taking the prenatal vitamins. When asked about her smoking and alcohol intake, Jessica reports that she is still smoking, but not as much. She tells Carol, "Casey smokes, so it is hard not to smoke, and I've only had a few beers since last visit." Jessica does not tell Carol about Ryan's recent illness or the social worker's visit ▤ ▽.

Jessica Riley   Season 2 Information

Episode 1

Jessica Riley is an 18-year-old single mother with a 1-year-old son, Ryan. She has had no contact with Ryan's father since before he was born. Jessica and Ryan live in a small, one-bedroom apartment with Jessica's boyfriend, Casey. She is now 6 months pregnant with Casey's child. Although Jessica works full-time at a restaurant, she struggles financially. She is glad Casey contributes to paying the bills and is not sure how she could make it financially without him. Although she was successful at completing her GED, Jessica dropped out of the community college she was attending when she learned she was pregnant with a second child. She didn't think she could afford to go to school with another baby and wanted to focus on working as much as possible.

Jessica has her 24-week prenatal visit. She continues to see Carol Ramsey, the nurse midwife, and likes her a lot because she makes her feel comfortable. She tells Carol that she tried to stop smoking, but hasn't been able to quit yet. When Carol asks about her alcohol intake, Jessica tells her that she is no longer drinking 🗒 📰.

Episode 2

Jessica drops Ryan off at her mother's home to be cared for by her sister Jenna so she can go to a party with Casey. Amanda Hardin, Robert's friend, is at the party and she tells Jessica that she has been staying with Robert after leaving her parents' house. She said she has been trying to get off drugs, but her parents are just too overbearing with rules. Amanda, only a couple years older than Jessica, is quite the party animal; she uses heroin at the party. She tells Jessica, "Don't get hooked on this stuff – it is a killer to get off of." Jessica is glad Casey does not use heroin.

Episode 3

After work one evening this week, Jessica picks up Ryan from her mother's home and visits with her for about 20 minutes. When she arrives back at her apartment, Casey yells at her for being late and demands to know where she was. When she tries to explain, he pushes her down, causing her to fall to the floor, and accuses her of lying to him. Shortly thereafter, he tells her he is sorry and treats her nicely for the next couple of days ✉.

Episode 4

Jessica sees Carol, the nurse midwife, for her 28-week prenatal visit. Jessica tells the nurse that her major complaint at this point is ongoing constipation. When asked about the types of fluids she consumes, Jessica replies that she mostly drinks soda. The midwife suggests that Jessica reduce the number of soft drinks she consumes each day and increase her fluid and fiber intake. She also encourages Jessica to consider signing up for childbirth classes, even though she has recently had a baby. An ultrasound is done during the visit, and Jessica is surprised to learn that her baby is a girl. Jessica tells Carol, "I thought I was going to have another boy, but having a girl is awesome! I love the clothes for baby girls and cannot wait to dress her up."

Later that same day, Jessica is surprised at Casey's reaction when she tells him they are having a baby girl. She knew he wanted a boy, but was surprised at his reaction. Jessica wonders what she can do to make him love her more 🗒.

Episode 5

Jessica wins free tickets to the Neighborhood Zoo in a drawing at work. During the weekend, Jessica and Casey use the tickets to take Ryan to the zoo. On this particular day, Jessica enjoys the attention she receives from Casey. She loves it when they are able to spend time together like a real family. It makes her sad when she thinks about Casey's comments about having a girl, but she is sure that he will love their daughter once she is born.

Episode 6

Jessica invites a female friend from work over to the apartment for lunch and a visit. They share a laugh about one of their male coworkers. After her friend leaves, Casey begins to yell at Jessica and accuses her of sharing secrets about him. Jessica denies this, telling Casey that she and her friend were just visiting. Casey grabs Jessica by the hair and threatens her. He tells Jessica that she is not to bring friends or her stupid mother to their apartment anymore. He also comments that Jessica is becoming a "fat whale."

Jessica has begun to experience leg cramps and heartburn. She does not recall having these symptoms when she was pregnant with Ryan and wonders if the stress of working, caring for Ryan, being pregnant, and trying to keep Casey happy is causing this. She frequently worries about making Casey angry and fears that he might leave her.

Episode 7

Jessica is very upset to learn that Casey lost his job. She worries about paying bills without his income and arranges to pick up additional shifts. She wishes he would not spend their money on beer.

Jessica is surprised when Casey tells her that he is going with her to her prenatal appointment. During the visit, Casey is very attentive and caring toward her. He dominates the conversation and tells Carol, the nurse midwife, that she is doing great and he wants to be sure everything is perfect. Jessica is pleased with his level of interest in her pregnancy, but she recognizes that his presence makes it difficult to talk with the midwife. Jessica doesn't really have a chance to tell the midwife about the heartburn and leg cramps she has been experiencing 🗒 ▶.

Episode 8

Jessica comes home from a long day of work to find Casey drinking and smoking pot. She asks Casey if he has been able to find a job yet because she is worried about making the rent payment. Jessica is surprised when Casey stands up and hits her on the left side of her abdomen, yelling that she is stupid and fat and has no right to tell him what to do. Jessica knows that she is not seriously hurt, yet she lies in bed all night crying. The next morning, she goes to work, hoping to have a good day in tips.

Episode 9

Jessica is confused by Casey's behavior. One day he is such a sweet guy, full of compliments and very apologetic about his occasional bad behavior – and then the next day he hits her. She tries to figure out what she is doing wrong that causes him to yell at her and hit her. She is relieved that Casey leaves Ryan alone.

Jessica has her 34-week prenatal visit. Carol talks with Jessica about fetal development and begins describing the birth process. During the exam, Jessica is scared when Carol asks her about the bruises on the side of her abdomen where Casey struck her. She tells the nurse that she bumped into a table, but Jessica can tell the midwife does not believe her story. She tells Jessica that sometimes she sees bruises like this on women who have been hit and asks her if that is what happened to her. Jessica denies being hit and again says she bumped into a table.

Episode 10

Once again this week, Jessica angers Casey and he strikes her just below the eye with his elbow. Jessica does what she can to conceal the bruise around her eye with makeup. She avoids direct eye contact with her coworkers and hopes nobody will notice. One customer by the name of Greg Ross does notice. He asks her about her pregnancy and when she looks at him, there is a moment of shared understanding. After he finishes his meal, the man leaves the following note for her written on a napkin:

Please do not hesitate to call if you ever find yourself needing help.

Greg Ross 987-1237

The man also leaves her a $150 tip on a $90 dinner. Jessica desperately needs the money and is very grateful for the generous tip. She throws the napkin away for fear that Casey will find it. She thinks it is weird that the man would want to help her anyway. She thinks about places to hide the money from Casey.

Episode 11

Jessica goes in for her 36-week prenatal visit, accompanied by Casey. Just before the exam, Casey tells the nurse midwife that Jessica has bruises on her abdomen because she is very clumsy and runs into things. Jessica quickly acknowledges that it's true.

Carol asks Casey to step out of the exam room so she can do a vaginal exam. Once he leaves the room she asks Jessica about bruises to her arms. She says to Jessica, "It has been my experience that many women who have

bruises like this have been hit." Jessica again denies that this is the case, telling the nurse midwife that she really is just big and clumsy. Carol shares with Jessica that shelter information can be found in the women's bathroom, but Jessica tells the midwife she does not need anything like that.

Episode 12

Jessica continues to work full-time, but it has become increasingly difficult, as she is very tired by the end of the day. She is so tired that she doesn't even have the energy to take care of Ryan. Several times this week, she has asked her mother to keep Ryan overnight for her and take him to daycare in the morning. Jessica misses Ryan, but she is relieved not to have to take care of him.

Jessica sees Carol Ramsey, the nurse midwife, for her 37-week prenatal visit. During the vaginal exam, the midwife tells Jessica that her cervix is thinning and beginning to dilate slightly. Jessica asks her how much longer it will be before the baby comes. She hopes to have the baby soon so she can be thin and look pretty again. Casey has been treating Jessica very well lately. In fact he surprised her with flowers and tells her how much he loves her.

Episode 13

Jessica takes the evening off from work because she is feeling very tired. While fixing dinner, Ryan begins crying in the other room, and she interrupts her cooking to attend to his needs.

When they all finally sit down to eat, Casey throws his plate against the wall and screams at Jessica for making a "lousy dinner." He then proceeds to yank her out of her chair and hit her in the back, knocking her down to the floor. She gets up, crying, and he hits her in the abdomen, saying, "You care more about that damn brat than me and what I want." She falls to the floor, and he kicks her in the abdomen. Jessica screams in pain. Somehow, she gets off the floor and makes it into the bedroom. The neighbor in the next apartment hears the commotion. Knowing that Jessica is pregnant and in an abusive relationship, the neighbor calls the police.

When the police arrive, they find Casey watching television and smoking a joint. Jessica is doubled over on the bed crying, and Ryan is in his crib crying. The police note that she is pregnant and call for an ambulance. They ask her if she was hit, and she denies it. The police tell Jessica that they are arresting Casey for drug possession and further questioning. Jessica calls her mother and asks her to come get Ryan and then meet her at the hospital. When the paramedics arrive, they start an IV, place Jessica on oxygen, and transport her to the hospital. At the hospital, the triage nurse sends her directly to the labor and delivery unit.

Jessica delivers a healthy female infant later in the evening. Because she suffered a small abruption to the placenta, the nurse midwife and physician suspect trauma from abuse. In the immediate postpartum period, Carol, the nurse midwife, talks with Jessica privately. Jessica is told that she had a small abruption, and that the placenta had an infarct. Carol explains that, in these situations, trauma is suspected. She also shares with Jessica that sometimes women in abusive relationships get hit or kicked in the abdomen. Jessica cries and admits that this is what happened, but she insists that Casey didn't mean to do it and will never do it again. Jessica tells Carol that she will not press charges.

Social work is called for a referral before Jessica is discharged. Jessica is told that a social work referral is required because of the risk of intimate partner violence and drug charges against Casey. Jessica worries about this, fearing that Casey will be angry if he finds out. The social worker makes a home visit the day after Jessica and the baby are discharged, and Jessica is relieved that Casey is not home. Jessica tells the social worker that everything is fine and that there really are no problems 🗐.

Episode 14

Casey and Jessica decide to name the baby Carrie. Jessica is happy because Casey is kind and sweet to her. She notices the efforts he seems to be making to be a good father. He tells her he is so sorry that he hurt her, but he is also glad she finally had the baby. Jessica knows how sorry he is and is glad that Casey didn't have to stay in jail. She anticipates that their problems are now in the past.

Jessica takes a few weeks off from work to be home with the baby. She would like to take more time off but cannot afford it. Casey agrees to pick up extra shifts until she can go back to work. Jessica's mother spends time at the apartment, helping with the baby. Jessica becomes angry with her mother when Evelyn suggests that she leave Casey and move back home with her children. Jessica does not understand why her mother cannot see that Casey has changed.

The social worker makes another visit this week to assess the home situation. Jessica once again tells her that everything is fine and that Casey is an excellent father.

Episode 15

Jessica has an appointment for a postpartum exam with Carol Ramsey, the nurse midwife. She takes Carrie and Ryan with her to the exam because Casey is sleeping and her mother is not available. Ryan is now 16 months old and has outgrown his car seat, so Jessica places Ryan in the front seat and straps him in with the seatbelt.

Carol tells Jessica that everything is normal, with the exception of a slightly low hematocrit level. She also notes that Jessica's breasts have reduced in size. Jessica explains that she has decided not to breastfeed. Carol starts Jessica on a contraception patch and explains that she should apply a new patch each week. Carol also explains the need to eat a healthy diet and take vitamins and iron. When asked about the situation at home, Jessica tells the midwife that everything is great and that Casey is a wonderful father. Carol admires how beautiful Carrie is and notes that she has contact dermatitis on her bottom. Carol suggests that Jessica use an ointment and change the brand of diapers she is using. She is delighted to also see Ryan and mentions what a big boy he is. She asks him if he helps Mommy take care of the baby.

Jessica Riley Season 3 Information

Episode 1

Jessica Riley is an 18-year-old single mother with a 17-month-old son, Ryan, and a 6-week-old daughter, Carrie. Jessica and her children share a one-bedroom apartment with Carrie's father, Casey. Jessica has not heard from Ryan's father since before he was born.

Jessica works full-time at a restaurant, but she struggles financially. She is glad Casey contributes to paying the bills and is not sure how she could make it financially without him. She has earned her GED, but she dropped out of the community college after she became pregnant with Carrie.

Jessica grew up in a single-parent home. Her father left the family when she was 7. She is the oldest child and has two younger siblings, Jenna and Jason. Her mother, Evelyn, helps by watching her baby in the evenings. Additionally, Jessica receives government assistance in the form of WIC coupons and Medicaid, and Ryan and Carrie attend a government-assisted daycare program.

This episode Jessica has a much-needed day off from work. She is very happy to stay at home with Casey and her two children. Because of his night-shift work schedule, Casey lies down for an afternoon nap. Jessica gets a phone call from her mother. While Jessica is on the phone, Carrie begins to cry. Before Jessica can get off the phone, Casey hangs the phone up on her, hits her on the left side of the face, and screams at her to keep the damn baby quiet. Crying, Jessica runs to get Carrie to protect her. She is thankful that Casey leaves the apartment. During the course of the next several days, Jessica develops a huge bruise on her face. She tells her coworkers and mother that she ran into a door.

Episode 2

Jessica's bruises are healing. She has a visit with the social worker this week and tells him things have been going well. When the social worker asks Jessica if the marks on her face are bruises, Jessica replies that she bumped her head on a door. Jessica is relieved that Carrie and Ryan look fine.

Episode 3

Jessica is thrilled when Casey tells her he is moving to the day shift. She is sure that if they can spend their evenings together, Casey will be happier and won't hit her anymore.

Episode 4

Casey tells Jessica he realizes he has not been very helpful the last several months and is going to change all that. He tells her he is going to quit partying and focus on being a good father to Carrie and a good husband to her. Casey says they should consider getting married. Jessica loves the idea.

Episode 5

When Casey fails to come home one night this week, Jessica stays up all night, concerned for his safety. When he finally comes home, Jessica asks him where he has been and why he didn't call. She also points out to him that he is late for work. She does not expect Casey's reaction. Casey strikes her in the head and throws her against the wall. Jessica hits the back of her head, resulting in a large, painful bump. He also strikes her on her left upper cheek with his fist. His behavior frightens her.

At work, Jessica again has to explain her facial bruises and swelling to her coworkers. Her mother Evelyn does not believe her explanations and attempts to talk with Jessica about getting away from Casey. Jessica tells her mother that she just sometimes makes him mad, but Casey does not mean to harm her ▶ ◢.

Episode 6

When Casey does not come home one night this week, Jessica thinks better than to ask him where he has been. She is afraid that he will hurt her again, or hurt her children. When they are at home together, she does everything she can think of to win Casey's approval. Because he is out of work again, Jessica is worried about money and hopes to work more hours at the restaurant.

The social worker makes a home visit to see Jessica, Carrie, and Ryan – partly because of a concern raised by Ryan's teacher, Miss Webb. The social worker again notes old bruises on Jessica's face, but he sees that the children appear well fed and unharmed. The social worker talks with Jessica about removing herself from her current situation. Jessica tells the social worker she will think about it, but that things are fine.

Episode 7

Jessica is thrilled to see all the money Casey pulls from his pants pocket. She asks him how he got so much money and wonders if he found a job. Her question is answered with a beating to the head and stomach. He yells at Jessica and asks her when she is going to lose some weight.

The next day, Jessica is confronted by several coworkers. They tell her that it is obvious what is going on and plead with her to get away from Casey. One of the girls tells Jessica about the battered women's shelter in town and asks her to go there if things get any worse. Jessica tells them it is all her fault, and Casey is not to blame. There is no way they could ever understand why she can't leave Casey. She loves and needs him, but at the same time, she is afraid of him. Jessica's mother Evelyn also pleads with Jessica to get away from Casey – if not for herself, then for the safety of her children. Jessica wants to talk to her mother but just can't figure out where to start [NEWS].

Episode 8

It has been a couple of weeks now since Casey hit Jessica. She is beginning to think that things are going to improve. He surprises her when he asks her to marry him. Jessica is thrilled and says yes. She knows they won't have money for a big wedding, but she hopes they can do something small. She wonders if her mother will help her pay for it; she calls her mother to share the good news!

Jessica picks up Carrie and Ryan from daycare and is told that Carrie feels hot. Jessica also notes that Carrie feels hot and is very irritable. Because it is after hours, she takes Carrie to the Emergency Department, where Carrie is treated by Dr. Gordon for an ear infection ◢.

Episode 9

At 2:15 a.m., Casey unexpectedly begins pounding on Jessica's head with his fists while she is asleep. She screams in pain and tries to get away. Casey yells at her for not waiting up for him. Jessica can tell that Casey has been drinking, and he is acting very strange. She is able to get out of bed, but he catches her and continues to beat her. She finally gets away from him, and he laughs at her, telling her she is fat and ugly. Shortly thereafter, Casey passes out on the couch.

Jessica quickly gathers a few belongings and her two children and leaves the apartment. She recalls what her friend told her about the battered women's shelter and goes there directly. At the shelter, Jessica is told that she and her children can stay there temporarily until other arrangements can be made. She is assured that it is unlikely Casey will find her. Jessica is told that the most dangerous time for women is when they have just left their abuser; for this reason, she must not reveal to Casey where she is.

From the shelter, Jessica calls her mother and explains the situation. Evelyn pleads with Jessica to come home, but Jessica knows that Casey will look for her there. Jessica doesn't even tell her mother exactly where she is, other than to say that she and the children are in a safe place. Jessica promises to get back in touch with Evelyn in a few days. She asks her mother to call her boss at work to let him know that she'll be out for a few weeks but to tell him nothing else.

Episode 10

Jessica, Ryan, and Carrie spend a long week at the shelter. She meets several other women who have had similar experiences. The shelter staff and professional counselors spend time with Jessica and the other women, talking with them about domestic violence and abusive situations, and helping them consider alternative long-term plans. They talk with Jessica about the possibility of pressing charges against Casey and getting a restraining order. During the week, Jessica experiences a range of emotions, from anger toward Casey for the way he has treated her, to sadness over missing him and wanting to work things out with him.

Jessica is able to talk with her mother during the week. Evelyn is so grateful that Jessica and the kids are safe. Evelyn tells Jessica that Casey came by and demanded to know where she and the children were. She warns Jessica to stay away from him.

Episode 11

Jessica calls Casey this week to talk and let him know that she and the kids are okay. She tells him she hopes they can patch things up. Casey tells Jessica that he loves and misses her and wants her to come back home. He asks Jessica where she is (something the shelter staff told her would happen), and when she refuses to answer, he becomes angry and threatens to kill her. Jessica hangs up, knowing now that she can never go back home to Casey.

A couple of days later, Jessica learns that Casey has been arrested and is in jail on armed robbery and vehicular homicide charges. She believes that, as long as he is in jail, she can return to her apartment and try to get back into a regular routine.

Episode 12

Jessica feels a huge sense of relief knowing that Casey is in jail, but at the same time she feels sorry for him and wishes there is something she could do for him.

Jessica's mother encourages her to attend church with her family. Jessica had attended the church regularly until she moved out and she has not been back since. After church, Evelyn takes everyone out for brunch. Jessica enjoys the company of her mother and siblings and is relieved that her mother doesn't use the opportunity to lecture her about not attending church.

Episode 13

Although she has returned to work, Jessica finds herself deeply in debt. Both of her credit cards are at their limits, and she is behind on paying her rent and utilities. She feels overwhelmed with the responsibility of trying to support her two children independently.

Jessica figures out that, even if she worked 24 hours a day for the next 2 months, she would still be in debt. If it were not for her WIC coupons and other government assistance, Jessica knows her kids would be hungry. She finds herself wishing that Casey were not in jail so that he could help her pay the bills ▼.

Episode 14

Jessica has an incoming call from Casey. She is frightened by it and decides not to answer the phone. She then gets a text from him asking her to come visit him at the jail. She tells her mother, Evelyn, about the call and text from Casey. Evelyn gives Jessica money to get a new phone number so that he can't call her anymore.

Jessica has been spending most of her free time with her children at her mother's house. She is comforted by the company of her mother and siblings as she continues to work through her feelings. Jessica feels reconnected to her family; in fact, she feels a connection with them that she cannot remember ever experiencing before. She has come to appreciate her mother's tireless efforts, not only for Ryan and Carrie, but also for her siblings, Jason and Jenna. She hopes to be as good a mother as Evelyn is.

It is during this week that Jessica makes the decision to move back home in the hopes of having the opportunity for a new start. Evelyn agrees to help her get back into school. Jessica knows this is the best chance she has to support herself and her children in the years to come ▼.

Episode 15

Jessica moves back to her mother's home this week. Her brother, Jason, is excited to have his big sister come home. Within a few days of moving, she receives a letter in the mail from Casey. She wonders how he knows that she moved back home with her mother. She feels uneasy and worries about her safety and the safety of her children in the future.

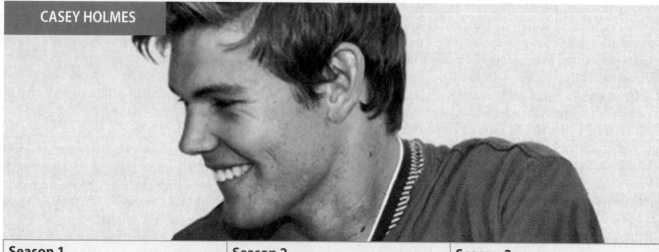

CASEY HOLMES

Season 1	Season 2	Season 3
Casey meets Jessica at a party and shortly thereafter moves in with her. He agrees to care for baby Ryan when Jessica is at work. Little does she know, he neglects Ryan. Casey parties heavily. He is a substance abuser and has difficulty holding jobs.	Casey becomes physically and verbally abusive to Jessica while she is pregnant. When she is near term he kicks her in the abdomen during a fight, causing her to go into labor. Because of all the commotion, neighbors call police. He is arrested for drug possession.	Casey continues a pattern of domestic violence and substance abuse. He gets arrested again and sent to jail. During this period of time, Jessica breaks off their relationship.

Casey Holmes Season 1 Information

Episode 1

Casey Holmes is a physically fit, 23-year-old male who had a troubled youth. His parents divorced when he was very young, and he bounced back and forth between parents, both of whom remarried. Growing up, he often saw his father hit his stepmother when he was angry. As an adolescent, Casey became involved with a gang and was arrested a few times for petty crimes, such as shoplifting and vandalism. He never finished high school and moved out on his own at the age of 18. Since that time, he has held a number of odd jobs and has made an effort to stay out of trouble.

For the past several months, Casey has been working as a basic laborer for a general construction company, performing tasks such as shoveling, raking, hauling mortar in wheelbarrows, and running a jackhammer to break up concrete. He has not been given an opportunity to learn more advanced skills because his supervisors and coworkers note that he often shows up late for work and displays little motivation. Casey is paid minimum wage and has health insurance as a job benefit. He feels that he is underpaid for the type of work he does. Casey also has a savings plan option as an additional job benefit, but he does not participate because he would rather just have the money to spend. On most days after work, Casey shares a 12-pack of beer with his buddies and smokes marijuana. He also uses other drugs when he can afford to buy them. He sometimes worries about the possibility of getting caught in a random drug screen, but he figures he can always get another job.

Episode 2

Casey goes to a party with his best friend, Robert. The party is hosted by Amy, a girl Robert recently met the previous weekend. Casey does not know anyone at the party, but is immediately attracted to Amy's friend, Jessica. Casey spends the entire time at the party talking with Jessica. He later leaves the party with Jessica and goes home with her to spend the night.

Episode 3

Casey has spent nearly every spare moment with Jessica since meeting her a few weeks ago. He has spent very little time around infants or children, so he thinks it is cool. He decides to move in with Jessica and offers to take care of Ryan in the evenings while she works. One day this week he has a hangover in the morning and is late to work. The superintendent emphasizes to Casey the need to get to work on time, but Casey thinks his boss is just giving him a hard time.

Episode 4

Casey takes care of Ryan in the evenings. He finds that he does not really like doing it. Because Ryan spits up a lot, he figures the kid must not be too hungry so he just quits trying to feed him. He does not often change Ryan's diapers because it is gross, and he knows Jessica will do it when she comes home anyway. The main reason Casey hates taking care of the baby is that Ryan cries a lot. When Ryan cries, Casey feels angry. Often, he copes by putting the baby in his crib, closing the door, and then playing video games or watching a movie with the volume up very loud so that he doesn't have to hear Ryan.

At work, Casey is disciplined by his supervisor for failing to wear ear protection while using a jackhammer. Casey tells his supervisor that he just forgets and that the ear protectors are uncomfortable ▶.

Episode 5
Casey has been busy and feels tired from working all day and needs to get out and hang around with his buddies. Sometimes, Casey leaves the baby alone in the apartment to get away from the crying. He figures that, as long as Ryan is in the crib, he should be okay. He is critical of how often Jessica holds her baby when she is at home. He tells her that she has turned Ryan into a spoiled brat, which is why he cries so much when she is away.

Casey is late to work once this week and is also written up for failing to use protective ear equipment again while using a jackhammer.

Episode 6
Casey has a party several nights in a row at the apartment while Jessica is at work. Casey, his best friend Robert, and some other friends use cocaine, smoke pot, and drink beer while they are partying. His friends poke fun at him for "babysitting." He puts Ryan in the bedroom with the door closed so that he doesn't bother them. Casey fails to show up for work 2 days in a row and is fired from his job.

Episode 7
Casey is looking for a job. Jessica has an appointment with the doctor for Ryan to get shots, and she has a test at school that she cannot miss. When she asks Casey if he will take Ryan, he tells her that Ryan is healthy, and "it is stupid to give shots to healthy kids unless they are living in a third-world country ✉."

Episode 8
Casey is still out of work. He tells Jessica he is looking for a job, but actually enjoys relaxing and spending time at home drinking beer and watching television. He borrows money from Jessica and his friend Robert to buy beer and gets drunk every day this week.

Episode 9
Casey gets a job with a landscape contractor. He works hard during the day and comes home very tired. Every evening, he drinks beer and smokes a joint to unwind. He also continues to take care of Ryan in the evenings.

Episode 10
Casey really hates his landscaping job, but he knows he needs the money. His truck needs some new repairs, and he wants to help Jessica with the rent. He also wants to have enough money to buy beer, pot, and cocaine.

Episode 11
Jessica tells Casey she is pregnant. He is happy with this news because this now means that Jessica is his. He asks Jessica if it is a boy and she tells him it might be. Casey tells her he hopes it is a boy, and they should name their baby Casey Junior. He celebrates by having his buddies over to drink beer.

Episode 12
Casey's friend Robert tells him about a huge party that was advertised on Facebook–to be hosted in a park near the University. At the party Robert introduces Casey and Jessica to his new girlfriend, Amanda Hardin, a 19-year-old girl who has attended the university. Jessica is feeling tired and goes home early. Casey, Robert, and Amanda stay at the party most of the night. Casey is impressed with what a party machine Amanda is. Amanda tells Casey and Robert that she is really in substance abuse rehab – but is "so done with it." They all laugh hysterically at the idea. The next day, Casey gets a call from Robert telling him that Amanda was arrested for drunk driving on the way home from the party. "That is such a drag," Casey tells Robert.

Episode 13
Casey is suspicious that Jessica is having an affair after she receives a phone call from a man. He screams at her and pushes her onto the couch, telling her that he'll hurt her if she ever leaves him. The next day, Casey feels badly about this and buys Jessica flowers ▶.

Episode 14
On her way out the door for an evening shift, Jessica tells Casey that Ryan has been sick and asks him to keep a close eye on him. After Jessica leaves for work, Casey puts Ryan in his crib, goes to the refrigerator, and opens a can of beer. He drinks beer and smokes pot most of the evening and only checks in on Ryan once. Casey is passed out asleep on the couch when Jessica comes home. He does not wake up until the following morning, when Jessica calls him from the hospital to tell him about Ryan.

Episode 15
Casey learns that a man from the hospital came by the apartment. Jessica tells Casey that the man came from the hospital to see how Ryan was doing. She also tells Casey that the man told her about free babysitting, so he will no longer have to watch Ryan in the evening. Casey is glad to hear this.

Casey Holmes Season 2 Information

Episode 1

Casey lives with his pregnant girlfriend, Jessica Riley, and her son, Ryan. He does not particularly like Ryan and thinks that Jessica spoils him. He is very proud of the fact that Jessica is pregnant with his baby. He is controlling of Jessica and does not want anybody else looking at her. On most days after work and into the evening, Casey drinks beer and smokes marijuana with his buddies. He is irritated that Jessica does not party with him as much as she did when they first met. Casey also uses other drugs when he can afford to buy them.

Casey and his buddies are partying in their apartment when Jessica gets off work one evening this week. Casey pops a beer open for Jessica and tells her to drink it because she has some "catching up" to do. He is happy that she takes the beer he offers her.

Episode 2

Casey's friend Robert is having a party. His girlfriend, Amanda Hardin, is at the party using heroin. Casey tells Robert, "That chic is intense, dude." Robert responds, "She's been staying here for a couple of weeks and she parties nonstop – but man, she is so hot!" Casey agrees she is good-looking but thinks that Jessica is lots better than that.

Episode 3

Casey is angry by the time Jessica arrives home from work nearly 30 minutes late one evening this week. He has had mental images of someone at work touching her, and he was sure she probably enjoyed it. As soon as she comes in the door, he begins to yell at her, wanting to know where she was and who she was with. He is so angry that he pushes her to the floor. Casey later feels sorry for what he did and vows to make it up to her. He treats her nicely for the next couple of days.

Episode 4

Casey is angry when Jessica tells him that they are going to have a girl. He tells her that she should be giving him a son and he doesn't know why anyone would want a girl ▶.

Episode 5

Casey has been late to work several days during the past couple of weeks. His boss tells him that he needs to be on time if he wants to continue to have a job. Casey does not like the fact that his boss hassles him so much. Over the weekend, Casey takes Jessica and Ryan to the zoo. He does not particularly like zoos, but he enjoys the outing. While at the concession stand, he notices a girl working behind the counter and thinks she is hot ✉.

Episode 6

Jessica has a girlfriend over to the house for lunch and a visit. Casey does not like the way her friend looks at him. He later overhears them laughing and talking about a coworker by the name of Michael. He becomes angry about the thought of Jessica being with Michael. After her friend leaves, Casey yells at her, asking who Michael is. He throws her to the ground, and kicks and punches her. He tells if he ever sees them together he will kill them both. Casey also tells Jessica that she is worthless. He thinks she resembles a fat whale, and he is not sexually attracted to her because of her weight gain ▶ ✉.

Episode 7

Casey is fired from his job this week. He had failed to check the hydraulic fluid level prior to operating the Bobcat and, because the fluid level was low, the pump burned out and significantly damaged the equipment. Casey buys a 12-pack of beer on the way home.

A few days later, Casey accompanies Jessica to her prenatal visit. He is curious about what goes on during her visits and wants to impress the medical personnel. He is very attentive to Jessica during the visit and asks many questions. He also wants to see if she is really going to visit the doctor, believing it's possible that she is meeting another man during these "appointments." ✉

Episode 8

Casey is enjoying listening to music, drinking beer, and smoking pot when Jessica starts hassling him about getting a job. He yells at her that she is not going to start bossing him around and telling him what to do. He hits her on the side of her abdomen. He is annoyed that she cries all night and wonders why she can't just get over it ✉.

Episode 9

While Jessica is out running errands, Casey agrees to care for Ryan. He prepares him lunch and Ryan refuses to eat it. Casey tries to force the food into Ryan's mouth, but he just spits it out. Frustrated, Casey yells at Ryan and tells him he is a bad boy. He puts him in his crib and tells him to take a nap. This sets Ryan off in a temper tantrum. Casey leaves the apartment for about 30 minutes so that he does not have to listen to the crying.

Episode 10

Casey knows the baby will be born soon and has new motivation to find a job. He recognizes his responsibility to his unborn child and thinks about wanting to be a good father. He goes to the public library to search online for job postings and completes several applications ✉.

Episode 11

Casey has found a night job working in a warehouse. The pay is okay, and at least he won't have to work all that hard. The worst part about the job, in Casey's opinion, is that the hours are not great for the party scene. However, he is told that a day position may open up in the near future.

Casey accompanies Jessica to her prenatal visit. Right before the midwife exposes Jessica's abdomen, he tells Carol that Jessica is clumsy and has some bruises on her abdomen from running into things. He steps out of the room during the exam and wonders if they will talk about the bruises. Before they leave the appointment, he asks Carol how long he will have to wait before he can have sex with Jessica after the baby is born and how long she will be moody.

Episode 12

Casey buys flowers for Jessica this week and tells her that she is wonderful. He also tells her that he will be glad when she is no longer pregnant.

Casey smokes cocaine with his friend Robert. They run out of cocaine and don't have the money to buy more, so Casey and Robert break into some cars and steal stereo systems, which they sell at a pawn shop for drug money. Casey misses work twice this week ▼.

Episode 13

Casey watches Jessica making dinner while he watches TV and thinks to himself that she is getting so fat! Ryan is in the other room crying, so Jessica stops what she is doing to attend to Ryan. When he finally sits down to eat, Casey

throws a plate against the wall and screams at her for making a "lousy dinner." He then proceeds to hit her hard in the abdomen, saying, "You care more about the damn brat than me and what I want." She falls to the floor screaming. Ryan is in the other room crying. Casey lights up a joint to relax. When the police arrive, they find Jessica doubled over and crying, Ryan in his crib crying, and Casey watching TV and smoking a joint. The police arrest Casey for drug possession and take him in for further questioning. Casey spends a couple of days in jail before his buddy, Robert, bails him out. He learns that Jessica had their baby and is anxious to get home to see her.

Episode 14

Casey and Jessica agree to name their baby Carrie. Casey wants to be a good father. He helps Jessica with some of the infant care duties but completely ignores Ryan. Casey does not like seeing the baby sucking on Jessica's breast. He thinks it looks ugly and tells Jessica she should feed the baby with a bottle. Jessica tells Casey that a man from the hospital will be coming by to see Carrie every once in a while ▼.

Episode 15

Casey does not like all the attention Jessica gives the baby. He also wishes that the baby was a boy. At the same time, he proudly tells everyone at work about his daughter because he enjoys the attention it brings him. Casey and Robert break into more cars for drug money this week. Casey considers it easy money, and it pays much better than his warehouse job [NEWS].

Casey Holmes Season 3 Information

Episode 1

Casey Holmes is a physically fit, 24-year-old male. He lives with his girlfriend Jessica Riley, their 6-week-old infant daughter Carrie, and Jessica's 17-month-old son Ryan. Casey does not particularly like Ryan and thinks that Jessica spoils him. He is proud to be a father, but wishes Carrie were a boy. During Jessica's pregnancy, he physically abused her on several occasions. Each time, he felt bad for hurting her and vowed to make it up to her. He has not injured Jessica since the night she went into labor.

Casey works the night shift at a warehouse as a stocker. He spends a lot of his free time with his buddies, drinking beer and smoking marijuana. Casey and his friend Robert have recently been vandalizing cars for drug money.

One afternoon after working a night shift, Casey is sleeping while Jessica is home with her children. When Carrie's cry wakes him up, he is angry. He walks out into the living room to find Jessica talking on the phone. He hangs

up the phone and strikes her on the left side of her face. He tells her that he is not to be disturbed while he is trying to sleep and to make the damn baby shut up. When Jessica starts to cry, he leaves the apartment for a couple of hours.

Episode 2

Casey and Robert spend most of their free time this week partying with friends. He talks about the new baby and how pretty she is. He is teased by some of his friends about being out at a party instead of taking care of his baby. "If you were a good Dad, you wouldn't be here," he is told. The comment really bugs Casey.

Episode 3

A day-shift position opens up at the warehouse where Casey works, and he applies for the position and gets it. He is happy to be able to get back to working during the day. Casey and Robert break into a home this week. Casey wants the additional money for his family.

Episode 4

Casey is making a concerted effort to be a good father. He wants his daughter to grow up and be proud of him and he wants to provide her a good home. He vows to party less and stay home more to help Jessica take care of the kids.

Episode 5

Robert convinces Casey to go to a party after work. Casey tells Robert he really should go home and help Jessica, but he agrees to go for just an hour or so. He ends up staying out all night, drinking and smoking crack. When he gets home the next morning, Jessica is hysterical; she was worried about where he might have been, whether he was okay, and that he might miss work. Casey hits Jessica in the face, throws her against the wall, and shouts, "You are not my mother, and I can do whatever the hell I want!" He goes to the refrigerator to pop open a beer. Casey is fired from his warehouse job.

Episode 6

Casey has been on a partying binge for the entire week. He has been staying out late and sometimes all night. At one party this week, he meets a girl by the name of Amber, and they end up having sex at the party in one of the back bedrooms. Casey thinks she is better looking than Jessica. He is glad Jessica has not asked him where he has been.

Episode 7

Casey is looking for a job this week. He applies at several places but is not very enthusiastic about any of the job leads. Casey and Robert steal a car and strip it of its parts to sell at a salvage yard. He becomes angry when Jessica asks him where he got the money. To punish her, he kicks her in the stomach and tells her to lose some weight ▼.

Episode 8

Robert and Casey continue to steal cars this week. They strip the cars of things they can sell. It is an easy way to make a lot of money and it is also very thrilling. His "success" has him feeling on top of the world! He goes home and apologizes to Jessica about getting angry with her, and he just can't stand the thought of ever losing her. He asks her to marry him and promises to be a good husband and father.

Episode 9

Casey comes home after partying and finds Jessica asleep. He wakes her up and begins to beat her because she did not stay up and wait for him. He later falls asleep. When he wakes up the next morning, Jessica and the kids are gone ▼.

Episode 10

Casey has been looking for Jessica all week. He is furious that she has left. He parks in front of Evelyn's house, expecting to find Jessica and the kids there, but sees no sign of them.

He asks Evelyn where they are, and she tells Casey that she really doesn't know. He frequently checks at the restaurant to see if she is at work, but he does not find her there ▼.

Episode 11

Jessica calls Casey this week, and he tells her to come back home. She tells him she misses him and loves him but that she can't come back right now. Casey promises never to hurt her again and asks Jessica where she is. When Jessica does not tell him, he threatens to kill her.

Later that same evening, Casey and Robert attempt armed robbery at a local business. While fleeing the scene, they are involved in an automobile crash that kills two innocent victims. Casey and Robert are booked in the Neighborhood Jail on charges of armed robbery and vehicular homicide ▼ [NEWS].

Episode 12

Casey experiences alcohol withdrawal symptoms within the first few days that he is in jail. He is transferred to a detox unit at Neighborhood Hospital and is seen by several mental health professionals. He has no use for them. He tells them he does NOT have a problem and that he is just fine. While at the hospital he looks for opportunities to escape. Unfortunately he has a guard posted outside his room, and no opportunities present themselves.

Episode 13

Casey goes to a legal hearing with a court-appointed defense attorney. He is formally charged with robbery and vehicular homicide. The prosecuting attorney presents evidence that Casey and his partner, Robert, have been responsible for a recent series of automobile thefts. Casey's attorney tells him he will do what he can to lighten the sentence, but given the homicide on top of the thefts, it will not be easy. Casey is angry and wonders how he is going to get out of this mess.

Episode 14

Casey remains in jail but has an opportunity to call Jessica's cell phone. He calls her in the hopes that he can convince her to come visit him. She does not answer the phone so he leaves her a text message. The message goes unanswered. He wonders where she is and what she is doing. He wants to get out of jail and go home to see Jessica and the kids ▼.

Episode 15

Casey remains in jail. He finds out from his buddies that Jessica and the kids have moved back to her mother's home. He writes a letter to Jessica, asking her forgiveness and begging her to come visit him.

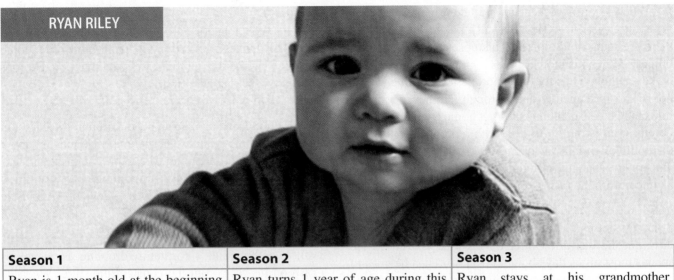

RYAN RILEY

Season 1	Season 2	Season 3
Ryan is 1 month old at the beginning of the story. Although he is healthy, he has colic and cries a lot. He receives good care at his grandmother's house, but is poorly cared for and neglected at his own home. He has a serious episode of RSV and dehydration, requiring hospitalization. Failure to thrive is diagnosed during hospitalization, and social services intervenes.	Ryan turns 1 year of age during this season. He spends less time around Casey and is mandated to go to a social services preschool. He spends an increasing amount of time in his grandmother's (Evelyn Riley) care. Ryan flourishes physically and mentally in this environment.	Ryan stays at his grandmother Evelyn's house more than with Jessica at this point. He is very happy to be with his grandmother, where he stays healthy and safe.

Ryan Riley Season 1 Information

Episode 1

Ryan Riley is a 1-month-old infant boy who was born to Jessica Riley, a 17-year-old single mother. Although his mother had minimal prenatal care, he was a healthy, 6-pound, 4-ounce infant at birth, and there were no complications during labor, birth, or immediately following birth. Ryan's grandmother, Evelyn, is his primary caretaker while Jessica is at work or at school, although many other people take care of him as well.

Ryan screams and cries almost nonstop for several hours every night this week. He is inconsolable. No matter what Jessica does, he continues to cry. He is taken to the Emergency Department (ED) twice this week. Both times, he is discharged with a diagnosis of colic.

Episode 2

Ryan spends one night with his grandmother. She has a small, warm, and comfortable bassinet for him to sleep in. He wakes up twice during the night in hunger. After he eats, he goes right back to sleep.

Episode 3

Jessica and Evelyn take Ryan to the clinic for his 2-month immunizations and well-child visit. He weighs 10 pounds at this visit, and his mother and grandmother are praised for his excellent weight gain.

Episode 4

Ryan cries when he is uncomfortable (such as when he has colic or is cold), when he is hungry, or when he just wants to be held. He has different cries for each of these needs that are detectable to an attentive parent. To a non-attentive caregiver, it is just crying. Ryan often feels cold and uncomfortable from a dirty diaper and often experiences hunger this week.

Episode 5

Ryan experiences inconsistent care. During the daytime, he goes to his grandmother's house. While there, his grandmother and Aunt Jenna hold him frequently, talk to him, and play with him. He is also fed consistently and kept clean. He finds his grandmother's voice comforting.

When Ryan is picked up and taken home, he has a different experience. He is usually put in his crib, and there are many loud noises. This upsets him and makes him cry. When his mother holds him, he finds it comforting, even though it is for only short periods of time. Casey holds him infrequently and is rough. He never looks at him, and he yells a lot. Feedings at home are inconsistent. Often, Ryan is put in his crib with a propped bottle, but the bottle often falls away, and Ryan can't get it. Ryan's diapers are changed infrequently, and he has developed an uncomfortable rash.

Episode 6

Ryan has not had a bath in several days. His clothes are dirty and he has dried milk on his face and chest. He spends most of his days lying in his crib. Then he goes to his grandmother's house. She gives him a bath and puts him in fresh, clean clothes. He is held by his grandmother until he falls asleep.

Episode 7

Ryan is now 17 weeks old. He is supposed to go for a well-baby check-up this week, but his mother cancels the appointment. He often feels hungry and is cranky. He is being fed about 4 to 5 ounces four times a day. He cries frequently and does not see his grandmother as much as before.

Episode 8

Ryan's mother spends a lot of time at work, and then when she is home she spends a lot of time partying. Ryan hears loud music and lots of people talking. There are many different smells when these people are around. Occasionally, his mother or some other person picks him up for a few minutes and then plops him back into the baby seat. On at least two occasions, Ryan spends the entire night in this seat.

Episode 9

Ryan barely sees his mother this week. She is either working or at school. He is cared for most of the week by Casey, which means he is ignored most of the time. Casey leaves Ryan alone in the apartment for short periods of time. He cries, but nobody hears him.

Episode 10

Ryan is now 6 months old. With Jessica's permission, Ryan's grandmother takes him to the pediatrician for a well-baby visit. He weighs 14 pounds. The pediatrician notes a change in his weight pattern and asks Evelyn about Ryan's home situation regarding feedings. Evelyn is able to describe her routine when she takes care of Ryan, but she admits it is only a few hours a day. She tells the physician that she is unable to describe Ryan's feeding patterns in the evening.

Episode 11

Ryan has developed a diaper rash. His skin is sore and itchy. This makes him very irritable. Ryan is often bored due to the lack of regular, purposeful stimulation. He cries frequently, seeking attention.

Episode 12

At $7\frac{1}{2}$ months of age, Ryan scoots around the carpet at his home and his grandmother's house. He puts anything within reach into his mouth to explore the taste and texture. He is not yet standing and holding onto furniture – he has not had many opportunities to develop leg muscle strength to do so.

Episode 13

Ryan is teething and is constantly drooling. He develops a rash on his face from the constant moisture. When he goes to his grandmother's house, she gives him many different things to eat. At his mother's home he primarily gets milk and baby cereal.

Episode 14

Ryan is now 9 months old. He has been sick for the past week with a cold. Because Evelyn is out of town this week, Jessica's friend, Megan, babysits Ryan for the day while Jessica works the first part of a double shift. Ryan does not feel good at all. He is not interested in eating or playing and has no energy.

Jessica picks up Ryan from Megan's house, takes him home, and leaves him with Casey for the evening while she goes back to work. Ryan is put in his crib and left alone all evening. During the course of the evening, Ryan gets worse and has nothing to drink. When Jessica comes home later that evening, Ryan is very sick and is having problems breathing. His mother immediately takes him to the hospital.

The Emergency Department physician, Dr. Gordon, asks Jessica how long Ryan has been sick, how many wet diapers he had in the past day, and when he last ate. Jessica tells Dr. Gordon that Ryan has had a cold for a week or so, but got sick just today. She admits that she doesn't know when he last ate or the number of wet diapers he has had. She tells Dr. Gordon that she has been working a lot of hours during the past several days.

Ryan stabilizes in the Emergency Department with oxygen and fluid support; his weight is measured at 15.2 lbs. After a workup, he is diagnosed with dehydration and bronchiolitis. He is admitted to the subacute pediatric unit. The admitting orders include an IV fluid infusion of D5 $\frac{1}{2}$ NaCl with 10 mEq KCl; urine bag for output measurement; O_2 by nasal cannula at 2 L/min; suction of nares and nasal pharynx; and oral electrolyte solution (Pedialyte) to encourage oral fluids while the respiratory distress resolves. After he is admitted, he is also diagnosed with respiratory syncytial virus (RSV) and failure to thrive.

Episode 15

Ryan spends the entire week at the hospital. As his respiratory syncytial virus (RSV) resolves, he starts taking oral fluids and eating baby food. His medical records are obtained from the pediatrician's office, and his weights at birth, 2 months, and 6 months are analyzed. A rapid weight gain is noted during his 7-day hospital admission, and Ryan now weighs 16 pounds. A diagnosis of failure to thrive is confirmed. The Social Services Department is consulted, and a home visit is planned shortly after discharge. Discharge teaching includes the topics of infant feeding and nutrition, general care, developmental milestones, and safety. Ryan is scheduled for a follow-up visit at the pediatrician's office 1 week after discharge.

A few days after discharge, a social worker makes a home visit and takes an extensive history. Issues regarding child care, feeding practices, and Casey come to light. Based on the visit, the social worker advises Jessica to take Ryan to Kangaroo Junction Preschool, a center for children at risk for domestic abuse or neglect, during the daytime and to Evelyn's home in the evenings. Specifically, it is recommended that Casey not care for Ryan.

Ryan Riley Season 2 Information

Episode 1

Ryan Riley is Jessica Riley's 1-year-old son. Ryan lives in a one-bedroom apartment with his mother and her boyfriend Casey. Ryan was hospitalized 3 months ago with dehydration, respiratory syncytial virus (RSV) and failure to thrive. Because he was found to be underweight and undernourished, Social Services made arrangements for him to attend Kangaroo Junction Preschool during the day and encouraged Jessica to take Ryan to his grandmother's home in the evenings when she is working.

Ryan has been attending the new daycare for a couple of months now. He has a very consistent routine and enjoys the social interaction with his caregivers at the center. His grandmother, Evelyn, takes Ryan in for his 12-month immunizations and well-child exam. On this visit, Ryan weighs 20 pounds. The pediatrician remarks to Evelyn that he is really starting to show some good progress. Evelyn is pleased and shares the good news with Jessica.

Episode 2

Jessica drops Ryan off at her mother's home to be cared for by her sister, Jenna. Ryan squeals in delight and says, "NaNa" when he sees her. He sits in Jenna's lap while she reads books to him. He points to pictures and says, "Da."

Episode 3

Ryan is picked up by his mother from Evelyn's home. When they get home, he is put in his crib. Then he hears yelling and his mother crying. The noises frighten Ryan, and he begins to cry. Casey comes into the room, yells at him loudly to shut up, and then slams the door.

Episode 4

Ryan has been actively crawling and loves to explore. He is regularly picked up and told "no" when he finds something interesting to touch, pull, or taste.

Episode 5

Ryan goes to the zoo with Jessica and Casey. He sits in a stroller nearly the entire time playing with paper. He gets cranky while in the stroller and wants to be held by his mother. Jessica gives him a bottle with Coke in it. Ryan is happy to drink the soda.

Episode 6

Ryan has started to pull himself up to a standing position while holding onto furniture. He takes a few careful steps while holding on, and manages to navigate his way down the couch. Evelyn tells him, "You will be walking soon!"

Episode 7

Fourteen-month-old Ryan is dropped off at his grandmother's house while his mother goes to a doctor visit. Ryan has been pulling himself up on furniture and walking while holding onto it for several weeks. While at his grandmother's house, he surprises everyone when he spontaneously lets go and walks across the room. His aunt Jenna and uncle Jason laugh and clap for Ryan. Ryan smiles broadly at their reaction.

Episode 8

Ryan has not seen his mother very much during the past week. He has been spending nearly all his time at the daycare center or with his grandmother. He loves his grandmother's home because Evelyn cuddles with him and Jenna and Jason are often there to play with him.

Episode 9

Ryan's appetite has fallen off. Not only is he not eating very much, but he has become a very picky eater. Casey gets frustrated with him when he prepares something for him to eat and Ryan refuses to eat it. Casey tries to shove food in his mouth and Ryan responds by spitting the food out. Casey roughly picks up Ryan, tosses him in the crib, and slams the door. This makes Ryan scared and angry! He screams and cries loudly with no response from anyone. At some point he falls asleep; he is later awakened by his mother who offers him a snack.

Episode 10

Because Ryan is now walking, he finds all sorts of things to explore at home. He does not like it when Casey is there because he yells at him often and puts him in his crib. Ryan does not like this because he gets bored in his crib. Although Casey has never hurt him, the yelling frightens him.

Episode 11

Fifteen-month-old Ryan has been running a fever and has a great deal of nasal drainage and congestion. He does not feel well at all. His grandmother, worried about how ill he was the last time he was sick, takes him to Neighborhood Pediatrics to be examined. Ryan is diagnosed with an upper respiratory infection. Evelyn is instructed to give him plenty of fluids and children's acetaminophen (Tylenol) for the fever. Ryan's weight on this visit is $21\frac{1}{2}$ pounds.

Episode 12

Ryan feels much better this week. He has spent nearly all of his time with his grandmother during the past few weeks because his mother has been working additional hours. He usually sees his mother between the time he is picked up from daycare and when she has to go back to work for the evening shift. Often he spends the night with his grandmother. Ryan misses seeing his mother, but he is very happy at his grandmother's house.

Episode 13

Ryan is picked up by his mother from daycare this week and she takes him home. As soon as they get home, he is put in his crib. He does not want to be in the crib. Ryan tries to climb over the rails to escape the crib, but is unable to. He cries until his mother comes into the room and spends some time with him. Later, he hears shouting and then hears his mother screaming. He is frightened and begins to cry. He then hears very loud music and his mother crying. Later, some strange men come into his room, which frightens him further. Ryan is not comforted until his grandmother picks him up and takes him to her home.

Episode 14

Ryan sees there is a baby in the house. His mother tells him this is his sister, and her name is Carrie. Ryan does not understand any of this, but he likes the baby.

Episode 15

Ryan goes with his mother and baby sister, Carrie, to see Carol, the nurse midwife. Ryan plays on the floor while Carol examines his mother. Later she talks to Ryan and she asks him if he helps his mother take care of the baby. He nods his head yes.

Ryan Riley Season 3 Information

Episode 1

Ryan Riley is Jessica Riley's 17-month-old son. As an infant, Ryan was diagnosed with failure to thrive, but this condition has improved over the past year.

Ryan has done well at the Kangaroo Junction Preschool program. He has come to understand the predictable and orderly routine at daycare and at his grandmother's home. At daycare, he has social interactions with many other children his age, primarily engaging in parallel play.

His world is not orderly and structured in his mother's home. There are no rituals for bedtime, mealtime, or morning routine. This week, Ryan sees Casey hit his mother, making his mother cry. He holds his favorite toy Boo Bear for comfort.

Episode 2

The social worker makes a visit to see Jessica, Carrie, and Ryan. The social worker sees that the living conditions are messy, but the children appear healthy and show no evidence of neglect or abuse. He watches Ryan at play talking to Boo Bear and playing with blocks on the floor, noting these behaviors to be age appropriate.

Episode 3

Ryan's baby sister goes with him to Kangaroo Junction. He watches as they put her in a room with other babies. Ryan goes with the older children to Miss Webb's room. Ryan is delighted to use crayons to draw a picture.

At home, Ryan protests when Jessica takes a marker away from him. He cries until she gives it back to him to keep him quiet. He makes marks on the wall and receives a spanking as punishment.

Episode 4

Ryan loves it when his mother places Carrie on the floor. He talks to her and makes silly faces. When Carrie cries, he gently pets Carrie's head.

Episode 5

Ryan cries when he sees Casey hit his mother and throw her against the wall. He is further frightened by the yelling. Casey tells Ryan, "You shut up, or I'll bust your chops." Later in the week, while at Kangaroo Junction, Miss Webb observes Ryan hitting stuffed animals with his hands and telling them to "shut up."

Episode 6

The social worker comes by to see 20-month-old Ryan this week. He observes a curious child who is very busy with purposeful behavior. He places his favorite stuffed toy Boo Bear under a pillow so that he can hide and stay safe. He goes into the kitchen and pulls pots and pans out of the cupboards, places various toy objects in the pots, and then puts the lids on the pots. Later he goes back to the kitchen to retrieve a specific toy from the pot. The social worker does not note evidence of physical abuse.

Episode 7

Ryan spends the night with his grandmother four nights this week. He enjoys being there because he sits on her lap before bed and looks at storybooks while she reads to him. When at home, he brings books to his mother for her to read, but is told no. He often gets angry and cries when he does not get his way.

Episode 8

When Ryan's mom picks him up from daycare, his sister is crying. His mother does not take them home. Instead, he goes with his mother to a bright room with strange people. He is told to sit still, but this is hard to do. A nice woman gives him a toy to play with while his mommy is busy with Carrie.

Episode 9

Ryan is very upset that his routine has changed again. He is taken by his mother to a strange home. There are other children there, but they are different from the children at his school. He wants to see his grandmother. He wants to see Miss Webb. He wants to go back home. He clutches Boo Bear for comfort.

Episode 10

Ryan remains at the new house. He has quickly learned a new routine here. He stays in a room with his sister and mother. The people at the house are nice to him. There are many toys to play with. He misses his grandmother and asks Jessica about her.

Episode 11

Ryan is very happy to go back to his home and return to his previous routine. He is also very happy to see his grandmother and Miss Webb. He notices that Casey is not at the apartment but does not ask his mother about him.

Episode 12

Jessica takes Ryan and baby Carrie to church this week along with his grandmother and his Aunt Jenna and Uncle Jason. Ryan has never been to a church and does not know what this place is. He has a hard time sitting still and staying quiet. He yells out in protest. His grandmother takes him outside and gently tells him he needs to stay quiet and then they will go out for "some yummy pancakes." Later at brunch, Ryan has his first pancakes and loves them.

Episode 13

With less commotion in the house, Ryan has really begun to blossom. He interacts regularly with Carrie and loves to play with her. He also gets very excited to see his grandmother, Aunt Jenna, and Uncle Jason. He especially likes to play with Jenna and Jason.

Episode 14

Ryan goes with his grandmother to the pediatrician's office so that his sister can get her shots. While there, the nurse weighs Ryan. He now weighs 25 pounds at $21 \frac{1}{2}$ months of age. The nurse and Evelyn are pleased with the progress he has made in weight gain, noting he is now just below the 25th percentile.

Episode 15

Ryan is happy to move to his grandmother's house. He watches his grandmother and mother set up a crib in the room for his sister and sees that Boo Bear has been placed on a bed in the same room. He knows they will stay here now.

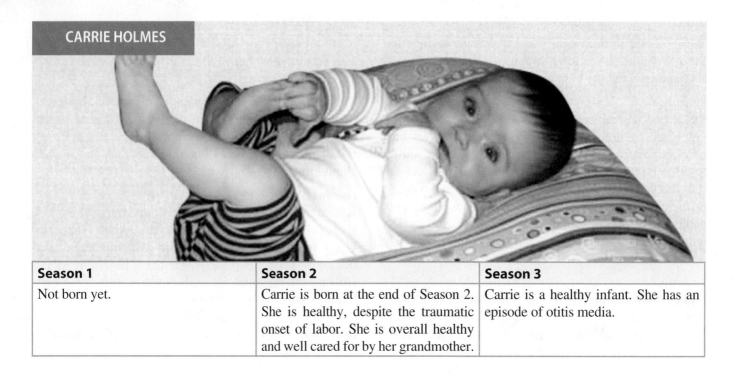

CARRIE HOLMES

Season 1	Season 2	Season 3
Not born yet.	Carrie is born at the end of Season 2. She is healthy, despite the traumatic onset of labor. She is overall healthy and well cared for by her grandmother.	Carrie is a healthy infant. She has an episode of otitis media.

Carrie Holmes Season 1 Information

Not born yet.

Carrie Holmes Season 2 Information

Not born yet.

Episode 13

Carrie Holmes is a newborn infant girl, daughter of Jessica Riley and Casey Holmes. She was born at 38 weeks' gestation by vaginal delivery after her mother went into labor following a small placental abruption from abdominal trauma. Carrie's Apgar scores were 7 at 1 minute and 9 at 5 minutes. Her initial assessment measurements were as follows:

- Birth weight: 6 pounds, 4 ounces
- Length: 49 cm
- Head circumference: 33 cm
- Chest circumference: 32 cm
- Ballard Scale: 38 weeks

The delivery occurs without fetal complications, and Carrie is perfectly healthy at birth. She is placed on Jessica's abdomen immediately after birth and covered with a warm blanket to maintain her body temperature. Shortly thereafter, Carrie is cleaned, examined, and has erythromycin ophthalmic ointment placed into her eyes. A dose of phytonadione (vitamin K) and hepatitis B vaccine are administered intramuscularly.

Prior to discharge, a heel stick is performed to obtain a blood specimen from Carrie for routine newborn metabolic screening. A urine sample is collected for a drug screen, which is negative. By the time of discharge (the day after she was born), she is breastfeeding about 7 times a day. She has 6 wet diapers and passes a large meconium stool. Her umbilical cord is drying, and the clamp is removed 目.

Episode 14

Carrie is settling into home life with her mother, father, and brother, Ryan. Sometimes she is breastfed, and other times she is given a bottle with formula. Jessica does not make it to the Neighborhood Pediatric office until Carrie is 1 week old. She weighs 6 pounds, 1 ounce. She is examined by the pediatrician and found to be in perfect health.

Episode 15

Carrie experiences a change in feeding; she is now getting a bottle with formula instead of her mother's breast for every feeding. Carrie sometimes experiences uncomfortable gas, and this makes her cry. She has also developed a sore rash on her skin. During Jessica's post-partum exam, the midwife examines Carrie and notes that she has diaper rash. Carrie is scheduled for a repeat PKU test this week, but Jessica fails to take her to the outpatient lab for the test.

Carrie Holmes Season 3 Information

Episode 1
Carrie Holmes is a 6-week-old infant girl, daughter of Jessica Riley and Casey Holmes. She was born at 38 weeks' gestation by vaginal delivery after her mother suffered a small placental abruption following abdominal trauma. She was perfectly healthy at birth. She is bottle-fed and has been in the care of her mother or grandmother, Evelyn, since birth. Carrie lives in a one-bedroom apartment with her mother, father, and brother, Ryan.

When her mother works, Carrie is in the care of her grandmother, Evelyn. She is kept warm and dry, is fed well, and is cuddled in a calm environment. She listens as her grandmother talks to her. When she is old enough, Carrie will go to Kangaroo Junction Preschool with her brother. At her mother's house, the care is less consistent. Often, there are strange, loud noises and angry voices. Carrie cries when she gets hungry or just wants to be held.

Episode 2
The social worker makes a visit to see Jessica, Carrie, and Ryan. The social worker sees that the living conditions are messy, but the children appear healthy and show no evidence of neglect or abuse. Jessica takes Carrie in for her 2-month well-baby exam and immunizations.

Episode 3
Carrie begins going to Kangaroo Junction Preschool with her brother, Ryan, on the days that Jessica works.

Episode 4
Carrie loves to lie on the floor and look at her brother, Ryan. She listens to him talk to her and he shows her his toys. When she gets hungry and starts to cry, Ryan strokes her hair.

Episode 5
Carrie is frightened by the loud voices and shouting at her mother's home. She cries, expecting her mother to pick her up and hold her. Casey picks her up, puts her in her crib, and slams the door shut. She cries herself to sleep.

Episode 6
The social worker comes by to see Carrie this week. Carrie has no markings on her body that suggest physical abuse and appears to be well fed. While interacting with Jessica, the social worker watches Carrie (who is lying on a blanket on the floor) and notes that she coos, raises her head and chest from a prone position, and expresses interest in objects that come into her visual field.

Episode 7
Carrie is rocked and cuddled by her mother. She studies her mother's face and coos. Later, while lying on the floor, she watches with great interest while her brother, Ryan, plays with toys.

Episode 8
Carrie is 17-weeks old. She has not been feeling well most of the day. She has been fussy and has not eaten well. Her right ear hurts, although she can't communicate this except by crying. When her mother picks her up from daycare, Jessica is advised that Carrie has a fever and perhaps should be seen by a doctor.

It is late in the afternoon, and Jessica knows that she can't go to the pediatrician's office at this point. She takes Carrie to the Emergency Department at Neighborhood Hospital, where she sees Dr. Gordon. Carrie is diagnosed with otitis media and sent home with a prescription for amoxicillin (Amoxil) and directions for Jessica to treat her fever with acetaminophen (Tylenol) and plenty of fluids. The Emergency Department nurse notes that Carrie has not yet had her 4-month immunizations and reminds Jessica to schedule an appointment to get those done.

Episode 9
During the middle of the night, Carrie's mother takes her from her crib, wraps her in a blanket, and takes her to a strange house. Carrie does not recognize anybody there. She is placed in a strange crib and goes to sleep.

Episode 10
Carrie is aware that she is in a new place. She listens and watches with great interest all the activity happening in the new place. Several people she has never seen before pick her up to hold her and talk to her.

Episode 11
Carrie and her brother, Ryan, return to their home. Carrie is delighted to see her grandmother.

Episode 12

Jessica takes Carrie and her brother, Ryan, to church this week along with her grandmother and her Aunt Jenna and Uncle Jason. Carrie has never been to this place before. She looks around with interest at first, and then falls asleep in her mother's arms.

Episode 13

Carrie is a very happy baby. She smiles regularly and is very playful. She loves to see not only her mother, but her grandmother, Aunt Jenna, and Uncle Jason. She makes Jason laugh when she rolls over from back to front and front to back. She squeals in delight when her brother, Ryan, plays with her.

Episode 14

Carrie is now 6-months old. Evelyn takes her in for a well-baby visit and learns that Jessica never took her in at 4 months for a visit and immunizations. At this visit, Carrie's weight is $15\frac{1}{2}$ pounds, and her head circumference is measured at 42 cm. The nurse observes that Carrie is able to roll over. She tells Evelyn that she can start giving the baby rice cereal. The nurse reviews Carrie's immunization records to determine what she needs to get on this visit.

Episode 15

Carrie and her brother move into their grandmother's home.

ROSS & JARAMILLO HOUSEHOLD

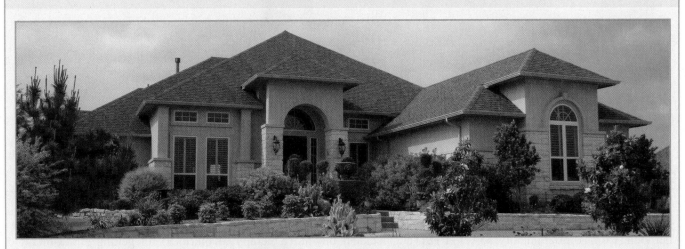

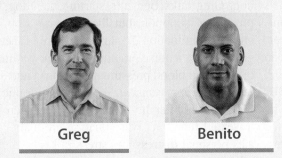

Greg   **Benito**

Housing	Greg and Benito live in an upscale single story home in Northwoods. They have a nice yard and live closer to town than to the lake
Parks and Recreation	There is a fitness center nearby where Benito works out regularly. There is a golf course located in the Northwoods area, as well as hiking trails near the lake where Benito sometimes runs.
Services	There is a shopping plaza in the area and the Neighborhood Hospital is located a few miles away.

Key: ▶ = video clip   ☰ = medical record   ▽ = journal entry   NEWS = news article

GREG ROSS

Season 1	Season 2	Season 3
Greg lives with his long-time partner Ben. He has inflammatory bowel disease (ulcerative colitis) that is managed with diet and medications. During this season, he has an exacerbation of colitis that is managed on an outpatient basis. Greg wants a child. He is frustrated when he tries to discuss this topic with Ben, because he avoids the discussion. Greg goes to the health fair and learns his blood pressure is elevated.	Greg and Ben read about a veteran with PTSD and decide to buy him a therapy dog. Greg talks Ben into starting the process of adoption, but they experience discrimination because they are gay. He sees a nurse practitioner about his elevated blood pressure and begins taking antihypertensive medications. Shortly thereafter he notices changes in sexual function. This situation creates personal distress and stress in his relationship with Ben.	Sal Lucero meets Greg and Ben to thank them for getting him a therapy dog. Greg figures out that the medication is contributing to his sexual dysfunction. He has an exacerbation of colitis requiring hospitalization. Greg and Ben continue to pursue adoption options and finally find a pregnant teen who agrees to give her baby up after birth.

Greg Ross Season 1 Information

Episode 1

Greg Ross is a 44-year-old Caucasian male who is in good health. He has inflammatory bowel disease, specifically ulcerative colitis, which was first diagnosed at age 28. His disease is considered mild in severity; it has not progressed, in his opinion, because of his strict adherence to diet therapies, including a low-roughage diet and avoidance of milk products. He takes no specific medication for the colitis when it is in remission, but he has medications to take when he has a "flare-up." It has been about $2\frac{1}{2}$ years since he last experienced active disease. Greg sees a gastroenterologist once a year or as needed for management of the colitis.

Greg is a sales representative for a large, national manufacturing company. His work requires that he travel 2–3 days a week. Because Greg is very intelligent and has excellent interpersonal skills, he is one of the most successful sales representatives in the company; he has been in the top 5% of sales reps nationwide for the past 7 years

in a row. His income is based on sales percentages, so he is earning a very high income.

Greg is gay and has been in a monogamous relationship for 10 years with his partner, Ben. They own a beautiful home that they share with their two pet dogs, Mitt and Bitt. Greg has been estranged from his family for most of his adult life. His parents and siblings have never accepted the fact that he is gay, so contact with his parents is usually limited to talking with his mother a few times a year. Greg has accepted this situation and gone on to lead his own life. He considers Ben and the dogs to be his family, although he dreams of having children. Greg's primary recreational activities are travel, fine dining, and golf. He has tried without success to get Ben interested in golf, so he plays regularly either with clients or the men at the country club. Greg is interested in helping others and is very charitable, providing financial help to various organizations and causes.

This episode Greg comes home after being out of town for 3 days this week. Over dinner he tells Ben that he won a 10-day trip for two to Italy because of his sales performance during the past year. He marks the trip dates on the calendar, noting it is only a few months away.

Episode 2

Nathan, one of the sales associates in Greg's company, and his wife Marta are expecting a baby soon. A baby shower for Nathan and Marta was held this week and Greg was invited to attend. He had never been to a baby shower before; growing up, this was something women would do and men never participated in such activities. Needless to say, Greg did not know what to expect, but he ended up having a great time. Nathan and Marta's excitement was palpable. Greg has always loved children and thought about how much happier he would be if he could raise a child. Greg finds it interesting that because he makes a great deal of money, people assume he is happy. Although he enjoys his lifestyle with Ben, he often finds himself wishing for a life with more purpose ▼.

Episode 3

Greg is a sponsor for a community fundraising event this week called Run for the Fish. Proceeds are used to reduce pollution at Neighborhood Lake. In addition to donating free t-shirts for participants, Greg helps with registration. His partner, Ben, also participates in the event [NEWS].

Episode 4

Greg is out of town for a week-long sales meeting this week. He plays several rounds of golf with senior sales associates and managers at the resort course where the meeting is held. In one of the golf rounds, two of the men in his golf group talk about their children's activities. Greg comments that he would love to be a dad someday. One of the men says, "You? A dad? What would that be … an immaculate conception?" This comment is followed by laughter from the group and Greg knows the laughter is because they know he is gay. "Yeah, whatever," responds Greg, and he says nothing more of it, although the comment stings ▼.

Episode 5

Greg's friend Nathan and his wife Marta recently had their baby, and Marta brings the baby to the office for everyone to see. He hears her describe the birth process in great detail and say how good the midwife was who delivered her baby. Greg wonders how a midwife differs from a physician.

Greg makes final plans for their upcoming trip to Hawaii by booking a number of interesting excursions. Many of the excursion advertisements depict families - parents with their children having fun. Greg thinks about all the interesting places he could take a child if he had one ▼.

Episode 6

Greg and Ben are in Hawaii this week on vacation following Ben's triathlon. They spend most of their time visiting local attractions and resting on the beach. Greg is glad that Ben is taking most of the week off from training. While on the beach, they watch a father playing in the surf with his young children. Greg comments to Ben that he thinks it would be great to have children together someday. Ben simply responds, "Yeah, kids are cool." Greg recognizes that although he and Ben have a good relationship, they really don't have that many activities that they share outside of taking vacations together. He is sure that if they had a child, they would spend more time together ▼.

Episode 7

Greg wanders into the health fair this week as he is passing by. He stops at the blood pressure screening table and is shocked to learn that his blood pressure is elevated at 138/94 mm Hg. The nurse at the screening writes his blood pressure measurement down and suggests that he have it checked again in the next week or so and to follow up with his primary care physician if it remains elevated. Greg elects not to mention the elevated blood pressure to Ben. He is sure Ben would tell him he needs to get more exercise and eat a healthier diet [NEWS].

Episode 8

Greg talks with Ben about the possibility of adopting a child or even perhaps fathering a child with a surrogate mother. Ben does not show much interest in the topic and questions Greg about how they will have enough time to raise children; he also points out that they already have everything they need. Greg is frustrated with Ben's lack of interest. His response underscores a character flaw he finds in Ben - that is, he is very self-centered and often selfish ▼.

Episode 9

After work, Greg drops by the pharmacy to pick up vitamins and dietary supplements for Ben. He sits down at the automated blood pressure machine and takes his blood pressure. The digital display reads 134/90 mm HG, and he decides that his blood pressure is probably not that bad after all. He also notices a pamphlet about HIV testing. He feels relieved that he is in a monogamous relationship, believing he doesn't have to worry about those issues.

Episode 10

Greg and Ben attend the annual Neighborhood Art Show this week. They go every year to support the community artists. Over the years Greg has developed friendships with many of the artists, so he is always happy to go. Greg buys several pieces of art in anticipation of donations for many silent auctions he supports throughout the year [NEWS].

Episode 11

In anticipation of his upcoming vacation to Italy, Greg has many loose ends to wrap up at work. He is not feeling as much excitement as he has in the past, realizing it is just another trip. Greg feels down, as he wonders what meaning his life has. What is his life's purpose? There has got to be more to life than making a lot of money, playing golf, and going on vacations. He finds himself thinking about having a child yet again. Perhaps he can talk with Ben about this again when they are relaxed and enjoying each other's company.

Episode 12

Ben and Greg are in Italy this week. They tour many places within Rome and are especially impressed with the Roman Coliseum. Greg enjoys being able to spend so much time with Ben. During the trip, he again tries to talk with Ben about having children. Ben points out that, if they had kids, they would never be able to take lovely vacations like this. Greg counters by commenting, "Yeah, but you know, this won't be fun forever." He is disappointed that Ben is closed-minded about the idea and worries that the relationship may never evolve to the point of raising a family together. He also wonders what will sustain their relationship over the years ▼.

Episode 13

Ben and Greg are finishing their vacation in Italy this week. Greg experiences abdominal pain and Diarrhea on the way home and blames it on the stress of travel and the lack of a controlled diet. The symptoms continue for a few days after he gets home.

Episode 14

Greg continues to have pain and diarrhea; he recognizes that he is having an acute exacerbation of colitis. He makes an appointment with the gastroenterologist, who gives Greg a prescription for oral Prednisone (deltasone) and sulfasalazine and advises him to drink plenty of fluids. The physician also comments that Greg's blood pressure is 146/96 mm Hg. The gastroenterologist explains that his blood pressure is higher than it should be, but his abdominal pain might have something to do with it. Greg is told to have his blood pressure rechecked when he is feeling better ▼.

Episode 15

Ben is out of town competing in another triathlon. Greg elects to stay home because of ongoing symptoms with his colitis. Because of the frequent episodes of diarrhea, he stays close to home, trying to rest his colon [NEWS].

Greg Ross Season 2 Information

Episode 1

Greg Ross is a 45-year-old Caucasian male who is in good health. He has inflammatory bowel disease, specifically ulcerative colitis, which was first diagnosed at age 28. His disease is considered mild in severity.

The recent exacerbation of Greg's colitis seems to have passed. He is feeling much better again and is able to resume his regular business travel.

Episode 2

While having dinner together, Greg talks to Ben again about considering having a child together—either through adoption or finding a surrogate parent. Greg explains how important it is to him and that he wishes Ben would at least give it some serious thought. He points out that, with their income, they can afford whatever they need to make things work. There's no reason to think they would be unable to continue doing the things they enjoy. Greg offers many suggestions, including hiring a nanny to stay in their home with their child while they work or travel out of town. For the first time, Greg feels as if Ben actually is listening to his point of view [▶] [NEWS]

Episode 3

Greg reads an article in the *News* this week that really catches his attention. He reads about a local man by the name of Sal Lucero, a veteran who suffers from post-traumatic stress disorder (PTSD). According to the article, it is thought that Sal would benefit from a therapy dog, but the VA no longer pays for this as a treatment. As attached as he is to his own two dogs and knowing the joy and companionship they offer, he can fully understand how a therapy dog could be helpful to somebody with PTSD. Greg and Ben talk about this after dinner and decide to offer to help the man get a therapy dog. They don't know exactly what it will cost, but they both think it is something they can do to help somebody who has given his time for military service. Greg contacts the newspaper to get contact information for Sal Lucero [▶] [▼] [NEWS].

Episode 4

Greg and Ben discuss the possibility of finding a surrogate mother as an alternative to adoption. Ben suggests asking his sister-in-law if she would consider being a surrogate parent for them. Greg likes the idea of having a child who is biologically related to Ben.

Greg follows up on the advice of the physician and checks his blood pressure at the drug store. He is surprised when 142/94 mm Hg is displayed on the monitor. He retakes the blood pressure and gets the same reading.

Greg is pretty sure the machine is inaccurate, but because of other readings that were elevated, he makes an appointment with Dr. Rowe at the family practice clinic.

Episode 5

Greg's friend Nathan and his wife Marta recently had their baby, and Marta brings the baby to the office for everyone to see. He hears her describe the birth process in great detail and say how good the midwife was who delivered her baby. Greg wonders how a midwife differs from a physician.

Greg makes final plans for their upcoming trip to Hawaii by booking a number of interesting excursions. Many of the excursion advertisements depict families - parents with their children having fun. Greg thinks about all the interesting places he could take a child if he had one ▼.

Episode 6

Greg has become obsessed with his blood pressure. He hates taking the medication because then he has to urinate frequently. At first he tries taking it in the morning, but this interferes with meetings and sales calls. Then he tries taking the medication at night, and he loses sleep because of the need to get up to urinate ▼.

Episode 7

Greg has been gone most of the past two weeks traveling for work and is very tired when he gets home. He has been taking the blood pressure medication for several weeks. At a follow-up visit with the nurse practitioner, his blood pressure is down to 136/88 mm Hg. When asked if he has experienced any problems with the medications, he says he does not think so. In reality, Greg is uncomfortable mentioning that his erections have recently not felt the same. He decides the symptom is probably related to being overly tired.

Episode 8

Greg and Ben have always had a very active sexual relationship, and Greg continues to notice a change in his ability to have an erection. Although Ben's sex drive has always been greater than Greg's, he has always been responsive to his partner. However, lately Greg can't seem to respond in the same way and he begins to worry about it. He is uncomfortable discussing it with Ben, hoping he does not notice.

After talking with a few of their gay and lesbian friends who have children, Ben and Greg decide to look into adoption. Greg spends hours on the internet learning as much as he can about the process. He learns of the many challenges that gay and lesbian couples face when they want to adopt, and this causes him to feel stressed. He learns that the first step is to find an agency to work with. Greg locates several agencies in the area and makes plans to contact a few of them to determine whether they will be able to help ▼.

Episode 9

This week Greg and Ben are in Spain for 5 days attending a festival as guests of one of Greg's influential clients. Greg has a noticeable problem with sexual performance this week – in fact, Ben asks him what the problem is. Greg is very distraught about this and worries about Ben's reaction. He tells Ben that he is just feeling tired from traveling, and it has nothing to do with him. This triggers a rare fight. Greg is shocked and offended when Ben asks him if he is seeing somebody else. Greg tells him he is not sure what the problem is, but he is not seeing anybody else. Ben barely speaks to him the rest of the week.

Episode 10

Greg continues to experience problems with sexual functioning He is now quite sure it is not due to fatigue. He reads about erectile dysfunction on the Internet and finds that some of the common causes include blood pressure medications and stress. He wonders if the blood pressure medication he is taking is the problem, but he can't specifically remember if the onset of the symptoms coincided with the time he began taking the medication. He makes a point to try to reduce his stress level and relax. He signs up for a massage once a week and decides to try to get more exercise to reduce his stress level. He is very embarrassed about the situation and avoids talking to Ben about it, but he also worries about how it is impacting his relationship with Ben. The one thing Greg has felt insecure about over the years is how attractive Ben is; Ben is regularly "hit on" by women and other men. Ben has a single gay friend in the cycling club that he has been spending more time with. Knowing Ben's strong sexual urges, Greg really begins to worry if Ben will have an affair with him.

Trying to maintain a positive attitude, he takes Ben out for a quick dinner. Greg notices their server, a young woman by the name of Jessica, is pregnant and he immediately wishes he could have a baby. Greg asks her when her baby is due and if this is her first pregnancy. When Jessica turns her head to respond, he can see she has a bruise near her eye. Their eyes meet and with a somewhat flat affect she responds, "Soon, and this is my second." Intuitively, Greg knows this young woman is troubled and he is sure she is being physically abused. He feels badly for bringing the subject up, especially as he watches her work. He can almost feel her pain. At the end of their meal, Greg leaves the young woman a $150 tip and a napkin with his phone number and the following message:

"Please do not hesitate to call if you ever find yourself needing help." Greg doubts he will hear from her, but wanted to reach out to her just the same ▽.

Episode 11

Greg is traveling this week and spends all week worrying about his sexual problems. He rents a gay porn movie and even that does not sufficiently arouse him. He finds himself obsessing over his erection issues and obsessing about the possibility of Ben spending time alone with Alex.

When he gets home from his trip Ben is sitting in the living room of their home looking sad and dejected. Greg is sure Ben is getting ready to admit to an affair with Alex or tell him he is leaving him. Instead, Greg is shocked to learn that Ben has lost his job due to company downsizing. Greg can tell how devastated Ben is and hopes he can console him. Things seem to be getting increasingly complicated for them.

Episode 12

Despite his concerns about the status of his relationship with Ben and the fact that Ben has recently lost his job, Greg and Ben continue to explore adoption options by meeting with the director of a private adoption agency. Greg learns that, although the agency works with gay and lesbian parents, they would not be considered a "priority" for infant adoption placements. The agency representative makes it clear that they would be more likely have a child placed with them if Ben and Greg were willing to consider a child with special needs or a "hard-to-place" child. Greg is frustrated by what he learns. This frustration is further aggravated by his ongoing sexual response issues.

Episode 13

It is a stressful weekend for Greg and Ben because of the adoption issues, Ben feeling depressed about his job loss and Greg's ongoing problems with sexual response. Greg goes out of his way to avoid physical contact with Ben, and Ben becomes angry with him. While having coffee, Ben is very direct with Greg and asks him what the issue is - and wants to know if there is "somebody else." Greg finally shares with Ben that, although he is not sure, he thinks the blood pressure medication he has been taking might be causing his decreased sexual response. Greg tells Ben that he quit taking the medication a few days ago to see if his "problem" would go away. Ben asks Greg why he did not feel comfortable talking with him about this. Greg feels badly that he did not open up more - but he continues to feel very embarrassed ▷ ▽.

Episode 14

Greg and Ben meet with another adoption agency this week. When they acknowledge that they are a gay couple, the agency claims it will not be able to help. Greg is disappointed in their closed-minded attitude toward them. He is beginning to wonder if he might have better luck trying to adopt a child as a single man and not mention that he is gay.

Episode 15

Greg and Ben go to the Neighborhood Arts and Crafts Fair over the weekend. While at the show, Greg buys a quilt from Pam Allen, a cancer survivor. He spends several minutes talking with the woman and her son Gary, who has Down syndrome NEWS.

Greg Ross　Season 3 Information

Episode 1

Greg has validated what he suspected might be wrong – the blood pressure medication was causing his sexual dysfunction! He quit taking the blood pressure medication several weeks ago and now has no problems with his sexual response. He is very happy to see that Ben is pleased as well. Greg is relieved that it was such a simple solution and decides that taking the medication is just not worth it. He makes another appointment with the family practice clinic to discuss alternative blood pressure management.

This week Greg gets a phone call from Sal Lucero, the man he helped to get a therapy dog. Sal lets Greg know he now has his dog. He says the paper would like to do a story about him getting a dog and wants to include Greg and Ben in the story. At first Greg declines and tells Sal

that is nice, but not necessary. However, realizing how important it is to Sal for this story to be told, he agrees.

Episode 2

Greg has an appointment with the nurse practitioner this week and admits he quit taking the blood pressure medication she previously prescribed "because it is messing with my sex life." The nurse practitioner, Margie, asks Greg in a very matter-of-fact way if he is experiencing problems having an erection. Greg finds her no-nonsense approach a relief, and his anxiety about talking about this is significantly reduced. He confirms this is the problem, and Margie tells him it is a side effect for some men. Greg's blood pressure is measured at 148/96 mm Hg. The nurse practitioner explains that having blood pressure this high is not acceptable, and not being able to have an erection is also not acceptable. She tells Greg they need a different treatment plan. Greg suggests that perhaps he can just avoid salt and increase his exercise. The nurse practitioner tells him that these changes alone are unlikely to reduce the blood pressure enough, but that those measures, in addition to taking medication, will be helpful. The nurse practitioner gives him a prescription for lisinopril (5 mg daily) and hydrochlorothiazide (25 mg daily).

Greg and Ben visit with another adoption agency and are again discouraged when told they should not get their hopes up about adopting an infant. Greg insists on knowing the reason for this. The agency representative tells them that Greg and Ben would not be considered as stable as a traditional married couple. They decide to continue exploring other agency options ▶ ✉.

Episode 3

Greg has a long stretch of travel; his work has taken him to Asia for 2 weeks. He is able to land an account that will surely put him at the top in company-wide sales this year – a coveted status he has been close to on several occasions, but has never earned. Given the fact that Ben has been out of work, Greg is especially happy about this!

Episode 4

Greg has a sudden and severe acute exacerbation of colitis this week. On one day, he passes several small, loose, bloody stools with cramping. On the following day, he has severe abdominal pain and nine episodes of bloody diarrhea stools with mucus by noon. He takes his temperature and notes that he has a fever.

Ben takes him to the emergency department, where he is treated by Dr. Gordon with IV fluids, oral Prednisone (deltasone), and sulfasalazine, and then sent home. He is told to follow up with his primary care provider if his symptoms do not improve. He cancels his out-of-town travel for the next 2 weeks to allow time to rest 🗏.

Episode 5

Greg follows up with his gastroenterologist, because he is still experiencing bloody diarrhea with mucus. The physician recommends admission to the hospital for IV prednisone, IV fluids, and bowel rest by maintaining an NPO status. Additionally, he recommends that Greg be evaluated for possible surgical evaluation. Greg does not even want to think about the possibility of a surgical intervention. This could mean a colon resection and even a colostomy. Greg can't think of anything more awful and worries, if it ever comes to this, how would Ben respond? After the recent sexual problems Greg experienced, he does not ever want to have to go through something like that. Greg tells the gastroenterologist he would like to

take a more conservative approach and hope this episode settles down again for a while.

Episode 6

Greg is back home and feeling much better. He goes with Ben to visit another adoption agency and is again told that gay adoptive parents are not given priority for infant placement. Ben suggests that they hire an attorney in order to be adequately represented through the adoption process. Greg is beginning to think that adoption may not be worth it, but he agrees with Ben that hiring an attorney might help ✉.

Episode 7

Greg is a major sponsor for the River Jazz festival this weekend. The purpose of the festival is to raise awareness of domestic violence and to raise money for a shelter for battered women. Greg is still not feeling 100% after his exacerbation of colitis, but he is well enough to attend the event for at least a few hours each day. He is very glad that Ben had agreed to help out and that he had turned over many of his tasks to Ben 📰.

Episode 8

Greg is back to his regular work and travel schedule, although he is still not feeling 100%. He is still passing several semi-formed stools with small amounts of blood every day. This makes holding meetings with clients and traveling rather difficult. Greg and Ben meet with an attorney, who suggests that they work with a private adoption agency or directly with birth parents. Greg and Ben decide to do this 📰.

Episode 9

Greg reads Pam Allen's obituary in the *News*. He recalls meeting Pam but can't quite place where – or any details about her. He knows he eventually will remember, so he places a copy in his desk. Greg gets a call from the family attorney that they have been working with, who says he has located a pregnant woman interested in putting her baby up for adoption. Greg learns she is about $7 \frac{1}{2}$ months along and is an unwed 16-year-old girl 📰.

Episode 10

Greg and Ben are thrilled to meet Terry Clark, a pregnant teen who has agreed to give her baby to them for adoption. Greg can see that she is very quiet and shy and perhaps uncertain about the process. Terry tells Ben and Greg that she is not ready to take care of a baby, but she hopes that they will let her see the baby. Greg assures Terry that they welcome her being involved. As part of the agreement, Greg and Ben agree to provide financial support to Terry until the baby is born and to help pay for medical expenses associated with the delivery. Later that afternoon, Greg receives a call from his attorney and learns that Terry really likes both of them and is glad they are going to be her baby's parents. Greg can hardly believe they will soon be parents! ▶ ▽

Episode 11
Greg has a follow-up visit to see the nurse practitioner this week and is glad to learn that his blood pressure is down to 134/86 mm Hg. The change in medications to lisinopril and hydrochlorothiazide seems to have done the trick, and Greg has no side effects. Greg proudly tells the nurse practitioner that he and his partner are adopting a baby and will soon be parents. He asks her for a recommendation for a good pediatrician in the community.

Episode 12
Greg accompanies Ben to an orthopedic physician's office to have his leg evaluated for another injury. He feels bad when he realizes that Ben will have to cancel another event. He wonders if Ben will finally give up his extreme (almost fanatical) training routine. Greg has always been supportive of Ben, but he wonders exactly what the point of it all is. Ben certainly is not improving his health.

Episode 13
Greg is out of town for nearly a full week of business travel. Although he has enjoyed success in his career, he wonders if he could make a career move that would not require extensive travel. Of course, he realizes it will impact his income, but Greg is highly motivated for a change if it means having more time at home once they have a baby. Greg knows better than to act impulsively on his emotions, but he does begin to contemplate alternatives ▽.

Episode 14
Greg and Ben are off to Alaska for a cruise. They have a wonderful time together and talk about the many plans they have for the baby. Greg is so happy that things seem to be coming together. He is excited about all of the changes that are about to occur in their life and dreams about being a father. They agree to have a live-in nanny so that the baby won't be exposed to illnesses at day care centers and so that the baby can have her complete attention. They place an ad and plan to do thorough interviews and background checks to find the perfect nanny ▽ NEWS.

Episode 15
While working in his home study, Greg receives a devastating phone call. Terry Clark, the pregnant teenager, changes her mind about putting her baby up for adoption. Greg learns that she was "forbidden" by her parents to give her baby to a gay couple. When he hangs up the phone, he puts his head on his desk and cries - he sobs harder than he has in a very long time. He did not even get the chance to hold the baby! As he collects himself, he notices the scrap of paper with Pam Allen's obituary that he had placed there months ago hoping he could recall how he knew the woman. As he rereads the obituary, he focuses on the name of her son - Gary. He suddenly remembers that Gary is the son with Down syndrome and that it was Pam Allen he bought the beautiful quilt from several months ago.

In his grief for the loss of a baby he will never meet, Greg gains an appreciation for a parent's love of their child. He remembers Pam and Gary and the love the two of them shared. Greg cries at the thought of Gary losing his mother. Because he feels Gary should have the quilt, Greg tracks down Gary's address and mails the quilt to him. The act of kindness lifts Greg's spirits ▽.

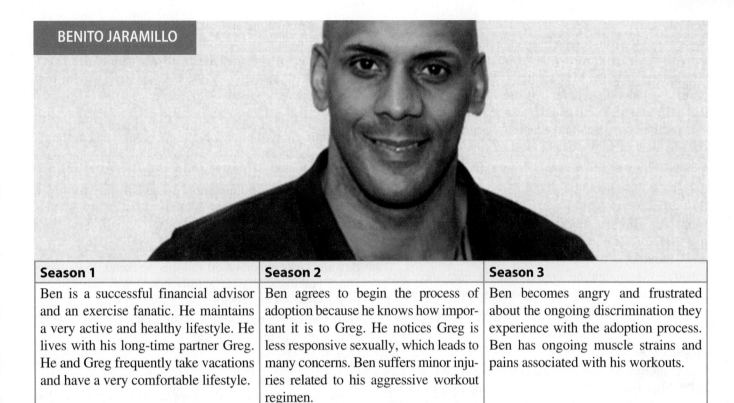

BENITO JARAMILLO

Season 1	Season 2	Season 3
Ben is a successful financial advisor and an exercise fanatic. He maintains a very active and healthy lifestyle. He lives with his long-time partner Greg. He and Greg frequently take vacations and have a very comfortable lifestyle.	Ben agrees to begin the process of adoption because he knows how important it is to Greg. He notices Greg is less responsive sexually, which leads to many concerns. Ben suffers minor injuries related to his aggressive workout regimen.	Ben becomes angry and frustrated about the ongoing discrimination they experience with the adoption process. Ben has ongoing muscle strains and pains associated with his workouts.

Benito Jaramillo Season 1 Information

Episode 1

Benito (Ben) Jaramillo is a 41-year-old Hispanic male in excellent health. He has a very successful career as a financial manager and consultant. He works long hours but has a great degree of flexibility in his schedule, allowing him to take time off whenever he needs to. His motto has always been, "Work hard, play hard." He has no medical problems and takes no prescribed medications.

Ben's primary outside hobby and interest is athletic training - in fact, many consider Ben to be an exercise and health fanatic. He participates in many athletic events, such as running, cycling, skiing, and triathlon events. To maintain his competitiveness, Ben trains several hours a day on most days. His training schedule includes a workout early in the morning and another after work. In addition to the aggressive training schedule, Ben eats a healthy diet and consults with a nutritionist regularly. He takes herbal preparations and vitamins to optimize his health. He has never been a smoker and has one alcoholic beverage almost nightly.

Ben lives with his longtime partner Greg and their two canine "children," Mitt and Bitt. Although Ben and Greg have very different personalities and interests, they get along very well, providing each other with companionship and balance. They particularly enjoy taking vacations together. Their relationship is monogamous. Ben gets along well with his parents and siblings. Although Ben's parents know that he is gay, they refer to Greg as Ben's "special friend." Ben's siblings consider Greg part of the family. He very much enjoys all of the things in his life that his comfortable income offers.

Ben has been training more aggressively this week for an upcoming triathlon in Hawaii. Ben and Greg had previously decided to spend one week there for vacation after the event. Greg announces that they are also going to go to Italy in a few months. Ben enjoys traveling but is secretly wondering if going to Italy for 10 days will interfere with training for another triathlon that he plans to compete in the following month ▼.

Episode 2

Ben has a frustrating week. With financial challenges seen at the state and national levels, several of Ben's investors are worried and want Ben to protect all of their money. Sometimes his clients get angry with him when their accounts lose money. As Ben sees it, he provides the best advice he can for the current market - but not even he can predict what will happen ▼.

Episode 3

Ben attends the Run for the Fish fundraiser this week with Greg. Ben elects to run in the "Double Trouble" race – which is a distance of 10 miles (two laps around the 5-mile Neighborhood Lake). He uses the race to train for the upcoming triathlon. Although Greg is one of the sponsors for the event, Ben finds himself wishing Greg would actually do more physical activity and run, instead of just helping with registration [NEWS].

Episode 4

Ben takes advantage of the fact that Greg is gone all week and uses the time alone to train for the upcoming triathlon. He spends 5 hours a day each day this week training, in addition to maintaining a regular work schedule. Although he enjoys Greg's company, Ben secretly loves it when Greg is gone for several days in a row so he can do the additional workouts without feeling guilty ▽.

Episode 5

Ben continues to train very hard this week until the day before they leave for Hawaii. He knows he won't win, but he hopes that he can improve on his personal best time ▽.

Episode 6

Ben competes in the triathlon this week in Hawaii. Although his time is a personal best, he is disappointed that it is an improvement of only 25 seconds. With the exception of early-morning runs on the beach, Ben decides to take a week off from training. He is annoyed when Greg talks about children and deliberately does not respond to Greg's comments. Although he likes children, he has never had a strong desire to have his own. Having kids would interfere with his training and work. He wonders why Greg keeps bringing up the subject.

Episode 7

Over the weekend, Ben goes on a day-long bike ride with a group from the cycling club. He invites Greg to come along but knows that he will decline. Ben bought Greg a high-end bicycle about a year ago, hoping to get him more involved, but Greg always prefers to play golf. He knows they don't spend as much time together as perhaps they should, but Ben finds golf to be a waste of time that does not provide enough physical challenge for him.

Episode 8

Ben is annoyed when Greg again talks with him about the possibility of adopting a child or fathering a child with a surrogate mother. Ben does not think Greg has any idea of the time commitment involved with raising children. Ben asks Greg, "Who would stay home to raise a baby? You

are always traveling and gone – so who would be stuck at home taking care of kids? How would I be able to keep up my training? If you want a baby to take care of, let's get a puppy." Ben does not understand why Greg would want to add such a complication to their lives.

Episode 9

Ben pulls a muscle in his groin this week while training. He is angry that this injury will keep him from running for at least a week - maybe two. He compensates by spending time in the swimming pool doing laps for swimming endurance. When he tells Greg about the injury, he gets little sympathy ▽ [NEWS].

Episode 10

Ben and Greg attend an art fair this weekend. Ben enjoys going but finds himself getting bored very quickly. "It is always the same people and the same stuff year after year," he tells Greg. Nonetheless, Ben picks out several gifts to give to his family [NEWS].

Episode 11

Ben continues to train by focusing on swimming. He knows he could potentially improve his overall triathlon times if he spends more time in this area.

Episode 12

Ben is in Italy this week with Greg. He has never been to Italy and finds the place fascinating. Greg brings up the "children" discussion again, so Ben points out that, if they have kids, they won't be able to take vacations like this. Ben wishes he would just drop the subject and not ruin the vacation. At the same time, Ben feels badly, because he can tell the comment hurts Greg ▽.

Episode 13

Greg experiences abdominal pain and diarrhea on the way home from Italy. Ben knows these symptoms tend to occur when he experiences stress, and he blames himself for not being more sensitive to Greg's feelings. This week, he begins an aggressive training schedule for an upcoming triathlon.

Episode 14

The triathlon is fast approaching and Ben steps up his exercise routine by spending 5 hours each day this week training. Between work and training he sees very little of Greg this week. "It is probably just as well," Ben thinks. He knows when Greg is having problems with his stomach he needs a lot of peace and quiet to rest ▽.

Episode 15

Ben participates in the triathlon this weekend. He is very pleased with his performance and is very happy to come in second place in his age group. He is disappointed that Greg is unable to come with him to watch ▽.

Benito Jaramillo Season 2 Information

Episode 1
Ben has been very happy about his progress in physical conditioning and performance at the various events in which he participates. He wishes he could pursue these activities on a full-time basis. However, recognizing the reality of lost potential in his highly competitive career, he decides it would be a poor decision on his part.

Episode 2
Ben is increasingly aware of how important it is to Greg to have children. Although he has never really thought it through, he comes to realize that it is logistically possible to raise a child together, and he agrees to give it serious consideration. He recognizes he has probably been selfish and unfair to Greg ▾.

Episode 3
Over dinner Greg mentions a story he read in the local newspaper about a veteran needing a therapy dog for post-traumatic stress disorder (PTSD). Ben tells Greg he also saw that article and thought how sad the situation was. Greg says to Ben, "Perhaps we could do something about it. What if we paid for the therapy dog for him?" Ben is immediately agreeable to the idea. He continues to be impressed with the level of Greg's empathy and generosity toward others and wishes he had those qualities naturally. "What a good man he is!" Ben thinks to himself ▾.

Episode 4
While visiting his brother's home, Ben asks his sister-in-law Shelly for her opinion about Greg's idea of having a baby. She says she doesn't think it is a bad idea but wonders just where they thought they would get a baby. Ben asks her if she would consider being a surrogate parent for them. She says she might consider it, but she is sure her husband would never go along with the idea and points out to Ben that it could be pretty complicated. She adds that, although Ben's parents are supportive of his sexuality, they might not be thrilled with this idea. Shelly says she will talk about it with her husband. She also suggests they either look for a surrogate who is not a relative or consider adoption ▶.

Episode 5
Shelly calls Ben this week to tell him that her husband is definitely against the idea of her being a surrogate parent. Ben is not surprised and wonders if it is because his brother is against the idea in general or against the idea for a gay couple. This bothers Ben, but he decides against taking it up with his brother. He has learned over time that many individuals superficially accept that he is gay, but when it comes down to it, they really are not fully accepting ▾ NEWS.

Episode 6
Ben calls Sam, a guy he knows from the gym, who is gay. Sam and his partner adopted a baby a few years ago. Ben asks Sam about the process and asked if anyone gave them a hard time because they were gay. He also asks Sam for his advice.

Episode 7
Ben has been training hard during the past few weeks for another upcoming triathlon event. He hopes to win this time and is trying a new high-protein nutritional supplement that he read about in a sports magazine to enhance his performance in distance events. The supplement purports to help the body convert its extra stored proteins into energy sources during distance races NEWS.

Episode 8
Ben competes in another triathlon this week. During the cycling portion of the event, he develops severe muscle cramps and is very disappointed when he is unable to finish the race. He tries to work through the cramps, but it is obvious that he is not going to be able to continue. Ben wonders if he failed to train adequately.

Episode 9
Ben is on vacation with Greg this week in Spain. He is glad to have a week off from training. Ben is aware of Greg's recent problems performing sexually and is not sure what to make of this change. He asks Greg what the problem is, but Greg obviously doesn't want to talk about it. Ben wonders if there is a problem between them that he does not know about.

Episode 10
Ben notices that Greg has been increasingly unresponsive to affection and almost seems to avoid sexual contact. This is a very dramatic change in their relationship, and Ben is frustrated with Greg's unwillingness to discuss it. Ben is pretty sure that Greg is not seeing somebody else because he keeps talking about adopting a child. Still, their ability to be close is somehow different.

Greg takes Ben out to eat, in what Ben perceives as an attempt to act like everything is fine and normal. While at dinner, Greg asks their pregnant server about her pregnancy and she responds, although it is clear to Ben that she is not interested in talking to him about it. Ben is almost embarrassed that Greg has asked her such personal questions. Greg tells Ben he is sure she is being abused and suggests they should do something to help her. Ben tells Greg he does not know that, and it is really none of his business. Just the same, he is not at all surprised to see Greg leave her a huge tip with a message and his name and phone number written on a napkin. "Even if she is abused, there is no way she is ever going to call you," he tells him. "She probably thinks you are some creepy old guy hitting on her." Greg responds to Ben by saying, "You are probably right, but at least she has a choice and knows someone cares about what's happening to her ▽."

Episode 11

Ben is shocked this week when he learns that his company is downsizing and he is being laid off. Ben cannot believe it! Never in a million years did he see this coming. He is relieved that Greg is out of town this week so that he can have time to process this loss. Ben thinks about how weird Greg has been acting lately. He isn't interested in sex anymore and seems to be constantly checking on him. What will Greg say when he tells him he no longer has a job? Ben feels very sad and insecure. Ben waits until Greg comes home at the end of the week to tell him - preferring to have that conversation in person as opposed to by phone. He is relieved that Greg is not angry and is accepting of his situation ▽.

Episode 12

Despite the fact that Ben has lost his job, Greg continues to talk about adopting a child. Ben accompanies Greg to an adoption agency. They discuss the various alternatives, such as adopting an older child as opposed to a very young child or infant. The adoption agency suggests that they consider adopting a young child or a child with special needs, because it can be a difficult transition for older children who have preconceived notions about homosexuality. They are told that younger children tend to adjust more easily to a home with gay parents. After listening to the discussion, Ben wonders if they should just forget about adoption.

Episode 13

Ben spends the weekend with Greg and finally comes out and asks Greg about his avoidance. He is relieved that Greg is willing to talk with him about his lack of sexual responsiveness. Ben was really beginning to wonder if their relationship was coming to an end and if the adoption idea was a last-ditch effort in Greg's mind to save their relationship. Ben talks with Greg about future employment options [NEWS].

Episode 14

Greg and Ben meet with another adoption agency this week. When they acknowledge being a gay couple, the agency tells them that it will not able to help them. Ben feels very angry. He knows they are capable of being good parents – in fact, better parents than many couples, especially considering the economic resources they have available. On the way home Greg comments that they should have told the agency that Ben could be a stay-at-home dad; perhaps that would have swayed her. "What would the point of that be?" says Ben. "They made up their minds already!"

Episode 15

Ben has been searching for a new job and has yet to find something that interests him. He is glad that he has the luxury of being choosy. He spends his additional free time exercising.

During the week he develops a significant amount of pain and swelling in his leg, despite the fact that he can't recall injuring it. Ben sees his family physician, Dr. Rowe, and learns he has developed a stress fracture. Dr. Rowe tells Ben that excessive exercise has most likely caused this injury. Ben is frustrated beyond belief. He has to wear a stupid plastic boot around for the next several weeks. Not only is he out of work, now he has to limit his exercise! ▶ ▽

Benito Jaramillo Season 3 Information

Episode 1

Benito (Ben) Jaramillo is a 42-year-old Hispanic male in excellent health. His motto has always been, "Work hard, play hard." Ben's primary outside hobby and interest is athletic training. He participates in many athletic events, such as running, cycling, skiing, and triathlon events. To maintain his competitiveness, Ben normally trains several hours a day on most days, but a recent stress fracture has caused him, to cut back.

This episode Ben is glad that Greg's sexual response has returned to its previous level. This has tremendously helped reduce the stress and insecurity he was experiencing within their relationship. Ben's recent stress fracture has healed; he has been told he can start exercising again, but to start slowly. Ben decides to withdraw from a triathlon he previously signed up for, knowing he is likely to get hurt. He surprises Greg by telling him he would like to play a bit of golf with him.

Ben is excited to see Sal Lucero again with his new therapy dog. Ben absolutely loves dogs and thinks Sal's dog is a beauty! Ben is also happy to be featured in the News because he knows this will help raise public awareness about the ongoing support veterans need. Perhaps this story will lead to good deeds by others.

Episode 2

Ben learns from Greg that his blood pressure is pretty high without blood pressure medication, and he needs to try other medications. Ben thinks to himself that Greg could probably treat the blood pressure problem with herbal supplements from the nutrition store and exercise.

Ben goes with Greg to visit another adoption agency. Although encouraged by the fact that the agency agrees to work with them, Ben and Greg are discouraged when told they should not get their hopes up about adopting an infant. Greg and Ben decide to continue exploring other agency options, but Ben feels underlying anger with the whole process.

Episode 3

Ben feels bored this week. Still out of work and on an abbreviated training schedule, he finds he really does not have much to do. His boredom is exacerbated by Greg's being out of town for an extended period of time. Ben continues to look for a job and is frustrated by the scarcity of work for somebody with his advanced skill set. Although he is glad Greg has a high level of income, Ben does not want to depend on him completely for financial support. His inability to get work also makes Ben feel a bit insecure – he worries that Greg will think less of him for not working.

Episode 4

Greg becomes very ill this week and Ben takes him to the emergency department. They are there for 20 hours between waiting to be seen, waiting for tests and treatments, and waiting to be discharged. Ben cannot understand how it could take so long to be seen and wonders what the wait would be for someone who is critically ill [NEWS].

Episode 5

Greg is admitted to the hospital this week due to ongoing issues with his colitis. Because he still does not have a job, Ben spends a great deal of time at the hospital with Greg. While at the hospital, Ben picks up a magazine with an article in it about gay and lesbian adoptions. The article reads:

"The adoption hierarchy places healthy infants and young children with white, married, middle- or upper-middle class couples first; the less preferred children then go to unmarried couples of all kinds, single individuals, and gay people. The children are less preferred, and the recipients are less preferred."

This makes him feel angry, but he finds that reading the article validates their experiences with various agencies. Ben feels he is not being discriminated against because he is gay, but because he is a Hispanic gay man ▼.

Episode 6

After being out of work for quite some time, Ben is happy finally to have a new position in another financial advising firm. He is very focused on getting a new client base established. He contacts former clients from his previous firm to let them know where they can find him should they choose to make a switch. Ben feels increasing anger and frustration about the lack of progress with the adoption agencies. He suggests to Greg that they hire a private lawyer who specializes in adoptions to help them through the process ▼.

Episode 7

Greg has obligated Ben's time to volunteer at the River Jazz festival this weekend. At first Ben is not happy about this. The festival (which supports shelters for battered women) is no doubt a good cause, but Ben wishes he did not have to use his time over the weekend in this way. When they get to the festival, Ben is given a sponsor's pin and is surprised and proud to see his name, along with Greg's name, on a large banner thanking major event sponsors. He had no idea that Greg had made a substantial donation to the event! People keep thanking him for his sponsorship and in doing so he meets several people who share a vision of providing supportive services for victims of domestic violence. He also sees many women with small children and thinks about what it might be like if he and Greg are ever successful with an adoption. At the end of the tiring weekend he reflects on Greg's genuine thoughtfulness and interest in making the world a better place for others.

Episode 8

Ben is back to training hard for a distance event, this time a mountain terrain extreme race. He has not competed since suffering a stress fracture and he hopes to avoid injuring himself this way again. This week, Ben and Greg meet with an attorney who agrees to help them find a child for adoption. The attorney suggests that they do a private, open adoption ▶.

Episode 9

Greg tells Ben that the attorney may have found them a baby. He goes on to tell Ben that they don't know for sure, but they should find out soon and hopefully will be able to meet the mother. Ben is shocked by this – not that he they might have found a baby, but at the idea of soon becoming parents. He is terrified and excited about this at the same time.

Episode 10

The attorney introduces Ben and Greg to a 16-year-old teenager named Terry Clark, who agrees to put her baby up for adoption immediately after birth. They agree to provide financial support to her until the baby is born and to help pay for medical expenses associated with the delivery. Ben is mesmerized when he looks at Terry's abdomen. He asks if he can touch her stomach to feel the baby and she agrees, although Ben can tell she is a bit uncomfortable. Ben tries to imagine the tiny baby curled up inside Terry's abdomen. When they get home, Ben finds a website showing pictures of what a fetus looks like at 32 weeks of gestation ▾.

Episode 11

Ben steps up the intensity of his workouts in preparation for the high-adventure event. He goes to the neighborhood high school football stadium and spends 2 hours running up and down the stadium stairs and running laps on the track. He also spends hours on the treadmill. He is very happy to be back to his high-level training again and is glad to be past all his injuries. While on a long run, he imagines running down the bike trail with a high-end stroller made specifically for runners. Ben thinks he will really like being able to take his baby out on runs with him.

Episode 12

Ben develops what he thinks is muscle pain that gets worse over several days. By the end of the week, his leg hurts when he walks on it. He sees an orthopedic physician specialist and is diagnosed with another stress fracture - this time in the other leg. He is also told he has significant inflammation in his surrounding knee joint space. As before, Ben is advised to rest his leg. When Ben asks the orthopedist why he keeps getting hurt, he is told that he has a 42-year-old body that does not tolerate the wear and tear to which he is subjecting it. The physician reminds Ben that an excess of anything - even exercise - can lead to health conditions or injuries. Depressed with this news, Ben has to cancel his plans to participate in the mountain terrain event ▾.

Episode 13

Ben feels frustrated by what the orthopedic specialist told him regarding his constant injuries. He does not understand, as healthy as he is, why these injuries keep occurring. Ben wonders if hiring a personal trainer would help him avoid further injuries and allow him to train at a level he desires.

Ben and Greg hear, through the attorney, that Terry's pregnancy continues to progress. He becomes increasingly excited about the baby that he and Greg will soon adopt. Ben has a blast buying baby clothes from the department store and is excited to show them to Greg when he gets home.

Episode 14

Ben and Greg are on a 2-week Alaskan cruise vacation. During the cruise, they spend a great deal of time talking about their plans for the baby. Although Ben at first was reluctant to commit to raising a child, he now is looking forward to his new role as a parent. Ben also reflects back on some of the recent challenges he and Greg have faced in their relationship and is relieved that all of their problems have resolved. He thinks to himself that things seem to be back the way they used to be ▾ NEWS.

Episode 15

Ben knows something is very wrong when Greg calls him, crying. Greg shares with Ben that their attorney called to tell them Terry has decided to keep her baby. How could she do this to them? How could she do this to her baby? He knows that he and Greg can offer the baby much more than Terry can. He feels as if all of their plans and dreams have vanished and even wonders if Terry was just trying to take advantage of them financially because they are very well off. He is also told that Terry's mother was against having the baby be adopted by a gay couple. Ben feels very angry at Terry's parents for forcing their views about homosexuality on her. In his anger, Ben strikes the wall, punching a hole in the drywall and breaking his hand in the process ▾ NEWS.

YOUNG HOUSEHOLD

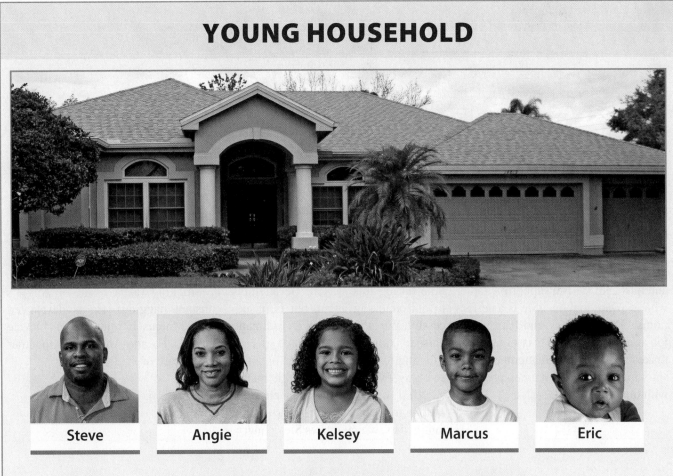

Steve **Angie** **Kelsey** **Marcus** **Eric**

Housing	The Youngs live in a large one story home in the Northwoods area close to the lake. They live in a nice housing development with sidewalks where Marcus can ride his bike.
Parks and Recreation	There are several parks in the area and a golf course on the far end.
Services	There is a shopping plaza near the area and the Neighborhood Hospital and Women's Health Services is located a few miles away in the downtown area.

Key: ▶ = video clip   ☰ = medical record   ▼ = journal entry   NEWS = news article

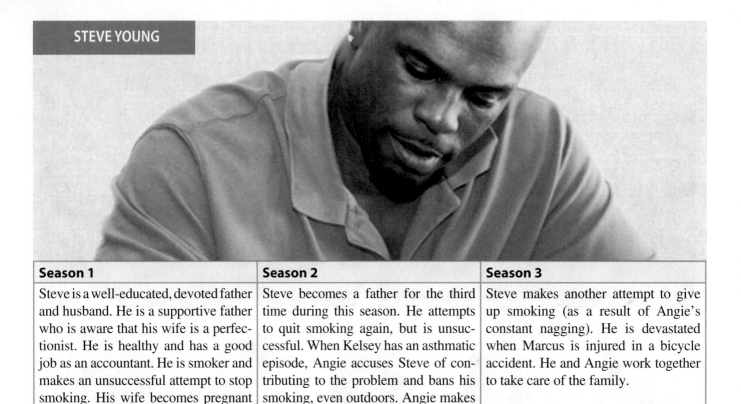

STEVE YOUNG

Season 1	Season 2	Season 3
Steve is a well-educated, devoted father and husband. He is a supportive father who is aware that his wife is a perfectionist. He is healthy and has a good job as an accountant. He is smoker and makes an unsuccessful attempt to stop smoking. His wife becomes pregnant with their third child.	Steve becomes a father for the third time during this season. He attempts to quit smoking again, but is unsuccessful. When Kelsey has an asthmatic episode, Angie accuses Steve of contributing to the problem and bans his smoking, even outdoors. Angie makes an effort to control for other environmental triggers by getting rid of the family cats, which makes Steve angry.	Steve makes another attempt to give up smoking (as a result of Angie's constant nagging). He is devastated when Marcus is injured in a bicycle accident. He and Angie work together to take care of the family.

Steve Young Season 1 Information

Episode 1

Steve Young is a 35-year-old African-American male who is in excellent health. Steve met his wife, Angie, in college and they have been married for 8 years. He has two children with her, Kelsey and Marcus. Steve graduated from college with a degree in accounting. Following graduation, he took the CPA exam and has worked for a large corporate accounting firm ever since. He has been extremely successful and has an income that easily supports his family. He is pleased that his wife is able to be a stay-at-home mother, but his success requires that he work very long hours at the office. Steve has few outside activities and rarely exercises. His world pretty much revolves around work and home. He recognizes that his inactivity has led to weight gain over the past few years, but is not concerned about it.

Steve began smoking at age 17 and, at this time, he has an 8 pack-year smoking history. He knows he should quit smoking, but he likes it and he figures he can probably get

away with it for a little while longer. Because he knows it is a source of irritation for his wife, he plans to quit smoking eventually.

Steve loves spending time with his wife and children in the evenings and on weekends. He is more than happy to help Angie with evening family activities, but he sometimes feels that her perfectionism is overbearing and secretly worries about the effect it may have on the children. He has attempted to discuss this concern with her, but she gets defensive, and he does not want her to perceive that he doesn't appreciate her efforts.

Steve goes with his family to the museum and out to lunch. He enjoys spending time with his children. He does not agree with Angie's demand that the children practice the piano and read as soon as they arrive home because he believes they should be given an opportunity to play. He does not voice his opinion and lets the issue go.

Episode 2

Angie discusses Marcus' lack of progress in playing the piano with Steve. He suggests to her that she "back off and let the kids be kids." She reminds him that the kids need discipline and structure. He notices she is a bit stand-offish the rest of the evening ▶.

Episode 3

Steve and Angie discuss having another baby. Although he is perfectly happy with two children, Steve is not opposed to the idea and believes their income can accommodate a third child. He tells Angie that he's in support of it and is pleased with how happy his response makes her [NEWS].

Episode 4

Steve decides this week that he is going to quit smoking, not so much because he wants to, but because he is tired of Angie nagging him about it. On Monday morning, he throws his cigarettes away and decides to quit smoking "cold turkey." ▼

Episode 5

Steve has not smoked for a couple of weeks now, and he feels miserable. He literally thinks about cigarettes from the time he wakes up until the time he goes to sleep at night. He even dreams about smoking. He feels very edgy and is in a bad mood all of the time. To satisfy his craving, he snacks constantly at work and at home and then finds himself worrying about weight gain. He tries nicotine gum, but ends up chewing the gum constantly ▼.

Episode 6

This week, one of the guys in the office announces his engagement. After work, Steve goes with a group from the office to briefly celebrate at a bar before going home. While having a beer with his friends, Steve has a cigarette, and it is one of the most pleasurable things he can imagine. The next morning he buys a pack of cigarettes ▼ [NEWS].

Episode 7

Steve takes Angie and the kids to the local Health Fair. He had wanted to stay at home to watch a sporting event on television, but he goes at Angie's insistence. He spots the American Cancer Society and American Heart Association booths and walks right past them because he does not want to be bothered with the smoking cessation information he'd find there. But when he gets home, Steve finds smoking cessation literature on the dresser in the bedroom. Steve knows that Angie picked it up for him.

Episode 8

Steve learns that Angie is pregnant this week and is very happy to know they will have another child together. Steve reflects on the news and knows that having children has been the best thing that has ever happened to him. He calls his mother to tell her the good news [NEWS].

Episode 9

Steve receives a phone call from Angie at 2 p.m. today, informing him that she is taking Marcus to the doctor. He will need to pick up Kelsey from school at 3 p.m. and get her to her art class by 3:45. Steve is able to cancel a couple of appointments so that he can take care of Kelsey [NEWS].

Episode 10

Angie tells Steve she ran into Rebecca Patterson and is worried about her husband Blake. Steve is aware that Blake Patterson recently returned from military conflict and recalls some of the challenges his own brother faced after coming home from deployment. Steve tells Angie that the readjustment can be difficult and everyone needs to let him have time to adjust ▶.

Episode 11

Steve goes with Angie and the kids to the open house at the elementary school. He is always interested in getting a report from the teachers about Kelsey and Marcus. He knows they are progressing academically (Angie would know if they weren't), and he really enjoys getting feedback about their social interactions.

Episode 12

Angie tells Steve that their friends Rebecca and Blake Patterson continue to have problems (based on what Kelsey described from a sleepover) and wonders what he thinks they should do. Steve reminds Angie that Blake might be experiencing some adjustment problems, but she does not know enough to do anything.

Episode 13

Steve is out of town all week on a consulting job with a potential new client. He talks with Angie two to three times each day, concerned that she might need his help.

Episode 14

Angie tells Steve that she is positive there are significant problems going on with Rebecca and Blake Patterson to the point that she suggested that the school nurse look into it. Steve tells Angie it is probably best to report the situation as opposed to trying to do something about it herself. If she is wrong, she could really damage her friendship.

Episode 15

Steve takes Angie and the kids on a weekend trip to his mother's house for a visit. Steve's mother is very pleased about the pregnancy and very excited for them. While there, Steve helps her take care of many house maintenance tasks that his mother can't do for herself. It also gives him a chance to spend time with his children away from the structured activities they have at home [NEWS].

Steve Young Season 2 Information

Episode 1

Steve Young is a 36-year-old African-American male who is in excellent health. He has been married to his wife, Angie, for 9 years. They have two children, Kelsey and Marcus, and are expecting a baby in the upcoming months.

This episode Angie reminds Steve about childbirth classes. He wonders why they have to go through all this, considering that they already have had two children. Steve thinks that he and Angie pretty much have childbirth figured out. Frankly, he would rather stay home after working all day [NEWS].

Episode 2

Steve continues to go with Angie to childbirth classes this week. Going to the classes has motivated Steve to stop smoking. He throws his cigarettes away and tells Angie he is going to quit ▼.

Episode 3

Marcus tells his Dad that he would like to have a bike to ride like all of his friends. Steve talks with Angie about the idea. At first she is resistant, voicing her concern that Marcus might get hurt. When Steve points out that Kelsey got her first bike at the same age, Angie reminds him that Kelsey is more attentive than Marcus. In the end, Steve gets Angie's approval and takes his son shopping ▶ ▼.

Episode 4

Steve retrieves the crib and other baby accessories from the attic for Angie so she can start putting a nursery together. Steve is very irritable because he wants a cigarette. He goes outside to have just one. One cigarette turns into two the next day and four the following day. Soon, he is back to smoking. He knows this disappoints Angie, but she just doesn't understand how hard it is to quit ▼.

Episode 5

Steve is concerned about Kelsey's coughing and wheezing and is relieved when she responds to the medications.

Episode 6

Steve has a rare fight with Angie this week. She yells at him for being a smoker and causing Kelsey's breathing problems. She tells him that his cigarettes are banned from the house; he may not even bring them inside. She also argues with him about getting rid of the cats because Steve does not share her belief that the cats are to blame. He is angry with her because she doesn't seem to recognize how devastating this decision is to the kids. Steve feels angry for several days following the argument.

Episode 7

Steve remains angry with Angie when she takes the cats to the animal shelter. He tells her that there is no evidence that the cats make Kelsey's condition worse, but he also knows that once she has made up her mind, there is little he can do. He does his best to comfort his children and wonders how his wife can have such a mean streak in her.

Episode 8

Angie tells Steve she ran into Rebecca Patterson today and learned that her husband, Blake, is being treated for depression. Angie says, "I can't believe he is having this problem taken care of by a nurse. If it were you, I would insist that you see a real doctor." Steve listens but does not respond. One of his colleagues at work is married to a nurse practitioner. To hear his coworker talk, nurse practitioners take care of many health problems very well.

Episode 9

Steve is awakened at 3 a.m. by Angie, who says she is going into labor. He asks her how often her contractions are, and she tells him every 20 minutes. Steve falls back asleep. He gets up at his usual 6 a.m. time and finds Angie in the shower. Her contractions have progressed. He gets the children up, makes them breakfast, and helps them get ready for school. He makes arrangements with their close friends to pick up the kids after school if needed, drops them off at school, and returns home to be with Angie.

In the late morning, Steve takes Angie to the hospital when she tells him it is time. He coaches her through her labor and accompanies her to the delivery room, where he is thrilled to watch the birth of his son.

Later that day, Steve brings his children to the hospital to see the baby. Kelsey and Marcus ask many questions about the baby and how it was born. Steve's mother and Angie's parents come by the hospital to see the new baby as well. Steve feels grateful for his wonderful family.

Episode 10

Steve goes back to work this week after taking time off to be at home with Angie and the new baby. Steve's mother-in-law has been staying at the house, so he is relieved to get away and go to work.

Episode 11

Steve is really ready for his mother-in-law to leave. She has been at their home now for nearly two weeks. He appreciates her efforts to help, but in his opinion, she has worn out her welcome. He asks Angie when she thinks her mother will be leaving, and Angie smiles and says,

"When she is ready to leave – but soon, I hope." Angie has always been very close to her mother, and although Steve gets along with her, she has a tendency to get on his nerves. She is very opinionated and seems to have to make a comment about everything.

Episode 12

Steve helps Marcus learn to ride his bike in the late afternoon before dark. He is excited when Marcus finally catches on and starts riding.

Steve makes another attempt to stop smoking. He had intended to quit smoking before the baby was born, but it did not happen, and he is angry with himself. He is smoking nearly a pack a day and knows it is time to stop! This time, he decides to follow a plan he read about in a magazine. He plans to cut his smoking down by half every week until he has quit completely ▼ NEWS.

Episode 13

Steve is still very committed to quitting smoking. He is in his second week. His plan has been to cut down his smoking by half each week until he quits. This week he is down to 8 cigarettes a day ▼.

Episode 14

Steve takes Kelsey and Marcus to the Bicycle Safety Awareness activity. He enjoys watching his children on the bikes. After they are finished, he takes them to McDonalds for a Happy Meal.

Steve continues his smoking reduction plan and is now down to four cigarettes a day. He has one after each meal, and then one more during the day when he most needs it. He tries to save it for the afternoon. Those 4 cigarettes are so nice ▼.

Episode 15

Steve takes his family for a long weekend visit to his mother's house. He is excited for her to meet her new grandson. Steve's mother lives about 4 hours away and has back problems, so she does not like to take long car trips if they can be avoided. While at her home, Steve takes care of a number of household chores for her, things she has problems doing herself. He is still trying to cut back on smoking and was cutting down by half each week. However, he knows he needs to pace himself, so he is still having 4 cigarettes each day ▼.

Steve Young Season 3 Information

Episode 1

Steve Young is a 36-year-old African-American male who is in excellent health. He has been married to his wife, Angie, for 9 years. He has three children with her, Kelsey, Marcus, and Eric. Steve met his wife in college. Steve graduated with a degree in accounting and has worked for a large corporate accounting firm ever since. He has been extremely successful and has an income that easily supports his family. He is pleased that his wife is able to be a stay-at-home mother, but his success requires that he work very long hours at the office.

Steve began smoking at age 17 and, at this time, he has an 8 pack-year smoking history. He has tried to quit smoking several times, but has just not been able to quit. He knows it is a serious irritation to his wife and is currently attempting to quit by gradually cutting back on the number of cigarettes per day.

This episode Steve has an incredibly stressful week at work because fiscal reports are due for several of his clients. He is at work from 6:30 a.m. until 9 p.m. several days this week, and feels bad about not being able to help Angie with the kids. He is down to just a few cigarettes a day, but has not been able to stop yet; he is just glad he has cut back as much as he has.

Episode 2

Angie tells Steve about the immunization issue. He is glad she agrees to the immunizations. Although he doesn't say it, he sometimes wonders what his wife is thinking and why she is so overly protective all the time NEWS.

Episode 3

Steven runs to the store at Angie's request to get an Oral electrolyte solution (Pedialyte) solution for the baby. Angie looks exhausted. He takes the kids to piano and swimming lessons, allowing her to stay at home with Eric and get some rest. He decides to stop and pick up a pizza on the way home so they will not have to hassle with dinner. The kids are thrilled with the idea of having pizza.

Episode 4

Angie tells Steve she needs to get out of the house. Since Eric was born, she has done very little away from the home. Steve offers to stay at home with the kids, but Angie decides she wants to take the family out to the mall for some shopping and a stop at the frozen yogurt store for a snack. Steve cannot think of anything less relaxing than to go to a crowded mall with two young children and an infant. He suggests a trip to the park as an alternative, but it is clear Angie wants to go to the mall.

Episode 5

Steve receives a phone call from Angie in a panic, telling him that Marcus was hit by a car. Steve tries to get some basic information out of her, but Angie is too upset to communicate clearly. Angie tells him to meet them at the Neighborhood Hospital Emergency Department (ED).

When Steve arrives at the ED, he asks the receptionist about his son. He is told to have a seat in the waiting room and that somebody will be with him. After 10 minutes, he gets up and again asks about his son. A nurse overhears him asking, clarifies that he is Mr. Young, and escorts him into the trauma room. Angie is relieved to see him; he holds her while they stand back and let the trauma team care for Marcus. On the way home that evening, Steve is so stressed out that he smokes 3 cigarettes, one after another [NEWS].

Episode 6

Steve tries to convince Angie to come home at night, offering to stay with Marcus himself. Angie insists that she needs to stay with her son. He is embarrassed by the way she treats the nurses and wishes she would just go home and get some rest.

Steve is thankful to have Angie's mother at the house to help with the kids. He realizes how difficult it would be to work full-time and manage all of their activities by himself. He wonders how families with two working parents do everything. Steve feels so tempted to start smoking regularly again, but resists the urge. He limits himself to between 2 and 4 cigarettes a day this entire week.

Episode 7

Steve is glad that Marcus is back at home. He sets a bed up for Marcus in the living room so that he can interact with the family during the day and evening. He is able to put him in his own bed at night so that he has a little variety in his surroundings [▼].

Episode 8

Angie comes up with a creative idea to have a puppet show for Marcus to lift his spirits. Angie and Kelsey have made very cute puppets, and they tell Steve he has to play both the mother and father puppet. He is very happy to see how much fun Marcus and Kelsey have with the puppet show. Marcus tells him they should do more family puppet shows and that next time he wants to make a puppet and be in the show [▼].

Episode 9

Steve has not had a cigarette in a week. He decides that he has been at 4 cigarettes a day long enough, and now it is time to take the final step and quit. He constantly craves cigarettes, but this time he wants to be successful.

He does not believe Angie has noticed yet. At least, she has not said anything.

Steve takes Marcus to physical therapy appointments twice a week to help him regain strength and agility. He is amazed at the ability of a child to adapt to obstacles [▼].

Episode 10

Steve continues to work very long hours at work. He has been able to stay away from cigarettes now for 3 weeks. Angie has not yet commented on the fact that he quit, and he wonders if she has noticed yet. Steve finds that he has more energy after quitting and vows never to start smoking again.

Episode 11

Steve accompanies Angie and the kids to the petition drive organized by Angie. He can tell many people are not interested in signing, but his wife has a way of getting their signatures just the same. Steve lets Angie do all the talking while he carries Eric or pushes him in a stroller and does his best to keep Marcus and Kelsey entertained on the outing.

Episode 12

Steve and Angie decide to take the kids to the zoo to see the baby elephant that is now on display. Fearing that Marcus might get overly tired from walking, Steve suggests renting a wagon at the zoo entrance so that Marcus can alternate between walking and riding in the wagon. The zoo is extremely crowded. Angie takes the baby into the restroom to change his diaper, and Steve sits on a bench with Marcus and Kelsey. Kelsey tells her Daddy she needs to go to the bathroom, too, and she takes off, running after her mother. A short while later, Angie comes back with Eric, but Kelsey is not with her. After a frantic search for his daughter, he eventually finds her at the "Kids Connection" facility for lost children at the zoo. Steve is so relieved Kelsey has been found and was not harmed. It is a situation he will never forget!

Episode 13

Steve believes his wife made a fabulous presentation to the Neighborhood Council; he knew, however, that there was no way they were going to place speed bumps on the street. He was not surprised at the opposition from other members of the community.

Episode 14

Steve recognizes that Angie has decided not to allow Kelsey to take a field trip out of concern for her asthma. Additionally, she is back to insisting that Marcus practice the piano. He advocates for his children and suggests she call the nurse practitioner to find out what the real risks are to Kelsey. She also eventually agrees to stop forcing Marcus to play piano. He is pleased that Angie actually backs down from her original position [▶] [NEWS].

Episode 15

Marcus asks Steve about getting a new bike and getting a dog. Steve knows he will have to work on Angie for a while to make that happen. It has now been a couple of months since Steve smoked a cigarette. He is so happy that he quit and now realizes that many of his clothes smelled like cigarettes. Angie has not said anything about his quitting, but he is quite sure she has noticed.

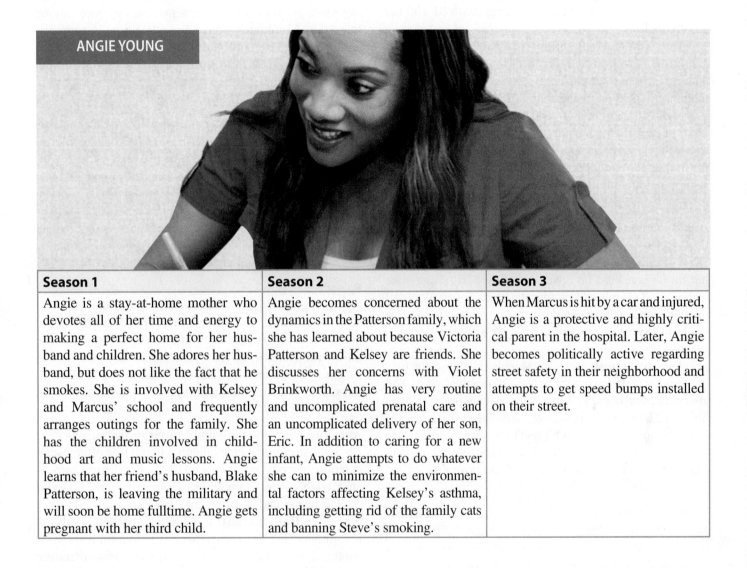

ANGIE YOUNG

Season 1	Season 2	Season 3
Angie is a stay-at-home mother who devotes all of her time and energy to making a perfect home for her husband and children. She adores her husband, but does not like the fact that he smokes. She is involved with Kelsey and Marcus' school and frequently arranges outings for the family. She has the children involved in childhood art and music lessons. Angie learns that her friend's husband, Blake Patterson, is leaving the military and will soon be home fulltime. Angie gets pregnant with her third child.	Angie becomes concerned about the dynamics in the Patterson family, which she has learned about because Victoria Patterson and Kelsey are friends. She discusses her concerns with Violet Brinkworth. Angie has very routine and uncomplicated prenatal care and an uncomplicated delivery of her son, Eric. In addition to caring for a new infant, Angie attempts to do whatever she can to minimize the environmental factors affecting Kelsey's asthma, including getting rid of the family cats and banning Steve's smoking.	When Marcus is hit by a car and injured, Angie is a protective and highly critical parent in the hospital. Later, Angie becomes politically active regarding street safety in their neighborhood and attempts to get speed bumps installed on their street.

Angie Young Season 1 Information

Episode 1

Angie Young is a 32-year-old African-American female who is in excellent health. She has been happily married to her husband Steve for 8 years, and they have two children, Kelsey and Marcus. Angie and Steve met in college. She graduated with a degree in nutrition. Following graduation, she worked for a nursing home facility as a dietician, but left this position shortly before her oldest child was born. Since that time, she has been a stay-at-home mother. Angie adores her husband, Steve, although she is annoyed by the fact that he is a smoker. She does not understand why he continues to smoke when it is so obvious that it is physically harmful.

Angie is a perfectionist. She strives to have a perfect home for her family and is committed to offering her children many opportunities to ensure that they excel in life. She has a highly structured routine that includes getting up in the morning and making a nutritious breakfast for the family and nutritious lunches for the children to take to school, getting the children to school, going to the gym to work out for two hours a day, taking care of errands and house cleaning, picking up the children from school, and taking them to after-school activities. In the evening, she makes dinner, helps the children with homework and piano lessons, makes sure they take baths, and gets them in bed by 9:00 p.m. Angie also volunteers at the school on a regular basis by helping in the classrooms and being available for field trips. She loves being involved with her children's lives.

This episode Angie arranges a family outing to the Natural History Museum on Saturday as an educational activity for her children. They spend a couple of hours at the museum and go to a restaurant for lunch. After lunch, Angie directs her children to read and practice the piano before being allowed to play. Shortly after Marcus begins to practice, she hears him talking and then finds him on the living room floor playing with the cats. She disciplines him by sending him to his room for 1 hour [NEWS].

Episode 2

Angie notices that Kelsey is experiencing seasonal allergy symptoms. Three times this week, she hears Kelsey coughing a little bit during the night, and she says her throat is a little bit "twitchy." Angie has experience managing Kelsey's symptoms; she gives her an albuterol inhaler (with spacer) and over-the-counter loratadine (Claritin) syrup. Over the course of a week, Kelsey's symptoms subside.

Angie gets frustrated with Marcus this week for failing to practice his piano for at least 30 minutes a day. She also notices he does not seem to be progressing as well as his sister, Kelsey. She is annoyed with Steve when he suggests that she lighten up a bit and tells her to "let the kids be kids." She responds, "Children need discipline, and Marcus will never improve if he does not practice [▼] [NEWS]."

Episode 3

Angie and Kelsey go to a homecoming party for Blake Patterson, the husband of Angie's friend Rebecca and father of one of Kelsey's friends, Victoria. Angie does not know Blake because for most of the two years Angie has known Rebecca, Blake has been away from home in military service. Rebecca has been talking about his homecoming for months and Angie is happy to attend the party. One of the women attending the party has a newborn infant. Angie has been longing for another baby for several months. Seeing and holding the baby at the party intensifies her interest. She talks with Steve about it, and they both decide to have another child. Angie decides that at the end of her next menstrual cycle, she will stop taking birth control pills [▶] [▼].

Episode 4

Angie talks with Ramona (the piano teacher) about the differences in progress she has noted in her children and asks if she thinks Marcus is progressing adequately.

Ramona tells Angie that every child's ability is where it lies and that every child is different; talent cannot be predicted or measured. She also tells Angie that boys do not focus as well as girls at this age. Angie asks Ramona if she should make Marcus practice more so that he will improve, but Ramona suggests just the opposite, saying that 10 to 15 minutes a day of practice time is appropriate for his age. Ramona adds that, if Angie puts too much pressure on him, Marcus might resist even more and not want to play at all [NEWS].

Episode 5

Angie has decided to reduce the practice time she requires of the children to 20 minutes. She sets the kitchen timer so they will know when practice time is over.

She is pleased that Steve has decided to quit smoking and encourages him, although she points out that his constant snacking will cause him to gain weight. She wishes he was not so crabby and tells him that his crabbiness is just another sign of how bad cigarettes are for him. Angie has her period this month and is disappointed that she is not pregnant [▼].

Episode 6

Angie sees her friend Rebecca Patterson at the store this week. She asks Rebecca how things are going with Blake home on a permanent basis after being away from the family for a number of years for military service. Rebecca laughs and indicates it is an adjustment for both of them, but says it is wonderful to have her husband back.

Episode 7

Angie arranges for the family to go to the Health Fair. They stop at a nutrition evaluation booth that offers a calculation of body mass index (BMI), bioelectric impedance analysis (to estimate lean body mass and body fat composition), and waist-to-hip ratio measurement. She is pleased to learn her BMI is 22 kg/m^2, her total body fat is estimated at 28%, and her waist to hip ratio is 0.62. At another booth, she picks up smoking cessation literature and places it on Steve's dresser when they get home [NEWS].

Episode 8

Angie has missed her period and notices fullness in her breasts. She buys a home pregnancy test kit, checks her urine, and finds the test is positive. Angie is ecstatic. She calls Steve at work and then calls her mother to share the news. She shares the news with her children when they come home later that day [▼].

Episode 9

Angie notices discharge around Marcus' eye while helping him get ready for school. She determines he must have had something in his eye during the night and thinks nothing more of it. In the afternoon, she receives a phone call from Violet Brinkworth, the school nurse, informing her that Marcus might have an eye infection. Violet advises Angie to pick up Marcus from school and take him to the family doctor. Angie calls Steve and asks him to pick up Kelsey from school and take her to her art class.

Angie takes Marcus to the pediatrician's office and is told he has conjunctivitis ("pink eye"). The nurse practitioner tells Angie it is very contagious and that he should stay home from school for the next day. She writes a prescription for eye drops and tells Angie to administer 2 drops every 2 hours for the first 12 hours, and then twice a day for 4 days. They leave the office, go to the drugstore to get the prescription filled, and then come home, where Angie makes dinner. All evening and into the night (until 5 a.m.), Angie administers the eye drops. She is very tired the following day and wonders if she'll be able to handle infant feedings during the night once the baby comes.

Episode 10

Angie spends time at Neighborhood Elementary School helping out in Kelsey's classroom. Her friend Rebecca Patterson is volunteering that day as well. Angie shares with Rebecca the news of her pregnancy. As she talks to Rebecca, Angie recognizes that something is not right; she specifically asks Rebecca what is wrong. Rebecca begins to cry and shares with Angie that something is wrong with her husband, Blake. He has not seemed interested in anything since returning home from military service, and there have been multiple arguments.

Later in the week, Kelsey and Marcus both come down with the flu. Angie has an appointment with her obstetrician, Dr. Howe, for her initial prenatal workup, so Steve comes home to stay with the kids while she goes for the appointment ▤ NEWS.

Episode 11

Angie attends the open house at school; she is very proud to know all of the teachers and office staff. Angie sees her friend Rebecca Patterson at the open house with her daughter Victoria, and she notices Rebecca's husband Blake is not with them. Rebecca seems very sad and disengaged. Angie also overhears Victoria telling Kelsey that

her Daddy did not come because he is mad at everyone. Angie wonders what is going on with the Pattersons NEWS.

Episode 12

Kelsey spent the night at Victoria Patterson's house as part of a sleepover this week. When Angie picks Kelsey up, she asks if she had fun. Kelsey tells Angie that Victoria's parents were yelling at each other and her Mom was crying. This information further confirms in Angie's mind that her friend Rebecca is struggling in her marriage. She wonders how she can help. Later in the week, Angie goes to the Neighborhood Women's Health Services for prenatal care ▤.

Episode 13

Kelsey has another episode with allergy symptoms; Angie can hear her coughing during the night three times this week. She manages Kelsey's symptoms with the albuterol inhaler and loratadine (Claritin) syrup. Angie also is a chaperone for Marcus' field trip to the roller rink this week. She is amazed at how quickly he learns to skate and wishes he would display the same natural talent on the piano NEWS.

Episode 14

Angie is at the Neighborhood Elementary School again this week to help in Kelsey's classroom. Angie sees Victoria Patterson (Rebecca Patterson's daughter) in the hall. Recalling how sad Rebecca looked a few weeks ago at the school open house, Angie asks Victoria how her mother is. Victoria looks up at Angie and says very matter-of-factly, "She cries a lot." This response concerns Angie a great deal. She sees the school nurse Violet Brinkworth and begins a conversation with her: "Maybe it is none of my business, but I am worried about the Pattersons… ▶."

Episode 15

Angie goes to the Neighborhood Women's Health Services for prenatal care. She goes with Steve and the children on a weekend trip to visit her mother-in-law. Angie enjoys an excellent relationship with her and is always glad to go visit ▤ ▼.

Angie Young Season 2 Information

Episode 1

Angie Young is a 32-year-old African-American female who is in excellent health. She has been happily married to her husband Steve for 8 years. They have two children, Kelsey and Marcus, and they are expecting a third.

Angie is a perfectionist. She strives to have a perfect home for her family and is committed to offering her

children many opportunities to ensure that they excel in life. She has a highly structured routine for herself and them. Angie also volunteers at the school on a regular basis by helping in the classrooms and being available for field trips. She loves being involved with her children's lives.

Angie has a prenatal visit this week. She has felt good, but has been annoyed with constipation and bloating. She also hates the fact that she is developing unsightly varicose veins. Through it all, she continues to keep the children in their regular school activities and is taking childbirth classes with Steve ▤ ▶.

Episode 2

Angie volunteers at Kelsey's school this week and runs into Rebecca Patterson. Angie asks Rebecca how things are going at home and she is told, "Everything is just fine." Angie can tell that things are *not* fine and Rebecca does not want to talk about it. She wonders if Violet, the school nurse, did anything with the concerns she shared with her. She goes to Violet's office to ask her what is going on with Rebecca but finds that Violet is at the middle school for the afternoon.

Later the same week, Angie hears about the argument Kelsey witnessed while at the Patterson's home working on a school project. Angie tells Kelsey she should stop hanging around with Victoria ⌗.

Episode 3

Steve talks with Angie about getting Marcus a bike. Angie is concerned that he might get hurt riding it, but Steve points out that Kelsey got her first bike at about the same age. Angie agrees to the idea.

Episode 4

Angie has her 32-week prenatal visit this week. She cleans out the guest bedroom (which has ended up being a "junk room") to make way for a nursery. She gets Steve to retrieve the crib and all of the baby accessories from the attic and decides the room needs a fresh coat of paint. Angie paints the room this week ▤ ▽.

Episode 5

Angie hears Kelsey coughing during the day and at night, and notes that the cough is worse than before. When she is awake, Angie can hear a faint wheezing sound with breathing. Angie treats her 4 mornings in a row with loratadine (Claritin) syrup and the albuterol inhaler before sending her to school. On the fourth day of her symptoms, Angie receives a call from the school nurse, reporting that Kelsey has coughed continually all day in class; the nurse recommends that she be seen by her pediatrician.

Angie takes Kelsey to the pediatrician's office. She is told the pediatrician is booked, but Kelsey can see the nurse practitioner (NP). Angie wishes she could just see a doctor instead. Angie tells Carolyn Marquette, the nurse practitioner, that Kelsey's symptoms only happen at this time of year; this time, it is just a little worse. Angie says, "With the air pollution this week, it is amazing anybody can breathe."

The NP tells Angie to give her daughter nebulizer treatments every 4 hours at home until tomorrow and check the peak flow. She also gives Kelsey a prescription for Prednisone (deltasone). Angie tells the nurse she is not in favor of her daughter being on steroids. The NP spends a great deal of time explaining current treatment guidelines to Angie. She assures her that the short dose of steroids will not have long-lasting effects and they will make her daughter feel much better. Angie asks the NP if this is what the doctor would prescribe. On the way home, Angie picks up the prescription and nebulizer and treats her daughter as directed ⌗.

Episode 6

On Monday morning, Angie takes Kelsey back to see Carolyn Marquette, the nurse practitioner (NP). Angie learns that Kelsey has asthma, rather than reactive airway disease. This news upsets Angie. She wants to know what caused the condition and wants to do everything in her power to keep Kelsey well. She is not happy about the prescribed treatment. However, after assurances from the NP and the pediatrician in the office, and after looking up information on the Internet herself, Angie realizes that the treatment prescribed follows the American Pediatric Academy's guidelines.

Angie becomes highly regimented in the treatment of Kelsey's asthma. She checks her peak flow religiously every day and gives her the control medications. Angie also looks for things at home that might trigger airway problems. She talks with Steve about needing to protect Kelsey from environmental triggers and tells him that he MUST quit smoking - even outside. She also decides that the cats must go ▶ ▽.

Episode 7

Angie has her 36-week prenatal visit. An ultrasound is done during the visit, and she learns that she will be having another boy. She had originally not wanted to know the sex of the baby until birth, but is very excited to think about her unborn son. Angie eagerly anticipates the birth, not only out of excitement for the baby, but also because she is tired of being pregnant. She has had increasingly more trouble sleeping because she can't seem to get comfortable. She also feels short of breath because the baby is pushing up against her lungs.

Angie takes the cats to the Animal Humane Center while the kids are at school. She knows they will be very upset, so she decides to take the cats away when the children aren't home to see it. Angie feels very badly for them and for herself. She hates being the "bad guy," but in her opinion, removing the cats is something that she must do for Kelsey's health ▤.

Episode 8

Angie is out doing a few errands and runs into her friend Rebecca Patterson and her daughter, Victoria. Rebecca can't believe that Angie is already almost at term. Angie tells Rebecca she hopes things are okay with her; Rebecca tells Angie that her husband is being treated for depression by a nurse practitioner. Angie says to Rebecca, "Why is Blake going to a nurse? He might get better faster if he saw a doctor."

Episode 9

In the early morning hours on Wednesday, Angie wakes up when she has a moderate contraction. She experiences another contraction about 20 minutes later, which lasts about 30 seconds. She wakes Steve up and tells him she has started her contractions and is annoyed when he falls back to sleep.

Several hours later, Angie's contractions are occurring regularly every 6 to 7 minutes. They are also becoming progressively stronger and lasting about 45 seconds. Steve takes Angie to the hospital, where she is admitted to the labor and delivery unit. Upon admission, her contractions are moderate to strong, occurring every 4 to 5 minutes and lasting just under 1 minute. Her cervix is 7 cm dilated, and her membranes are ruptured. About 45 minutes later, she delivers a son in an uncomplicated birth. Angie stays at the hospital overnight and is discharged with her infant, Eric, the following day.

Episode 10

Angie is adjusting to caring for a new infant, along with keeping up with all of her other obligations. Her mother has stayed for the better part of the week to help her with the baby and kids while Steve is at work. Angie doesn't remember feeling so tired after the births of her other children.

Episode 11

Angie has a postpartum follow-up visit with her physician this week. She reports that she is feeling good and that breastfeeding is going well. She also takes Eric for his 2-week well-baby check-up at Neighborhood Pediatrics.

Episode 12

Angie takes Eric for his 1-month well-baby checkup. He has gained an appropriate amount of weight, and his immunizations are given to him. Angie encourages Kelsey and Marcus to help her take care of Eric with age-appropriate tasks. Kelsey is always willing to help, but Marcus is less interested ▼.

Episode 13

Kelsey has a mild cough this week. Angie monitors her peak flow several times a day to keep an eye on her status. She is pleased when Kelsey's symptoms do not progress. In her mind, this provides justification for her decision about the cats, as unpopular as it was.

Episode 14

Steve takes Kelsey and Marcus to a bicycle safety awareness activity at the local school. Angie is glad to have the house to herself with Eric. She is hopeful that she can take a nap while everyone is gone, but Eric is awake the entire time, requiring her attention.

Episode 15

Angie and Steve visit his mother for a long weekend. She can tell that Steve is excited for his mother to see the baby. Steve's mother lives alone and cannot easily visit because of ongoing back pain. Angie loves Steve's mother; she finds her very sweet and considerate. Bearing in mind that her mother-in-law lives 4 hours away, Angie wonders if things would be easier if she were to move closer to them at some point.

Angie Young Season 3 Information

Episode 1

Angie Young is a 33-year-old African American female who is in excellent health. She has been happily married to her husband Steve for 9 years, and they have three children, Kelsey, Marcus, and Eric.

Angie is a perfectionist. She strives to have a perfect home for her family and is committed to offering her children many opportunities to ensure that they excel in life. Although she likes to maintain a highly structured routine, she has found it to be much more difficult with a new baby. Angie is enjoying her infant son, but finds that it is more work than she remembered with her other two children. Angie has stopped volunteering at the school for the time being, but plans to do it again when Eric is a little older.

Angie has registered Kelsey and Marcus for swimming lessons at the Neighborhood Pool. She likes the facility because it can accommodate indoor and outdoor swimmers, thus allowing for year-round swimming. Neither Angie nor Steve ever learned to swim, but she wants her children to have this skill. It is her belief that all children should be taught to swim.

Episode 2

Angie takes Eric in for his 2-month well-baby exam. The nurse practitioner (NP) tells Angie that he is due for his Immunizations. Angie tells the NP that she is not so sure about immunizations after reading about some of the problems they cause. She tells the NP that she has heard about babies who develop autism as a result of immunizations.

The NP reinforces the benefits of immunizations and explains that thiamazole is no longer used in vaccinations; she emphasizes that there really is no evidence to support the connection to autism anyway. Angie agrees to the immunizations. She is not sure if she likes the NP or not ▶.

Episode 3
Eric becomes very fussy and quits eating. Angie notices that he has very frequent, watery stools. She tries to give him water over the course of the day, but the diarrhea continues. She asks Steve to run to the store for an oral electrolyte solution in the evening.

Eric continues to have diarrhea throughout the night, so in the morning, Angie takes him back to the pediatrician's office. The NP sees Eric and reassures Angie that she is doing everything right. Eric is a little dehydrated, but it is nothing that can't be treated at home with the oral electrolyte solution. The NP reminds Angie to monitor his diapers for evidence of adequate urinary output. Angie tells the nurse that she thinks this whole situation probably resulted from the immunizations he received the previous week. The NP attempts to explain that viral diarrhea is not something that is caused or prevented by immunizations. Angie is relieved when Eric's diarrhea stops later that evening ▶.

Episode 4
Angie is out of milk and makes a quick trip to the store. While there, she sees her friend Rebecca Patterson and her daughter, Victoria. Rebecca is thrilled to see the baby and talk with Angie. Rebecca tells Angie that their family has been getting family therapy as part of Blake's treatment. Rebecca tells Angie things are getting much better.

Angie is beginning to feel stir-crazy. Since Eric was born, she has done very little away from the home other than healthcare appointments, a few trips to the store and one trip to Steve's mother's home. Steve offers to stay at home with the kids so she can go out and do anything she wants, but Angie feels guilty for not wanting to spend time with her family. She decides it would be nice to go to the mall for some shopping and perhaps a stop at the yogurt store for a snack. They load the kids into the car and spend the afternoon there. Despite the fact that the mall is very crowded, Angie enjoys being out.

Episode 5
Angie is breastfeeding Eric in the front room of their home when she hears screeching tires outside. She doesn't give it another thought until, a short while later, she hears sirens. A neighbor knocks on the door to tell Angie that Marcus has been hit by a car. Angie runs outside, leaving Eric in the house with Kelsey. She sees Marcus' body lying in the median of the street and begins to scream, believing he is dead. Paramedics have just arrived and are assessing Marcus when she reaches him. A large man holds Angie back while the paramedics attend to her son until she calms down. Angie then spots two teenage boys standing to the side. One of them is crying, and she knows that these are the boys who hit Marcus. She begins walking toward them, screaming, and asking them how they could hurt an innocent little boy. The large man again holds her back, saying, "Not here, not now." After Angie is able to see that Marcus is stable, she runs back to the house to call Steve. She asks one of the neighbors to attend to Kelsey and Eric. Angie gets into the ambulance to go to the hospital with Marcus.

Angie and Steve are permitted to be in the trauma room in the Emergency Department while the trauma team stabilizes Marcus. Angie is thankful to be allowed to be with her son during this time and is grateful that Steve is so strong throughout the ordeal.

Episode 6
Angie's mother comes to stay with them to care for Kelsey and Eric so that Angie can spend as much time as possible with Marcus at the hospital. Angie watches everything the nurses do and questions them constantly, checking to make sure they know what they are doing. She insists that everyone wash his or her hands on entering the hospital room because she doesn't want Marcus to get an infection. She is persistent with the orthopedic team about letting her take Marcus home as soon as possible.

Angie finds that all the time spent at the hospital makes it challenging to maintain a breastfeeding routine with Eric. She gets a breast pump and makes sure she keeps a supply for her infant at home while she is away. Although Angie spends most nights at the hospital with Marcus, she leaves periodically during the day when Steve can be there so she can spend time with Kelsey and Eric.

Late in the week, Charles, the young man who almost killed her son, comes to visit Marcus with his friend. Angie is furious at first - how dare he come to see Marcus? However, as the two young men talk, she can see that Charles is deeply sorry about what happened. As it turns out, Angie appreciates their efforts ▼.

Episode 7
Angie is able to convince the physicians to send Marcus home this week. He requires a great deal of care, but Angie is sure she can take care of him and her other children better if Marcus is home. Angie's mother has agreed to stay as long as she is needed.

Kelsey comes home from gymnastics lessons with a cough that is easily treated with the rescue inhaler. Angie tells Kelsey that she might have to stop taking gymnastics because it seems to be bad for her breathing.

Episode 8

Angie can see that her son, Marcus, is happier at home, but his limited activity has him a bit depressed. Angie has an idea to create a family puppet show for Marcus. Angie and Kelsey come up with a story about a boy who is lost in the woods and is helped by the animals. She helps Kelsey make animal puppets, and she makes a little boy puppet and mother and father puppet. Angie is very happy about how much fun the entire family has with the puppet show. Because the puppet show was so much fun, Angie contemplates the possibility of taking this idea to the Neighborhood Elementary School as a learning project.

Episode 9

Angie is angered by news that the boy driving the car that hit Marcus got off with a charge of recklessness and the loss of his driver's license until age 20. She believes she needs to do something to prevent other people from getting hurt. She writes to her Congresswoman to complain about speed limits in the Neighborhood and to determine what she can do to slow down speeding cars.

Episode 10

Angie is surprised by the quick response from the Congresswoman. She encourages Angie to follow up with local officials regarding speeders, but claims that there is nothing that she can do officially on the state level. The Congresswoman wishes Marcus a speedy recovery. Angie begins making phone calls to city officials.

During the week, Eric develops a runny nose, cough, and fever. He is very fussy and not interested in eating. Angie takes him to Neighborhood Pediatrics and again sees the NP. She cannot believe the NP won't give Eric a prescription for antibiotics and questions the NP about the reason. Angie has read about the overuse of antibiotics, but is concerned that, in Eric's case, he might really need them ▼.

Episode 11

Angie learns that there is nothing she can do to get the speed limit changed on their street. She is told that one option for her is to get signatures on a petition asking for speed bumps to be placed on the streets. Angie organizes a neighborhood petition campaign and takes her entire family on an outing with her to help her collect signatures [NEWS].

Episode 12

Angie suggests taking the kids to the zoo because there is a new baby elephant on display. She carries Eric in a front infant pack, and Steve gets a wagon to pull Marcus and Kelsey when they want to ride. Angie is aware that the zoo is extremely crowded and tells Steve that they need to watch the kids closely.

Angie takes the baby into the restroom to change his diaper and asks Steve to wait for her at a nearby bench. When she returns, Angie is horrified to find Steve only with Marcus. "Where is Kelsey?" she asks in a concerned tone. Steve replies, "I thought she was with you! She ran to catch up with you!" Angie tries to stay calm, but soon panic ensues. She is sure Kelsey has been abducted! Angie and Steve are screaming for Kelsey when a zoo employee comes up to assist. She radios a lost-child alert, and all zoo staff keep an eye out for the little girl. After about 30 minutes, Kelsey is located, and Angie reunites with her at the Kids Connection, a facility for lost children. She is relieved that Kelsey is unharmed and furious with Steve for not keeping an eye on her ▼.

Episode 13

Angie takes the signed petition to the Neighborhood Council Meeting this week. She is disappointed when several people come to the meeting to speak out against her proposal, citing that speed bumps will damage their cars' suspensions. She does not understand why people are more concerned about their cars than about the safety of their children.

Kelsey brings a permission slip home from school for a hayride on a farm 20 miles south of the Neighborhood. The hayride is part of a pioneer learning experience with her class and will be held later in the month. Angie tells her Kelsey that she should not go because of her asthma [NEWS].

Episode 14

Angie asks Marcus if he is ready to start taking piano lessons again. She is not surprised when he tells her that he doesn't want to do it. Steve intervenes on his behalf and tells her that they really need to stop pushing the children and Marcus should be allowed to drop that activity. He also talks to her about letting Kelsey go on the hayride. After much discussion, Angie agrees to call the nurse and ask her opinion. The NP suggests that Angie should premedicate Kelsey with Albuterol inhaler and loratadine (Claritin) before the hayride ▼.

Episode 15

Angie takes Eric to Neighborhood Pediatrics this week for his 6-month visit. She sees the NP again, whom she has come to trust. On this visit, she does not argue about the immunizations and is just happy to talk to the nurse about her son. Angie appreciates the fact that the nurse asks Angie how Marcus has been doing.

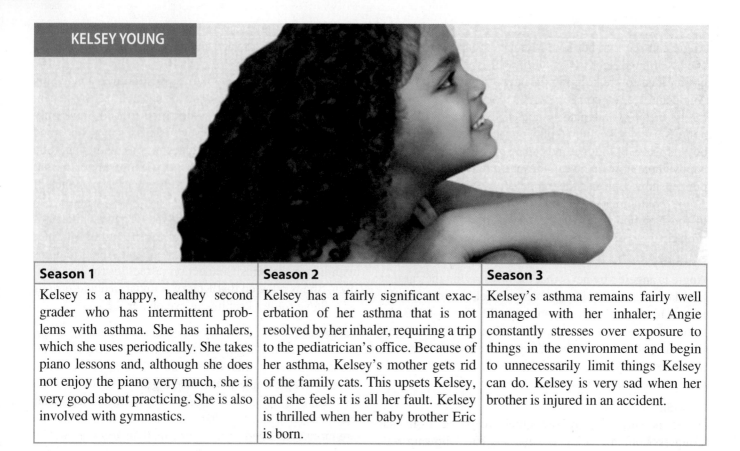

KELSEY YOUNG

Season 1	Season 2	Season 3
Kelsey is a happy, healthy second grader who has intermittent problems with asthma. She has inhalers, which she uses periodically. She takes piano lessons and, although she does not enjoy the piano very much, she is very good about practicing. She is also involved with gymnastics.	Kelsey has a fairly significant exacerbation of her asthma that is not resolved by her inhaler, requiring a trip to the pediatrician's office. Because of her asthma, Kelsey's mother gets rid of the family cats. This upsets Kelsey, and she feels it is all her fault. Kelsey is thrilled when her baby brother Eric is born.	Kelsey's asthma remains fairly well managed with her inhaler; Angie constantly stresses over exposure to things in the environment and begin to unnecessarily limit things Kelsey can do. Kelsey is very sad when her brother is injured in an accident.

Kelsey Young Season 1 Information

Episode 1

Kelsey Young is the 7-year-old daughter of Angie and Steve Young. She is a typical girl who is in enrolled in second grade at Neighborhood Elementary School. She likes her teacher and has many friends, especially Keisha and Victoria. She has a very stable home life and is close to her parents and brother, Marcus. Kelsey loves animals, especially the family cats, Chico and Kiekie. Her favorite places to visit are the pet store and the zoo. She loves to read stories and see movies that involve animals. She has never been particularly active physically, but after watching gymnastics on TV, she has taken an interest in this activity. She takes piano lessons, but has little interest in them.

Overall, Kelsey is healthy, but she has ongoing problems with reactive airway disease. This condition does not make her feel bad except when she has periodic episodes, which seem to be seasonal. Her mother typically manages her symptoms with an albuterol inhaler with a spacer and over-the-counter loratadine (Claritin) syrup. She is up-to-date on her immunizations and sees a dentist every six months.

This episode Kelsey goes with her family to the Natural History Museum and then out to lunch on Saturday. Kelsey likes the mammal display the best. In the afternoon, her mother insists that she practice the piano for 30 minutes and then read for 30 minutes before going outside to play with Keisha. She complies with her mother's demands and is glad she didn't make her mother angry, like Marcus did.

Episode 2

Kelsey experiences allergy symptoms this week and coughs periodically during the night three times this week, although the coughing is not severe enough to wake her. Her mother gives Kelsey the albuterol inhaler to use and gives her another medication to treat her symptoms. She feels well enough to go to school.

Episode 3

This week Kelsey and her mother go to her friend Victoria's home to celebrate Victoria's father's homecoming. Victoria's dad has been in the Navy for a number of years and has not been home very much. Kelsey and Victoria quickly lose interest in the adults' conversation and retreat to Victoria's room to play with dolls.

Episode 4

Kelsey is invited to a birthday party for her friend Samantha at Big Red's Pizza Parlor this week. The party conflicts with her music lesson. Kelsey wants to go to the party, but her mother insists that she go to the lesson instead. Angie compromises by taking Kelsey to the birthday party late, after the piano lesson. By the time she arrives, the children have already eaten pizza and opened presents and are playing the arcade games. Kelsey feels very disappointed and is angry that she missed most of the party.

Episode 5

After school, Kelsey goes to Keisha's house to play. Keisha has a kit of princess makeup and she gives Kelsey a "makeover." Kelsey does not have any makeup and does not really find it all that much fun, but she goes along with it anyway.

Episode 6

Kelsey goes to the zoo on a field trip with her second-grade class. She is very excited to see all of the animals. Because her mother is one of the chaperones, she makes sure that her best friend, Keisha, gets to ride to and from the zoo with her. Before they leave the zoo, Kelsey's mother buys her *Animals of the Jungle,* a coloring poster kit with markers. As soon as she completes her homework that evening, she spends time with her father coloring a lion poster.

Episode 7

Kelsey goes to a Health Fair with her family this week. Her favorite activity is an apple puzzle game at a booth that teaches children about healthy snacks. She notices her brother is not interested in the game and instead eats the apple slices.

Episode 8

Kelsey is told by her mother that she has a tiny baby growing in her stomach, and Kelsey will soon have a new brother or sister. Kelsey tells her mother that she hopes she gets a baby sister.

Episode 9

Kelsey is surprised and delighted to see her father at school to pick her up; she is used to only seeing her mother at school. He tells her that he is taking her to art class, and on the way he stops at an ice cream store for an after-school treat. Kelsey thinks she has the very best daddy in the world.

Episode 10

Kelsey comes home from school and tells her mother she has a headache and a stomach ache. She is not interested in playing the piano and instead lies down on the bed in her room. A short time later, Kelsey throws up. She stays home from school the next two days with the flu. She hears her mother tell her daddy that she probably caught the flu from the other kids at school.

Episode 11

Steve and Angie attend the open house at the grade school this week. Angie, of course, knows Kelsey's second-grade teacher very well, but Kelsey is especially excited for her daddy to meet her teacher.

Episode 12

Kelsey and her friend Keisha are invited to Victoria's house for a sleepover. Early in the evening, they spend most of their time in Victoria's room playing. Kelsey feels envious of the numerous new toys and other things Victoria has been given by her father since he returned home from military service. Later in the evening as the girls play a game in the den, they hear Victoria's parents arguing loudly and then hear Victoria's mother crying. The girls look at each other, but say nothing ▶.

Episode 13

Kelsey has another week with allergy symptoms and has episodic coughing three nights this week, although the coughing does not wake her up. Her mother gives her the inhaler and the loratadine (Claritin) syrup.

Episode 14

Kelsey asks her mother if she can go to Victoria's house to play. Her mom tells her it may not be a good idea to go to her house right now, but suggests that she invite Victoria to play at their house. When Kelsey invites Victoria, she is told that she can't come over. Kelsey invites Keisha over to play instead.

Episode 15

Kelsey goes with her family on an out-of-town trip to see her grandmother. Every time they go there, she gets to make cookies with her grandmother; this is their special activity. Her grandmother also has a dog that Kelsey loves to play with, and a man who lives down the street has horses. Her father takes her on a walk each day to give carrots to the horses.

Kelsey Young   Season 2 Information

Episode 1

Kelsey Young is the 7-year-old daughter of Angie and Steve Young. She is a typical girl who is in enrolled in second grade at Neighborhood Elementary School. She likes her teacher and has many friends, especially Keisha. She has a very stable home life and is close to her parents and brother, Marcus. She knows there will be a baby in the house soon and looks forward to taking care of it.

The weather turns cold this week, and Kelsey has a "flare-up" of her reactive airway disease. Her mother gives her the albuterol inhaler and the cough syrup, but she does not feel well for several days. She coughs frequently day and night for 3 days. Although she feels well enough to go to school, she does not feel like running around on the playground. She and Keisha sit on the swings and talk about horses until some boys start to throw sand at them. Instead of chasing the boys, Kelsey just gets off the swings and walks away with Keisha, informing the boys that she is going to tell the teacher.

Episode 2

Kelsey goes to Victoria Patterson's house after school to work on a school project. While there, Victoria's father, Blake, comes home and begins yelling at Victoria for failing to do her chores after school. Victoria runs to her room crying, and Mr. Patterson tells Kelsey she needs to go home. Kelsey calls her dad to come pick her up. While waiting for him, Kelsey hears Mrs. Patterson yelling at Mr. Patterson about the fact that the girls were doing a school project. Later at home when Kelsey tells her mom what happened, Angie tells Kelsey to stop hanging around with Victoria.

Episode 3

Kelsey talks with her mother about the baby. She is fascinated by the fact that the baby is inside her mother's stomach and tries to imagine what the baby looks like and what it is doing in there. Kelsey likes to touch her mother's stomach, especially when she can feel the baby move. She asks her mother how the baby breathes inside, but she does not understand her mother's explanation. She hopes the baby will be a girl.

Episode 4

During recess, Victoria Patterson approaches Kelsey and Keisha and invites them for another sleepover. Kelsey tells Victoria that her mother says they can't be friends anymore. Kelsey and Keisha then turn around and run to the swings. Keisha asks Kelsey why they can't be friends with Victoria. Kelsey shrugs and says, "I don't know, but I think it is because her dad is mean."

Episode 5

Kelsey has another round of allergy symptoms, but this time they are worse. Her coughing keeps her (and the rest of the family) awake at night. When she is awake, she has a subtle wheeze with breathing. Her mother gives her loratadine (Claritin) and the inhaler before school each morning. By Friday (the fourth day of her symptoms), her classroom teacher sends her to Violet Brinkworth, the school nurse, who then calls her mother. She hears the nurse tell her mother, "Kelsey should be seen by her primary care provider."

Kelsey is seen by a nurse practitioner. Her peak flow is assessed and found to be in the yellow zone, prompting an immediate nebulizer treatments. Kelsey thinks the treatment is strange. It makes a weird sound, and white smoke comes out the end. She thinks it looks like she is smoking a funny pipe.

Following treatment, Kelsey is better, but her peak flow shows that she is still in the yellow zone. She gets a second nebulizer treatment, and this improves her breathing significantly. Kelsey feels much better. On the way home, she and her mother stop at the drugstore to pick up medications ▤.

Episode 6

On Monday, Kelsey returns to see Carolyn Marquette, the nurse practitioner. It has been a few days since her breathing episode. She has been feeling well all weekend and has slept well. Her mother gives her another breathing treatment a little while before going to the office. Her peak flow is checked by the NP and found to be 200, which is in the green zone.

Kelsey is devastated when she hears her mother announce that the family cats must go to prevent Kelsey from getting sick again. She believes this situation is all her fault. She loves the cats and cannot bear the thought of giving them away. She is also upset by the fact that her mother and father are fighting. She is not used to having them argue like this. Kelsey is very sad and cries for hours ▤.

Episode 7

The family cats are gone when Kelsey gets home from school. She goes into her room and cries. She tells her mother that she doesn't mind having problems breathing; she just wants her kitties to come home. Kelsey is angry with her mother and angry that she has a problem with breathing.

Episode 8

Kelsey sees her former friend, Victoria Patterson, sitting by herself at recess. Kelsey remembers how her dad yelled at them last time she was at Victoria's house. Kelsey knows none of the girls play with Victoria anymore. She wonders if Victoria's dad is still being mean to her.

Episode 9

Kelsey is excited when she learns that her new baby brother is born. She talks to the baby and tells him she is his big sister and she will take care of him. Kelsey asks her mother if she has changed the baby's diaper yet. She is intrigued by the appearance of the umbilical cord.

Episode 10

Kelsey looks forward to coming home each day to see the baby. She likes it when her mother lets her sit in a chair to hold Eric. She stands on a chair next to the changing table to watch her mother or grandmother change the diapers. She also enjoys watching the baby get a bath in the tiny bathtub. She thinks about her cats often and wonders how they are.

Episode 11

Kelsey has a show-and-tell assignment at school this week. She asks her mother if she can bring Eric to school to show the class her new baby brother. Angie tells Kelsey it might not be a good idea to expose Eric to all the germs at school, so instead she takes several pictures of Eric including one with Kelsey holding Eric. The pictures are enlarged and placed on a poster board so Kelsey can tell the class different things about Eric.

Episode 12

Kelsey plays with Eric as he lies on a blanket on the floor while her mother takes a shower. Kelsey loves playing with the baby.

Episode 13

Kelsey has a mild cough this week, but it does not progress any further. Angie tells Kelsey that it is a good thing that the cats no longer live with them or she might have ended up in the hospital.

Episode 14

Kelsey goes to the Bike Safety Awareness class with her brother and father. She has fun but thinks she is a little "old" for the activity. She perceives it as an activity for little kids. The best part of the outing is that her daddy takes them to McDonalds for a Happy Meal.

Episode 15

Kelsey is very excited to visit her grandmother this week because they have a new baby. She tells her grandmother all about the baby and how she helps her mommy take care of Eric. Kelsey's grandmother tells her, "Eric is very lucky to have a big sister like you." This makes Kelsey feel very proud!

Kelsey Young Season 3 Information

Episode 1

Kelsey is the 8-year-old daughter of Angie and Steve Young. She is a typical girl who is enrolled in third grade at the elementary school. She likes her teacher at school and has many friends, especially Keisha. She has a very stable home life and is close to her parents and her brothers, Marcus and Eric. Kelsey loves her new baby brother and enjoys helping her mother take care of him. She also loves animals and is still angry with her mother about getting rid of their cats. She loves to read stories and see movies that involve animals. She takes gymnastics, swimming lessons, and piano lessons.

Overall, Kelsey is healthy. She has asthma and takes Fluticasone propionate and salmeterol (Advair Diskus 100/50) in the morning and evening. If she has an acute breathing problem, she takes a rescue medication, Albuterol metered-dose inhaler (MDI) with a spacer. She takes 2 puffs, waits 15 to 20 minutes, and then repeats. She has not needed to use her albuterol in months. She is up-to-date on her immunizations and sees a dentist every 6 months. Kelsey and her brother, Marcus, are taking swimming lessons at the Neighborhood Pool starting this week. Kelsey enjoys swimming but does not like getting in the cold water.

Episode 2

Kelsey plans to spend the night with Keisha. This is her first time spending the night away from her home since the overnight at Victoria Patterson's house. Kelsey does fine all evening until it is time to go to bed when she starts to feel very sad and wants to go home. After a call from Keisha's mother, her father drives to Keisha's house to pick up Kelsey and bring her home.

Episode 3

Kelsey is aware that the baby is sick, and she is worried. Kelsey's father takes her to her piano and swimming lessons so that her mother can take care of the sick baby. Kelsey experiences some coughing after being in the pool. When she gets home, her mother checks her peak flow. It is found to be 200, so her mother does not give Kelsey albuterol. The coughing subsides shortly thereafter.

Episode 4

Kelsey goes to the large shopping mall with her parents and brothers. Kelsey loves to go to the mall because there are so many interesting people and things there. Her mother buys her a new pair of shoes and a new outfit to wear to school. Kelsey can't wait to show Keisha her new clothes.

Episode 5

Kelsey hears her mother screaming outside and runs to the door to look. She is unable to see anything but an ambulance down the street. She becomes frightened, thinking that Marcus is hurt. When Eric begins to cry, Kelsey does not know what to do and tries to comfort him. Finally, a neighbor comes to the house and tells Kelsey that her brother was injured and is on the way to the hospital. The neighbor makes Kelsey supper and helps her with her with homework. Kelsey is relieved when her daddy comes home several hours later.

Episode 6

Kelsey has been to the hospital to see Marcus, but only once in the lobby. She is told she is not allowed to go into his hospital room because she is too young. She feels sorry for her brother when she sees his casts and the pins in his hips. She asks Marcus if it hurts, and he tells her yes. Kelsey is happy that her grandmother is at the house this week. Because she has watched her mother over the past few months, Kelsey knows the routine and helps her grandmother take care of Eric.

Episode 7

Kelsey goes to her gymnastics lessons with her dad. After the lesson, Kelsey starts to cough. When she gets home, her mother checks her peak flow and finds it is 190. She administers the rescue medication (albuterol with spacer). A few minutes later, her peak flow is 220, and Kelsey stops coughing. Kelsey's mother tells her that she might have to quit gymnastics because of the asthma. Kelsey responds by saying that she likes gymnastics.

Episode 8

Kelsey feels sorry for her brother Marcus because he still has to lie around so that his bones can heal. She has great fun with her mother and father preparing a puppet show for Marcus. Kelsey makes three puppets, all animals: a bear, a lion, and a giraffe. In the puppet story, her animals help rescue a little boy who is lost.

Episode 9

Kelsey is disappointed when her mother decides to take her out of swimming lessons. She hears her mother talk about her asthma to other people on a regular basis and decides that she must have a bad disease, yet she does not feel too bad. Kelsey is still in gymnastics class and hopes she does not have to quit gymnastics, too. As she practices the piano at home she finds herself wishing the asthma would prevent her from being able to play.

Episode 10

Kelsey is happy that Marcus is back at school with her. She helps him get to his class and tries to take care of him. She often sits with him at recess. At home, Kelsey reminds her mother that Marcus has his cast off now and wants to know when he is going to have to practice the piano.

Episode 11

Kelsey accompanies Marcus, Eric, and her mother and father on a petition-signing event to get speed bumps placed on the streets. She is not happy about going because she wants to play at Keisha's house.

Episode 12

Kelsey learns at school about a new baby elephant at the zoo. She tells her mother she would like to see the baby elephant. On the day her family goes to the zoo, there are many people there, and it is sometimes hard for Kelsey to see the animals. After visiting the elephant exhibit, her mother says she is taking Eric to the bathroom for a diaper change. As her mother walks away toward the bathroom, Kelsey tells her father she needs to go too and takes off running to catch her mother.

As she is running toward her mother, Kelsey trips and falls. Not injured, she quickly gets up and continues running, but she can't see her mother anymore. She heads toward a building she thinks is the bathroom, but it is a concession stand. She runs to the next building, and it is a gift shop. Kelsey is swallowed in the sea of people and can't find the bathroom. Her parents have taught her not to talk with strangers, so she is afraid to ask anyone where the bathroom is. Before long, Kelsey is completely lost. She tries to go back to the bench where her father and Marcus were, but she can't find that either. Kelsey is very frightened and just keeps walking. Eventually, she sits down and starts to cry. A woman with two children asks her if she is lost; Kelsey nods her head. The woman finds a zoo employee who takes her to a building called "Kids Connection" and is told her parents will meet her here. Kelsey is so happy when her parents, brother, and the baby find her at the building. She tells her mother that she wants to go home.

Episode 13

Kelsey's teacher at school announces to the children that they will be going on a hayride for a learning activity as part of the Pioneer Unit later in the month. Permission slips are distributed, and the children are instructed to return the signed slips by next week. Kelsey is angry when her mother tells her she should not go on the hayride because of her asthma. Kelsey feels like asthma ruins everything for her.

Episode 14

Kelsey is delighted when her mother gives her the signed permission slip for the hayride. She can't wait to tell Keisha that she is going on the hayride after all [NEWS].

Episode 15

Kelsey goes on the hayride with her class at school. They learn about shoeing a horse, milking cows, and building log homes. Kelsey likes the hayride the best because she is able to watch the horses as they pull the wagon.

MARCUS YOUNG

Season 1	Season 2	Season 3
Marcus is a healthy 6-year-old boy in the first grade. During this season he is sent home from school with "pink eye." He takes piano lessons, but is really not interested in playing the piano—this is his mother's idea. Practicing the piano causes conflict between Marcus and his mother.	Marcus learns to ride a bike and rides his bike most days after school. He continues to have battles with his mother over practicing the piano. He loves to go to Saturday art classes. Marcus is excited about the birth of his brother Eric.	Marcus is hit by a car while riding his bike. He is admitted to the Pediatric Intensive Care Unit with skeletal trauma. Pain management and dealing with a frantic, perfectionist mother are the issues facing nurses at the hospital.

Marcus Young Season 1 Information

Episode 1

Marcus Young is the 6-year-old son of Angie and Steve Young. He is a typical boy who is in enrolled in the first grade at the elementary school. He likes his teacher at school and has many friends. He has a stable home life and is close to his parents and sister, Kelsey. Marcus loves his pet cats, Chico and Kiekie. He also enjoys going to the park and playing on the playground equipment. He is very interested in sports and wants to play football and baseball someday. He takes piano lessons but is not interested in this activity at all. Marcus has no health-related problems; he is up-to-date on his immunizations and sees a dentist every 6 months.

Marcus goes with his family to the Natural History Museum and then out to lunch on Saturday. He likes the dinosaur and volcano displays the best. In the afternoon, his mother insists that he practice the piano for 30 minutes and then read for 30 minutes before he can go outside to play. He sits in front of the piano and plays for about 10 minutes before getting distracted by his cat, Chico. His mother finds him playing with the cat and sends him to his room for 1 hour for failing to practice.

Episode 2

As soon as Marcus comes home from school this week, his mother makes him sit down to practice the piano before he gets to play a computer game, believing this approach might motivate him more. Marcus protests, but sits down to practice. He practices for about 10 minutes before he gets distracted by his sister. He is sent to his room without a snack until dinner for failing to practice.

Episode 3

Marcus' mother tells him they will be going to Mr. and Mrs. Patterson's house to celebrate Mr. Patterson's coming home after being gone a long time. Marcus hates going to their house because the only toys there are for girls. He tells his mother he does not want to go. He is very happy when he hears his father tell his mother that Marcus can stay home with him and they can find something to do together.

Episode 4

After his piano lesson, Marcus overhears his mother talking to Ramona (his piano teacher) about his practice habits. Marcus and his sister see a lady walking her dog on the sidewalk and run out of the house to pet the dog and talk to the lady.

Episode 5

Ever since Marcus started first grade, he has been jealous of the things other kids get to eat for lunch. He tells his mother that he would like to have cookies, chips, or snack cakes in his lunchbox, like the other kids get. His mother tells him that those foods are not nutritious, and he should be happy to have the lunch he gets.

Episode 6

Marcus goes on a field trip to the children's art museum, where they draw pictures of their families with finger paints. Marcus proudly shows his mother the picture he brings home and is happy to see the picture placed on the refrigerator.

Episode 7

Marcus goes to a Health Fair with his family this week. Overall, he has fun, especially in the children's section. They visit a booth that teaches children about healthy snacks (but his mother already serves these at home), a place where they are weighed, and a place where they learn to take care of their teeth. Marcus is happy to get a new red toothbrush. His favorite booth involves jumping rope and then counting his heartbeat in his wrists. He used to think jump ropes were only for girls, but decides after trying it at the Health Fair that it is fun.

Episode 8

When he arrives home from school, Marcus is told by his mother that she has a tiny baby growing in her stomach, and he will soon have a new brother or sister. He looks under Angie's blouse at her stomach and is unimpressed. He tells his mother that he would like a snack.

Episode 9

Marcus wakes up in the morning with a sticky sensation and crust around his left eye. His mother cleans his eye before he goes to school. While at school, his eye is itchy, and he rubs it frequently. As the day progresses, his eye begins to hurt. He is sent to the nurse's office by his teacher, and the nurse then calls his mother to come pick him up.

His mother takes him to the pediatrician's office where he is seen by a nurse practitioner. Marcus is told that he has conjunctivitis (pink eye), but he doesn't think his eye is pink. A prescription for Ciprofloxacin (Ciloxan) ophthalmic drops is written. On the way home from the office, they stop at the drugstore to fill the prescription. When they get home, Kelsey tells Marcus, "Daddy got me ice cream today on the way to art class." Marcus feels sad and wishes his father would have taken him to the doctor so he could have had ice cream on the way home.

Episode 10

Marcus hears his sister throw up. A few hours later, Marcus throws up too. His mother tells him he has the flu, and he stays home the next two days from school. Marcus does not feel like playing or eating anything. He does not enjoy the cartoons either. He has been sick and home from school twice now in the last few weeks.

Episode 11

Marcus continues to take piano lessons with Ramona at his mother's insistence. He has come to really hate playing the piano and admits this when Ramona (the piano teacher) asks him if he enjoys it. Marcus tells Ramona that she'd better not tell his mother because she might get angry with him. He tells Ramona that he wants to play on a baseball team instead.

Marcus goes to the school open house with his parents. While there, he goes outside to play with a basketball with his dad and sister. They have fun until Angie puts a stop to it.

Episode 12

Marcus has his daddy all to himself one evening this week when Kelsey goes to spend the night with her friend. While Marcus picks out a movie for them to watch, Steve makes a glass of extra chocolaty chocolate milk to drink.

Episode 13

Marcus goes to a roller skating party with his first-grade class this week. He is not so sure he wants to go because he thinks roller skating is for girls. After he puts on the skates and figures out how to keep his balance, he decides he likes it. He spends most of his time with his friend, Darren, acting like monsters and chasing the girls around the roller rink.

Episode 14

Marcus overhears his mother talking about having a baby. He still can't understand how the baby got in her stomach, and he does not know how it will breathe.

Episode 15

Marcus goes with his family on an out-of-town trip to see his grandmother. He loves his grandmother and wishes that she lived closer. There is a fort in the backyard that he loves to play in, and there is no piano.

Marcus Young Season 2 Information

Episode 1

Marcus Young is the 6-year-old son of Angie and Steve Young. He is a typical boy who is in enrolled in first grade at the elementary school. He likes his teacher at school and has many friends.

Marcus goes to a birthday party at his friend's house. They play on a trampoline. Marcus thinks it is the best thing ever. When he comes home from the party, he asks his mother if they can have a trampoline. His mother says trampolines are dangerous and reminds Marcus to practice the piano before dinner.

Episode 2

Marcus is aware his sister, Kelsey, called daddy to pick her up from Victoria Patterson's house. He later overhears Kelsey tell their mother that Victoria's daddy was yelling at her and it made Kelsey scared to be there. Marcus hears his mother tell Kelsey to stop spending time with Victoria. Marcus wonders why Victoria's daddy yells. He is glad his daddy is nice.

Episode 3

Many of Marcus' friends are getting bikes, so he asks his father if he can get a bike, too. His father takes him to the store and gets a bike with training wheels. He tells his father that he doesn't want the training wheels but is told that he must first learn to ride safely with the training wheels, and then they can take them off.

Episode 4

Marcus has new motivation to practice the piano as soon as he gets home from school every day. He knows that after he practices, he can ride his new bike. For now, Angie restricts Marcus to riding in the backyard on the patio and on the sidewalks around the house. Marcus does not like the fact that his bike has training wheels. He imagines himself riding down the streets like the people he sees when he is in the car with his parents.

Episode 5

Marcus knows his sister had to go to the doctor because she had a bad cough. He watches with interest when his sister breathes in white smoke while having a treatment. He tells his mother that he would like to do that, too, and he is disappointed when he learns the machine is just for Kelsey. Angie suggests that he practice the piano instead.

Episode 6

Marcus is upset when he hears his mother say that they need to get rid of the family cats to prevent Kelsey from getting sick. He hears his mother and father arguing about it, which makes him feel very sad. He goes to his room to pet Kiekie.

Episode 7

Marcus is very sad when he comes home from school and learns that the cats are gone. He is told that they went to another home to live and that they will be well cared for. This does not comfort Marcus one bit. He wants his cats. Although he was told to practice his piano lesson, he goes to his room instead and spends the rest of the afternoon lying on his bed feeling very sad. His father later comes into his bedroom and attempts to comfort him.

Episode 8

Marcus is out running errands with his mother when they see Mrs. Patterson and Victoria. Marcus knows that Victoria has been Kelsey's friend, but they are not friends anymore. Kelsey tells Marcus that she can't play with Victoria anymore because her dad is mean and yells a lot. Marcus looks at Victoria but does not talk to her.

Episode 9

Marcus is excited when his father picks him up from their friend's home after school and announces that he has a new baby brother. Marcus is intrigued when he meets his new brother at the hospital. He knows the baby was in his mother's stomach, but has a hard time understanding just how it got out. Marcus touches the baby's head and hands; he is surprised at how small the baby is.

Episode 10

Marcus has adjusted to having a new baby in the house. He likes having his grandmother at the house and likes looking at the baby. He is a little disappointed that the baby is too small to play with. Marcus is glad that his mother has been too busy with the baby to notice that he has not been practicing the piano. Marcus misses the cats and asks his father about getting a dog.

Episode 11

Marcus becomes jealous of the fact that Kelsey gets to take a poster with pictures of Eric to school for show-and-tell. He tells his mother he wants to make a poster, too. Angie has extra poster board at home and she helps Eric assemble a poster to take to school. Eric is very excited to show the poster to his teacher and other students in his class [NEWS].

Episode 12

Marcus learns to ride a bike without training wheels this week. He had been working very hard to learn to ride and suddenly figured out how to keep his balance. He spends every day after school riding his bike up and down the sidewalk in the front of their home. Marcus stays on the sidewalk because his mother told him that, if she catches him in the street, she will take his bike away.

Episode 13

Ramona (the piano teacher) has sensed complete disinterest and lack of concentration in Marcus during the past several lessons. She talks with him about what kinds of things are going on with him. He tells her about learning to ride a bike without training wheels, about the cats, and about the new baby. Having this information is helpful to Ramona, who now has a better understanding of his lack of focus.

Episode 14

Marcus, Kelsey, and Steve go to the Bike Safety Awareness class. Marcus loves the activity because he gets to demonstrate his skill by riding through orange cones and around other obstacles. Marcus is proud of the fact that he is able to do this more efficiently than his sister, even though his training wheels just recently came off.

Episode 15

Marcus loves seeing "Grandma Young" and looks forward to the car trip. Marcus has learned some of the key landmarks along the way and points them out to his father as they approach "Turn here, Daddy," he says. When they get there, Marcus is proud to show his Grandma his new brother. Marcus comments that Eric is still too little to play with, but he will play with him when he gets bigger.

Marcus Young Season 3 Information

Episode 1

Marcus Young is the 7-year-old son of Angie and Steve Young. He is a typical boy who is in enrolled in the second grade at the elementary school. He likes his teacher at school and has many friends. He has a stable home life and is close to his parents, his sister, Kelsey, and his new baby brother, Eric.

Marcus and his sister, Kelsey, are now taking swimming lessons at the pool. Marcus likes swimming and wishes he could just take swimming lessons instead of piano lessons. Marcus occasionally sees a dog that belongs to some people up the street. He asks his parents about getting a dog.

Episode 2

Marcus rides his bike after school nearly every day. He has learned how to navigate over the curbs along the sidewalk. Because his mother makes him practice the piano before he can ride, Marcus is highly motivated to get this done as soon as possible after school. His friend, Darren, also now has a bike.

Episode 3

Marcus is happy that his father is taking him to after-school swimming and piano lessons this week while his mother stays home with the sick baby.

Episode 4

When Marcus' mother announces that they are going to the mall, Marcus protests and asks if he can stay at home. Marcus hates to go to the mall. He gets bored every time they go because all his mother does is look at clothes. Not even a promise of a trip to the frozen yogurt store interests him. Despite his protests, he ends up at the mall with his family. Fortunately, Marcus is entertained for a short while at the mall's arcade with his father.

Episode 5

One day after school this week, Marcus and Darren are riding their bikes up and down the sidewalk. A big black dog runs out of its owner's yard and begins to chase them. The boys get scared and ride faster. Marcus darts off the sidewalk and around a parked car to get away from the dog. He never sees the speeding red car driven by Charles (Randall Johnson's best friend). Charles sees Marcus at the last minute and attempts to miss him.

Marcus is struck from behind. The impact throws him through the air more than 30 feet. He is fortunate to land in a grassy spot in the median of the roadway, but sustains a pelvic fracture, a right leg fracture, a left leg laceration, and a left arm laceration. He briefly loses consciousness but does not sustain a head or spinal cord injury.

Marcus does not remember much about the incident. He wakes up in the intensive care unit at Neighborhood Hospital with his mother and father at his side. He has tremendous pain in his hips, legs, and arm. He is very frightened.

Episode 6

Marcus remains at Neighborhood Hospital. He has a weird metal frame around his hips with the metal going into his body. His mother and father tell Marcus he had surgery and those pins are holding his bones in place so that he can heal. Marcus does not like the fact that he can't wear underwear or go to the bathroom normally.

He wants to go home and misses going to school. He is very happy that his mother stays with him at the hospital and even happier when his dad comes by. His dad shows him pictures and tells him silly stories about what his sister and baby brother are doing, making him laugh. His dad then takes pictures of Marcus making silly faces to show to Kelsey. He giggles when he imagines Kelsey looking at his pictures.

Marcus is still restricted to bed rest and is bored. He has lost interest in watching cartoons on TV. The nurses and other hospital staff attempt to keep him occupied by providing a variety of activities for him, such as coloring and other crafts. He gets cards and balloons from his classmates at school. He watches as his mother decorates the hospital room with the colorful cards.

Two teenage boys visit Marcus at the hospital. One of the teens tells Marcus that his name is Charles, the driver of the car that hit him. He tells Marcus that he feels very bad about hurting him, but is glad to see that he is going to get better. Charles gives Marcus a handheld video game to play with. Marcus likes Charles and his friend, Randall.

Episode 7

Marcus is now home from the hospital. His leg remains in a cast, and his pelvis is still pinned; he remains confined to bed. A home health nurse comes to see him every couple of days. Marcus is miserable being stuck in bed, but he is much happier at home than he was in the hospital. He is very happy to eat his mother's cooking and see his sister and brother, Eric. His father moves a bed into the family area so that Marcus can be involved in all the family activities.

A lady from the school comes to see Marcus every day so he does not fall behind in school. Fortunately, he is right-handed, so he is able to complete writing assignments with assistance. Several of his classmates make a surprise visit to see Marcus, and he is very happy to see them. When they leave, he feels sad for missing out on going to school.

Episode 8

Marcus has been feeling down because he remains mostly confined to bed while his bones heal. He feels much better being home, but he hates not being able to get up and go out to play. He is delighted when his family has a *Young Family Puppet Show* for him. The puppet show is about a little boy who is lost in the woods. The animals help him by finding him a place to sleep and food to eat. Eventually they help him get back to his family. He tells his parents that they should do more family puppet shows.

Episode 9

Marcus still has pins in his pelvis and a splint on his leg. He is able to get up out of bed a little bit now and is so happy to be out of bed and moving around. He takes great interest in some comic books his father has brought home. The lady from school continues to come to his house to help him with school work. Although he likes her, he misses being at school and is looking forward to going back soon. He goes to a clinic a couple of times a week to do exercises with hospital people. He likes to go because they make the exercises fun. Marcus has some pain in his leg and pelvis with the exercises, but not as much as before.

Episode 10

The pins are now out of his pelvis, and Marcus is finally able to go back to school. He is unable to run on the playground at this point, but he is happy to go outside at recess and watch the kids play. He shows the kids at school the scars from where the pins were and tells them the pins went all the way into the bones. The kids at school think the scars are gross. He is very tired when he comes home from school and needs to take a nap. He is glad that his mother does not make him practice the piano.

Episode 11

Marcus is quickly regaining his agility with his movement. Anyone watching him would not know he had been so severely injured a few months ago. Although he fell a little bit behind in his school work, the teacher has developed a plan that will help him catch up within a few weeks. Marcus goes around the neighborhood with his mother to collect signatures for speed bumps. He wishes he could stay home.

Marcus loves to play with Eric. He likes to put his face near Eric's and make noises because this makes Eric laugh.

Episode 12

Marcus is very excited to go to the zoo. His Dad gets him a wagon to ride in when he gets tired. Even though he is not tired, he wants to ride in the wagon because it is fun. While at the zoo, Kelsey gets lost for a while. Marcus can see how worried his parents are. In fact, his mother starts to cry when they can't find Kelsey. Eventually they find Kelsey at a building that has some toys. Shortly thereafter they leave the zoo. Marcus is disappointed that they have to leave before he can see the bears.

Episode 13

Marcus is embarrassed when his teacher asks him in front of the class about his mother being in the newspaper regarding the speed bump issue at city hall. He did not know she was in the paper and wonders why they put her picture there [NEWS].

Episode 14

Marcus dreads it when his mother asks him if he is ready to take piano lessons again. He has not played in several months and has not missed it one bit. He wishes his mother had forgotten about it. Marcus is so glad when his father talks his mother out of making him start the lessons again.

Episode 15

Marcus has been thinking about bikes and dogs non-stop. All of his friend have dogs and bikes and he wants to have both. He tells his Dad that he wants to get another bike and a dog. His dad promises to talk with his mother about it [▶].

ERIC YOUNG

Season 1	Season 2	Season 3
Not born yet	Eric is born in an uncomplicated birth. Most of the story describes infant care and age-appropriate behaviors in the context of the family and daily routine.	During this season, Eric has a bout of diarrhea that requires a trip to the pediatrician's office. Later he has a viral upper respiratory infection. Most of the story describes age-appropriate behaviors in the context of the family and daily routine.

Eric Young   Season 1 Information

Not born yet.

Eric Young Season 2 Information

Not born yet.

Episode 9

Eric Young is born this week in an uncomplicated labor and delivery. He is placed on his mother's abdomen immediately after birth and covered with a warm blanket to maintain his body temperature. His Apgar scores are 8 and 10 at 1 and 5 minutes, respectively. He weighs 3.3 kg (50th percentile), is 51 cm long (50th percentile), and has a head circumference of 35.2 cm (50th percentile). Shortly after birth, Eric is cleaned and examined, and erythromycin ophthalmic ointment and tetracycline ophthalmic ointment are placed into his eyes. A dose of phytonadione and hepatitis B vaccine are administered intramuscularly.

Eric has no problems or complications following birth and is discharged home with his mother and father the next day. Prior to discharge, a heel stick is performed to obtain a blood specimen for routine newborn screening. By the time he is discharged, he is breastfeeding about eight times a day and has had seven wet diapers and a large meconium stool. His umbilical cord is dry, and the clamp has been removed.

Episode 10

Eric continues to adapt to his new surroundings. He is comforted by his mother's smell and voice. He breastfeeds well, and then he sleeps.

Episode 11

Eric is seen at Neighborhood Pediatrics for a 2-week well-baby visit. His weight is 3.6 kg.

Episode 12

Eric lies on a blanket and listens to his sister talk to him. He is unable to focus on her face, but he can see her general shape and knows intuitively this person is not his mother. Eric is seen for his 1-month well-baby visit.

Episode 13

Eric is 4 weeks old now. When he is hungry, he cries and his mother responds by breastfeeding him. After he eats and is satisfied, he falls asleep. He has a strong grasp reflex and his hands are usually in a closed position.

Episode 14

Eric is spending noticeably greater amounts of time awake than before. He is a happy baby who is rarely fussy. He is comforted when held by his mother and father.

Episode 15

At six weeks of age, Eric is taking his first trip away from home to meet Grandma Young. Eric is placed in the car seat by his father. He quickly falls asleep and stays asleep most of the way. He is held by a lady he has never seen before. Eric studies her face as she talks and sings to him. Eric hears an unfamiliar sound – a dog barking – but he is unable to see what is making the noise.

Eric Young Season 3 Information

Episode 1

Eric Young is the newborn infant of Angie and Steve Young. He was born at 38 weeks' gestation in an uncomplicated birth. He is 7 weeks old and is in perfect health. He is a breastfed infant who lives in his home with his parents and two siblings, Kelsey and Marcus.

Eric is spending a little more time awake now. For short intervals he is quiet and alert. During these times, Eric's mother talks and sings to him. Her voice and the sounds interest him. She sometimes holds things close to his face for him to see and she touches his skin with various objects.

Episode 2

Eric is now 2 months old, and his mother takes him back to Neighborhood Pediatrics to see the nurse practitioner (NP) for a well-baby check. He weighs 5.0 kg (45th percentile), his head circumference is 38.6 cm (48th percentile), and his length is 55.6 cm (50th percentile). The NP notes that he smiles responsively and holds his head well when in an upright position. He gets immunizations during this visit (HBV, DTaP, Hib, IPV, PCV). He experiences pain and cries when given an injection in the leg.

Episode 3

Eric spends time this week at the nursery at the local fitness club while his mother works out. A few days later, he has an emesis and then very watery diarrhea. He becomes cranky and cries a lot, more than usual for this typically happy baby. He is given water throughout the day by his mother and continues to have diarrhea. In the evening, his mother gives him an oral electrolyte solution (Pedialyte) During the night, he continues to have diarrhea. By morning, Angie recognizes that he just does not look right.

The following morning, Angie takes Eric to the pediatrician's office, and he once again sees the nurse practitioner (NP). His weight is down only a little bit, but he has an elevated temperature, and his skin has decreased turgor. His diaper is dry. The NP suggests that Angie continue to give the baby the oral electrolyte solution (Pedialyte) and monitor his fluid output. She explains to Angie that he should have at least four wet diapers a day.

Over the course of the next 12 hours, the diarrhea slows down and eventually returns to his normally loose stools. Eric eagerly breastfeeds for the next few days.

Episode 4

Eric goes to the mall with his family. He spends the afternoon in his stroller or being carried around by his father. He hears many new and different sounds.

Episode 5

Eric has become quite the chatterbox. He is very happy and babbles and coos, to the delight of his parents and grandmother. He is completely unaware of events that have occurred within his family.

Episode 6

Eric is now 14 weeks old. He is aware he is not seeing his mother as much as usual and cries more frequently when she is away. She does not come to him when he cries.

Episode 7

Eric is now aware of his surroundings to the point where he recognizes when he is in a strange place away from his home. He is highly interested in looking around at things and actively babbles when his sister talks to him.

Episode 8

Eric's mother takes him to Neighborhood Pediatrics for his 4-month well-baby check. On this visit, he weighs 6.4 kg (40th percentile), his head circumference is 42 cm (50th percentile), and his length is 63 cm (40th percentile). He gets immunizations during this visit (DTaP, Hib, IPV, PCV). He experiences pain when given an injection in the leg and cries.

The nurse practitioner (NP) notes that Eric actively grasps objects when offered to him and inspects his hands. She also notes that he lifts his head easily when in the prone position and looks around the room; she does not observe head lag when she pulls Eric to a sitting position.

Episode 9

Eric has learned to roll from his back to his side. He gets frustrated when he is left alone too much and demands attention from his siblings or his parents when he becomes bored. Eric also drools a lot now, making the front of his shirt wet, cold, and uncomfortable.

Episode 10

Eric develops a runny nose, cough, and fever this week. He is very fussy and does not eat well. His mother takes him to Neighborhood Pediatrics and, once again, he sees Carolyn Marquette, the nurse practitioner (NP). The NP examines Eric and tells Angie that he has a viral upper respiratory infection and that she just needs to give him acetaminophen (Infant Tylenol) and keep him well hydrated.

Episode 11

Eric's father puts him in a stroller and takes him out with the family to gather signatures for Angie's speed-bump campaign. Eric watches with interest the changes in his surroundings, but eventually gets bored. Steve tries to please him with a pacifier and various toys, without luck. Eric is only happy once he is carried by his father. He eventually falls asleep during the outing.

Episode 12

Eric is now able to distinguish various members of his family. He loves it when his siblings play with him. He smiles regularly and makes many sounds now, to everyone's delight.

Episode 13

Eric has been very fussy of late because his teeth are just about to start coming in. He is now sitting and loves to grasp toy objects that are on the floor around him. He cries if Marcus takes something away from him.

Episode 14

To the delight of his family, Eric has begun to "talk" when he is interacting with Steve and says "Ma" or "Da." When Steve or Angie appears, he recognizes them and often holds his arms up to be picked up. He has now also begun to search for items that he drops.

Episode 15

Eric's mother takes him to Neighborhood Pediatrics to see the nurse practitioner for his 6-month well-baby check. On this visit, he weighs 7.4 kg (37th percentile), his head circumference is 44 cm (50th percentile), and his length is 67 cm (40th percentile). He gets immunizations during this visit (DTaP, Hib). He cries when the injection is given in his leg.

HEALTH CONNECTIONS CLINIC

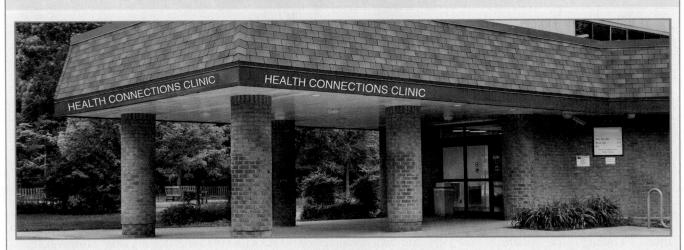

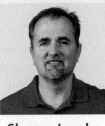

Shawn Jacobs

Housing

Parks and Recreation

Services There is regular bus service in the area, both to the Downtown and to residential areas. There are several convenience stores and small eating establishments within 3 blocks of Health Connections Clinic.

Key: ▶ = video clip ▤ = medical record ▽ = journal entry NEWS = news article

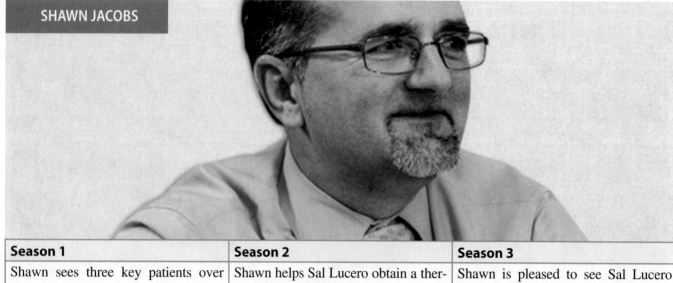

SHAWN JACOBS

Season 1	Season 2	Season 3
Shawn sees three key patients over time, including Matt Nolan, a veteran with substance abuse issues; Sal Lucero, a veteran with post-traumatic stress disorder; and Amanda Hardin, a college student with substance abuse issues. Shawn is currently involved in a substance abuse research study in the role of site investigator.	Shawn helps Sal Lucero obtain a therapy dog and continues to work with Amanda Hardin and Matt Nolan. He follows two new patients — Aaron Hidalgo, who also has substance abuse issues, and Blake Patterson, a veteran who is experiencing depression. Shawn presents at a national conference as a keynote speaker and he is involved in a patient satisfaction project to improve access for patient care services.	Shawn is pleased to see Sal Lucero obtain a therapy dog. However, he is very sad to learn one patient has died and another one is unable to stay substance free. Shawn also treats several new patients, including Clifford Allen, Helen Martin, Mark Martin, and Anthony Martin. Shawn continues to be involved in scholarly projects to improve patient care outcomes.

Shawn Jacobs Season 1 Information

Episode 1

Shawn is a 34-year-old White male who works as a mental health nurse practitioner. He has been a psychiatric mental health nurse practitioner for 6 years and recently completed a doctor of nursing practice (DNP) degree. Shawn has been working at a federally and state-funded community-based health clinic called Health Connections Clinic for 2 years. The clinic provides mental health services, as well as women's health and health promotion/disease prevention services. The clinic employs three physicians, 4 family nurse practitioners, and 2 mental health nurse practitioners. The clinic sees an average of 20 adult patients a day for mental health services. Pediatric mental health services are managed by providers in another clinic. The large majority of cases seen by the mental health providers include substance abuse and depression.

Shawn is involved in a multisite interdisciplinary collaborative research study related to substance abuse. This opportunity arose as a result of his doctoral work as a DNP student. He is very happy to be involved as a site investigator at one of twelve sites in the regional study.

This episode Shawn has a new patient referred from the family practice side of the clinic. The patient, 29-year-old Matt Nolan, was brought in by a friend who said, "He is messed up and needs help." After completing a thorough history and examination, Shawn learns that Matt is a recently divorced veteran who served two tours in the Middle East. Matt admits to using marijuana, methamphetamines, and alcohol whenever he can get enough money for them, but he does not think his problem is all that bad. When asked about the friend who brought him in for help, Matt replied, "He is just on my case. "Shawn asks Matt if HE wants help (as opposed to others wanting him to get help). Matt replies, "I guess." Shawn gives Matt his card and tells him to give it some thought and says he would be willing to work with him, but he stresses to Matt that substance abuse recovery is hard work that he would need to commit to.

Episode 2

Amanda Hardin is a 19-year-old student at the nearby university. She comes to the clinic with her parents after a referral from a provider at the student health services. When Shawn asks Amanda about the reason for her visit, Amanda's mother, Barbara, gives Shawn a long story about Amanda going to school, partying too much, and getting hooked on drugs. She also adds that she can't understand how this happened because Amanda was raised in a good home. When Shawn attempts to redirect questions back to Amanda, her mother does all the talking. Amanda remains quiet and looks at the floor. Shawn asks the parents to step out so he can talk to Amanda alone. Amanda's parents agree, but Barbara states, "Just keep in mind that Amanda can't be trusted to provide accurate information."

Once alone with Amanda, Shawn conducts a mental health assessment. He is unable to get Amanda to share much on this first visit, but she does confirm she has a problem with oxycodone and alcohol and she wants help. Shawn asks her to return in a week and to take measures not to use between now and her next visit ▶ ▼.

Episode 3

This week Shawn sees Matt Nolan again. Matt had been in a few weeks previously for substance abuse. This time Matt is seeking help after his ex-wife filed a restraining order against him, claiming he had threatened to hurt her and his children. When Shawn asks Matt to provide further details of the events, Matt admits he does not recall what happened. He remembers partying with friends and then going to her house to pick up the kids. He awoke at a friend's house the next day but does not remember anything else. Matt thinks she made everything up, but he recognizes that perhaps he had a black out. Shawn acknowledges having a blackout is a possible explanation.

Matt tells Shawn he is ready to start a program. Shawn gives him some things to work on, and asks Matt to return next week, but knows it is unlikely he will be back anytime soon. Shawn has become very good at recognizing the mixed messages of what addicted patients say and what they actually do.

Episode 4

Amanda Hardin has returned to the clinic after two weeks. On this visit she is not accompanied by her parents. Amanda tells Shawn her parents are looking into sending her to a substance abuse treatment facility for intensive therapy. When asked about her missed appointment from last week, Amanda tells Shawn she wanted to have one last binge before getting serious about treatment and was probably drunk and high and did not remember to come to an appointment. She said her last use was "about" 4 days ago.

When asked why she wants treatment, Amanda tells Shawn that she has failed school and has had to move back home with her parents. Her parents won't let her drive any of their family cars, and she knows she needs to get cleaned up or her parents might throw her out. Amanda also mentions that the "oxy's cost a lot" and she is pretty short on money. She wants to get away from the ongoing expense. Shawn points out to Amanda that her motivation is externally driven and that, for long-term success, internal motivation is necessary.

Episode 5

A 47-year-old homeless patient by the name of Joyce Rollins is seen by Shawn this week. She was brought to the clinic by staff from the homeless shelter asking for some help on her behalf. Shawn is able to access her medical record and learns that Joyce was treated by other providers in the clinic in the past, but she has not been seen in about 2.5 years. According to the record, Joyce is bipolar, has post-traumatic stress disorder (PTSD) associated with sexual abuse, and has addictions to alcohol and methamphetamine. She also has hepatitis C, is HIV positive, and is malnourished.

Shawn has 15 minutes on the schedule and wonders how he is supposed to provide any kind of quality care to this complex patient. Knowing he will be behind schedule the rest of the day, he takes the time needed to complete a comprehensive health assessment, including a comprehensive mental health assessment. He notes that Joyce has significant cognitive challenges not noted previously on the health record. She is unable to provide specific information, but Shawn is able to glean that she has been living in a distant state for the past few years and has recently returned to the Neighborhood community.

Shawn notices a foul smell coming from Joyce's large bag. He asks Joyce if he could see what is in her bag. She replies, "Sure," and she dumps the contents of her entire bag onto the floor. Among the many random items from the bag are spoiled food and a dead mouse. Joyce does not seem to recognize anything wrong with the contents of her bag. Shawn makes a call to Dr. Jacobe, a local psychiatrist, and makes arrangements for Joyce to be admitted to the Neighborhood Psychiatric Unit under his care NEWS.

Episode 6

This week Shawn picks up another new patient. Salvador (Sal) Lucero is a 38-year-old Hispanic male. He is single but has a steady girlfriend. Sal's girlfriend Giovanna comes with him to the clinic. Sal's primary complaint is trouble sleeping. Shawn completes an intake assessment and learns that Sal works in a warehouse for a distribution company and is a veteran who returned home from active duty four months ago. Since arriving home he has been adjusting to life outside of the military. In exploring his symptoms further, Shawn learns that Sal has frequent nightmares (2-3 times a week) causing him to wake up and then not be able to go back to sleep - leading to sleep deprivation. He is also easily agitated to the point of feeling like "he is going to explode." The symptoms started while he was on active duty and have become more troublesome after arriving home. They have been going on for several months now. Shawn recognizes his symptoms as consistent with post-traumatic stress disorder (PTSD); Shawn also suspects Sal has an underlying anxiety disorder but decides to explore this further in another session. Shawn prescribes prazosin as a treatment for his night terrors. He asks Sal to return to the clinic the following week and to consider joining group therapy ▼.

Episode 7

This week Shawn begins serving as a preceptor to a DNP student named Rachel from the university. Rachel tells Shawn she is a Family Nurse Practitioner doing a post-masters DNP program in behavioral health.

Shawn leads a group therapy session this week. He is pleased to see that Sal Lucero has come to the meeting. Sal shares with the group that he has had many challenges getting along with people. He feels irritable, has frequent nightmares, and has occasional episodes of panic. Listening to Sal describe his symptoms again in the group setting helps Shawn understand his situation better. He is sure that Sal has PTSD with hyperarousal symptoms with anxiety.

This week Shawn initiates a 4-week assessment project in his clinic to evaluate the ways patients get into their clinic system and the barriers they face getting follow-up appointments. Many of the providers agree with Shawn that the system is not efficient, but they also tell him things are "political" and he should not waste his time ▶.

Episode 8

Shawn sees on the schedule that Amanda Hardin has an appointment with him again, the first one in over a month, and he is glad to see she is on the schedule. During her visit, she tells Shawn that she has been through intensive inpatient treatment and is feeling great. She proclaims that she has "gotten cleaned up." She said her parents have given her car back and she is looking for a job - with a goal of getting back into school. Amanda tells Shawn that, as part of ongoing treatment recovery, she was advised to continue to work with a mental health professional and continue with group therapy. She also needs ongoing treatment with methadone. She provides documentation of her treatment so Shawn can provide appropriate follow-up care.

Shawn tells Amanda he is glad she is following through with ongoing treatment, because long-term success requires ongoing effort and extends far beyond any month-long intensive treatment. Shawn makes arrangements for Amanda to attend a substance abuse therapy group at the Health Connections Clinic. He also gets her a referral to the methadone clinic. Amanda tells Shawn going to the methadone clinic once a day will be a "real hassle" and she would prefer it if he could just give her a prescription for it. She is not happy when he tells her that is not possible.

Episode 9

Shawn is happy to meet with Sal Lucero again this week. Sal continues in group therapy and has opened up a great deal. Sal confirms the nightmares have lessened, although he is still easily startled and has a hard time responding appropriately - meaning he is still having significant anger issues. Shawn reminds Sal how far he has come since they first met. Sal mentions a recent article in the local newspaper and asks Shawn about the possibility of getting a therapy dog.

Shawn is aware that there has been a reduction of funding from Veterans Affairs about use of therapy dogs for PTSD, because of the lack of evidence of its effectiveness. Shawn wonders if the issue is lack of effectiveness or lack of studies that evaluate effectiveness. Based on his own anecdotal experience, therapy dogs are very effective in the right situation ▼ [NEWS].

Episode 10

Amanda Hardin, the 19-year-old former college student, continues to make good progress with her treatment for oxycodone and alcohol addiction. She has been attending group therapy sessions regularly and going to the methadone clinic every day for her methadone treatment. Amanda's mother leaves messages for Shawn on a regular basis, asking for information about Amanda's progress - as though she is checking up on her daughter. Shawn knows her intentions are probably good, but he is not able to have a conversation with Amanda's mother without Amanda's permission ▼ [NEWS].

Episode 11

Shawn was surprised to hear that Matt Nolan (the 29-year-old veteran) came back to the clinic this week. Matt tried to make an appointment and became angry when he was told there were no openings. He yelled at the schedulers and told them he had an emergency. Before anyone could do anything else, Matt stormed out of the clinic.

This week Shawn finishes his project studying how patients enter the clinic system and the barriers they face in getting follow-up appointments. His next step is to analyze the data. He has made arrangements to work with the school of public health to assist in analyzing and interpreting the data ▶ ▼ [NEWS].

Episode 12

The leader of the substance abuse group therapy session tells Shawn that one of his patients, Amanda Hardin, attended a session the previous evening and was asked to leave because she was acting erratically. When she was asked to leave, she became very disruptive and upset other group members. The therapist suspected she was under the influence of something.

Shawn tries to reach her on her cell phone but does not get an answer. He calls her home phone number listed in the chart and her mother, Barbara, answers the phone. Barbara tells Shawn she has not seen Amanda since yesterday and was planning to file a missing person's report. An hour later, Shawn gets a phone call from Barbara who informs him Amanda was arrested during the night for driving under the influence. Barbara suggests that Shawn's therapy is not as good as the intensive therapy Amanda went through earlier. Shawn does not comment and simply thanks her for the update. Shawn does not hear anything else the rest of the week ▼ [NEWS].

Episode 13

Matt Nolan shows up at the clinic again without an appointment. He again makes a scene at the reception desk and demands to see Shawn. Shawn happens to have an available slot and is able to work him in that afternoon.

Matt confides he really wants help now. He was recently arrested for driving under the influence for the third time and lost his license. He can't see his children and he is running out of places to stay after being evicted from his apartment. Matt tells Shawn it is time to get his life back on track.

Matt admits to recent use of methamphetamines and alcohol. Shawn tells Matt there is not a pharmaceutical treatment for methamphetamine addiction, but there are several treatment options including Cognitive behavior therapy, a 12-step program, family education, and contingency reinforcement plan. He arranges for Matt to get admitted into a substance rehabilitation unit for treatment of his alcohol and methamphetamine addictions.

Deep down, Shawn still is doubtful that Matt is fully committed to treatment. Perhaps he will be surprised ▶ ▼.

Episode 14

Shawn contacts the rehabilitation unit to get a status report on Matt Nolan. He is told that Matt checked himself out of the unit after 6 days. Matt reportedly told the staff, "I've had enough and am good to go."

Amanda Hardin comes into the clinic this week and tells Shawn she had been doing great with her treatment until she ran into some of her friends and ended up hanging out with them. She tells Shawn, "I would have been fine but they wanted me to party with them. I've been at it, smoking heroin, taking oxys, and drinking for the last two weeks." When asked about the arrest, she tells Shawn that she really did not do anything wrong but the "stupid cop" that pulled her over "had an attitude" and accused her of driving erratically. She is furious with her parents because they took her car away again.

Based on Amanda's responses Shawn recognizes she is not taking responsibility for her actions. He asks her what she wants to do at this point. Amanda replies that she wants to get clean. Shawn doesn't believe she has hit bottom yet and is not really ready to commit to treatment ▶ ▼.

Episode 15

Shawn sees Sal Lucero as a follow-up to treatment for PTSD. Shawn is very pleased at the progress Sal has made. He states his nightmares are not as frequent, and he has better coping skills as evidenced by being able to "talk himself down" when he wakes up in a sweat from a nightmare.

Sal continues to talk about getting a therapy dog but knows he can't afford it without the Army paying for it. Shawn has a connection with some dog trainers in the NBH community and tells Sal he will see if anyone can estimate the cost of dog training for a service dog.

Shawn writes an editorial for the newspaper about the need for funding support for therapy dogs. He is contacted by the editor of the Neighborhood Newspaper hoping to get further information for a special interest story regarding the lack of funding for animal therapy for veterans. With Sal's permission Shawn gives the editor Sal's contact information for the story ▼ [NEWS].

Shawn Jacobs Season 2 Information

Episode 1

Amanda Hardin makes a visit to the clinic this week and tells Shawn she had a good week. She says she is now living with her friends because her parents were always "on her case." Shawn tells Amanda that he noticed she has been missing group therapy and appointments with him. Amanda tells Shawn he sounds like her parents. She explains she was pretty busy last week moving and she tried to change her appointment but was told there were no other appointment times available. She promises to attend next week.

Shawn asks her to provide a urine sample for drug screen and she tests positive. Shawn reinforces to Amanda that he can't help her unless she is motivated ▽ NEWS.

Episode 2

For a second week in a row, Amanda Hardin tests positive for drug use when she is in the clinic. She admits to using oxycodone, heroin, and alcohol this week. Shawn is firm and tells her he can't help her at this point. Amanda simply says, "OK, whatever," and leaves the clinic.

In collaboration with colleagues from the school of public health, Shawn has finally finished analyzing his project data related to how patients enter the clinic system and barriers they face getting follow-up appointments. He writes a 1-page brief and makes an appointment to discuss the findings with the medical director and clinic administrator ▽.

Episode 3

Shawn smiles when he sees in the News a story about Sal and his desire for a therapy dog for PTSD. What Shawn did not expect was the public response. Moved by his story, two wealthy businessmen from the community (Greg and Ben) offer to pay for a service dog. Shawn helps Sal make contact and complete the paperwork needed to begin the process of getting a dog.

Shawn has a meeting this week with the clinic's administrator and the medical director. Shawn presents compelling evidence that the current processes used for scheduling appointments result in a lack of reconciliation for no-show or rescheduled appointments and making it hard for patients to find appointment times. Shawn also is able to show that the current time-frame allocated for the intake of a new patient is completely inadequate for optimal care and leads to a chronic back-up of appointment times. The administrator and medical director are very impressed with the findings and agree that the next step would be a review of current policies with the possibility of policy updates ▽ NEWS.

Episode 4

A new patient is seen by Shawn this week. Blake Patterson is a 30-year-old White male who has recently been discharged after serving 8 years in the United States Navy. He is referred to the clinic by Dr. Rowe from Neighborhood Family Practice for possible depression. Shawn completes a comprehensive history and assessment, including a thorough mental health assessment. Mr. Patterson scores a 24 on the Center for Epidemiologic Studies Depression (CES-D) Scale, indicating moderate depression.

As a result of completing the assessment, Shawn learns that Blake has no history of mental health problems and is not contemplating suicide. He seems to be suffering from situational depression. Shawn learns that shortly before he was discharged from the Navy, Blake was driving a vehicle with his closest friend when they were involved in a traffic accident. His friend was killed and Blake walked away without a scratch. Blake has been dealing with extreme guilt and has become progressively more depressed since returning home. Blake is a smoker and describes occasional use of alcohol; he denies drug use. Blake's depression has negatively impacted his relationship with his wife and daughter. They had all been looking forward to his homecoming after being gone for the better part of 8 years, but things have not worked out as planned. Shawn prescribes Bupropion hydrochloride (Wellbutrin) XL 150 mg once a day for Blake and asks him to return to the clinic in a week.

Episode 5

Blake Patterson returns to the clinic to see Shawn in a follow-up visit and comments what a challenge it was to get an appointment. Shawn asks Blake how he is feeling; he responds that he feels about the same. Shawn completes a mental status assessment. Although Shawn finds Blake to be stable and coping reasonably well, he increases the dose of bupropion XL to 300 mg once a day. Blake is reminded that the medications take 3-4 weeks to reach full effect ▽.

Episode 6

Shawn sees Matt Nolan in the clinic again this week. Matt, a 29-year-old veteran, has been into the clinic on several other occasions seeking help for substance abuse, but he has yet to get far with treatment. Shawn reminds Matt he is very happy to help, but that he (Matt) needs to be committed. Shawn tells Matt he has yet to see commitment. Matt says, "I have finally hit rock bottom and am ready to get serious this time." He goes on to tell Shawn his girlfriend recently broke up with him because he was too "messed up" and kicked him out of her apartment. He now has no place to live and has also lost his job. The inpatient rehabilitation unit was full, so Shawn told Matt they would start with an outpatient program and he would need to return to the clinic next week. Shawn works directly with the schedulers to ensure that Mat can get an appointment ▶.

Episode 7

Shawn is not surprised that Matt Nolan does not show up for his appointment this week. It is very clear to Shawn that Matt needs help. However, until Matt decides he wants help, Shawn knows there is little he can do for him.

At monthly grand rounds, Shawn presents to his colleagues the findings of his study regarding problems getting patients into the clinic and barriers for follow-up appointments. In the conclusion of his presentation, he proposes changes to some of the operation policies at the clinic, including new procedures for managing new patients. He is disappointed that his colleagues - the ones who live with the inefficiencies on a daily basis - are less than enthusiastic about some of the changes he proposes. Rather than sharing his enthusiasm for making positive changes to improve patient services, most are reluctant to consider changes or offer alternative suggestions ▽.

Episode 8

A new patient, Aaron Hidalgo, is seen in the clinic this week. Aaron, a 52-year-old male, has multiple arrests for driving while intoxicated (DWI). As part of his sentence agreement, Aaron agrees to undergo mandatory treatment for his substance use in a relatively new program for habitual DWI offenders. Shawn is part of a clinical trial research team tracking data for this treatment as part of a state-wide assessment for possible legislation in the future. Shawn is well aware that individuals addicted to alcohol are among the most challenging to treat and, even with best intentions, their drop-out rate is high.

Because Aaron agrees to take part in the program, Shawn gives Aaron details about what the program entails. Aaron will be taking a drug called Vivitrol (naltrexone) that is used to treat alcohol addiction by blocking receptor sites. This drug is given once a month by injection and it is very important that individuals undergoing this treatment avoid alcohol and other street drugs while taking the medication. Shawn also tells Aaron that Vivitrol is only part of the addiction treatment plan. He needs to attend all counseling, group therapy, and education sessions ▽.

Episode 9

Aaron Hidalgo surprises Shawn when he shows up for group therapy and his individual appointment this week. Aaron tells Shawn it was a tough week, but he remains committed to "giving up the booze." Shawn is hopeful that Aaron keeps up with the treatment plan.

Shawn has an appointment with the medical director to discuss the reaction of his colleagues at the clinic to his study findings and proposed changes. After some discussion, Shawn and the medical director decide to collect a patient satisfaction survey. Perhaps having the perspectives of the patients would give them a better idea how to proceed ▽.

Episode 10

Blake Patterson makes a return visit to the clinic. He states he is beginning to have more energy, is sleeping better, but continues to struggle with relationship problems with his wife and daughter. His wife wants everything to go back to "the way things used to be" and he just can't get there. He finds they argue regularly, making him feel more depressed. He also tells Shawn that the nurse at his daughter's school told his wife Rebecca that their daughter has become increasingly withdrawn and her school performance is affected. Shawn talks with Blake about the possibility of family therapy.

Shawn works with a consulting group to conduct a patient satisfaction survey. They agree to a one-month data collection period. The consulting group will summarize the findings in a report ▶ ▽.

Episode 11

This week Shawn attends a national meeting of mental health nurse practitioners. He was selected as the plenary speaker to feature his work on the interdisciplinary collaborative research project related to substance abuse. His presentation receives high praise from attendees. After the presentation, Shawn is invited to join a national task force related to behavioral health initiatives for underserved populations. Shawn is very excited to have this opportunity! ▽

Episode 12

Shawn is pleased to see that Aaron Hidalgo continues to stay fully engaged with his treatment plan for alcohol abuse by attending group therapy, counseling sessions, and education sessions, and by getting his monthly injections. At a session led by Shawn this week, Aaron proudly tells the group he has now been sober for 6 weeks - longer than he has been in the past 10 years. As part of the group therapy they are asked to describe how they are feeling. Aaron says he thinks about drinking and admits he could not stay sober without the support of the group ▽ [NEWS].

Episode 13

Shawn sees Blake Patterson this week. He and his wife agree to try family counseling as a way to address some of the ongoing anger and relationship problems that linger. Shawn makes arrangements for them to attend a family counseling session with a family expert in the community ▽.

Episode 14

Sal Lucero makes a visit to see Shawn this week. He told Shawn he continues to go to the group therapy sessions and has made some progress, but he has not yet overcome many of his PTSD symptoms. He also shares with Shawn that he will be getting a therapy dog soon. The dog is in the final stages of training and he will begin learning to work with the dog.

Episode 15

Shawn and the medical director review the results of the patient satisfaction survey conducted by the consultant group along with several e-mails and letters received from patients. The information reflects a relatively high level of patient dissatisfaction with the Health Connections Clinic. The dissatisfaction is across all service lines - not just behavioral health. Although the quality of providers is rated high, the overall patient dissatisfaction was related to making appointments, the clinic chronically running behind schedule, and challenges in getting prescriptions refilled. This information mirrors some of the findings from Shawn's study. The medical director asks Shawn what his plans are for implementing changes to the clinic ▼.

Shawn Jacobs Season 3 Information

Episode 1

Shawn is a 35-year-old White male who works as a mental health nurse practitioner. He has been a psychiatric mental health nurse practitioner (PMHNP) for 7 years and completed a doctor of nursing practice (DNP) degree two years ago. Shawn has been working at a federally and state-funded community-based health clinic, called Neighborhood Health Connections Clinic, for 3 years.

Shawn has recently joined a national task force related to behavioral health initiatives for underserved populations. He has also been working with the clinic's medical director attempting to elicit change at the clinic based on findings from a study related to patient access and a recently completed survey on patient satisfaction.

Shawn gets a call to come to the front lobby. When he gets there he sees Sal Lucero proudly standing with a beautiful therapy dog. Sal thanks Shawn for paving the way for him to get his dog. Shawn anticipates this will be good for Sal. He asks him to keep in touch and let him know how it goes ▼.

Episode 2

The medical director holds a mandatory patient improvement retreat for all employees of Health Connections Clinic. The medical director talks about the need for a strategic plan that is patient-focused and provides high-quality care. He challenges all employees to work together to consider evidence collected and best practices to improve clinic operations.

Shawn presents the data from his study again, but this time it is presented along with collaborating evidence from the patient satisfaction survey. Using direct quotations from the patients, the information is transformed into a powerful call to action. The clinic providers become engaged in working toward new processes.

Episode 3

One of the clinic schedulers tells Shawn that one of the patients they had seen from time to time, Matt Nolan, is dead. Shawn looks up the story online in the local newspaper, which simply says he was found dead outside a bar with traumatic injuries. The death was ruled a homicide and is under investigation. Shawn feels intensely sad that he was unable to help Matt and wishes there could be more effective treatment options for patients like Matt. Shawn presents at a regional substance abuse conference this week ▼ [NEWS].

Episode 4

Shawn and his colleagues at the clinic present the proposed policy changes for clinic operations to the board of directors as well as to the state agency. The directors are impressed with the presentation and tell Shawn they will review the proposed policies further and will follow up with them ▼.

Episode 5

Shawn sees a familiar name on the clinic schedule for today - Amanda Hardin. It has been many months since he last saw Amanda, the former university student who fell into substance abuse. He is saddened when he sees her. She has lost a great deal of weight and looks pale. Amanda is tearful as she tells Shawn that she is homeless and is "working the streets" to get her fix. She is "owned" by a man named Ronald and has become fearful of what might happen next. She has not talked to her parents in months and needs his help fixing things. When asked about her recent drug use, Amanda tells Shawn she has been smoking a lot of heroin and marijuana because it is cheaper than using "oxy's." After a long discussion, Shawn agrees to help Amanda arrange a meeting with her parents.

Shawn meets with Amanda and her parents for a family session. Her mother is angry and tearful; she can't believe her daughter has ended up on the street as a prostitute. She also feels remorseful for kicking Amanda out of the house and wonders if this is all somehow her fault for driving Amanda away.

Amanda's parents are willing to help her again and all agree another try at an intense inpatient treatment would be Amanda's best option where she can focus on getting better without the fear of retaliation from Ronald. Shawn makes the appropriate arrangements, and Amanda leaves for the treatment facility with her parents. It would be the last time he sees Amanda ▶ ▼.

Episode 6

Shawn gets a call from Neighborhood Rehabilitation Hospital requesting a mental health consultation for a patient by the name of Mark Martin, a 27-year-old male who is reportedly depressed. Shawn reviews the medical record and learns that he suffered a spinal cord injury resulting in paraplegia a few weeks ago.

On the initial visit, Shawn conducts a comprehensive history and assessment, which includes a mental health assessment. Shawn does not find Mark particularly interested in discussing things, but he is easily able to determine that Mark is clinically depressed and would benefit from an antidepressant. After consulting with Katy, a pharmacist at the rehabilitation hospital, the decision is made to start Mark on duloxetine (Cymbalta) because it not only treats depression but also helps neuropathic pain ▼.

Episode 7

Shawn makes a trip to Neighborhood Rehabilitation Hospital to follow up with Mark Martin. Mark is still feeling very depressed and tells Shawn he had a fight with his fiance and feels angry with her. Shawn validates that there is significant change in roles and relationships with an injury like this. Although Mark still shows little interest in discussing things, Shawn believes he has made some progress in establishing trust with Mark.

Shawn asks the clinic's medical director if they have heard anything from the state agency related to their proposed policy changes. Shawn is told that they are still "under review."

Episode 8

During a visit to NBH rehabilitation hospital, Shawn has a worrisome conversation with Mark Martin. His fiance broke up with Mark and he has made statements of his life being over. He is concerned about the possibility of self-harm now, and especially when Mark is discharged. He encourages the nursing staff to check frequently on Mark and provide plenty of opportunity for him to talk.

Shawn sees a new patient, Clifford Allen, this week. Mr. Allen has a terminally ill wife and an adult son with Down syndrome. Because this is a first visit, Shawn completes a comprehensive history and assessment - including a thorough mental health assessment. Mr. Allen scores a 20 on the Center for Epidemiologic Studies Depression (CES-D) Scale, indicating moderate depression.

Based on the history, Shawn learns that Mr. Allen has not been sleeping well. Mr. Allen states he can't shut his mind off; his mind is constantly racing because he is worried about Pam, Gary, and finances. Mr. Allen admits to using alcohol to help him relax and fall asleep, but he still wakes up throughout the night ▼.

Shawn prescribes Bupropion hydrochloride (Wellbutrin) 150 mg orally each morning for depression and trazodone 100 mg orally at bedtime to help him sleep. He decides on trazodone because of Clifford's addictive personal traits. He also advises Clifford to stop drinking, because taking the medication in combination with alcohol could be dangerous. and because drinking alcohol actually interferes with sleep. Shawn asks Clifford to come back again later in the week.

Episode 9

Shawn sees Mr. Allen again this week and learns that his wife passed away two days ago. He acknowledges the significance of the loss and is glad Clifford kept the appointment. Shawn specifically assesses Mr. Allen for activating symptoms and increased depression, and asks if he has slept since his wife died. Shawn reminds Mr. Allen that he has not been taking the antidepressant long enough to reach full therapeutic effect, but confirms that he has been taking the medication and asks about any side effects. The dose has been increased to 300 mg a day. Shawn recommends Hospice Grief Counseling for both Mr. Allen and his son. Clifford tells Shawn he had been told about this by another nurse and that he might have to check into it, but he wonders if he needs this in addition to his appointments with Shawn. Shawn explains that there are different benefits from group therapy that cannot be gained from one-on-one appointments. He encourages Clifford to do both and to return next week.

A new patient, Helen Martin, is seen in the clinic this week. Shawn learns about recent events and Mrs. Martin's referral from cardiology for a possible anxiety disorder. Shawn completes a comprehensive history and assessment, including a thorough mental health assessment. When Mrs. Martin mentions a paraplegic step-son, Shawn wonders if Mrs. Martin is related to Mark.

Mrs. Martin tells Shawn that she has been taking Ativan (lorazepam), but she feels like she is on a "see saw" - going from feeling good to feeling anxious. Based on the history and exam, and after reviewing Mrs. Martin's medical records from the emergency department visit and cardiologist, Shawn orders laboratory work to check her thyroid function. He also starts Mrs. Martin on buspirone 10 mg every day and Zoloft (sertraline) 50 mg daily. For now, Mrs. Martin is advised to take the Ativan as needed only if she feels anxious.

A few days later, Shawn learns that Mark Martin will be soon discharged and a different medical group will be following Mark for his depression. Shawn has a phone conversation with the psychiatrist to go over Mark's care thus far NEWS.

Episode 10

Mr. Allen is in for a visit early in the week. Shawn again conducts a mental health assessment and determines Clifford is not declining following his wife's death. Mr. Allen confirms he is not drinking and is still taking the medications; Clifford thinks the medications are making a difference. When he mentions that he hates how the medications seem to make his mouth so dry, Shawn recommends drinking water, hard candy or chewing gum to minimize the symptoms. Mr. Allen tells Shawn that he has signed up for grief counseling and will be attending his first session next week.

On the same day, Shawn sees a new patient by the name of Anthony Martin. According to the medical records, this young man has major depression and psychosis and has been in and out of mental health systems. His story seems familiar, but Shawn can't quite remember from what context. Shawn attempts to complete a comprehensive mental health examination but has a hard time getting cooperation from Anthony. He does not say much and declines the option for Shawn to get a history from his parents. Shawn tells Anthony he is aware of the challenges he has had taking medications and wants him to think about the option of a long-acting injection of risperidone that would only require a shot once every two weeks as opposed to taking pills every day. Anthony tells Shawn he will think about it.

Later in the week, Shawn also sees Mrs. Helen Martin in the clinic. He learns that Mrs. Martin has had a very stressful week between having her paraplegic son discharged from the rehabilitation hospital to the home and her daughter moving out of the house. Shawn suddenly understands the complexity of the situation when he realizes Mrs. Martin is Anthony Martin's mother and Mark Martin's step-mother. This is truly a family in crisis! Mrs. Martin cries as she describes how overwhelmed she feels. She feels as though she has no control over anything. Mrs. Martin states she is using the Ativan "a lot" to help her make it through each day. Shawn increases the buspirone dose to 20 mg every day and the Zoloft dose to 100 mg daily. For now, Mrs. Martin is advised to take the Ativan only if she is feeling very anxious. He advises Mrs. Martin to return in a week. At the conclusion of the visit, Mrs. Martin says, "You know, my son Anthony is now being seen at this clinic. Do you know him?" Knowing the need for honesty and balancing this with maintaining confidentiality, Shawn responds by saying, "Mrs. Martin, the clinic sees many patients and all encounters are confidential ▶ ▼."

Episode 11

Mrs. Martin is in the office again this week. She tells Shawn that she is feeling exhausted from the stress of caring for Mark and worried sick because her son Anthony stormed out of the house after an argument and she has not seen or heard from him in several days. Shawn recalled that Anthony was a "no show" for an appointment this week. This news is very worrisome to Shawn because things can get very dangerous for Anthony if he is not taking his medications.

Despite all the issues Helen faced this week, she tells Shawn that she believes the medications (buspirone and wellbutrin [Zoloft]) are helping and that she is still taking Ativan. Shawn gives Helen several referrals for caregiver assistance and suggests that Helen consider family counseling. Shawn asks Helen to come back to the clinic in a week ▼.

Episode 12

Shawn sees Mr. Allen in the clinic this week. He asks Clifford how he is feeling and completes a mental status assessment. Shawn finds Clifford to be coping reasonably well. Shawn praises Mr. Allen for establishing a set routine and for making special time to spend with his son. He encourages Clifford to continue the grief counseling, and specifically advises Clifford to eat regularly, avoid alcohol, get plenty of sleep, and continue taking his medication. When Mr. Allen mentions that he is considering retiring to focus his attention on Gary, Shawn points out that retiring right now represents another loss and he might want to hold off on making any major decisions right now.

Shawn does a presentation on mental health issues among veterans this week at a local Sigma Theta Tau meeting. He meets Violet Brinkworth, a nurse from the Neighborhood School System, who tells him she has heard good things about his work. Shawn is happy to have his efforts positively acknowledged ▶ ▼.

Episode 13

Mrs. Martin makes another visit to the clinic this week. Helen tells Shawn that things have settled down a little bit in her household.

She tells Shawn that Anthony is living at a friend's house but he has not returned her messages. Helen asks if Anthony has been coming to the clinic for his appointments; Shawn tells Helen he is unable to comment. Helen says she worries about him but is at least glad to know where he is. At the end of the visit Mrs. Martin mentions that she ran out of Ativan last week and wants to get a refill; Shawn tells Helen that probably won't be necessary since her other medications are helping her at this point.

Episode 14

Mr. Allen meets with Shawn this week and reports he is really beginning to feel better. He states he is sleeping well, eating well, has given up alcohol completely, and has more energy now than he has had in months.

Mr. Allen also tells Shawn that he made a decision to retire. He is sure this is the right decision and hopes Shawn is not angry with him for making this decision. Clifford also asks Shawn when he can stop taking the bupropion (Wellbutrin) ▼.

Episode 15

Shawn is very glad Mr. Allen kept his appointment this week. He was a bit worried that Mr. Allen might have decided to stop all his treatment measures, which could have had significant consequences. Mr. Allen stated he had his retirement party and was actually feeling a bit down now that his retirement is official. Mr. Allen verbalized an understanding of the risk of stopping treatment and recognizes his need to stay healthy not only for himself, but for Gary.

Shawn learns from Mrs. Martin that Anthony Martin is on the streets. He keeps an eye out for him every morning and evening on his commute from home to work. Just maybe he will see Anthony so he can reach out to him.

HOSPITAL

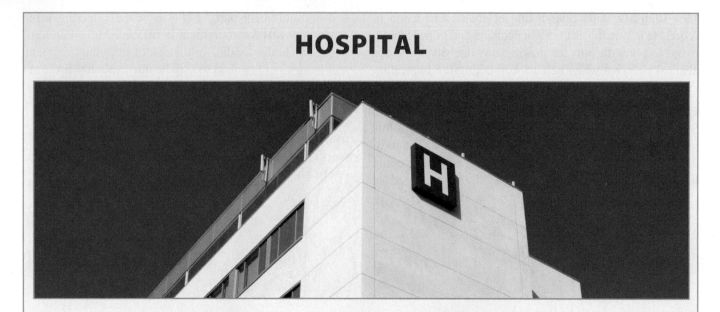

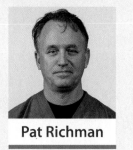

Pat Richman

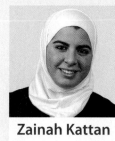

Zainah Kattan

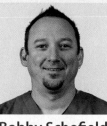

Bobby Schofield

Housing

Parks and Recreation

Services
There is regular bus service to the Hospital from all sections of The Neighborhood. There are many convenience stores and a variety of eating establishments within 6 blocks. There is one grocery store located 2 blocks from the Hospital. There is a corner park within 1 block.

Key: ▶ = video clip   ☰ = medical record   ▽ = journal entry   [NEWS] = news article

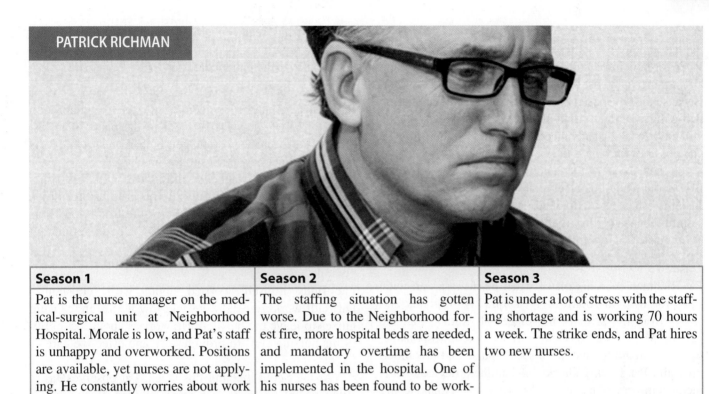

PATRICK RICHMAN

Season 1	Season 2	Season 3
Pat is the nurse manager on the medical-surgical unit at Neighborhood Hospital. Morale is low, and Pat's staff is unhappy and overworked. Positions are available, yet nurses are not applying. He constantly worries about work and his staff's ability to provide safe, effective care to their patients. In fact, a medication error by a student nurse nearly causes a patient's death. Pat receives a complaint from a patient about one of his nurses.	The staffing situation has gotten worse. Due to the Neighborhood forest fire, more hospital beds are needed, and mandatory overtime has been implemented in the hospital. One of his nurses has been found to be working under the influence of drugs.	Pat is under a lot of stress with the staffing shortage and is working 70 hours a week. The strike ends, and Pat hires two new nurses.

Patrick Richman Season 1 Information

Episode 1
Patrick Richman is a 47-year-old nurse manager who works on the general medical-surgical unit at Neighborhood Hospital. He has been a nurse for over 20 years and has been the unit manager for the past 8 years. He originally earned an associate degree in nursing and went back to school to earn a bachelor's degree in nursing about 10 years ago. Pat considers himself to be a laid-back person and feels he has a good rapport with his staff. He is married and has two sons. He serves as an Assistant Scoutmaster for his son's Boy Scout troop.

Although Pat has been a successful nurse manager for years, lately he has been feeling like he isn't doing a good job. The staff is overworked and unhappy, and overall morale is low. He has tried to solve the problems with the staff, but the bottom line is that the unit needs more employees, but no one is applying for the empty positions. The morale is low not only on his unit, but also throughout the hospital. The chief nursing officer hires an outside agency to conduct an employee survey to understand the source of the low morale ▼.

Episode 2
Pat talks with Bobby, the acting charge nurse on the unit. Bobby informs him that they are short a nursing tech, and that the nursing supervisor won't find them any help. Bobby seems very upset with Pat when he explains that he will do his best to get help from an agency, but he can't promise him anything.

Episode 3
Debbie Koch, the nursing instructor from the local nursing program, has a meeting with Pat to review the goals and objectives of the clinical course she is teaching and asks Pat to be sure his nursing staff are aware of this information. Pat often wonders if he would enjoy a teaching position - especially on days when he feels worn down from the challenges associated with running a nursing unit ▼.

Episode 4

Pat has another stressful week at work. Mandatory in-services for new intravenous pumps must be scheduled, and all nursing staff must be educated by the end of the week. Because the unit-based educator recently quit, Pat ends up doing much of the training himself. Pat also learns that he will have to take an advanced degree and wonders how he can possibly find the time.

A new boy by the name of Jason Riley joins the Boy Scout troop this week. Pat can immediately see that Jason is a boy who is picked on by his peers. He puts a stop to the teasing during the meeting, and lets the senior Scoutmaster know of the situation.

Episode 5

Pat Richman is in his office when he hears a unit-wide page for help in room 547. Pat quickly responds and learns from the primary nurse, Zainah Kattan, that the patient, Mr. Larson, has suddenly become unresponsive, but he is breathing and has a strong pulse and low blood pressure. Pat quickly checks his handheld device for his medical information and sees Mr. Larson is a diabetic and recently received a dose of insulin. Pat suspects he has acute Hypoglycemia and suggests checking his blood glucose level. After confirming that it is low, Pat administers 50% Dextrose in water IV push per the standard unit protocol. Mr. Larson quickly recovers.

Later in the afternoon, he debriefs with Zainah and Jennifer. After asking them both questions, he asks Jennifer to show him on the syringe how much insulin she gave and determines the problem was caused by an incorrect dose. Pat learns from Jennifer that her instructor, Debbie Koch, was with another student doing a procedure with a patient, so she asked Bobby to help her. Pat later talked with Bobby about the incident. Bobby told Pat he only watched the student give the medication - that the student led him to believe the instructor had already checked the dose. Bobby also told Pat he does not know Mr. Larson and can't possibly know everything about all the patients. Pat helps Zainah complete the documentation reporting the incident for the Quality-Safety Committee ▶ ▼.

Episode 6

Pat always takes his two children to the annual Neighborhood Rodeo, but he can't make it this year because he has been working so many hours. In addition to his regular managerial duties, this week, he even had to pick up a shift on the floor because of staff calling in sick. It was the first shift he had worked in 8 months, and it was exhausting. His staff members have also been working far more than they should, with some nurses working five 12-hour shifts a week and others working extra-long shifts. He has real concerns about the long hours and patient safety, but knows they have to have nurses on the floor to cover the patient care [NEWS].

Episode 7

Pat reads about the problems with the Neighborhood Hospital Emergency Department in the paper. The last thing he needs is the hospital getting bad press while he is trying to attract new nurses to his unit [NEWS].

Pat enjoys a weekend hiking trip with his son's Boy Scout troop. He continues to observe Jason Riley's interactions with the other boys in the troop and wonder what kinds of problems he might be experiencing at school.

Episode 8

Pat finds himself worried about work constantly. Difficult working conditions and low wages are causing nurses to leave the hospital. He worries about the ability of his nursing staff to provide safe and effective care to the patients.

At the Scout meeting this week, Pat observes Jason Riley go into a rage after being scolded by the senior Scoutmaster for his behavior. Pat talks with Jason to settle him down. He then talks to the head Scoutmaster about his perceptions regarding Jason and ways to redirect the boy's behavior positively, but the frustrated Scoutmaster simply says, "We are not babysitters, and I don't need troublemakers in this troop ▼."

Episode 9

Pat receives a report from the Quality-Safety Committee regarding the Root-cause analysis conducted from a significant medication error that occurred on the unit months ago. The finding from the analysis was a procedural failure with the administration of a medication involving a nursing student, nursing instructor, and two staff nurses. It is recommended that Pat meet with the nursing instructor to review the situation and follow recommended guidelines when nursing students are passing medications on the unit. He is also advised to review the process with his nursing staff. No disciplinary actions are recommended by the committee ▼.

Episode 10

Pat has received a complaint about Bobby, filed by Dr. Ocampo, the husband of a patient. Dr. Ocampo states that Bobby was rude and was not taking care of his wife properly. Pat knows he needs to address the issue, but will not have time this week ▼.

Episode 11

Pat has a meeting with Bobby this week to discuss the complaint filed by Dr. Ocampo. Bobby is quick to point out that when you have nurses like Zainah Kattan and the student nurses spending all their time in Mrs. Ocampo's room, anybody else just going in and getting the work done is going to seem pretty rude. Bobby tells Pat that Zainah is really disorganized and suggests he look at her time management. Pat does know that Bobby seems more efficient with his time and wonders if there is not some truth to what he has to say. Still, Pat knows Bobby is a bit of a manipulator and recognizes these two nurses just don't get along ▶.

Episode 12

The hospital executive leadership team, that includes the Chief Executive Officer and the Chief Nursing Officer, has announced an interest in getting a new medication administration system. They appoint Pat to an interdisciplinary committee, led by the pharmacy division to develop a request for proposals from vendors regarding their systems. Pat agrees to serve on the committee because he knows nursing needs to be represented, but he wonders how he will fit yet another obligation into his schedule.

Episode 13

Pat attends a meeting for nurse managers. The managers are informed that the hospital administration is implementing mandatory overtime for nurses in the near future. Pat is told not to say anything to his staff.

Pat missed the Boy Scout meeting last week, but was disappointed to learn that Jason Riley had been kicked out of the troop by the Scoutmaster. He realizes Jason has problems, but wishes he could have had a positive experience in the troop.

Episode 14

Pat meets with the interdisciplinary committee to begin discussions about developing a request for proposals for a new medication administration system. The committee chair, Dr. Lee Dykes, PharmD, is the pharmacy manager. He presents an overview of the type of new systems available and the new systems on the horizon. Pat is amazed at how much change is taking place – particularly as it relates to technology.

Episode 15

Pat reads about the plans for a new cancer treatment facility that will be built at the hospital. He wonders where the administrators plan to get nursing staff for the facility and worries that it will attract nurses away from his unit. He agrees that the new facility is a good idea, but does not think the administration is reality-based in their decision.

The interdisciplinary committee Pat is serving on for the new medication administration system completes the request for proposals and sends this back to the hospital executive team. Despite the work involved, Pat enjoys interactions with members of the committee. He finds he learns so much when working with professionals from other disciplines 🟦NEWS.

Patrick Richman Season 2 Information

Episode 1

Lately, Pat has been very concerned about nursing shortages on his unit.

Pat meets with Zainah Kattan, whom he considers an ideal employee. She has been doing a great job, and Pat reluctantly agrees to her request to start cross-training for the sub-acute care unit. Although Pat wants to allow Zainah other opportunities, he does not want her to leave his unit. He decides to start the cross-training slowly so that he doesn't lose her anytime soon.

Episode 2

The unit is going to be short on staff again. Pat is relieved when Bobby agrees to pick up extra night shifts. Earlier in the day, Zainah Kattan had complained to him that a student and Bobby were flirting a lot; Pat decided that was the least of his concerns - he needed the unit covered and Bobby was helping him out a great deal by working the extra shifts 🔽.

Episode 3

The clinical nursing instructor, Debbie Koch comes by Pat's office, closes the door and asks to speak with him. She tells Pat about her concerns that one of his nurses, Bobby is flirting too much with one of her students. She also tells Pat she suspects they might be involved in a relationship. Pat tells Debbie that he is not about to get involved with the personal lives of his nurses and there is not a rule against such relationships. He tells Dr. Koch that one nurse mentioned there was some flirting going on, but there was no evidence that patient care was being negatively impacted. Dr. Koch is obviously not happy with his position and leaves his office. Pat decides he should probably monitor the situation ▶🔽.

Episode 4

Pat makes a point to be out on the unit this week to assess concerns about excessive flirting or unprofessional behavior among his staff. He observes Bobby off and on during over two consecutive days while the students are there and sees no evidence of flirting - in fact, his assessment of Bobby is that he acting like he always does. Pat wonders why he is spending his time on silly unfounded issues and decides Dr. Koch and Zainah are probably being overly sensitive. He hears no additional complaints and does not think about it further.

Episode 5

The Neighborhood forest fire has made the entire hospital crazy. There are far more patients needing hospital beds than are available, and the nurses in the Emergency Department keep calling to the unit, demanding that they make beds available.

Pat becomes really angry when he attends an administrative meeting in which the managers are informed that mandatory overtime will be instituted at the hospital beginning the next pay period. He can't believe how bad their timing is [NEWS].

Episode 6

Pat holds a staff meeting that he has been dreading the whole week. He announces mandatory overtime to the staff and can feel the tension in the room. He has brought muffins and coffee to try to improve the staff's mood, but he can see that this clearly has not helped. The person he thought would be most negative about the news was Bobby. Pat is surprised that Bobby says little during the meeting [NEWS].

Episode 7

Pat is working to revise the budget when Debbie Koch, the clinical nursing instructor walks into his office with Jacob McCain, the nursing student, and closes the door. Pat thinks to himself, this can't be good! Debbie asks Jacob to share with Pat his concerns. Jacob tells Pat that one of the patients he is caring for this week, Mr. Alden, was recently seen by social services for possible elder abuse. He tells Pat he knows this because of his previous clinic rotation at the Neighborhood Senior Center. He goes on to tell Pat that the social worker asked to be informed of additional suspicious injuries. He tried to tell Bobby but was pretty sure Bobby was not going to act on it. Jacob gives Pat the contact information for the nurse at the Senior Center Clinic, Karen Williams.

Pat thanks Jacob and Debbie Koch for coming forward with this information and says that he will be sure to follow up on it. After they leave, Pat makes a call to the social services director for a consultation and passes along Karen Williams contact information. He later talks with Bobby about this and Bobby denies that the student mentioned this to him [NEWS].

Episode 8

Pat is pulled off the unit for two full days to attend strategic planning meetings for the Neighborhood Hospital system. Pat recognizes the need for strategic planning, but he also gets frustrated when excessive time is spent doing these activities. New mission and vision statements are created, new strategic goals are identified, but then it seems that there is little visible change in the actual day-to-day activities at the point of patient care. Pat wonders if the hospital executive leadership team (the Chief Executive Officer, the Chief Operating Officer, the Chief Nursing Officer, and the Chief Financial Officer) are aware of how poorly big ideas from strategic planning filter down to the unit level ▼.

Episode 9

Pat gets a page from Zainah Kattan requesting immediate assistance with one of her patients. Mr. Alden's condition has become critical and the physician wants to intubate him and send him to the medical intensive care unit. Pat makes the necessary calls to get Mr. Alden transferred and then helps Zainah complete the transfer. After the event, Zainah talks to him about the fact that she should have called sooner - she just knew something was wrong, but did not know what. Pat assures Zainah that developing clinical judgment takes time and the fact that she was aware reflects her growing expertise. In the future, with a similar set of circumstances she will know to take action sooner. Pat is not sure he provided much comfort to Zainah, but he was very proud with the way she managed things.

Episode 10

Pat learns that Mr. Alden, the patient who was recently on his unit, died in the intensive care unit from respiratory failure. He feels badly that Mr. Alden never got out of the hospital following his injuries. He wonders what the status of the abuse investigation is and hopes that none of his staff will have to testify.

Episode 11

Pat is surprised when Zainah makes an appointment with him to talk about Bobby. Zainah tells Pat that she suspects Bobby may be working under the influence of drugs. Although Pat has never seen Bobby as a model employee, he certainly never suspected anything like this. He wonders if this is just the latest episode in the Bobby versus Zainah feud ▼.

Episode 12

Pat has decided to keep a close eye on Bobby without letting anyone know. He spends more time on the unit when Bobby is working. Additionally, Pat interviews some of Bobby's patients to learn about their perceptions of his care ▽.

Episode 13

Pat continues watching Bobby. He has not actually caught Bobby doing anything wrong, yet he strongly suspects he is taking narcotics. Pat knows what he must do, but is feeling overwhelmed with all that has been going on lately. Pat contacts his supervisor, the area director of nursing, and the human resources department, to make sure he handles this situation appropriately ▽.

Episode 14

Pat receives a phone call from Zainah Kattan at 7 a.m., informing him that she thinks Bobby is "messed up." After observing Bobby for a few minutes, Pat relieves him of his duties and orders Bobby to submit a urine sample for a drug screening. Pat is extremely disappointed, but not surprised, when he is notified that Bobby tests positive for several types of drugs. In addition to having to deal with this, Pat is now down yet another nurse. Because Bobby belongs to the nursing union, he also fully expects they will get involved. He just hates having to deal with that ▽.

Episode 15

Pat learns that Bobby has decided to enter the diversion program. He is hopeful that Bobby will be successful and will be able to return to work, although he knows it is unlikely he will come back to his unit because of the high volume of narcotic drugs and ease of access ▽ [NEWS].

Patrick Richman Season 3 Information

Episode 1

Pat considers himself to be a pretty laid-back person, but the past several months have been very stressful. He has seen a lot of changes at the hospital in the past 5 years, but has a feeling that bigger changes are still to come.

While attending a nurse manager's meeting, Pat becomes anxious and angry about an announcement made by the hospital's chief nursing officer (CNO). Supporting a national move for a more educated workforce, the CNO announced that all future staff nurse hires would be for BSN-prepared nurses, and that all staff nurses will be required to get a BSN degree within the next four years. She went on to report that nurse managers will be required to have a graduate degree. The CNO also offered tuition assistance and flexible scheduling for nurses needing to go back to school for the advanced degree.

Pat feels frustrated with this decision. How will he work around the scheduling issues among nurses on his unit so that they can attend class? He also feels anxious because he is one of the nurse managers employed at Neighborhood hospital without a graduate degree. "Have I not been doing a good enough job?" he wonders. He originally got an associate degree and already went back to school once to get a BSN degree. Going back to school yet a third time is not something he really ever planned to do ▽.

Episode 2

Pat, the employee health nurse, and the human resources representative meet with Bobby to discuss his treatment plan. Bobby tells them that the meetings are going well, and he hopes he can go back to work as a nurse soon.

Episode 3

Pat feels like he just can't get a break. In addition to the nursing shortage and the situation with Bobby, now a disgusting pervert who raped and killed a 6-year-old child has been admitted to his unit. He starts to wonder if life really needs to be this stressful and resolves to think about looking for a new position with less responsibility. He laughs to himself when he thinks about what a position at the new cancer treatment facility would be like ▽ [NEWS].

Episode 4

Although he knows he will have to deal with it, Pat must suppress the anger he feels toward a patient on his unit. After the way he has treated some of the nurses, Pat feels angry that the accused rapist has complained about the care he has received from nurses on his unit. Does he expect to be treated like royalty? As far as Pat is concerned, any pain he has experienced is only a fraction of the pain that the little girl's family must be feeling ▽ [NEWS].

Episode 5

Just when Pat thought things couldn't get any worse, the nurse's union is threatening to strike. Among other things, the union is upset about the mandate that staff nurses must get a BSN degree. He really can't blame them for being angry. As a leader he maintains confidence and optimism when talking with the nursing staff, but when alone in his office he ponders how he will keep things together during the strike [NEWS].

Episode 6

Pat has gotten over the shock of having to go back to get a graduate degree. He talks with the nursing instructor, Debbie Koch, and learns she recently completed a doctoral degree - and survived. After checking around, he realizes many nursing programs offer MSN and doctoral degrees online. The flexibility of "attending" class online is very convenient, although he realizes he will have a significant learning curve while getting used to an online learning platform.

Pat completes an application at three colleges - all offering concentrations in nurse executive and organizational leadership. Two of the programs offer a master's degree, but his first-choice program is a doctor of nursing practice degree that admits students with a bachelor's degree. Pat decides if he is lucky enough to be offered admission to the doctoral program, he might as well "go for gold" and earn the doctoral degree ▶ ▾.

Episode 7

Pat has not heard anything further about the strike. He figures no news is good news. Unfortunately, he has heard news about Bobby. His license has been suspended, and there is nothing Pat can do about it. He has been under so much stress that he has been getting stress headaches. He has to take an analgesic to help reduce the pain [NEWS].

Episode 8

This week, the nurses at Neighborhood Hospital stage a walkout. Pat had to work on the unit again and calls in anyone not involved in the strike who might be willing to come in. He cannot believe that the nurses would neglect the patients and is disappointed by their lack of commitment! The hospital responds by closing the hospital to admissions and discharging any patient they can. Also, several agency nurses and traveling nurses are hired to help. Pat is grateful for the help, but it is hard to manage the unit with temporary help ▾ [NEWS].

Episode 9

The nursing strike continues, and Pat finds himself working 70-hour weeks. He finds it stressful crossing the picket lines with some nurses, whom he considered friends, taunting him. He is barely able to get enough nurses to cover the unit, but does so between some of his own nurses, like Zainah Kattan, working additional hours and the temporary agency and traveling nurses. Pat wonders if the chief nursing officer thinks forcing nurses to get higher educational degrees is worth the additional tension [NEWS].

Episode 10

Pat is relieved that the nursing strike is over and that he has more staff available to cover shifts. Pat has four interviews lined up for nursing positions on his unit. The hospital has offered a sign-on bonus, which has attracted nurses from nearby communities ▾ [NEWS].

Episode 11

Pat is surprised at the number of applications for nursing positions the hospital is receiving. Word that the hiring preference is for BSN-prepared nurses has gotten out, and many nurses are applying from other hospitals because of the improved benefits for nurses who have a BSN degree. Pat recognizes his reaction to the new hospital mandate was emotionally based and that he was wrong ▾.

Episode 12

Pat is surprised to get a phone call from Bobby Schofield this week. It has been a while since he heard from him. Bobby tells Pat he would like to meet him for coffee and a talk. The next day, Pat meets Bobby for coffee and they talk for hours. Bobby tells Pat about his friend Jim and that he is off the booze and drugs, but needs to continue working on his problem. Pat can see the Bobby has changed. He agrees to write a letter of support for Bobby to reenter the diversion program.

Episode 13

Pat is pleased with the applicants he has interviewed during the past few weeks. He decides to hire a new BSN graduate nurse from the local university and a BSN-prepared nurse with many years of experience.

Episode 14

Pat is pleasantly surprised to receive notification of acceptance to the doctor of nursing practice (DNP) program in nurse executive and organizational leadership. Never in his wildest dreams did he ever think he would be working on a doctoral degree. Although he feels intimidated and nervous, Pat is very excited and looks forward to the beginning of his first class ▾ [NEWS].

Episode 15

Pat is happy when Zainah Kattan accepts the charge nurse position on his unit. Because of her high standards and enthusiasm for nursing, he knows she is just the right person for the position.

Pat is pleasantly surprised when he hears that Bobby has been attending AA meetings regularly and seems to be turning his life around. Pat is also relieved that things finally seem to be turning around at work.

ZAINAH KATTAN

Season 1	Season 2	Season 3
Zainah Kattan is a 23-year-old nurse who has lived in a tight-knit Muslim community in The Neighborhood her whole life. She recently completed orientation on the medical-surgical unit at Neighborhood Hospital. Due to increased patient loads and staffing issues, Zainah stays late to do patient charting and picks up extra shifts. She is anxious about being assigned two nursing students, including Jennifer Porter. Zainah becomes extremely fatigued and overwhelmed at times, but her confidence gradually increases.	Zainah receives good feedback from her nurse manager, Pat. Her confidence as a nurse continues to build, yet she is still exhausted at the end of the day. Zainah trains student nurses again, including Kayla Sharif, who questions the kind of clothes Zainah wears. She has problems with another nurse on the unit who flirts with Kayla instead of working. He seems unstable and she suspects substance abuse. As her long work hours continue, Zainah also has problems within her relationship with her fiancé.	Zainah expands her nursing experience by joining a state-level work group. She faces sexual and cultural harrassment from an accused rapist and finds it very hard to care for this patient. The nurse's union goes on strike, leaving Zainah to work many extra shifts. She continues to have problems in her relationship and decides to call off the wedding.

Zainah Kattan Season 1 Information

Episode 1

Zainah Kattan is a 23-year-old nurse who graduated from nursing school seven months ago with a BSN degree. Since graduation, she has been working on a general medical-surgical inpatient unit at Neighborhood Hospital, and has recently come off orientation. She has been told she will primarily work 12-hour day shift, but all staff are expected to work "off shifts" when the need arises. Zainah has a long-term goal of working in an adult Intensive Care Unit. She has been saving her money and looks forward to buying her first new car.

Zainah has lived in The Neighborhood her entire life - in fact she was born at Neighborhood Hospital. Her parents are originally from Syria and raised Zainah and her older brother and sister in a tight-knit Muslim community. Zainah lives alone in an apartment and follows traditional Muslim practices. She recently entered into an Islamic engagement with Abdul Salan, a man she has

known since childhood. To stay healthy, Zainah watches what she eats and maintains a regular workout routine consisting of walking, running, and riding a bicycle.

Zainah has a busy week. Because of increased patient admissions, she has seven to eight patients of her own. She finds it a challenge to document all the patient care she does within the electronic medical records. Zainah's manager, Pat, talks with her about this and gives her advice about time management and point-of-care charting. The feedback he gives her is generally positive. He also asks Zainah if she is available to cover extra shifts. Zainah agrees to take a night shift next week and also volunteers at the immunization clinic [NEWS].

Episode 2

A new group of nursing students has begun a clinical rotation on the unit this week. Zainah is very anxious about the possibility of working with the students because it has only been seven months since she graduated and she is sure she does not know enough to be working with them. She hopes that no students are assigned to work with her patients, because she doesn't think she can manage her own work and a student. The clinical instructor, Dr. Debbie Koch, was one of her instructors when she was in her first year of school. Zainah asks her former instructor several questions during the two days she is on the unit and is really happy to have access to her expertise ✉.

Episode 3

Zainah covers an extra shift again this week. She and her fiance, Abdul, participate in the "Run for Fish" event in the community. She has not been exercising as regularly as she used to because she can't seem to find the time. She has started to gain a little weight and is feeling self-conscious. The run is a fun opportunity to be active again ⬛.

Episode 4

Zainah was relieved the past few weeks when no nursing students were assigned to any of her patients. Her luck ran out this week when Zainah realized she had not one, but two, nursing students assigned to her patients. Zainah feels very nervous about working with students, yet she vows to be as helpful as possible. She knows how discouraging it is to be in a clinical setting, trying to learn, and have the nurses be unkind or ignore you.

Even though the clinical instructor is on the unit, Zainah feels responsible and double-checks everything the students do. Fortunately, everything goes well with the students, but Zainah feels exhausted and emotionally drained after they leave the unit.

Episode 5

A nursing student by the name of Jennifer Porter is assigned to take care of one of Zainah's patients this week. Jennifer is a first-year student in Debbie Koch's clinical group. Her assigned patient, Mr. Larson, is an elderly diabetic patient. Zainah reviews Mr. Larson's care with Jennifer to be sure there is clarity about what care is needed. When Zainah goes to lunch, she lets Jennifer know that Bobby, one of the other nurses, is covering for her. When she returns from lunch, Jennifer reports to Zainah that she just administered 3 units of regular insulin to Mr. Larson because his blood glucose was 232 mg/dL. Zainah was able to confirm the correct dose was given as described by looking at the medication administration record and noting Bobby's co-signature.

About 40 minutes later, Jennifer rushes out of Mr. Larson's room yelling for help. Zainah and several staff respond and find Mr. Larson unresponsive, yet breathing. He has a pulse and his blood pressure is 100/57. Zainah

is frightened and does not know what to do. Fortunately, Pat Richman is there and calmly suggests checking the blood glucose level. While Zainah and Jennifer check the glucose, Pat pages the attending physician. Zainah and Jennifer find the level to be at 36 mg/dL. Pat says, "Well, that would make anyone unresponsive! Let's give him a bolus of dextrose IV." Mr. Larson is given the Dextrose and shortly thereafter the physician arrives to assess the situation. Mr. Larson recovers without further incident.

In a debriefing about the situation, Zainah is devastated as Pat asks her questions about what might have happened. She feels the situation is entirely her fault. Zainah tells Pat about the student giving insulin before lunch and can't understand how his glucose level dropped from 232 mg/dL to 36 mg/dL in such a short period of time. Pat asks Jennifer to show him on the syringe how much insulin she gave Mr. Larson. When Jennifer shows Pat, it immediately becomes clear that Jennifer made an error in reading the insulin syringe. She gave Mr. Larson 30 units of regular insulin - 10 times the appropriate dose. Jennifer begins to cry because she is sure she will be kicked out of nursing school for making a medication error. Zainah is angry with Bobby because he was the one to sign off on the medication. Pat tells Zainah not to worry, and that he will deal with Bobby. He then shows Zainah how to fill out the necessary documentation for the Quality-Safety Committee ✉.

Episode 6

Zainah stays to cover part of a second shift and is at the hospital for 17 hours. She is exhausted and must return the following morning at 7 a.m. She wonders if this impacts the quality of her care. Zainah often feels very irritated with her coworker, Bobby, who always seems to have time to take long breaks. After the medication error incident from the previous week, Zainah has little respect for him.

Episode 7

The Quality-Safety officer contacts Zainah this week to review the medication incident that occurred in recent weeks. Zainah is told they are conducting a root-cause analysis (RCA) of the situation. Zainah is very nervous about the meeting, fearing she will be found negligent in her supervision of a student. Instead, Zainah finds the discussion very positive and helpful. She finds the process is not one in which they are attempting to establish fault but rather to gain a better understanding of the system failures with intent to minimize the possibility of a similar situation happening again ✉.

Episode 8

Zainah is feeling more comfortable at work. She is working with Jennifer Porter again this week and no longer dwells on the medication incident that occurred previously. Zainah is finding it easier to work with nursing students and realizes she does know enough to help them learn. Zainah is really impressed with how much Jennifer has learned since starting her rotation.

Zainah has also decided to start taking action with Bobby when he is not following through with things. Specifically this week she says something to Bobby when she notices that his call lights are frequently on when he is in the break room. Although he does not respond to her in a kind way, Zainah decides she will take the high ground and be professional in all her interactions with him ▶.

Episode 9

Zainah reads about increased alcohol and drug use in the Neighborhood Newspaper. As a practicing Muslim, she does not drink alcohol or use any drugs. She sometimes finds herself feeling angry with alcohol- and drug-abusing patients. She thinks that they have brought many of their problems on themselves [NEWS].

Episode 10

One of Zainah's patients this week is Mrs. Ocampo, an elderly woman who was admitted to the unit following surgery for a hip fracture. She has Alzheimer's disease and is extremely confused. She yells frequently, and speaks in a language that Zainah can't understand. At the start of the day shift, Zainah and Jennifer find that Mrs. Ocampo pulled her IV out. Zainah has to get the IV restarted before she does anything else - and this makes her feel behind for the rest of the day. Fortunately, the nursing student, Jennifer Porter, is assigned to take care of Mrs. Ocampo, and she is able to help keep a close eye on her to keep her safe. Zainah is so happy to have the extra help! Zainah notices that Mrs. Ocampo seems to be calm only when her husband is present. Zainah takes a special interest in Mrs. Ocampo and works hard to provide exceptional care to her.

Episode 11

Mrs. Ocampo is still on the unit this week. She has calmed down but is still combative at times. Zainah has formed a rapport with her husband, Dr. Ocampo. She feels proud of the care she's been able to give Mrs. Ocampo and finds other nurses' comments and complaints inappropriate. Bobby, another nurse on the unit, is particularly rude. Zainah feels indignant and resolves to take even better care of Mrs. Ocampo.

On one of her days off this week, Zainah volunteers at the Senior Center for the annual flu shot clinic. She also buys her first new car this week ▼ [NEWS].

Episode 12

Zainah and the nursing student, Jennifer Porter, see Dr. Ocampo sitting in Mrs. Ocampo's room. He looks very tired and short of breath. Zainah asks Dr. Ocampo how he is feeling, and he replies (referring to his wife), "*She* is your patient, not me." Later in the day, Zainah

sees the discharge planner and mentions to her that she has concerns about Dr. Ocampo and his ability to manage his wife's care after discharge. Zainah then talks with Jennifer about the need for nurses in the inpatient setting to provide input related to the long-term care needs for the patient. Zainah suggests that Jennifer attend the case management meeting with her later in the day.

Episode 13

Zainah is glad to see that Mrs. Ocampo has finally gotten well enough to be transferred to the rehabilitation hospital. Zainah can see the toll this hospitalization has taken on both Dr. and Mrs. Ocampo and hopes that Mrs. Ocampo can go home soon.

Episode 14

Zainah and her fiance, Abdul, go out for a romantic dinner. Abdul mentions their parents would like to see them get married soon and suggests they plan their wedding celebration. Zainah is thrilled when Abdul gives her a ring she previously looked at a few months ago. She can't help wondering, though, how she is going to find the time to plan a wedding with all of the extra hours she has been working ▼.

Episode 15

Zainah gets a call from the Emergency Department (ED) about a new admission. She is told by the ED nurse that Mr. Robert Jackson, a 70-year-old African American male is being admitted to the medicine service with a diagnosis of bacterial pneumonia, dehydration, and emphysema. She is told that Mr. Jackson has had a chest-x-ray and labs completed. He is on oxygen, 2 liters by nasal cannula, he has an IV of D5W 0.45% NaCL running at 100 cc/hour, and he has had one dose of ceftriaxone (Rocephin). He is scheduled to have respiratory therapy treatment every 6 hours.

Zainah takes a nursing history on Mr. Jackson as part of the admission process and learns he is divorced and is a retired veteran. He has two grown daughters who live in distant states and he sees them only occasionally. He tells Zainah he took a job as a shuttle driver for the Neighborhood Senior Center because money has been tight and his benefits were not sufficient to make ends meet. When Zainah asks Mr. Jackson about sources of social support, he mentions the staff at the Senior Center as his primary network. Mr. Jackson also tells Zainah he is in extremely good physical condition but just caught this bad cold. From Zainah's perspective, Mr. Jackson is quite ill, fatigued, very thin, and having significant respiratory compromise. She smiles as she thinks about the differences in their perceptions.

Over the course of a few days, Mr. Jackson's condition improves and Zainah is able to spend time with Mr. Jackson, teaching him about measures to improve his respiratory capacity and other measures to for health promotion. She does not try to talk him out of smoking, but she emphasizes that smoking increases his risk. While having this conversation with him, an elderly woman walks into the room and tells Mr. Jackson he needs to listen to the nurse and give up those "damn cigarettes." A huge smile comes across Mr. Jackson's face as he says, "Mary Martin - did you come all the way over here to harass me?" Zainah is pleased to see Mr. Jackson has a visitor and leaves the two of them to chat ▶.

Zainah Kattan Season 2 Information

Episode 1

Zainah Kattan is a 24-year-old nurse who graduated from nursing school last year with a BSN degree. She works on a general medical-surgical inpatient unit at Neighborhood Hospital. She usually works the 12-hour day shift, but also picks up additional shifts when the need arises. Zainah has a long-term goal of working in an adult Intensive Care Unit.

Zainah continues to receive positive feedback from her unit manager, Pat Richman, and continues to gain confidence as a nurse. She still plans to eventually become an intensive care nurse and wants to start getting experience with more complex patients. She and Pat agree that she will start cross-training for the sub-acute unit.

Zainah is usually very happy to work with nursing students, but one student, Kayla, is pretty much a "flake" and a flirt. While on the unit she is chatty with Bobby and Zainah is surprised to see him engage so much with her. By the end of the second day she is working with him, it is all Zainah can stand to listen to Kayla giggle when talking with Bobby. Zainah reports to the nursing instructor, Dr. Debbie Koch, that Kayla needs to focus more on her nursing care and less on Bobby.

Episode 2

Zainah starts her morning shift in a great mood, but her mood changes when she realizes Kayla, the nursing student, is assigned to care for one of her patients. After getting a report from Bobby (who worked the previous night shift), Zainah observes Bobby hanging around on the unit for a little while talking with her. Zainah is glad not to have to endure another shift with the two of them on the unit together. Kayla is nice enough, but Zainah questions her clinical preparation. Throughout the shift, Zainah continually has to remind Kayla to do things; she just seems to lack focus. Kayla asks Zainah why she always wears the scarfs on her head - and asks if she gets hot always wearing long sleeves. Zainah wonders about Kayla's level of maturity, and recognizes she is just curious about her hijab. Kayla does not seem to recognize Zainah's practice is very normal to her ▼.

Episode 3

It is another long week at the hospital. Zainah takes a night shift and has to work with Bobby. She hasn't gotten along with him since he was rude to Mrs. Ocampo, and she doesn't like working with him. He's competent, but patients often complain about him. She wishes her manager, Pat, would do something about Bobby, but because of the nursing shortages, even Bobby is better than having no nursing coverage.

Zainah is a volunteer organizer for the "Walk for Life" fundraiser. She spends all of her free time this week on final preparations and then the whole weekend at the event. She is so fatigued by Sunday evening that she cancels plans with her fiance, Abdul, and spends the evening at home watching TV [NEWS].

Episode 4

Zainah is working with nursing student Kayla Sharif when they get report from a nurse in the post anesthesia unit for a patient by the name of Vincent Matsui, a 32-year-old male who had a debridement and stump revision for an infected stump of the left lower leg. She learns that his procedure was without complications. When Mr. Matsui arrives on the floor, he is accompanied by his wife, Amy, and Mr. Matsui's parents. After completing a postoperative assessment and giving him pain medications, Zainah talks with Amy and learns that Vincent lost his leg as a result of military combat about 4 years ago. He had made great progress by learning to walk again with a prosthesis. However, about 10 weeks ago he fell (when he was not wearing the prosthesis). This resulted in significant trauma to the stump. The stump would not heal and then became infected. She tells Zainah that he has been depressed due to the loss of independence during this time and due to the fact that his leg will need to be shortened for the stump revision. To Zainah's surprise, Kayla has an incredible ability to interact with the Matsui family. It is clear Mr. Matsui, his wife, and parents enjoy having her involved in their care. Although Zainah does not care much for Kayla and initially found her immature because of the way she acted around Bobby, she recognizes Kayla certainly has strengths with interpersonal skills with patients.

The following day, Zainah is again assigned to work with Mr. Matsui. During morning shift report, Bobby Schofield (who worked the night shift) tells Zainah that Mr. Matsui was stable throughout the night, but he was constantly asking for pain medication. Bobby tells Zainah it is a classic case of drug-seeking behavior. Zainah is surprised to hear this, as this was not her experience with him on the previous day. At the beginning of the shift while doing her morning assessment, Mr. Matsui tells Zainah he had a "bad night" because he was in a lot of pain most of the night. Zainah looks at the Medication Administration Record and Narcotic Records and sees that Bobby gave Mr. Matsui appropriate doses of pain medication.

This is the second time Zainah has followed Bobby on a shift where a patient complained about poor pain control. Zainah can't quite understand this situation, because when she gives pain medications to her patients, they report adequate pain control ▶ ▽.

Episode 5
The unit is full of patients with emphysema and asthma because of the Neighborhood forest fire. The Emergency Department keeps calling for beds. Because beds are not available, there is pressure to get patients discharged. Zainah is kept very busy admitting new patients as soon as others are discharged or transferred to other units. The entire staff is stressed, and morale is low on the unit NEWS.

Episode 6
At the monthly staff meeting, a new mandatory overtime policy is announced. This angers most of the nurses, and even Zainah feels demoralized. She doesn't know how she can possibly work more than she already does, but she feels uncomfortable with all the complaining. She's nervous about the antagonism on the unit and trusts that administration will find a good solution. She resolves not to get involved in the issue and is determined just to focus on taking care of her patients.

Zainah and Abdul haven't been able to spend enough time together lately. It seems like they never go out anymore, but just end up watching movies and falling asleep on the couch ▽.

Episode 7
Zainah takes care of an 88-year-old man by the name of Mr. Alden this week. Mr. Alden was admitted after an apparent fall at home; he has a fractured arm and ribs. Zainah notices how frail Mr. Alden is and that he appears underweight. When talking to his son, Zainah learns that Mr. Alden has become very unsteady on his feet and that he does not eat very much. Zainah can tell Mr. Alden is in quite a bit of pain and is not very motivated in his own care. When Zainah asks Mr. Alden, "Don't you want to get better quickly so you can go home?" she is surprised when Mr. Alden says, "No." NEWS

Episode 8
Zainah cares for Mr. Alden again this week. She is surprised to see that he is still on the unit, expecting that he would have been discharged by now. She learns that Mr. Alden has developed pneumonia while hospitalized and attributes this to the fact that he was not moving much. She is surprised how much worse he looks this week. She checks him regularly during her shift and never sees his son.

Episode 9
Zainah works day shift and gets report from Bobby who has worked the night shift. He gives her a very superficial and uninformative report. Zainah is assigned to care for Mr. Alden again. At the beginning of her shift she assesses him. He seems stable, but something does not seem right, although she does not know what. Over the next several hours he becomes less responsive, and his respiratory rate and pulse rate creep up. Becoming worried about his condition, Zainah calls the attending physician. After a short evaluation, he tells her they need to get him intubated and admitted to the Intensive Care Unit. Zainah quickly calls Pat Richman for additional help, gets the equipment, and assists the physician with getting him intubated. Shortly thereafter Mr. Alden is transferred to the Medical Intensive Care Unit.

Zainah is upset with the events, thinking that she should have called the physician earlier. She reflects on the experience, knowing something did not seem right at the beginning of the shift and wonders what it was that she was sensing ▽.

Episode 10
This is a bad week for Zainah. She learns that her patient, Mr. Alden, died, and she is sure it is her fault. And if that were not enough, Zainah cries when she reads about Dr. Ocampo's death in the *News*. She found him to be such a caring man and wonders what will become of his wife Lydia.

Zainah and Abdul decide they need to make more time for each other. They go out for dinner and a movie and have a wonderful evening together. Zainah decides to focus on wedding plans instead of problems at work ▽ NEWS.

Episode 11
Zainah just can't shake the feeling that something is going on with Bobby. She observes that he moves slowly, is tired all the time, and seems to be spending a lot of time in the medication room. She worries that Bobby may be using drugs or alcohol and schedules an appointment with her unit manager, Pat Richman, to discuss her concerns ▽.

Episode 12
When Zainah begins her shift and gets report, she recognizes the name of one of her patients as somebody she recently cared for - Mr. Robert Jackson. She learns Mr. Jackson was admitted to the hospital yesterday afternoon on the Cardiology Service. His admitting diagnosis

is syncope and second-degree (Mobitz II) heart block. His other conditions are hypertension and emphysema. Mr. Jackson has been on cardiac monitoring with transcutaneous pacing pads applied. Zainah learns the cardiologist is evaluating the potential need for a permanent pacemaker.

When she goes in to see Mr. Jackson, he immediately recognizes her and is clearly happy to see her. Zainah can see Mr. Jackson is worried and distressed about what happened and about his condition. He says to her, "It happened so fast. One minute I was out in the parking lot cleaning the windows of the shuttle van, and the next thing I know, I am in an emergency room. What if I had been driving when that happened? I might have killed some folks!" ✉.

Episode 13

Zainah takes an extra night shift this week. When she leaves the hospital in the morning, she discovers that someone hit her brand-new car. She breaks down crying at the sight of it. Everything has been so overwhelming and tense lately. She just can't handle one more thing and knows the repairs to her car will be expensive. To make matters worse, Zainah and Abdul get into an argument. Zainah feels like everything is falling apart ✉.

Episode 14

Zainah is shocked when she observes Bobby at the beginning of the shift. She decides he is really wasted and calls Pat Richman, her nurse manager, to report his condition and shares her concerns. She later learns that Bobby tested positive for drug use. She is disappointed, but not really surprised. Zainah wonders if the other nurses on the unit will know she is the one who reported Bobby to Pat - and if they find out, she wonders how the other nurses on the unit will perceive her ✉.

Episode 15

Zainah's good friends, Nicole and Ramon, both nurses at Neighborhood Hospital, get married. The wedding is beautiful, but Zainah and Abdul get into another argument at the reception. Things are tense and distant between them. Recently they have had many arguments over little things. She begins to wonder if she should marry Abdul ✉.

Zainah Kattan Season 3 Information

Episode 1

Zainah Kattan is a 24-year-old nurse who works the 12-hour day shift on a general medical-surgical unit at Neighborhood Hospital. She occasionally works on the sub-acute unit as well. Tension is high among the nursing staff due to nursing shortages and mandatory overtime. Zainah does not mind an occasional extra shift, but not only does this occur often, but it is expected. Zainah is trying to remain positive at work.

Zainah and her fiance, Abdul Salan, a man she has known since childhood, have recently had many arguments. Zainah wonders if marrying him is the right thing to do.

The hospital chief nursing officer (CNO) announces this week that all staff nurses are expected to have a BSN degree within the next four years. Zainah is so glad she earned a BSN degree when she went to nursing school. She would hate to be in the shoes of some of her colleagues.

Episode 2

Zainah joins a state-level professional nursing work group around improving nursing education through university-hospital collaborative residency programs. Reflecting on her own experiences as a new nurse, Zainah thinks a residency program would have helped her make the adjustment from school to the workforce. Zainah agrees to be a liaison between the group and her hospital. She talks with Pat Richman about the ideas shared at the meeting ✉.

Episode 3

Zainah learns that Alvin Cromwell, a man who is accused of raping and murdering a local 6-year-old girl, is in the hospital and on her unit. She overhears her colleagues talking about withholding his pain medication and joking about his code status. Zainah initially feels strongly about caring for each patient with equal care and feels her coworkers are behaving inappropriately. When she goes to his room to do an initial assessment, she finds he has a guard in his room and he is handcuffed. Zainah feels uncomfortable around Mr. Cromwell and the guard, especially when Mr. Cromwell looks at her and smiles. Later in the shift, Zainah goes to Mr. Cromwell's room to administer medications. He tells Zainah, "You seem nervous around me. Don't worry; I did not kill that stupid little girl. I am a good boy. Why don't you take off that ugly scarf and let me see your head and face. Better yet, why don't you take all your clothes and dance for me." He then begins to laugh hysterically. Zainah is so furious that she almost loses control and this makes Mr. Cromwell laugh even harder. The guard smiles, seemingly amused by Zainah's reaction, but he says, "Knock it off, Alvin." Zainah feels complete disgust toward this man and also thinks he is crazy! He does not deserve the care he has been receiving! She never considered herself to be the kind of person who would allow her emotional reactions to influence the quality of her care.

Episode 4

Zainah is assigned to take care of the accused rapist and murderer, Alvin Cromwell, again. She talks to the charge nurse and asks for a reassignment. When asked why, Zainah tells the charge nurse that Mr. Cromwell is evil and says inappropriate things to her. The charge nurse just laughs and says, "Yeah, well, join the club - he does that to everyone. You should be used to this by now!" Zainah decides she will just have to deal with it. Throughout the shift she remains impassive and barely interacts with him. Mr. Cromwell is irritated with Zainah and says to her, "Why don't you go back to your own country." She thinks to herself, "THIS IS MY COUNTRY!" She does not take his reports of pain seriously and does not make answering his call light a high priority. Zainah has always prided herself on caring for people equally, but finds it is difficult to do so this week ▶ ▽ [NEWS].

Episode 5

The nurse's union is threatening to strike, and Zainah doesn't know what to think. Many of the older nurses who work on her unit encourage her to join the union to be protected, but Zainah has never believed that professional nurses should join a union. She also knows many want to protest the chief nursing officer's new mandate for advancing educational degrees. She is concerned that if she does not join the union, some of the nurses will turn against her [NEWS].

Episode 6

Some of Zainah's colleagues on the nursing unit complain about the new hospital mandate for staff nurses to earn a baccalaureate degree. While retrieving a few things from a supply cart, one of the nurses on Zainah's unit complains to her about the policy as unfair "because they do the same job that other nurses do, and the degree does not matter." Zainah is very well aware of the national goals, but stays silent on the matter. Zainah does not want to become their target as she has seen happen in the past. Zainah hates how stressed out she feels while at work! ▽

Episode 7

Zainah attends a national nursing conference for professional development. Her fiance, Abdul, was invited to go, but he ended up staying home because he could not get away from work. Zainah wishes they could just spend some quality time together ▽.

Episode 8

Zainah and Abdul have another big fight. Zainah tells him, "I don't understand how you can be treating me like this. We are supposed to be getting married." He does not respond and just leaves the house. They barely speak for the next several days. Zainah agrees to work extra shifts because of the strike and also to keep her mind off of her problems with Abdul [NEWS].

Episode 9

Zainah works two extra shifts this week because of the nursing strike. She is so busy that she would even be happy to see Bobby. She disagrees with the union and cannot imagine abandoning patients. At the same time, it is difficult to walk past many of her striking coworkers when she goes to work. She never imagined that her job would be like this ▽ [NEWS].

Episode 10

Zainah is relieved when the strike ends this week. Pat Richman, the unit manager, asks Zainah to consider applying for a charge nurse position on the unit. Zainah tells Pat that she'll think about it ▶ ▽ [NEWS].

Episode 11

Zainah's relationship with Abdul continues to be strained. She comes to realize that he is not the man she wants to spend her life with. She meets with her parents and tells them she would like to end the engagement. They are disappointed, but want what is best for her. Zainah and Abdul have dinner that night, and both agree to end the engagement. She is sad, but hugely relieved by this decision ▽.

Episode 12

Zainah is glad to be busy at work this week so that she does not have to think about her breakup with Abdul. Having a lot of time alone, she thinks about the next steps she might take in her own career ▽.

Episode 13

Zainah joins a gym this week and takes an aerobics class. She feels renewed and rejuvenated, and realizes how poorly she has taken care of herself lately. She calls her sister and talks her into going with her on a Caribbean cruise. She has never done anything like that and decides it would be a great way to get over her disappointing breakup from Abdul. She begins to search the Internet for cruise specials ▽.

Episode 14

All of the recent issues that have arisen as a result of the new education mandate by the hospital CNO have caused Zainah to begin considering graduate school. She realizes that she will continue to improve her opportunities if she gets a graduate degree. She wonders what focus she wants an advanced practice nurse, such as a nurse practitioner, or in a leadership track, or even an education track. She makes an appointment at the local college to speak with an adviser to better understand her options ▽.

Episode 15
Zainah learns of an opening in an adult intensive care unit (ICU) at another hospital in a nearby community.

Although she eventually may want to work in an ICU, she is committed to Neighborhood Hospital and her peers. She accepts the charge nurse position on her unit. Despite the ups and downs of this past couple of years, she realizes how much she has grown professionally and looks forward to beginning this challenging new position ▽.

BOBBY SCHOFIELD

Season 1	Season 2	Season 3
Bobby is frustrated with the staffing problems on the unit. He also becomes fed up with his coworkers and gets into an argument with one nurse when comments are made about the way he cares for his patients. To relieve his stress and unwind, Bobby drinks beer, gets stoned, and parties with friends. One day, he shows up to work drunk and stoned. No one seems to notice, and Bobby takes great pleasure in knowing that he was not caught.	Bobby begins to regularly take narcotics from work. He takes a brief interest in Kayla Sharif, a student nurse. He worries that another student, Jacob McCain, will pick up on his drug use. Bobby's coworkers notice his constant mood swings and report his questionable behavior to Pat. Finally, Bobby is asked to provide a urine sample for drug screening, tests positive, and is reported to the Board of Nursing. He must go through the Diversion Program to keep his nursing license.	Bobby does not believe he has a substance abuse problem, but he pretends to go along with the Diversion Program in order to keep his job. Eventually Bobby's license is suspended. He finally realizes he needs help and makes a serious effort. He knows he has a long recovery ahead of him, but he feels truly committed this time.

Bobby Schofield Season 1 Information

Episode 1
Bobby Schofield is a 32-year-old staff nurse on the medical-surgical unit at Neighborhood Hospital. Bobby has been a nurse for 5 years. He got into nursing because he thought it would be an easy, flexible, and exciting career with job security and good money. Overall, he likes his job, but lately he has gotten bored. He applied for a position with the flight nurse team, but was not offered the position.

Bobby is single and, although he has a few close friends, he considers himself a loner. He has never had a close relationship with his family. Although he dates, he is not in a serious relationship. He loves to party and have a good time.

Bobby's nurse manager, Pat Richman, tells Bobby he will need him serve as acting charge nurse for the shift over the next few weeks because the regular charge nurse will be out on annual leave. Bobby is not too thrilled with the idea, but likes the fact he gets paid a bit more - and this gives him the opportunity to take a lighter load of patients. Bobby does not hesitate to delegate many things to other people that are typically taken care of by the charge nurse.

Episode 2

Bobby is the acting charge nurse on the unit again this week. On one of the days, he becomes frustrated when a nursing tech calls in sick. Because the unit is full, he contacts the nursing supervisor on call and asks if she can send a nursing aide to the floor to cover the shift. The supervisor tells Bobby he will have to do without, at least until noon. Bobby also talks with his nurse manager, Pat, who isn't any more helpful than the supervisor. To make matters worse, there are nursing students on the unit and they ask so many questions.

After a long, 4-day stretch at the hospital, Bobby is glad to have some time off. He spends his days off partying with friends ▼.

Episode 3

This week, Bobby gets into an argument with another nurse on the unit who made a sarcastic comment about his "caring way with patients." Bobby is fed up with all of the pathetic nurses on his unit and tells Pat Richman several of the nurses need an attitude adjustment. Who are they to tell him how to do his job? After work, he really feels a need to unwind. He picks up a six-pack on the way home from work, kicks back in front of the TV, drinks beer, and gets stoned ▼.

Episode 4

Bobby hates it when students are on the unit. He finds them to be annoying, especially when they ask what he perceives to be dumb questions. The nursing instructor, Dr. Debbie Koch, has been coming to the unit for a number of years with students. Bobby recognizes that she is a good instructor, be he really does not care for her; she seems to be so "by the book"-oriented and he believes she is a bit unrealistic about what direct patient care is like. His general approach to students is to let them do the care for his patients and it is up to Debbie and the students to let him know if they need help.

Episode 5

Zainah tells Bobby she is going to lunch and asks him to watch her patients while off the floor. While Zainah is at lunch, Jennifer Porter, one of the nursing students, asks Bobby if he would watch her give insulin to a patient.

Bobby says to Jennifer, "You should do that with your instructor or your primary nurse," and Jennifer tells him they are both unavailable. Annoyed, Bobby asks her if she has already drawn the medication up and she tells him yes. He goes to Mr. Larson's room and watchers Jennifer give the injection. He then co-signs the medication administration; shortly thereafter he goes to lunch.

When Bobby returns from lunch, he learns Mr. Larson had a hypoglycemia episode. Pat Richman, the nurse manager, asks Bobby about his role with the student giving the insulin. Bobby tells Pat the student had already drawn up the medication and was led to believe the instructor or Zainah had checked it. He tells Pat he can't read people's minds and that the student is just unreliable. He tells Pat the instructor should probably fail the student. Later, when Zainah Kattan verbalizes her frustration with him, Bobby tells Zainah, "Well, next time you should not go to lunch until your meds are passed." Bobby hates it when other people try to blame him for their mistakes.

Episode 6

Bobby partied most nights this week. On one night, he got really wasted. He was out until 4 a.m. and had just enough time to go home, take a nap, and get a shower before getting to work at 7 a.m. He had never gone to work stoned or drunk before and was nervous that someone would notice. Fortunately, the unit was short-staffed, and the charge nurse did not seem to notice. Bobby felt a certain pleasure in getting away with it.

Episode 7

The Quality-Safety officer meets with Bobby this week to discuss the incident in which a student administered an incorrect dose of insulin. Bobby tells the officer that Zainah Kattan was the primary nurse supervising the patient and it was his understanding that she checked the dose with the student and that he only was ensuring the student gave the medication correctly. Bobby mentioned to the Quality-Safety officer that Zainah is a new nurse and is often very scattered - and adding students into the mix was probably a contributing factor. Bobby was glad when the meeting was over because it was cutting into his break time.

Episode 8

Bobby has worked several shifts this week. He feels irritable and unfocused at work. All of the whiny patients get on his nerves. He can't stand all of the stupid requests they make constantly, as if he is their personal servant. He is also very annoyed with Zainah Kattan, who bothers him when he's on his breaks to tell him that his patients need him, and a nurse aid who wants help lifting a patient. He wishes they would all just get off his case ▶ ▼.

Episode 9

Bobby reads in the paper about the possibility of companies banning smoking on company property. He feels like smoking is the only thing that keeps him sane at work. If Neighborhood Hospital administrators take away the ability to smoke while on a break, that would be the last straw! ✉ [NEWS]

Episode 10

Mrs. Ocampo is one of Bobby's patients this week. She is confused and disruptive, and he finds her behavior to be incredibly frustrating. Bobby initiates the paperwork to get her restrained because she attempts to pull out her tubes. He also obtains an order for lorazepam (Ativan) to settle her down. Her husband is demanding and rude, and keeps interfering. Bobby is completely fed up with both of them. They just don't get it ▶.

Episode 11

Mrs. Ocampo is still on the unit, and she really annoys Bobby. He gives her lorazepam (Ativan) to quiet her down whenever she gets too agitated.

Bobby's manager, Pat Richman, calls Bobby into his office to discuss a complaint filed by Dr. Ocampo about his rude behavior. Bobby denies treating Mrs. or Dr. Ocampo rudely, but instead suggests that the real issue is that he gets in and gets the work done - while the nursing student, Jennifer Porter, and Zainah Kattan are in Mrs. Ocampo's room all the time to appease the family. So by comparison, he probably seems rude - but is just doing his job. Bobby tells Pat, "You should really take a close look at how Zainah Kattan uses her time - you will find she is very inefficient ✉."

Episode 12

Bobby attends team meeting with the hospital discharge coordinator, Zainah Kattan, Jennifer Porter, the student nurse, and Dr. Ocampo. Bobby is annoyed that the student is in the meeting - this is the same student who gave the insulin overdose. Dr. Ocampo has this idea that he should take his wife home. Bobby can't understand how Dr. Ocampo is unable to see what a bad decision this is. Frankly, he hopes she will be transferred soon.

Episode 13

Bobby has grown very tired of dealing with Dr. Ocampo. He is always asking Bobby questions, which annoys him. Bobby wishes Dr. Ocampo would just stay home once in a while. He is glad when he hears that Mrs. Ocampo is being transferred to the rehabilitation unit.

Episode 14

One of Bobby's post-operative patients, Pamela Allen, was just diagnosed with colon cancer. When her family is not around, she cries all the time. Bobby can hardly stand to go into her room. He is completely fed up with all of his needy patients.

Episode 15

Bobby takes care of Robert Jackson, a 70-year-old male with emphysema and pneumonia. Bobby takes a liking to Mr. Jackson. He is "a tough old dude that doesn't complain," Bobby thinks to himself. When conducting a shift assessment, Bobby can see that the intravenous (IV) catheter in the left antecubital space (inserted in the Emergency Department) does not look quite right and seems a bit puffy. He palpates the area and Mr. Jackson confirms it is pretty sore. Bobby discontinues the IV catheter and inserts a new one in the right forearm.

Bobby Schofield   Season 2 Information

Episode 1

Bobby has always been smart and fiercely independent. He loves to party and have a good time. Bobby's recreational drug use has progressively increased, but he thinks he can handle it. He often feels restless and dissatisfied.

This episode when Bobby arrives at work and gets report, a student nurse by the name of Kayla Sharif introduces herself to Bobby and tells him she has been assigned to care for two of his patients. Bobby rolls his eyes and says "Ok, fine," and gives her report. Ordinarily, Bobby does not care to interact much with the students and generally ignores them. However, he thinks Kayla is pretty cool and before long he is flirting with her and she flirts right back. Bobby thinks about her quite a bit the rest of the week.

Episode 2

Bobby agrees to work a night shift this week. During the shift, he keeps the morphine from a discontinued PCA vial instead of wasting it and slips it into his pocket. In the morning before leaving, he sees Kayla Sharif again during morning report. After report he spends a few minutes hanging around the unit so that he can talk with her. He tells her they should party sometime; she gives him her phone number and Bobby tells him he will call soon. When he gets home, he injects the morphine into his vein and finds that it is a great high. It relieves all of his tension and anxiety - and it was remarkably easy to get.

Episode 3

Bobby calls Kayla Sharif, the nursing student, and tells her about a great party he is going to and wants to know if she is interested in going. Kayla tells him she has clinical the next day and Bobby tells her, "No problem - just don't stay late." Kayla and her girlfriend meet Bobby at the party and they spend most of the evening hanging out and flirting more. Kayla is pretty drunk by midnight and her friend takes her home. Bobby agrees to call her in the morning to make sure she wakes up in time for clinical. The next morning when Bobby calls her, Kayla tells him she has a hangover but it was worth it because she had a blast at the party. Kayla is a few minutes late to the hospital and misses the first part of the morning shift report.

Episode 4

Bobby works several night shifts this week and begins to regularly take narcotics from work. His strategy is that for most of the shift he collects a portion of the dose of a patient's pain medication and hides it in his locker. He administers a partial dose to the patient and documents that he administered the full dose. Then, during the final hours of his shift, he administers a full dose so the patients are not in pain when the day shift nurses arrive, or he will tell people that the patient is just drug seeking and won't be satisfied regardless of how much pain medication they receive. Bobby thinks his plan is brilliant because it is unlikely anyone will notice. He looks forward to going home, using the drugs, and relaxing. Bobby experiments with a wide variety of drugs, but discovers that he enjoys morphine the most.

Kayla has been spending more time with Bobby - to the point where she has stayed overnight with him a couple of times. He has to be careful because he is not sure he can trust Kayla enough to tell her what he is doing. He likes Kayla, but he likes the drugs more. Kayla tells Bobby she got in trouble with her nursing instructor for flirting with him too much and was told that her behavior was unprofessional. They agree to try to "cool it" while at the hospital ▽.

Episode 5

Kayla is at Bobby's house partying with some of his friends when one of his friends asks Kayla if she wants to get high. Kayla tells his friend she does not use marijuana or other drugs. He tells her, "That's cool - but maybe you should try." As Bobby observes this conversation, he can tell Kayla is uncomfortable with the idea of drug use; this confirms for him that she can't know about his drug use. A few days later, Bobby tells Kayla he wants to take a break from seeing her. When Kayla becomes upset and cries, he knows he is done with her. He is glad her clinical group is about done with the rotation on his unit so that he does not have to see her anymore. After about a week of not returning her calls or texts, he quits hearing from her. He is glad not to have to deal with her after that ▽.

Episode 6

Bobby attends a staff meeting where Pat Richman, the unit manager, announces the new mandatory overtime policy. All of the nurses are angry and discouraged. In some ways, Bobby is annoyed with the administration's demands, but he also sees it as an opportunity. After all, he only has access to morphine when he is at work. He volunteers for a couple of extra night shifts, because it's easier to take narcotics on night shifts with fewer people working and less supervision ▽.

Episode 7

Another group of nursing students start a clinical rotation on the unit. One student, Jacob McCain, is assigned to one of Bobby's patients this week. Early in the shift, Jacob tells Bobby that one of the patients, Mr. Alden, may be a victim of elder abuse. Jacob tells Bobby about seeing him at the Senior Center previously and the concerns that were raised at that time. Bobby tells Jacob, "Take a chill pill! Mr. Alden said he tripped and fell at home. Besides, his son is here with him and seems like a cool dude." Bobby decides Jacob has a "super nurse" mentality that reminds him of Zainah Kattan.

Episode 8

Bobby becomes increasingly creative in finding ways to steal morphine without getting caught. He removes morphine from pre-filled syringes and replaces it with saline, draws narcotics directly out of IV lines, volunteers to go to the pharmacy, and alters the narcotic count. Bobby no longer waits to go home before injecting - he sometimes does it on his breaks. He feels smarter than everyone else; the people he works with are so busy and dumb that they don't even notice ▽.

Episode 9

Bobby's drug use continues to escalate both while at work and when he is home. On one night shift this week, he "shoots up" three times in 12 hours and all but ignores his patients. He does a limited assessment on each patient at the beginning of the shift and periodically checks with the nursing techs to make sure the patients are okay. The only thing he really takes care of is getting the medications administered to the patients - and he does this from a task-based approach. When the day shift nurses come in, he hates the fact that Zainah Kattan is following his group of patients because she is so damn picky about everything and everyone. He tells Zainah that all the patients had a great night and they are all doing well.

Episode 10

Jacob McCain is on the unit again this week. Bobby is still annoyed with him about the Mr. Alden situation, but he also recognizes Jacob is very smart and seems to notice everything. For the first time in months, Bobby does not try to take any narcotics at work. He is afraid Jacob or his instructor might notice something. Instead he pretty much hangs out in the break room and tells Jacob to let him know if he needs help with something.

Episode 11

Bobby has been feeling particularly edgy and unfocused at work lately, and avoids conversations with coworkers. He is unaware that some of his coworkers are beginning to notice his evasiveness and mood swings ▼.

Episode 12

Bobby's narcotic use continues to escalate; he rarely works a shift now without using a narcotic at least once. He finds he physically feels better when he uses the drugs and is sure nobody notices. Bobby sees Mr. Jackson has been admitted to his unit again and, although he is not assigned to care for him, he goes in to see how he is doing. Mr. Jackson is one of the few patients Bobby actually likes to care for 🔲.

Episode 13

Bobby begins to think about stopping narcotic use - at least at work. Although he thinks of quitting, he feels very anxious and depressed. He decides he is okay for now, but vows to quit soon ▼.

Episode 14

Bobby reports to work one day this week impaired. He is looking forward to beginning his shift so that he can get a narcotic fix. Bobby is surprised when, out of nowhere,

Pat Richman, the unit manager, approaches him, relieves him of his patient care assignment, and tells him he needs to give a urine sample for a drug screening. Bobby knows he will test positive and wonders which of the nurses has been watching him.

A formal complaint against Bobby is filed to the Board of Nursing by Neighborhood Hospital and he is placed on administrative leave without pay. Bobby receives notification from the Board of Nursing about the complaint filed and he has one of two options: he can keep the matter confidential if he chooses to go through a diversion program, or he can fight the allegation and then this becomes public record. After consulting with a legal advisor, Bobby decides he will admit to the substance abuse and go through a diversion program. Deep down, he knows that he does not need this, but sees that this is the path of least resistance. In order to get accepted into the diversion program, Bobby has to submit a formal written request. He does this and hopes to get through this quickly so that he can get back to work ▼.

Episode 15

Bobby receives a response from the Board of Nursing diversion program director. He is told that in order to be accepted in the diversion program, his next step is to be interviewed by the director. His appointment is scheduled for the following week.

Bobby Schofield   Season 3 Information

Episode 1

Bobby Schofield is a 33-year-old nurse who has recently had a complaint filed at the Board of Nursing for drug impairment. He agreed to enter the Diversion program for substance abuse. He must agree and adhere to a 5-year contract that includes abstinence, treatment, frequent meetings with a supervisor, and drug testing to make sure he has not relapsed. If he follows through with the contract, he will be able to keep his nursing license, and his treatment will remain completely confidential.

Bobby hates the diversion program. He is supposed to admit that he has a substance abuse problem, which he doesn't truly believe. He resents all of the supervision and thinks the Alcoholics Anonymous (AA) and Narcotics Anonymous (NA) meetings are idiotic ▶ ▼.

Episode 2

Bobby has a meeting with his nurse manager, Pat Richman, the employee health nurse, and the human resources representative to discuss his treatment plan.

Bobby knows he has to pretend to go along with the diversion program to keep his job, but he still believes he has everything under control. He thinks abstinence is a joke and that he could probably get away with some very limited use ▼.

Episode 3

After hitting the bars with his buddies, Bobby goes in for a treatment session. Because it is obvious to everyone that Bobby is intoxicated, the leader of the session asks Bobby to submit a urine sample. A few days later he is notified by the diversion program director and told he tested positive for drugs. Bobby admits to "mild use" and had a few beers prior to attending but assured the director he can quit whenever he wants.

Episode 4

Bobby tests positive for opiates again. He quits the diversion program because he thinks it doesn't do anything for him.

Episode 5

Bobby receives a letter from the Board of Nursing (BON), stating that they have received official notification that he has dropped out of the diversion program. He is offered another opportunity to go through the diversion program. If he declines, he must attend a disciplinary hearing. Bobby is sure he will convince the stupid people on the BON that he is not a drug user anymore and that he is clean. He is sure he can convince them to let him keep his license so that he can avoid the stupid meetings. He elects to attend the hearing.

Episode 6

Bobby is burning through the little savings that he has, since he is on administrative leave without pay. He hopes to get back to work soon so that he can start generating some income. Bobby does enjoy having all the time off to party and sleep, but he misses having access to the drugs. He can't afford the street cost of the drugs he was stealing at the hospital.

Episode 7

Bobby has his disciplinary hearing this week before the Board of Nursing (BON). His license is suspended. Bobby is in a state of disbelief. He asks the BON members what options he now has. He is told that, if he wants to try the diversion program again, and if he shows some real recovery, he may be able to get his license reinstated after 2 years.

Bobby feels shocked by the decision. He wonders how he will be able to make his rent and car payments. He is furious and goes to a bar and drinks there until it closes. He wakes up in a stranger's house, doesn't know where his car is, and has to walk home ✉.

Episode 8

Bobby feels depressed. He does not have any income coming in. No money for drugs, no money for alcohol, and he is challenged to come up with rent payments. With very little money he contacts his friends for help - and suddenly they don't seem to be interested in hanging out with him. Bobby realizes he needs to get his act together. He sees there is a nursing strike going on at the hospital and he actually wishes he could go back to work ✉ [NEWS].

Episode 9

The Board of Nursing hearing was a real wake-up call. Bobby continues to feel depressed and is concerned about making his house and car payments. He goes to an Alcoholics Anonymous (AA) meeting, where he meets an older gentleman named Jim. Bobby immediately likes him and learns that Jim has been in the program for 30 years. Jim takes Bobby out for coffee after the meeting, and they end up talking for three hours.

Episode 10

Bobby goes to the AA meetings three nights this week. His new friend, Jim, tells him that anytime he wants a drink or needs to smoke, he should call him. Bobby calls Jim frequently for support because he finds that Jim understands what he is going through ✉.

Episode 11

Bobby gets a job this week working in retail for seasonal work. He gets about 20 hours a week and he finds his paychecks barely cover the rent. He wonders how people working in these jobs can make it. Bobby recognizes he had taken his good income as a nurse for granted. Bobby's friend Jim tells him that you can't make a recovery until 1) you really come to grips with the fact that you have a problem, and 2) you really want to do something about it. "Until you get to this point," Jim tells Bobby, "you will waste your time in treatment ✉."

Episode 12

Through Jim's encouragement, Bobby calls Pat Richman and asks him to meet him for coffee. To his surprise, Pat agrees. Bobby is very nervous about meeting with Pat, but what he really wants to do is say that he is sorry and that he now understands that he needs help. Pat is very understanding of Bobby's situation and lets him know there are always opportunities for second chances, but he really needs to commit. Pat offers to write a letter of support should he choose to apply to the diversion program again ✉.

Episode 13

Bobby contacts the diversion program director and asks for a meeting. He tells the director he has hit bottom and wants a second chance. He agrees to a new contract and feels committed this time. He knows it is his only chance at getting his nursing career back. The diversion program director accepts his request and for the first time in a very long time, Bobby feels happy and is looking forward to something ✉.

Episode 14

Being back in the diversion program, Bobby feels encouraged about the possibility of getting his license reinstated. He knows he may have some challenges getting a job in the future because his dismissal case is public, but he also feels confident that Pat Richman will help him get another job when the time is right.

Episode 15

Bobby attends meetings regularly and is working closely with his diversion program supervisor. He knows he has a long road ahead; every day is a struggle, but he feels a sense of hope ▶ ✉.

PUBLIC SCHOOL

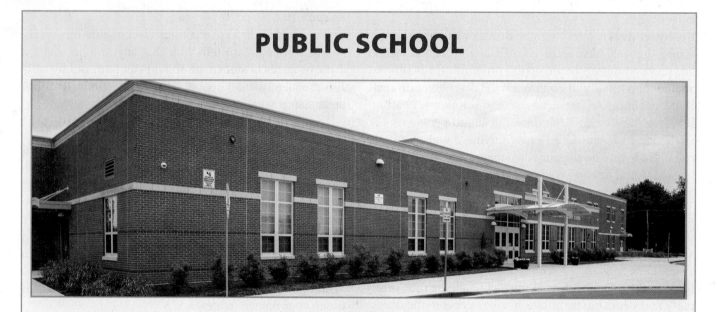

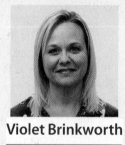

Violet Brinkworth

Housing	The schools are located in several areas within the Neighborhood.
Parks and Recreation	There is a YMCA and a recreation park located close to the middle and high schools. There are small parks located near the elementary school

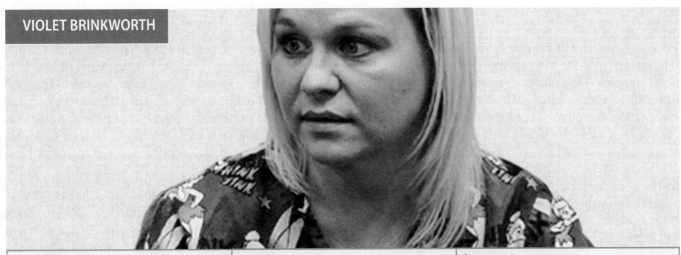

VIOLET BRINKWORTH

Season 1	Season 2	Season 3
Violet is the nurse at the elementary, middle, and high schools. She observes the unhealthy foods that the children are buying at school and talks to the principals about offering more nutritious choices. She is also concerned about substance abuse among students. Violet hears that Jason Riley got in a fight and is having trouble with schoolwork; Violet wonders if he has a learning disability. Marcus Young comes to school with pink eye. Jacob McCain, a nursing student, does clinical rotation with Violet this season. Violet meets with the mother in a veteran's family whose daughter is at the school.	Violet has student nurse Kayla Sharif join her for rotation and finds her a great help. Violet continues to interact with Jason Riley. She has been asked to complete a questionnaire that will help to assess whether Jason has a learning disability. Kelsey Young comes into the nurse's office coughing and having trouble breathing. Violet also interacts with Jenna Riley and becomes concerned about her weight gain. The school board announces a ban on all "junk" food sold at the schools. Two new health aides are hired to help Violet with the three schools.	Because many parents and students are angry about the "junk" food ban, the principal tells Violet that she is considering bringing back some of the more popular items. Violet calls Jenna Riley's mother when she is concerned about her need to see a physician. Violet has a run-in with the middle school principal about a sexuality unit she is planning to teach. A female student is found on the floor with difficulty breathing. Violet defends her decision to call an ambulance to come to the school.

Violet Brinkworth Season 1 Information

Episode 1

Violet Brinkworth is a 41-year-old nurse who works for the Neighborhood Public School System. She has been married to her husband Richard Brinkworth for 15 years. Because Richard is often away on business trips, Violet decided to become a school nurse 6 years ago so she could be on the same schedule as her son, who is now 12 years old. For the first few years, Violet worked fulltime at Neighborhood Elementary School. However, because of budget cuts, Violet now also covers Neighborhood Middle School and Neighborhood High School. Fortunately, the schools are close to one another. Despite this, Violet finds it difficult to be an effective nurse because each school has so many needs.

Violet has organized an alcohol and drug abstinence event at the Neighborhood High School. She partners with Sheriff Shuster and the Neighborhood law enforcement agencies to help the high school students understand the risks of alcohol and drug intoxication. Although Violet has nearly all students attend the mandatory event, she is disappointed to see that many of the students don't seem to take the information very seriously. She follows up with substance abuse experts to determine the best follow-up strategies for the event.

Episode 2

While heating her lunch in the teacher's lounge at the Neighborhood Elementary School, Violet overhears two teachers talking about Jason Riley, a fifth grader. One teacher comments that Jason was in another fight this week and that his mother Evelyn must be out of touch with her son's behavior. Violet knows Jason well; he often tries to get out of class and come visit her. Because she knows that Jason has trouble with his peers and schoolwork, Violet is interested to hear the perceptions of the teachers.

This week Violet has a nursing student by the name of Jacob McCain working with her. He will be completing a school-based nursing rotation with her for the next few months. Violet finds Jacob to be a very mature young man who genuinely seems interested in learning. She reviews her general scope of practice for her job and comments that trying to cover all three schools is a challenge. Violet suggests that Jacob join her in a meeting with the Neighborhood administration next week as she proposes a plan for additional help.

Episode 3

Violet and Jacob present a proposal for the Neighborhood District School Board to request an additional school nurse within the Neighborhood Elementary, Middle, and High Schools. Violet discusses the problems associated with trying to "cover" three schools. There is just not enough time to address the needs of all of the students. The board members tell Violet that they understand the challenges she faces and remind her of the serious budget shortfalls experienced by the school system. The administrators agree to take Violet's proposal under advisement and tell her that they will also explore other solutions, including hiring a health aide. Violet does not think this is a very good idea because the district does not require health aides to have any training other than first aid.

After the meeting, Violet and Jacob debrief about the discussion in the meeting. Jacob thanks Violet for including him. He tells her the experience was good because previously he thought that being a school nurse was "a boring position" but he now realizes it is much more complex than he ever imagined.

Episode 4

Violet and student nurse Jacob McCain screen all of the Neighborhood Elementary School students for vision and hearing problems. When Jason Riley comes in to be screened, Jacob tests his vision and tells Violet that Jason can only read the 20/100 line of the eye chart in both eyes. Violet tests Jason again to confirm the findings. She then tests Jason's hearing, which is within normal parameters. Violet calls Jason's mother, Evelyn Riley, and suggests that Jason be taken to an optometrist for a vision exam.

Episode 5

While watching the evening news, Violet is upset to learn that two high school students, Amy Price (a sophomore) and Carrie Rivera (a junior), were charged with drunk driving after causing a crash that left a mother and her young son dead. Violet knows the girls are considered "party girls." Violet reflects on the alcohol and drug abstinence program she held at the school a few months ago and wonders if such events are a total waste of her time. She wishes the education could have prevented this tragedy. The following day at the high school, students are talking about the wreck. Violet takes the time to talk with students about what was discussed at the drug and alcohol workshop held at the school several weeks ago [NEWS].

Episode 6

Violet tells Jacob McCain (the nursing student) that in addition to substance abuse at the middle and high school, she is very concerned about obesity among students from elementary to high school. She and Jacob spend two days during the lunch hour observing the middle school students and documenting what they buy for lunch.

At the end of two days, Violet and Jacob compare their notes and learn that most students buy foods such as pizza slices, French fries covered with cheese sauce, nachos with cheese sauce, cheeseburgers, and fried burritos from the snack bar. Potato chips and other snack foods are also popular. She notices that dill pickles are the only food offered at the snack bar that represents the vegetable food group. Violet talks with the food services supervisor and asks him if fresh fruits and vegetables could be offered. Violet is told that those food items are expensive and end up being thrown away because so few of the students buy them. Violet posts a nutrition poster in the hallway near her office as one way to perhaps gain some awareness among students.

Episode 7

Violet sees Jason Riley in the hallway and notices that he is wearing new glasses. She asks him if he is happy with the change. Jason shrugs his shoulders and says that his headaches are better, but he still is too "dumb" to do his schoolwork. Violet wonders if Jason has ever been tested for learning disabilities [NEWS].

Episode 8

This week the Neighborhood Elementary School went on lockdown after a third-grade student brought a gun to school with intent to scare some of his classmates who reportedly bullied him. Violet discusses some of the latest literature on bullying with the principal of the elementary school and the District Superintendent. They tell Violet that the issue will be discussed further at the School Board meeting and they will let her know if they need her to come.

Also this week the two girls (Amy Price and Carrie Rivera) who were involved in an alcohol-related car crash that claimed the life of a mother and her young son are back in school. Their legal problems are far from over, but the girls have been allowed to return to school while on house arrest with strict supervision. Violet is shocked and disappointed that the message sent to the other students is that what they did was okay [NEWS].

Episode 9

Marcus Young, a first-grade student at the Neighborhood Elementary School, is sent to the nurse's office by his teacher. The teacher is concerned because Marcus has been rubbing his left eye all day and now complains that it hurts. Violet examines Marcus' eye and sees that it is red, irritated, and has discharge. She calls Marcus' mother, Angie Young, and explains that Marcus could have an infection in his eye and that it might be contagious. She asks his mother to pick Marcus up from school as soon as possible and take him to his healthcare provider for treatment. Violet sends a note to the classroom teacher to keep an eye out for other children with similar symptoms and to ask all of the students to wash their hands. Violet downloads a consumer-friendly information sheet about pink eye from a government health website and sends it home with all the students to give to their parents [▼].

Episode 10

Violet sees Sam, a fifth-grade student, with scrapes and bruises after a fight with Jason Riley on the playground. Sam tells Violet that Jason is "such a loser." Violet asks Sam what caused the fight, and he tells her that Jason just started to beat him up for no reason.

Violet spends one evening this week at the Neighborhood High School open house.

Episode 11

Violet makes herself available two evenings this week for the Neighborhood Elementary and Middle School open houses. Only a few people stop to say hello, making Violet feel somewhat invisible.

Episode 12

Violet talks to the Neighborhood Middle and High School principals about stocking the student snack bar with more nutritious choices of food and drinks, citing several studies that link childhood obesity with childhood onset type 2 diabetes. The principals agree that the food could be more nutritious and say that they will review the foods sold in the snack bars. However, they explain that the school district has a contract with a company that will provide each school with a $3,000 donation plus a percentage of sales if the school sells its products for the school year. The principal of the high school tells Violet that the girls' soccer team desperately needs new

uniforms, and the donation has been earmarked to cover that expense [▼].

Episode 13

This week Violet oversees the conversion of the student health records to an electronic records system. Fortunately, the systems administrator and information technology team from the school district lead the conversion process, but she is directly involved as well. Because she has three schools to cover and no help, this takes all week to complete [NEWS].

Episode 14

Angie Young, one of the mothers who regularly volunteers at Neighborhood Elementary, stops in to see Violet. Mrs. Young tells Violet that she is very worried about Victoria Patterson's family and proceeds to share her concerns. Violet knows Victoria's mother, Rebecca, pretty well because she also volunteers at the school. Violet recalls Rebecca mentioning that her husband recently retired from active military service. As Violet reflects on what Ms. Young said, she realizes that she has not seen Rebecca much recently and that last time she saw her, she had a flat affect. Violet has a conversation with Victoria's teacher and learns that in recent weeks, Victoria has not been completing her homework and has been having behavior issues. Her teacher also has begun to wonder if there are problems at home.

Violet decides to call Rebecca and asks if she would mind coming to the school to talk with her. When Rebecca comes in that afternoon, Violet shares her concerns and asks if she might be able to help. To Violet's surprise, Rebecca opens up and tells her that Blake, her husband, has become increasingly withdrawn and irritable, causing a significant disruption within the entire family. After listening further, Violet wonders if a mental health referral would be helpful for Blake. Violet urges Rebecca to consider talking with their family healthcare provider and getting some professional help [▶].

Episode 15

Jenna Riley, an eighth-grade student at Neighborhood Middle School, comes to the nurse's office and asks Violet if she can sleep for a while. She says that she is very tired and not feeling well. Violet does not know Jenna but recognizes that she is Jason's sister. Violet assesses Jenna for fever and finds that she does not have one. She asks Jenna if she feels bad enough to call her mother and go home, but Jenna says she'll be okay if she can just nap for a while. Violet lets her stay in the office for an hour and then sends her back to class [▼].

Violet Brinkworth Season 2 Information

Episode 1

Violet Brinkworth is a 41-year-old nurse who works for the Neighborhood Public School System. Violet decided to become a school nurse 6 years ago. For the first few years, Violet worked fulltime at Neighborhood Elementary School. However, because of budget cuts, Violet now also covers Neighborhood Middle School and Neighborhood High School. Violet finds it difficult to be an effective nurse because each school has so many needs.

The superintendent of the Neighborhood School District meets with Violet to inform her that the School Board approved a plan to hire two health aides to help her cover the elementary, middle, and high schools. Violet appreciates the fact that her request for help was heard, but tells the superintendent that what is really needed is another nurse because health aides really are of little help. The superintendent tells Violet that they cannot afford another nurse, and they could not justify the expense when they could hire two health aides for far less money. They recommend that with two aides, a health provider will be staffed at each school all day every day. Violet becomes angry and says to the superintendent, "A health aide is NOT a licensed health provider!" She knows her comment does not please the superintendent and wishes the meeting could have been more positive. Back in her office, Violet reviews the salary range for health aides and knows that it will be difficult to find good help.

Episode 2

Jason Riley comes to the nurse's office for the third time this week, claiming to have a stomachache. As Violet talks with Jason, she learns that he has been kicked out of Boy Scouts for biting another Scout. She also learns that he has been in another fight this week. She asks Jason about his glasses. Jason tells her that his glasses are in his backpack and sometimes he does not wear them to avoid being teased. Violet sends a note to the school counselor, letting her know of her concerns about Jason.

Episode 3

The school counselor consults with Violet about Jason Riley. He asks Violet to complete an assessment questionnaire. Two other school staff members have been asked to complete the questionnaire as well. The questionnaires will be used to assess Jason for learning problems.

Rebecca Patterson, one of the volunteer parents, drops in to thank Violet for her advice about her husband, Blake. Rebecca tells Violet that she was able to get Blake to see their family physician, Dr. Rowe, who recommended that Blake see a mental health professional for possible depression. She says that she knew something was wrong and is grateful that Violet cared enough to have that initial conversation with her. Blake has his first appointment soon, and Rebecca tells Violet that she'll keep her posted. Violet is relieved to know they are getting help NEWS.

Episode 4

Violet is disappointed, but not surprised, that there are no applicants for the school health aide positions this week. She calls the district Human Resources Department and asks if there are other options for hiring – perhaps another type of provider position such as an emergency medical technician or a paramedic. The HR Department tells Violet that they cannot change the job posting without going back to the superintendent. Violet wishes that she had not lost her temper the last time they met. She is pretty sure that she will not have any sympathy from the superintendent NEWS.

Episode 5

A teacher sends Kelsey Young, a second-grade student, to the nurse's office because she has been coughing. Violet notices that Kelsey has an increased respiratory rate, is coughing frequently, and is wheezing. Kelsey tells Violet that she has problems breathing. Because Kelsey does not have an inhaler at school, Violet calls Mrs. Young to pick Kelsey up from school and suggests that she be seen by her doctor. When Mrs. Young arrives, Violet encourages her to send an inhaler to school that can be kept in the nurse's office, but Mrs. Young seems reluctant to do this. A few days later, Violet contacts Mrs. Young and asks her to help her develop an asthma action plan to ensure that Kelsey gets appropriate and prompt treatment at school as needed. Violet notices that Angie is much more cooperative with this approach and recognizes her need to be in control of situations. By asking Mrs. Young to help develop the plan, she is able to get an improved and helpful response NEWS.

Episode 6

A teacher at Neighborhood Middle School tells Violet that one of her students, Jenna Riley, has gained a lot of weight recently and wants to know if she has any medical conditions. Violet vaguely remembers Jenna, but does not recall anything specifically, so she tells the teacher that she will look into the matter. When Violet reviews Jenna's file, she sees that there is no history of any medical problems and that she is up to date with her immunizations.

Episode 7

This week Violet has another nursing student assigned with her for a clinical rotation. The student, Kayla Sharif, tells Violet that her sister is a junior at the Neighborhood High School. Violet does not believe she has ever met Kayla's sister. Violet finds that having nursing students assigned to work with her is a two-edged sword. On the one hand, she finds them to be somewhat helpful after they get oriented, but on the other hand, it seems that just about the time they get oriented and to a point of being helpful, the clinical rotation is over.

Rebecca Patterson stops in and tells Violet that her husband, Blake, has been seeing a nurse practitioner at the Neighborhood Health Connections Clinic and has been on a depression medication for a few weeks now. She tells Violet that she has not seen any difference yet. She hopes the medication works soon because he is difficult to live with and she does not want this to negatively impact her daughter, Victoria. Violet reminds Rebecca that the benefits of medication and other treatment for depression take time; she promises to keep tabs on how Victoria is doing with her classes and will let Rebecca know if any issues worsen [NEWS].

Episode 8

Violet gets a phone call from the School Board President, wanting to know how Violet feels about the food choices at school. The president explains that she is tired of seeing children eating "crappy" food. Violet says that she previously attempted to get more healthy alternatives into the school snack bar but was unable to get the food services supervisor to make any changes in the menu choices. The School Board President asks Violet to gather information on the nutritional value of some of the more popular snack bar items and to create a presentation for the next School Board meeting in three weeks. Violet agrees to this and hopes this will also give her leverage to get the School Board to agree to hire another nurse - especially since the school health aide positions have yet to be filled. Violet asks Kayla Sharif, the nursing student who is completing a clinical rotation with her, to help her prepare the presentation. They use information gathered from a survey conducted earlier in the year as a starting point for their report [image].

Episode 9

Violet talks with Victoria Patterson's teacher to inquire how things are going. The teacher tells Violet that although she is still passing, Victoria's academic performance has dropped off. He also states that Victoria has become less engaged with school and friends. In fact, she often walks around the playground alone now, whereas she used to spend all of her time with her two friends, Kelsey Young and Keisha Reynolds. Violet calls Victoria's mother, Rebecca, and shares this information with her. She offers a few referrals for family counseling. She also suggests that Rebecca could discuss family counseling with her husband and get a referral from his mental health provider.

Episode 10

Violet and Kayla go to the School Board meeting to present the findings on the nutritional value of the popular items that are sold at the snack bars at Neighborhood Middle and High Schools. Violet stresses to the board that there are not enough healthy items, such as fresh fruits and vegetables, available to the students.

Violet is reminded of the contract the schools have with a supplier. As a recommendation, Violet suggests that the vending machines in the schools be filled with bottled water or juice, as opposed to soda, since the supplier carries both. The food services supervisor, who is also at the meeting, disagrees with Violet and claims that the snack bar would lose a large amount of money if he were to sell fruits and vegetables as opposed to popular foods. He says that students won't buy those items and there would be significant waste. No decision is made at the meeting, but the board says it will study the issue further.

Episode 11

At long last, two health aides have been hired. Violet spends the week orienting them to their new jobs. She clearly explains to them the scope of their job duties, teaches them basic first aid measures, and reviews the medication policies. She explains that they can only dispense prescription medications to students who have supplies at school, but they may not give any student over-the-counter medications, such as Tylenol or cold medicines. Kayla is really surprised at the limited level of understanding these health aides have and is surprised that they are considered acceptable alternatives to having another school nurse.

Episode 12

Amy Price and Carrie Rivera, the two high school students arrested last year after causing an automobile crash that killed a mother and her young son, are once again the talk of the school. Because Carrie was driving while intoxicated at the time of the accident, she was found guilty of vehicular manslaughter. Amy Price, also intoxicated at the time of the accident, was found not guilty, because she did not yet have a driver's license (only a driver's permit) and was a passenger in the vehicle. Although Carrie recently dropped out, Amy has continued to attend school.

Kayla tells Violet that her sister (also a high school student) knows Amy Price and that since the accident she has continued to drink regularly and is rumored to be using drugs. Violet talks with the school counselors about this situation and they inform her that they have attempted to reach out to Amy but have had no luck. They state that they really have no recourse as long as she is not using drugs on school property or coming to school impaired. Violet and Kayla think about ways to reach out to Amy.

Episode 13

The School Board appoints Violet to a task force charged with reviewing food choices at the schools. The task force is directed to submit a recommendation to the School Board within 2 weeks.

Kayla tells Violet that, according to her sister, Amy Price was really drunk at a party over the weekend and ended up in the Neighborhood Emergency Department with acute alcohol poisoning. She had been doing shots of tequila, one after another. Kayla tells Violet that many of Amy's friends are really worried about her partying, but her parents don't seem to care. Violet confirms that Amy was absent on Monday, but she was back in school on Tuesday. Violet sends a note to Amy asking her to come by the office, but she does not respond. She also attempts to contact Amy's parents, but her calls go unanswered.

Episode 14

Violet sees Rebecca Patterson this week. Rebecca thanks Violet for keeping tabs on her daughter, Victoria. Rebecca tells Violet that her husband, Blake, told the mental health nurse practitioner about the changes noted in Victoria at school, and now they are seeing a family counselor. Rebecca really wants to save her marriage and hopes the family sessions will help everyone [NEWS].

Episode 15

Based on recommendations from the task force to which Violet belongs, the School Board announces a ban on all "junk" food sold at the schools. The supplier agrees to switch drinks from sodas to water, tea, lemonade, and fruit juice. Many of the students and parents at the school are furious about the ban and vow to fight it. One angry mother and her daughter learn that Violet was on the task force and share their displeasure with her. Violet is surprised by the response ▼ [NEWS].

Violet Brinkworth Season 3 Information

Episode 1

Violet Brinkworth is a 42-year-old nurse who works for the Neighborhood Public School System. She has been married to her husband Richard Brinkworth for 16 years. Because Richard is often away on business trips, Violet decided to become a school nurse 7 years ago so she could be on the same schedule as her son, who is now 13 years old. She sometimes feels frustrated with her job because of the lack of support from the school principals.

This episode Violet sees Jason Riley in her office at lunchtime so that he can take his amphetamine and dextroamphetamine (Adderall). He tells Violet that he doesn't want anyone to know he takes medication because he doesn't want to be teased.

Meanwhile, several angry students and parents have signed a petition demanding that the Neighborhood schools bring back the original menu items in the snack bars and vending machines. The students and parents argue that the kids are old enough to make their own decisions and don't need the school deciding what they should or should not eat. The principal tells the parents that she will consider their demands and determine if a compromise can be reached. She explains to Violet that she wants to support the task force and the decision that was made, but since many parents are upset, they should probably bring back the most popular items that have been removed from the menu ▼ [NEWS].

Episode 2

Jenna Riley comes into the nurse's office this week complaining of a twisted ankle. Violet does not see any indication of an ankle injury, so instead she talks to Jenna about other things. Jenna tells Violet that she is unhappy about her weight, which reminds Violet of Jenna's teacher's remarks about her weight gain. She asks Jenna if she has been really thirsty or hungry lately, and Jenna admits that she's been drinking a lot more soda because she's "always thirsty." Violet tells Jenna that she should see her family doctor and gets Jenna's permission to call her mother [NEWS].

Episode 3

Violet contacts Evelyn Riley to find out if Jenna was seen by a physician. Mrs. Riley shares with Violet that Jenna is having a lot of tests done by Dr. Rowe. She is a little worried about there being a problem because of all the lab tests ordered, but does not know for sure what the problem is yet [NEWS].

Episode 4

Violet visits with Mr. Keller, the principal of the Neighborhood Middle School, about her intention to include information about sexually transmitted infections and pregnancy in a health unit that she is preparing. The principal is resistant to the idea, because he knows that there is a local group of churches that is mounting a campaign against books and materials that they deem to be too inappropriate and immoral to be allowed in the schools. Violet wonders how much of this argument is really coming from the community groups as opposed to Mr. Keller himself. Violet reminds the principal that the school requires each student to turn in a signed permission slip before he or she is eligible to be present when she teaches on these topics.

Episode 5

Violet sees Rebecca Patterson this week at the school with her daughter, Victoria. Violet asks Rebecca how things are going and is told that things at home are much better. Rebecca tells her that the family therapy has been fabulous and Shawn Jacobs, the nurse practitioner at Neighborhood Health Connections Clinic, is outstanding. "I honestly thought I was headed for a divorce," she tells Violet, "but I think I finally have my husband back." Violet smiles when she hears this, grateful this family has been helped by another nurse.

Mrs. Riley calls Violet this week to let her know that Jenna was diagnosed with type 2 diabetes and that she will be taking her to an endocrinologist to decide how best to treat it. Violet thanks Mrs. Riley for the update and asks her to keep her posted so that she can be informed of the treatment plan.

Violet also learns that Marcus Young, one of the students attending the Neighborhood Elementary School, was struck by a car while riding his bike. She learns that he is in the hospital and is expected to recover. Violet thinks that Angie Young is probably going crazy about now.

Episode 6

Mr. Keller, the Neighborhood Middle School principal, informs Violet that the School Board is not comfortable with the topics of presentations that she has been planning, and that she needs to limit her focus to abstinence only. Furthermore, he asks Violet not to discuss sexually transmitted infections and instead to create a brochure that will be made available to the students. Violet is furious and argues that she is doing the students a disservice by withholding information that they need to keep themselves safe. Grudgingly, she agrees to focus on abstinence.

Episode 7

Out of 120 seventh-grade students, only six have returned notes from parents asking that their children not participate in the sexuality unit. As an alternative assignment, Violet gives these students a packet to work on that focuses on obesity and nutrition. These students are sent to the library to work on the packets during class time. During this same week, Violet notices a large stack of the sexually transmitted infection brochures that she created for students in the trash can in the teachers' lounge. She knows that only teachers and staff have access to the lounge and is distressed that someone would intentionally throw away important information that the students need. Violet suspects that Mr. Keller, the principal, is behind this, but says nothing.

Violet also meets with Jenna Riley and her mother this week to discuss her diabetes management plan. Violet stresses the importance of notifying her if there are any changes in her treatment plan. That way Violet will be able to provide appropriate care should Jenna need it while at school.

Episode 8

Two eighth-grade students come to Violet's office this week to ask her how to get condoms or birth control for "their friends." Violet tells them to let their friends know that the Neighborhood Health Department Clinic offers birth control and exams for sexually transmitted infection for free or at a reduced cost. She wishes that she could give this information to all of the students and hopes that the students who came to her are able to pass along the information to the others.

Episode 9

Violet receives a call from Mr. Anderson at the Neighborhood Hospital with a job offer. She is well aware that the nurses are currently on strike, citing increased patient loads and unsafe working conditions. She is offered considerably more money than she earns at the school, but turns down the offer in order to keep her schedule and take care of her son.

Episode 10

This week Violet writes a letter to the parents of all of the eighth graders, asking for official copies of shot records and reminding them that their children will not be allowed to begin high school if their immunization records are not up to date. As she reviews the records, she finds several students who are missing one or more of their scheduled immunizations. She makes a list of these students' names and waits to see if they bring in new or updated records.

Episode 11

Violet notices a sudden increase in students with flu-like symptom across all three schools. At first there were a few cases in each school each day, but by the third day the number has skyrocketed and Violet notifies the Public Health Department. The Health

Department confirms that there is a flu outbreak that is being monitored. Violet sends a notification home to all parents about the outbreak and encourages them to keep children home from school if they have any symptoms at all.

Episode 12

Violet attends the local Sigma Theta Tau meeting this week and is pleased to see that Shawn Jacobs from Neighborhood Health Connections Clinic is doing a presentation on mental health issues among veterans. She recognizes that he is the same nurse practitioner who has been working with Blake Patterson, the father of Victoria Patterson, a student from the elementary school. After his presentation, Violet introduces herself and lets Shawn know that his work has made a difference for one of her students.

Episode 13

While working at Neighborhood High School, a student comes running into Violet's office and tells her that one of the students is sick in the hall outside the girls' locker room. Violet hurries out and finds Amy Price, a student with alleged drug and alcohol problems, lying on the floor awake. When Violet asks her what happened, Amy does not respond. Violet notices that Amy's pupils are dilated, and she has labored breathing. Violet checks Amy's pulse and notes it is very weak and rapid. She sends a student to the main office to tell someone to notify the principal and then Violet calls 9-1-1 on her cell phone. She asks Amy if she has taken any medicine or drugs recently. She does not respond, but Amy's friend tells Violet that she took a "whole bunch" of pills but nobody knows what the pills were. The paramedics arrive and take Amy to Neighborhood Hospital. Violet writes up a detailed incident report and submits it to the office.

Episode 14

Violet is called into the principal's office at Neighborhood High School and is reprimanded for calling an ambulance to come to the school. The principal tells Violet that in the future she needs to allow her to decide whether or not an ambulance is needed and make the call ▶ ⌄.

Violet has a heated exchange at this point, telling the principal that there was no time to try to find her, and that she used her professional judgment and decided to call an ambulance based on her assessment of the situation. She also tells the principal that she is very willing to inform her of the need to call for emergency help if she is easy to find, but will not put a student's life in jeopardy to appease her need to control the situation. The principal tells Violet that she is expected to follow the school policy. Violet responds that emergency situations trump policies, and that in the future she will continue to use her professional clinical judgment to prioritize actions needed in emergency situations. It is on days like this that Violet wonders if she would be better off working at Neighborhood Hospital.

Episode 15

The school year has come to an end. Violet spends the last week of school chaperoning students as they engage in various end-of-year activities. She also spends time reorganizing her files and preparing her year-end reports. She is very tired and is looking forward to several weeks of rest before the next school year starts ⌄.

SENIOR CENTER

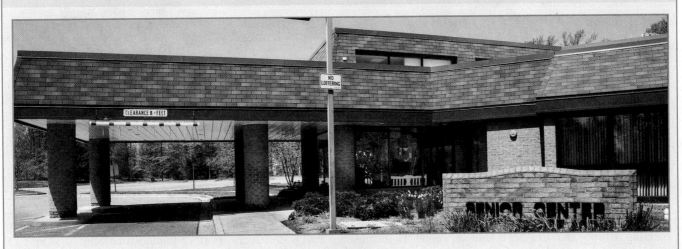

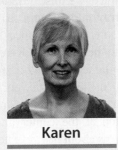

Karen

Housing

**Parks and
Recreation**

Services   There is regular bus service in the area, both from the downtown and residential areas. There is a grocery store within 2
blocks and several small convenience stores and locally run
eating establishments located within a 4-block radius.

Key: ▶ = video clip   ☰ = medical record   ▼ = journal entry   [NEWS] = news article

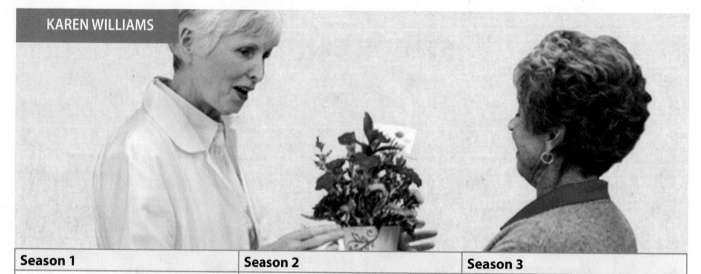

KAREN WILLIAMS

Season 1	Season 2	Season 3
Karen works at the Senior Center Nursing Clinic and interacts with a variety of older adults who visit there. Student nurses Kayla Sharif and Jacob McCain do clinical rotation with Karen at the Senior Center. They become acquainted with Mrs. James during this season. Karen attempts to educate Mrs. James about her medications and how to manager diabetes, but she seems disinterested. Suspecting elder abuse involving Mr. Alden, Karen contacts a social worker from Adult Protective Services to evaluate Mr. Alden's situation at home. Veteran Robert Jackson, the center's van driver, is admitted to the hospital.	The number of seniors coming to the center is increasing, and Karen feels overwhelmed. Eloise Saunders, a retired army nurse, begins to visit the Senior Center and announces her willingness to help Karen. Karen learns that Mrs. James has had a stroke and visits her in the hospital, encouraging her to get better. Mary Martin visits with Karen at the center and voices her concerns about having cataract surgery. Karen reassures her that she will have great improvement in her vision. Karen hears from Jacob McCain that Mr. Alden is injured and in the hospital, and she calls the social worker on his behalf. Robert Jackson collapses at the Senior Center.	A new nursing student, Jennifer Porter, joins Karen this season and quickly proves to be a valuable asset. Karen and Jennifer do a presentation on medication management. Because the Senior Center Nursing Clinic is very busy, Karen writes a letter to the City Council requesting an increase in funding. Mrs. James is now at home recovering from her stroke. She comes to the center to visit with Karen and allows her to check her blood pressure and glucose level.

Karen Williams Season 1 Information

Episode 1

Karen Williams is 57 years old. She has been a geriatric nurse for 30 years and has worked at the nursing clinic at the Neighborhood Senior Center for five years. Karen's position is supported by funds from the city budget. In addition to providing health screenings and information to seniors, Karen also supervises nursing students who come to the center for their clinical experience. The clinic is open from 10-12 a.m. and 1-3 p.m., Monday, Wednesday, and Friday. The clinic is very small, consisting of a check-in station, an examination room, and a supply room. In addition, Karen has a small office in the back.

In the past, Karen would see an average of 20 people per week, but she has noticed an increase in numbers during recent years. She believes the increased number of patient visits to the clinic is directly related to the increased number of elders who come to the Senior Center. Karen is on a first-name basis with most of the individuals who regularly come to the center. They often come to her with their questions and concerns. One thing that Karen enjoys about geriatric nursing is that the seniors are eager to talk, and most of them are very appreciative of her help.

Karen is a widow; her husband died suddenly two years ago of heart disease. She finds working at the clinic rewarding, and it provides an opportunity for regular and interesting interactions.

Karen currently has a nursing student by the name of Kayla Sharif who will be with her for the next several weeks. Kayla is in her second semester of nursing school. Karen reviews the general operating procedures with Kayla and suggests that Kayla shadow her for the first few days.

George Murphy, a regular visitor to the clinic, shares with Karen that his son and daughter are trying to force him to sell his home and move into an assisted living facility. It makes him angry to think of leaving the house where he and his wife lived for 20 years, but he admits that he can't take care of the house anymore. Karen encourages George to talk with his children about how he feels. When asked if he has visited the assisted living facility, he tells Karen that he refuses to live in a place like that. She encourages him to consider making a visit just to see what it is like. Betty Marks, another Senior Center regular, overhears the conversation George is having with Karen. Trying to be helpful, she suggests that George come to live with her [NEWS].

Episode 2

Kayla Sharif, the nursing student, helps Karen check equipment and order supplies for the clinic. Kayla tells Karen that it never occurred to her that many supplies have an expiration date and need to be checked periodically.

Robert Jackson, a divorced 70-year-old African American and Vietnam veteran, is a regular face at the Senior Center. He has worked for the Senior Center as the shuttle van driver for the last 5 years after retiring from a job as a government security supervisor. Although many people who are at the clinic are of similar age as Mr. Jackson, he is in far better physical condition than most of his peers. A lifelong smoker, he suffers from mild emphysema. He sees himself in the role of "helping the elderly." Karen notices he is really the center of attention and is well liked by nearly all who attend the Senior Center. He checks in regularly with Karen and Kayla to see if they need his help.

Episode 3

Karen and Kayla see Mrs. James, a first-time visitor to the Senior Center Nursing Clinic. As Kayla attempts to get baseline information and a history from Mrs. James, Karen overhears the conversation and recognizes that Kayla is intimidated by this patient and is struggling to get a good history. Karen joins them and facilitates the discussion so that Kayla can complete the history.

Mrs. James's primary concern is a sore on her leg that is painful and getting worse. Upon examination of the wound, Karen can see she has an infected ulcer on her leg that needs treatment. Karen determines that Mrs. James needs to be seen by her primary care provider. She helps Mrs. James get an appointment and arranges for Robert Jackson, the shuttle van driver, to take her there.

When he returns from taking Mrs. James to her appointment, Mr. Jackson stops back in the clinic and starts talking with Kayla about Mrs. James. Karen overhears Mr. Jackson say, "That lady really has an attitude," followed by Kayla's laughter and agreement. Kayla says, "Yeah, she is really weird too… and the wound on her leg was really disgusting!" When Mr. Jackson goes outside to smoke a cigarette, Karen gently reminds Kayla that talking about patients in this way is not appropriate. Kayla attempts to justify the conversation by mentioning that Mr. Jackson is just one of the staff; Karen corrects her and tells her Mr. Jackson is not a provider and does not work directly in the clinic. Karen can see that Kayla is embarrassed about the situation and hopes that she was not too hard on her ▶ ✉.

Episode 4

Mr. and Mrs. Simmons, who have been coming to the Senior Center Nursing Clinic for many months, stop in to ask Karen to check Mr. Simmons' blood pressure. Mrs. Simmons explains to Karen that her husband's blood pressure was elevated at a recent visit to the physician, and he was told that, if it stayed elevated, he would need to take "blood pressure pills." Karen asks Kayla to take his blood pressure; she reports to them that it is 128/72 mm Hg. Karen also takes the blood pressure and confirms Kayla has taken an accurate reading. Karen talks with Kayla about emerging technology that allows patients to send blood pressure measurements and other information directly to their providers and medical records.

Episode 5

Mr. Alden, a widower of a few years, is usually at the Senior Center once a week. Karen has tried to have a conversation with him on several occasions, but he does not interact much. She wonders about him and knows that Robert Jackson, the shuttle driver, seems to talk with him more than anyone. Karen asks Mr. Jackson what he knows about Mr. Alden and is told, "Not much – he's not a talker." Later in the morning, Karen notices that Kayla (the nursing student) is playing a game of cards with Mr. Alden and has him laughing. Karen is impressed with Kayla's ability to connect with the older adults who come to the Senior Center.

Episode 6

Karen sees Mrs. James again this week at the Senior Center Nursing Clinic. Mrs. James is proud to show Karen that her leg is healing. Karen attempts to talk with her about her medications and give her information about managing her diabetes, but Mrs. James shows little interest. Karen encourages Mrs. James to bring a list of the medications that she takes on her next visit. Mrs. James is in a hurry to leave so that she can get her free lunch.

Karen and nursing student Kayla discuss the upcoming health fair. Karen tells Kayla that the Senior Center Nursing Clinic has a table each year and suggests that perhaps Kayla would like to be in charge of this. Kayla talks with her nursing instructor and agrees this would be an excellent activity as part of her clinical assignment. Kayla and two other nursing students work with Karen to gather appropriate materials. They decide that the theme will be *The Benefits of Social Engagement for Elders* ▶ ▼.

Episode 7

Kayla does not come to the clinic this week because she is at the Health Fair representing the Senior Center and Nursing Clinic. When Karen goes to help Kayla and the two other nursing students set up, she is pleasantly surprised and very impressed with the quality of their work.

Back at the clinic, Karen encourages the seniors at the center to attend the Neighborhood Health Fair. Many of them ask her if they will be giving away any free food or medical supplies at the fair. She has arranged transportation to the health fair with Mr. Robert Jackson, the shuttle driver for the Senior Center.

When they return from the Health Fair, Mr. Jackson tells Karen that he is in perfect health because he passed all the screening tests. He then proceeds to flex his biceps and says, "I am a picture of perfect health!" Karen is amused by his antics ▼ NEWS.

Episode 8

Mary Martin stops in the Nursing Clinic and tells Kayla and Karen all about her bone density screening results at the Health Fair and the recommendation that she follow up with her healthcare provider to get a full bone scan. Mary asks Kayla and Karen about the bone scan test and if they think this is a good idea. This is Kayla's last week at the Nursing Clinic with Karen ▶.

Episode 9

This week a new nursing student, Jacob McCain, starts a clinical rotation with Karen. Jacob is a third-semester nursing student. Karen reviews the general operating procedures with Jacob and suggests that he shadow her for the first few days.

As one of his first learning activities, Karen assigns Jacob to help a group of women from the Neighborhood Senior Center develop a presentation for Smoking Awareness Week. Their goal is to teach individuals about the hazards of smoking. Jacob helps them assemble a plastic "smoking lung" prop from the Lung Cancer Association. Jacob helps another woman make a chart of the number of cigarettes her husband smokes per day, per week, and per year, and the cost of all of those cigarettes over a 20-year period. Another group member plans to talk about how she developed asthma from second-hand smoke in her home.

Episode 10

Mrs. James comes into the clinic to see Karen this week. Karen checks her vital signs (blood pressure, 126/92 mm Hg; blood glucose, 124 mg/dL) and asks Mrs. James about her medication list. Mrs. James pulls out a bag from her purse and dumps out a large supply of pills. Jacob, the student nurse, does an inventory of the pills she has brought in while Karen examines Mrs. James's feet. While performing this exam, Karen notices that Mrs. James's shoes are in poor shape. One shoe has been cut down, and the edges are covered with cotton balls and tape. She talks to Mrs. James about the need to wear shoes that fit and suggests that she check at the Senior Center for help obtaining properly fitting shoes. Karen also notes that the wound on Mrs. James's leg has nearly healed. While Karen is assessing her feet, Mrs. James talks about her frustrations with her doctors and all of her appointments, and Karen listens quietly. It seems to her that Mrs. James is quite isolated and does not have many opportunities to talk about her feelings. Karen listens attentively and encourages Mrs. James to call her physicians to inquire about the appointments.

After Karen is finished with the foot examination, Jacob comments to Mrs. James that many of the drugs are expired and it is not clear which medications Mrs. James is supposed to be taking. Mrs. James grabs all of her medications and puts them back in her bag. Clearly annoyed, she tells Jacob she knows what they are for, and she is not going to take the time to explain it all to him ▶.

Episode 11

This week, the Neighborhood Senior Center Nursing Clinic is offering flu vaccinations. Karen and Jacob review the immunization clinic procedures and check to be sure that an adequate number of vaccines are stocked. As they are preparing for the shot clinic, one of the staff members from the kitchen knocks on the door and asks if her daughter can get a flu shot. Karen encourages her to bring her daughter to the clinic and tells her the cost is $20.

Four first-semester nursing students are scheduled to help give flu vaccines at the center. Karen asks Jacob to orient the students to the clinic, and reviews the procedures for the day. Karen is very impressed with Jacob's ability to get these students oriented and is amazed at the difference between a first- and third-semester student. One student admits to Karen that she is nervous about giving vaccinations to some of the ladies because their arms are so thin. Karen reviews the injection techniques with the student and reassures her that she will be supervising the entire time and available should she have questions NEWS.

Episode 12

Karen sees Mr. Alden sitting alone at the Senior Center with disheveled hair and unclean clothes. She encourages him to come into her clinic to have his blood pressure checked. When she asks him to pull up his shirt sleeve, she notices that his arm is purple and appears freshly bruised. He tells her that he thinks he fell down, but when she looks closely at his face, she sees another bruise that is turning yellow. She asks him if he has any other bruises. He reluctantly agrees to show her his abdomen, and it too is very bruised. Karen asks Mr. Alden if he lives with anyone, and he tells her that he lives with his son. When she asks him if he remembers how he got all of the bruises, his reply is, "I don't know."

Karen talks to Jacob McCain, the nursing student, and explains that, based on her observations and Mr. Alden's vague answers, she suspects elder abuse, which they have a professional obligation to report. Karen contacts Naomi Carson, a social worker at Neighborhood Adult Protective Services, and shares her concerns about elder abuse. Naomi agrees that the circumstances warrant a home visit to evaluate Mr. Alden and his living situation. Later in the week, Jacob talks about this case in his clinical seminar at school and discusses how it links to the concept of advocacy ▶ 📰.

Episode 13

Mary Martin comes into the clinic this week. She shares with Karen that she has been recently diagnosed with Osteoporosis and wonders if she will get hurt during the exercise class at the Senior Center. Karen asks if Mary talked about exercising with her doctor; Mary confirms that she saw Dr. Rowe, who said it was fine. Karen explains to Mary that exercising helps to strengthen her bones and can increase her bone density. Karen provides positive encouragement for Mary's participation in the exercise class and tells her that aerobics is an excellent form of weight-bearing exercise.

Karen and Jacob see Mrs. James in the clinic again this week. Mrs. James is clearly annoyed with Jacob's presence and only directs her conversation to Karen. She tells Karen that she can't get her medication for her Blood glucose filled. When Jacob tells her that he would like to check her blood sugar level, she looks at him and says, "Do you know what you are doing?" Jacob rather enjoys Mrs. James and does not get intimidated or take offense to her comments or behavior. He holds out his hand and she complies by placing her finger in his palm. He measures her blood glucose level and tells her it is 192 mg/dL and that she is right about needing to get the prescription filled.

Karen is able to arrange a refill for Mrs. James. While on the phone with a pharmacist, Karen also get a more comprehensive understanding of her medical conditions and her list of her medications - something they have been unable to do up to now ▼.

Episode 14

Naomi Carson, the social worker from Neighborhood Adult Protective Services, drops by the Senior Center Nursing Clinic and talks with Karen and Jacob McCain as a follow-up to Karen's concerns regarding Mr. Alden. Naomi tells Karen and Jacob that the visit was inconclusive but agrees with Karen that there is reason for concern. Naomi asks them to keep an eye out for Mr. Alden and to call her if they observe additional findings that are concerning.

Mary Martin is back at the Senior Center this week and sees Jacob McCain, the nursing student, sitting at a desk. She walks in, sits down and tells him all about her appointment with the eye doctor and the eye drops and the cataract surgery. She asks Jacob many detailed questions about cataract surgery that he attempts to answer by searching on the internet. Karen sees that Jacob is not looking at a reliable website and inserts herself into the discussion. Karen tells Mary that many of the questions she is asking are better answered by her doctor.

After Mrs. Martin leaves, Karen talks to Jacob about finding a balance between answering general health questions and attempting to answer detailed questions such as those Mrs. Martin was asking. Karen also reminded Jacob about the reliability of sources for health information on the web.

Episode 15

Jacob McCain, the nursing student, sees Mr. Jackson, the shuttle driver, in the Senior Center getting some coffee. He hears him coughing and senses that he is not feeling well. Jacob asks how he is feeling and Mr. Jackson replies, "Just caught a cold." Jacob encourages Mr. Jackson to come into the clinic to see Karen. Karen quickly realizes Mr. Jackson is quite ill. He has a fever, appears dehydrated, and has a bad cough. Karen makes arrangements for him to be seen at the Neighborhood Hospital Emergency Department. Karen is impressed with Jacob and praises him for not only recognizing Mr. Jackson's condition, but also encouraging him to get seen. Later in the day they learn Mr. Jackson has been admitted to the Neighborhood Hospital with bacterial pneumonia.

Karen Williams Season 2 Information

Episode 1

Karen Williams is 57 years old. She has been a geriatric nurse for 30 years and has worked at the nursing clinic at the Neighborhood Senior Center for five years. In the last few years, the number of visits has grown from 20 per week to 34 per week.

Next month the Senior Center will be sponsoring a weekend trip by bus to a nearby national park. Although a fee is required, the cost is minimal. Karen tells Mrs. James about the trip and suggests that she go on the outing.

A group of nursing students is at the Neighborhood Senior Center Nursing Clinic for just one day to check blood pressures. Karen overhears one of the students agree to give Mrs. Marsh, a 78-year-old woman, a ride home from the center. Karen pulls the student aside and talks with her about the situation, explaining that Mrs. Marsh consistently asks for rides and special favors from the staff. Karen gently points out that the student should not offer to give rides to Mrs. Marsh or any other senior. The student tells Karen that she was overwhelmed and didn't know what to do, so Karen reassures her and tells her that talking and listening to Mrs. Marsh is perfectly fine, but she should not become involved beyond that point [NEWS].

Episode 2

In order to qualify for funding, Karen maintains a log of the number of individuals she sees. By looking through her records, she recognizes that the numbers have definitely increased, despite the drop in nursing hours. Karen is glad to see that elders in the community use the service, but she is concerned about the time constraints she faces in trying to connect with so many individuals. She also finds that she has limited time for teaching the seniors at the center, which is a part of her job that she enjoys a great deal [NEWS].

Episode 3

The Senior Center Planning Committee organizes a trip to a national park for sightseeing. Karen agrees to go and ensures that the bus has an updated first aid kit. She reminds everyone to bring plenty of water, as well as hats and sunscreen. Most of the seniors attending are fairly healthy, so Karen does not anticipate problems. After arriving at the park, the seniors take a short walk. Mr. Dallion, who has emphysema, returns to the bus, feeling short of breath after the walk. Fortunately, he brought his oxygen pack on the bus just in case he needed it. Karen assists Mr. Dallion with the oxygen. On the way home, she sits with George Raley, who talks to her the entire way home about his stiff knee and shows Karen the scars from his knee replacement surgery [▼].

Episode 4

Mr. Jackson, the veteran who drives the shuttle van for the Neighborhood Senior Center, is finally back to work. He was hospitalized with pneumonia several months ago and had a very slow recovery because the pneumonia exacerbated his underlying emphysema. Karen notes that Mr. Jackson has lost some weight, but other than that, he looks good and is truly happy to be back to work. Despite his recent respiratory ailments, Mr. Jackson goes right back to taking his smoking breaks outside the Senior Center.

Episode 5

Karen can see the effects of the forest fire on many of the individuals at the Neighborhood Senior Center Nursing Clinic. Mr. Jackson calls Karen and asks her opinion about whether he should come to work. Karen is glad he called; she suggests that he stay at home – especially considering his recent bout with pneumonia. Karen talks with Mr. Jackson's supervisor on his behalf. Many of the seniors, including Mr. Dallion, have needed to use oxygen more often this week. She advises these individuals to stay indoors to avoid respiratory irritants [NEWS].

Episode 6

This week Karen meets a new visitor to the Senior Center, Eloise Saunders, a 72-year-old former Army nurse who worked in military field hospitals in Vietnam. She recently moved to the Neighborhood to live near her daughter Andrea after the death of her husband. On this first visit, Ms. Saunders is accompanied by her daughter to scope out the Senior Center and determine if this would be a place she would like to spend time. Mrs. Saunders quickly spots the Senior Center Nursing Clinic and walks in to check it out. She announces to Karen, "I'm an old Army nurse and I'll be able to help you take care of sick folks." Karen can see that she appears to be in very good physical health.

Episode 7

Karen receives a call from Jacob McCain, the nursing student who completed a clinical rotation with her earlier this year. Jacob tells Karen he has some important information about a patient he saw at the Neighborhood Senior Center Nursing Clinic and hoped that by calling her he was not breaking confidentiality policies. He went on to say that Mr. Alden, the elderly man who they suspected was being physically abused, was at the Neighborhood Hospital with a fractured arm and several fractured ribs. He also was malnourished. Jacob told Karen that he mentioned the previous concerns of abuse to the primary nurse but he was pretty sure nothing would be done. Jacob remembered that the social worker asked them to report back to her if there was any further indication of potential abuse. Karen tells Jacob to let his instructor and nurse manager on the unit know, and that she will notify the social worker, Naomi Carson. Karen had noticed that Mr. Alden had suddenly stopped coming to the Senior Center after she reported her concerns to social services and had wondered if there was something to that ▾ [NEWS].

Episode 8

Mary Martin is in Karen's office talking about her great-grandson, Tyler, when a man by the name of Brian James walks into the clinic. He tells Karen and Mary that his mother, Norma James, had a stroke a few weeks ago. Karen tells Brian that she had noticed his mother had not been in for a few weeks and appreciated knowing why. Mary tells Brian that she is very good friends with his mother and she will pray for her. Mary proceeds to tell everyone at the Senior Center all about Mrs. James and her stroke.

Karen decides to visit Mrs. James at the Rehabilitation Hospital. Mrs. James looks exhausted and complains that the nurses aren't taking good care of her; they make her walk every day and go to "stupid classes." Mrs. James makes it clear that she feels there is no point to any of this. Karen encourages Mrs. James to get better so that she can get home to care for her cats. Mrs. James was unaware that her cats were still alive and being cared for, and now has renewed interest in her own care.

Episode 9

Karen walks through the Senior Center and spots Eloise Saunders (the former Army nurse) taking a blood pressure on Mr. Simmons. Mr. Simmons has hypertension and regularly asks Karen to take his blood pressure as a way to monitor it. Eloise tells Mr. Simmons the blood pressure is a bit high. Concerned that Mrs. Saunders might be giving Mr. Simmons incorrect information, Karen later asks Mr. Simmons to stop in the clinic so she can record the blood pressure in his clinic record. Privately, Karen talks with Mrs. Saunders about the situation. Eloise tells Karen, "Mr. Simmons wanted his blood pressure checked and you were busy with another patient, so I found the blood pressure cuff and stethoscope and checked it." Karen realizes she will need to find a way to let Mrs. Saunders "help her" without jeopardizing care. Later, when Mr. Simmons stops by, Karen checks the blood pressure - and sure enough, Mrs. Saunders had been correct - the blood pressure was a bit high.

Mr. Jackson stops in and says to Karen, "I noticed that crazy old lady Mrs. James had stopped coming to the clinic and I was actually kind of happy about that. But then I heard from Mary Martin that she had a stroke and is at the Rehabilitation Hospital. Did you know about that?" Knowing Mary had told everyone at the Senior Center about Mrs. James, Karen simply says, "Yes, I heard that too," but did not offer any additional information. The following day, Mr. Jackson tells Karen that he went to see Mrs. James and reports, "She actually was kind of glad to see me. Imagine that! ▶ [NEWS]"

Episode 10

Mr. Andrews at Neighborhood Hospital calls to offer Karen a job with excellent pay, which would mean a salary increase of over $25,000 per year. Although Karen is flattered by the offer, she is not surprised, given the well-publicized staffing shortages at the hospital. Karen feels committed to her work with the elders in the Neighborhood community and is really not interested in going back to work in a hospital setting.

Episode 11

Naomi Carson contacts Karen this week to inform her that Mr. Alden recently died. He had been in the hospital for several weeks, got pneumonia (probably as a result of the fractured ribs and lack of mobility), got progressively worse, and then died. An autopsy was ordered and there was evidence of multiple abuse injuries. Naomi said Mr. Alden's son was being charged with elder abuse and not to be surprised if she is subpoenaed. Karen feels awful that this happened to Mr. Alden and wonders if there was more she could have done for him.

Eloise Saunders, the former Army nurse, comes by the clinic three times during the week, asking Karen if she needs her help. She lets Karen know which people at the Senior Center probably need to see her. Ms. Saunders ends up having a friendly exchange with Mr. Jackson regarding the Vietnam War. They take an immediate liking to each other ▶ ▾.

Episode 12

Mr. Jackson (the 70-year-old Vietnam vet who works at the Senior Center as the shuttle bus driver) is rushed into the clinic on a gurney by several Senior Center staff. He was reportedly doing some work outside on the shuttle van when he suddenly collapsed to the ground. Although he is nonresponsive, he is breathing. Karen notes his pulse is slow and his blood pressure is 86/50. Karen calls 9-1-1 and then places low-flow oxygen on him. Somehow, Eloise Saunders (the former Army nurse) slips into the treatment room and is at Mr. Jackson's side, holding his hand and gently talking to him, telling him, "Hold on!" and "Everything will be okay." Determining she is doing no harm, and is perhaps calming Mr. Jackson, Karen allows her to stay by his side until the paramedics take Mr. Jackson to the hospital.

Later in the day, Karen learns Mr. Jackson had a cardiac arrhythmia and will be in the hospital a few days getting a workup. Mrs. Saunders hangs around the clinic with Karen the rest of the day "helping her." ⌵

Episode 13

Karen discusses with the Senior Center project director ways to let Mrs. Saunders, the 72-year-old former Army nurse, help in the clinic. Karen believes that if Mrs. Saunders has some sort of designated nurse role, it might be easier to keep track of what she is doing, as opposed to her just randomly trying to help. The project director and Karen decide to give Mrs. Saunders a title of volunteer nurse; Mrs. Saunders is thrilled with the idea. Karen outlines specific hours she can help in a volunteer capacity and the types of things she can do to assist. Even though Mrs. Saunders will have a very limited role, Karen believes it will make her feel useful. Karen and the project director give Ms. Saunders a white lab coat to wear when she is "on duty," so that everyone in the Senior Center will know when she is working in that capacity ⌵.

Episode 14

The Neighborhood Senior Center Nursing Clinic is very busy and crowded this week, and Karen is overwhelmed by the number of individuals who want to see her. She is concerned that a few of the seniors are not being seen by their primary care physicians because they are reluctant to go or unable to get appointments. Karen's plan with Mrs. Saunders works like a charm. People in the center refer to her as "Nurse Ellie," and she wears the white lab coat with great pride. Karen is also pleased that Eloise stays within her designated role quite well and is actually helpful with all the people being seen.

One of the seniors, 91-year-old Betty O'Dowd, stops by the clinic complaining of ongoing pain throughout her lower abdomen for the past few weeks. Eloise tells Karen that she is sure something is wrong with Betty. After talking with Betty, Karen is also concerned. Karen tells Betty that she really needs to see her physician about the abdominal pain. That is the last time Betty is in the clinic.

Episode 15

Mary Martin visits with Karen and talks about needing cataract surgery. She shares with Karen her fears about the surgery – specifically that she heard that she could go blind. Karen tells Mary that cataract surgery is very common, and the risk of blindness is very low. She also tells Mary that many of the seniors have reported great improvement in their vision since having the same surgery. Mary tells Karen that she needs to be able to see well so that she can take care of her great-grandson Tyler, going on to say that her daughter-in-law doesn't take good care of him. Karen suggests that Mary talk with some of the other women at the center about their cataract surgery experiences.

Karen Williams Season 3 Information

Episode 1

Karen Williams has been a geriatric nurse for 31 years and has worked at the nursing clinic at the Neighborhood Senior Center for six years. Karen is very committed to her work and believes the center helps to foster healthy community relationships for those individuals who come. The volume of visitors continues to increase at the center and in recent months there have been an average of 50 patients per week. Despite the fact that she now has a "volunteer nurse" working with her a few hours three times a week, Karen recognizes the need for an additional nurse. She begins to explore funding options to meet this need.

This episode, after being off for several months, Mr. Jackson comes in to the Senior Center to let Karen know that he is retiring from being the shuttle driver for the center. He tells Karen that he has "a bunch" of new medications and a pacemaker. He was advised by his doctor not to go back to work as a shuttle driver. Karen can see that Mr. Jackson is disappointed, and she encourages him to continue coming to the Senior Center whenever he has time.

Karen calls Mrs. James at home to see how she is doing and talks with her son Brian. He shares with Karen that his mother has become very dependent on him, but he will soon need to return home. Karen asks Brian if there are any resources that his mother may need that she could help him to obtain. Brian assures her that he has had plenty of help, and it is now up to his mother to demonstrate her independence. Karen asks Brian to encourage Mrs. James to come back to the Neighborhood Senior Center once she feels up to it.

Episode 2

Karen has another nursing student, Jennifer Porter, who is assigned to the Neighborhood Senior Center Nursing Clinic for the next several weeks as a clinical rotation. Jennifer is in her final semester of nursing school and is completing her capstone clinical (the final senior-level clinical rotation). Jennifer tells Karen that she specifically wanted to do her capstone in this setting because of her interest in geriatric care with a goal of becoming a geriatric nurse practitioner. Karen is thrilled to have a senior student. She reviews the general operating procedures with Jennifer and tells her that she can start seeing patients immediately.

Eloise Saunders tells Jennifer she is the volunteer nurse and explains her role as well. Eloise tells Karen that since she has some extra help right now, she will be off for a few weeks visiting a son in another state.

Episode 3

Karen quickly sees that the senior nursing student, Jennifer, will be a real asset to her. She is very knowledge-able and has good common sense – she knows when to ask questions. For example, Margaret Herrera, a 64-year-old woman who frequently comes to the Neighborhood Senior Center Nursing Clinic, tells Jennifer that her doctor prescribed a "water pill" for her a few days ago, but she did not also get a prescription for potassium pills, like her friend Loretta Sparks has. Margaret asks Jennifer if she should go back and demand to receive potassium pills. Jennifer looks at the prescription bottle and notes that Margaret has been prescribed spironolactone. Jennifer confers with Karen and concludes that Margaret has no reason for alarm because spironolactone is a potassium-sparing diuretic. Jennifer reinforces with Margaret the same patient information previously shared by her physician and the pharmacist, and suggests that she follow up with her physician or a pharmacist if she has further questions about her medication.

Episode 4

Karen has been asked to collaborate with William, a pharmacist from the Community Health Center, to do a free presentation for the general community about medication management among the elderly. Karen sees this as a perfect opportunity to get the nursing student involved with patient teaching and presentations. Karen tells Jennifer that one of the critical things they do is present accurate information in a way that the average lay person can understand. Jennifer tells Karen that she just recently had a patient teaching assignment in which they had to consider health literacy; she knows of a good resource to cross-check the information they prepare. Karen is very glad to have Jennifer's help on this project ▽.

Episode 5

Karen and Jennifer – in collaboration with William (a pharmacist who works at the Community Health Center) – conduct a presentation entitled *Medication Management for the Elderly* this week at the Neighborhood Senior Center. Because it was publicized in the Neighborhood newspaper, there is a very large turnout. Karen is acutely

aware of the challenges that many elderly people face with medication management and adherence. After the presentation, many individuals personally thank Karen, Jennifer, and William for the helpful information. Many of the regulars at the center comment about how pleased they were that "their nurse" was in the newspaper [NEWS].

Episode 6

With the permission of the Senior Center project director, Karen writes a letter to the City Council requesting an increase in funding for the Senior Center Nursing Clinic, specifically to hire another nurse to assist her during the busiest hours and to extend the hours of service. Karen also encourages the seniors who regularly visit the center to write letters. Karen explains to Jennifer, the nursing student, that it is often a challenge to get adequate resources for publicly funded clinics.

Mary Martin announces to everyone at the Senior Center that Betty O'Dowd, one of the seniors frequently seen in the clinic, just died of cancer. Karen recalls that the last time Betty was in the center, she said she had been experiencing abdominal pain for about a month. Karen is very sad to hear of that outcome, as Betty was one of her favorite people. She attends Betty's funeral a few days later.

Episode 7

Mrs. James makes her first visit to the Senior Center following her stroke. When she meets Jennifer, the student nurse, Mrs. James tells her that she only wants to see Karen. Mrs. James comments to Karen that things have changed with "that other nurse" being here. Mrs. James tells Karen that she is glad she still works at the clinic. Karen checks her blood glucose level and blood pressure while Mrs. James talks about her cats.

Mrs. James becomes visibly annoyed when Mr. Sanchez stands in the doorway waiting to talk with Karen. Mrs. James gets up and leaves in a bit of a huff. Karen invites Mr. Sanchez to sit down and asks how he is doing. Mr. Sanchez is 80 years old and lives alone. His wife died last year, and he has had a difficult time adjusting to being widowed. He explains that he has been coming to the center less often because transportation has been an issue for him. Karen gives him information about the shuttle service offered by the Senior Center ▶.

Episode 8

Eloise Saunders, the volunteer nurse, is back from visiting her son. She is more than ready to resume her role as "Nurse Ellie." Jennifer and Eloise hit it off immediately. Eloise is delighted to tell Jennifer all about her nursing experiences as an Army nurse working in field hospitals. She feels that she is giving this student an important lesson in nursing history.

Karen receives a letter from City Council about her request for additional funds. She is told to write a formal proposal with justification for additional funding. Karen wonders aloud how she will find time to write a proposal. Eloise tells Karen that she thinks she can help her do that. Jennifer also offers to help Karen write the proposal as part of her capstone course. Jennifer tells Karen that she is currently taking a course involving health policy; she can see connections between what she is learning in that class and the actions that they need to take to get funding. Karen is impressed that Jennifer has such exposure in her program; she can see that nursing education has certainly changed since she went to school.

Episode 9

Mr. Jackson, the recently retired shuttle driver for the Senior Center, makes a visit to see Karen and Eloise. Karen is with another patient and Eloise is not yet "on duty," so Jennifer signs him in. He tells Jennifer that he had to recently retire because of a heart condition and has been trying to figure out what to do next. Jennifer learns that he is a divorced 71-year-old Vietnam veteran and is a bit lost without having the regular routine of a part-time job. He tells her he did not mind hanging around the center when he had a job, but he does not see himself coming just to kill time. Jennifer suggests he contact some of the Neighborhood city agencies to see about volunteer work. Mr. Jackson tells her, "That would be fine, but I really need the income."

Episode 10

Mrs. James sees Karen at the Senior Center again this week. Although she has become quite a regular participant, she would never admit that she enjoys it. She is visibly annoyed when Jennifer tries to "check her in" and she tells Jennifer that she wants to see the "real nurse," not some student. Karen asks her about her medications and glucose measurements; Mrs. James responds by saying that everything is fine. Still, she allows Karen to check her blood pressure and glucose.

Episode 11

Karen sees Mary Martin this week. Mary explains to Karen how stressful the situation is at her son's home. She describes trying to help care for her grandson Mark, who was recently in an auto accident and was left paralyzed. She also describes all of the problems with Anthony and how his mother has driven him away. Karen reminds Mary that she needs to take time for herself to rest, both physically and emotionally.

Episode 12

Jennifer, Eloise, and Karen spend a significant amount of time preparing the funding proposal and justification for a second clinic nurse. Karen knows that once Jennifer has completed her capstone clinical, she will really be back on her own, with limited help from Eloise. She uses this experience to articulate the need for another nurse. Karen also realizes that the capacity can be better met by having two examination rooms rather than one. Although it was never the intent, the demand for services would best be addressed by offering full primary care services. However, members of the Board of Directors are not interested in changing the focus of services provided.

Episode 13

This week, fitness guru Jack Blaine is hosting a free seminar at the Senior Center. In addition to the public seminar, Karen has arranged for Mr. Blaine to meet informally with the seniors during their lunch hour. Karen is pleased with the response Jack receives from the seniors. They are receptive to his suggestions and ask many questions about their own fitness routines.

Episode 14

Mrs. James stops in to see Karen early in the week to inform her that she will be leaving to visit her son Brian for a few weeks. Mrs. James explains that she knew Karen would wonder what happened to her, and she didn't want Karen to worry about her absence. Later in the afternoon, Mary Martin stops in for a brief moment to give Karen some flowers to thank her for being so helpful. Although Karen leaves the center feeling tired and sometimes burdened, she feels content.

Episode 15

This is Jennifer's last week of her clinical rotation. She is very excited to be graduating and invites Eloise and Karen to her graduation ceremony. Jennifer tells them both how much she has enjoyed the experience and how she has learned so much from them both. Karen makes plans to attend her graduation at the end of the week.

WOMEN'S HEALTH SERVICES

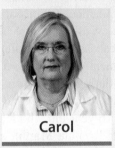

Carol

Housing

Parks and Recreation

Services There is regular bus service in the area, both from the downtown and residential areas. There are several small upscale stores and eating establishments within 3 blocks of Women's Health Services. There are also convenience stores and a grocery store within 6 blocks.

Key: ▶ = video clip   ☰ = medical record   ▽ = journal entry   [NEWS] = news article

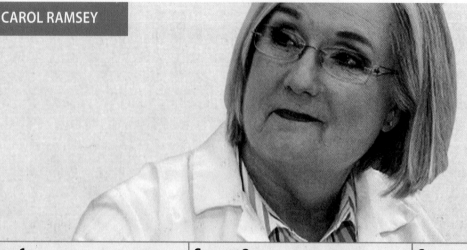

CAROL RAMSEY

Season 1	Season 2	Season 3
Carol is a nurse midwife. She loves her career, but because her patient load has recently increased, she is feeling overwhelmed and run down, spending time after hours to finish her work. Carol notices that more teenage girls are coming to the Community Health Clinic seeking birth control. She participates in the community health fair, providing information and promoting sexual health. Carol detects a mass in the abdomen of a patient, which is later diagnosed as cancer. Jessica Riley comes to the clinic for her first prenatal exam.	Student nurse Jennifer Porter joins Carol for clinical rotation. Initially reluctant to bring a student into this type of practice, Carol comes to see the value of this exposure in developing clinical assessment skills and clinical judgment. Carol is sees a variety of patients during this season, including a woman with severe preeclampsia; Terry, a 16-year-old who learns she is pregnant; Kristina Martin, a 15-year-old requesting birth control pills; and Jessica Riley, who is receiving prenatal care. She suspects that Jessica is the victim of domestic abuse. After delivery of her baby, Jessica finally admits to the abusive relationship that she has with Casey, but refuses to press charges. Carol contacts a social worker to follow up on Jessica's case.	Carol's patient load continues to increase, so she is thrilled to hear that another nurse midwife has been hired. Nancy, one of Carol's older pregnant patients, wants her daughter to be present during the birth of her son. Kristina Martin presents to the Community Health Clinic with Chlamydia. Carol gives her a prescription and talks with her about STD prevention. Carol begins to think about opening her own clinic for midwifery and gynecological care. In this season, her nursing student is Jacob McCain, and Carol initially finds herself unwilling to allow him to assist in examinations. This conflict leads Carol to re-evaluate her assumptions.

Carol Ramsey Season 1 Information

Episode 1

Carol Ramsey is a 51-year-old certified nurse midwife who works at Women's Health Services, seeing her own patients. She has been a midwife for 21 years, after spending the first 8 years of her career as a labor and delivery room nurse. In addition to working four and a half days a week at WHS, Carol works one afternoon each week at the Neighborhood Community Health Department where she sees a variety of patients, many of whom are seeking contraception, pregnancy testing, or screening and treatment of sexually transmitted infections.

Carol is not feeling well this week. She has been trying to recover from a mild cold, but it has really zapped her energy. She has a full caseload this week, because one of the midwives in the practice is out on medical leave for the next few months. Carol and the other nurse midwife at the Neighborhood Women's Health Services are working extra patients into their schedule. This is a bit tough for Carol, because she feels as if she is already working at full capacity. Carol finds it hard to see extra patients in addition to working at the Community Health Department.

Episode 2

A new computer upgrade that has been in the works for several months is finally implemented this week. Carol and the other providers feel overwhelmed because of multiple system problems, including the fact that the medical office personnel are unable to transfer the old medical records into the new system. Carol ends up documenting her patient care visits on a legal pad, knowing she will have to spend time after hours getting the data entered into the system ▼.

Episode 3

Carol has been following two patients, Donna and Marta, throughout their pregnancies. This is a first pregnancy for both. Carol sees Donna for her 39-week visit and she sees Marta for her 37-week visit. The two women have become friends as a result of attending prenatal classes and have pledged to help one another during labor and after their babies are born. Both women are interested in natural childbirth and desire the use of no analgesics or other pharmacologic agents. Carol finds both women to be progressing perfectly. Carol anticipates that Donna will be going into labor soon [NEWS].

Episode 4

Carol spends most of her day at Neighborhood Hospital with two of her patients, Donna and Marta. The two women are friends and both happen to be in the labor unit at the same time. Donna presented to the hospital after her membranes spontaneously ruptured. Marta presented with contractions. Neither woman has progressed in over 12 hours. Carol attempts to get them to progress through nipple stimulation, walking, and warm baths. Eventually Marta begins to progress actively, and Carol successfully delivers her baby several hours later. The next morning, Carol finds that Donna has still failed to progress, so a Pitocin drip is initiated. After a few more hours without adequate progression, Carol consults with Dr. Tito, the obstetrician. Dr. Tito decides to perform a cesarean section in order to achieve the best outcome for Donna and her baby. Donna is devastated, verbalizing that she "failed" to give birth naturally. Carol feels as if she let Donna down ▼ [NEWS].

Episode 5

Carol sees Donna and Marta for a postpartum visit. The two friends scheduled their appointments back to back so they could go together. Marta had a minor laceration that is healing nicely. Her fundus is at an appropriate size and she is describing a typical amount of post-birth bloody vaginal discharge. Marta tells Carol she is breastfeeding and her only issue is nipple soreness.

Because Donna had a cesarean section, Carol evaluates her incision. She finds that it is healing nicely. Donna tells Carol she wishes she did not have to have a cesarean, but she also knows it was necessary to have the best outcome for her baby. Carol is relieved to see that she is coping with that disappointment appropriately.

Episode 6

Carol sees an increase in the number of teenage girls who are coming to the Community Health Department's Family Planning Clinic seeking birth control. She often feels frustrated when she tries to talk with them about safe sex practices and protecting themselves against sexually transmitted infections. Most of the girls are only interested in obtaining birth control pills ▼.

Episode 7

Carol participates at the community health fair this week. She is involved with a display promoting sexual health that is sponsored by the Community Health Department. At her table she has information regarding safe sex practices, contraception, and sexual abuse, as well as a container filled with free condoms. Carol notices several middle-aged women pass by the table and give her dirty looks, as if she is promoting evil behavior. By the end of the afternoon, the container of free condoms is empty ▼ [NEWS].

Episode 8

Carol is invited to be involved with recruitment of participants and data collection for an interdisciplinary study involving determinants of prenatal care among pregnant adolescents. Carol is very excited to be involved with this study. She has always had an interest in clinical research but has not had the time, let alone the expertise, to conduct studies independently. Carol's role will be to identify potential participants based on predetermined guidelines and to recruit them to participate in the study. She also will be involved in providing data related to their prenatal care. Carol knows she has several patients who may be potential participants for the study. She successfully recruits her first patient this week ▼ [NEWS].

Episode 9

Marcie, a 42-year-old woman, comes into the clinic this week to be evaluated for pregnancy. She is sure that she is pregnant because she has not menstruated for "two or three months," she has gained ten pounds, and she reports fullness in her abdominal area. Marcie has never been seen at the clinic before, and she tells Carol that she moved into the Neighborhood about one year ago. A pregnancy test is negative, and a pelvic exam reveals that her ovaries and uterus are normal in size and shape. Carol palpates a mass in her abdomen, just above the ovaries. She also notes that a guaiac test of her stool is positive for occult blood. Carol asks Dr. Tito, one of the gynecologists in the office, to evaluate Marcie. Dr. Tito agrees with Carol's findings. Marcie is scheduled for a Computed tomography (CT) scan of the lower abdomen and asked to return to the office the following week ▼ [NEWS].

Episode 10

This week, Marcie has a follow-up appointment at the Neighborhood Women's Health Specialists office. Carol is sickened when she reads the radiology report and shares the information with Dr. Tito. The CT scan shows a large mass in the colon that extends into the pelvic area. Although Carol knows a pathology report is necessary to confirm the diagnosis, she feels certain that Marcie has advanced colon cancer. Carol and Dr. Tito talk with Marcie and refer her to a surgeon for follow-up. Carol knows she is unlikely ever to see Marcie again but cannot stop thinking about her ▼.

Episode 11

Carol has had great success in recruiting participants for an interdisciplinary study looking at determinants of prenatal care among pregnant adolescents. This week alone, Carol identifies four patients who meet the predetermined guidelines. She explains to the women that participating in the study involves completing a survey, participating in an interview and focus group, and completing the prenatal care visits. All four women agree to participate and complete paperwork providing their written consent ▼.

Episode 12

Seventeen-year-old Jessica Riley comes to the clinic for her first prenatal exam. Carol asks her about previous pregnancies and learns that she already has one son. Carol asks Jessica if she drinks alcohol or smokes. When she finds that Jessica does both, she explains that both are extremely harmful to the developing fetus. She encourages Jessica to try to stop, or at least to cut down drastically on her intake. She conducts an initial prenatal exam. Based on her last menstrual period, size of her uterus, and symptoms, Carol

determines that Jessica is about 16 weeks pregnant. Carol tells Jessica about the research study she is involved in and asks her if she would be willing to be a participant. Jessica tells Carol that she is not interested ▶ [NEWS].

Episode 13

Carol joins a state-level professional nursing work group focused on increasing the education level of nurses. Carol has been concerned about the need for increasing the number of graduate-prepared nurses who provide primary care in advanced practice roles. At the meeting, the discussion centers on facilitating doctoral education of nurses by supporting the Doctor of Nursing Practice degree for advanced practice nurses. Carol has a master's degree and wonders if she is going to have to go back to school again.

Episode 14

It has been a busy week for Carol. She has delivered eight babies in 6 days and has had a full schedule all week. She is feeling really exhausted. Sometimes a week or two goes by without a delivery, and at times all of her patients deliver at the same time. It is never easy to predict what a week will look like. The practice is still down one midwife, because the midwife on medical leave recently resigned, and Carol wonders when another person will be hired. She wonders just how long the physicians will expect her to carry the additional workload ▼.

Episode 15

Carol has a vacation scheduled beginning next week. The office manager asks her if she would consider canceling her plans because the practice will really be shorthanded if she is gone for a week. Carol has already made plans to be gone and purchased her airline tickets months ago. She refuses to feel guilty about saying no ▼.

Carol Ramsey Season 2 Information

Episode 1

Carol Ramsey is increasingly busy at Women's Health Services (WHS) because the practice recently lost a nurse midwife and has been down one position for months.

This episode Jessica Riley comes to the clinic for her 24-week prenatal visit. Carol asks her how she feels, and Jessica reports that she is less tired than before. Carol asks Jessica if she has given any more thought to quitting smoking and drinking. Jessica says that she has cut back, but her boyfriend Casey gives her a hard time if she doesn't party with him. Carol is beginning to wonder what kind of relationship Jessica has with Casey.

Carol begins teaching another childbirth class this week through Neighborhood Hospital. She donates her time to this effort for community service [NEWS].

Episode 2

Carol recently agreed to work with undergraduate nursing students in clinical rotations. Although she agreed to this, she is not sure if it is a good use of her time, or if her clinical role is too advanced for undergraduate students. Carol prefers to work with nurse midwifery students but, because of limited clinical sites for undergraduate students, Carol agreed to do this on a trial basis. Debbie

Koch, a clinical nursing instructor from the university nursing program, and Jennifer Porter, a third year nursing student, meet with Carol to discuss clinical objectives for a clinical rotation.

Episode 3

This week Carol and nursing student Jennifer Porter see Sandra, a 28-year-old woman in her 23rd week of pregnancy. Sandra complains of swelling in her hands and face that does not go away, as well as headaches. Carol notes that her blood pressure is 142/96 mm Hg, and her urine protein is 2+. Recognizing the symptoms as preeclampsia, Carol asks Dr. Tito, the obstetrician in the office, to follow Sandra for the remainder of her pregnancy. As they debrief about the situation, Carol uses this clinical case to help Jennifer understand the role of the advanced practice nurse and the need to recognize when referral is in the best interest of the patient.

Episode 4

Carol sees Jessica Riley again this week. When Carol asks her how she is feeling, Jessica reports less fatigue, but ongoing constipation. Carol asks her what kinds of fluids she drinks, and Jessica replies that she mainly drinks soda. Carol encourages Jessica to drink at least 8–12 glasses of water a day and eat more fiber, such as raisins, oatmeal, or bran cereals. When Carol asks Jennifer Porter about the reasons Jessica may be constipated, she is surprised that Jennifer's answer is right on the mark. Jennifer also states that, depending on Jessica's activity level, mild exercise might also help.

Episode 5

Carol is very impressed with the undergraduate student, Jennifer Porter. Although she was reluctant to work with undergraduate students, she can see the value of exposing them to advanced practice roles. Carol is a member of a state Nursing Action Coalition group that is working to increase the number of primary care providers in the state. Working with Jennifer Porter makes Carol wonder about other ways to increase exposure of undergraduate students to advanced practice nurses so that they will consider this as a future career option.

Episode 6

As part of an interdisciplinary research team evaluating determinants of prenatal care among pregnant adolescents, Carol attends a national meeting to present their work. Carol is delighted to be part of this team and hopes to be involved in future studies.

Episode 7

Jessica Riley comes in for a visit along with her boyfriend Casey. Carol finds Casey to be dominant, as he insists on answering questions for Jessica. Carol mentions Casey's

visit in her case notes and writes a note to remind herself to question Jessica alone at her next visit. After they leave, Jennifer Porter (the nursing student) says to Carol, "There is something about him that makes me nervous, but I know I should not judge people."

Later in the week, Carol meets 15-year-old Kristina Martin, who presents to the Community Health Department requesting birth control pills. Kristina admits to Carol that she has been having sex and is afraid of getting pregnant. Before writing a prescription, Carol confirms with a pregnancy test and menstrual history that Kristina is not pregnant. She teaches Kristina how to take her birth control pills and reminds her that the pills will prevent pregnancy, but will not protect her against sexually transmitted infections.

Episode 8

Carol and Jennifer see many patients this week; visits range from prenatal workups to postpartum checks. Jennifer has become increasingly confident and competent at checking patients in, identifying the correct care protocols, and providing appropriate initial care before Carol sees the patient. Carol can see the value of this clinical rotation in building clinical assessment and clinical judgment skills.

Episode 9

Jessica Riley comes to the clinic, accompanied by her boyfriend, for another prenatal visit. Casey waits in the waiting room for Jessica. Student nurse Jennifer Porter talks with Jessica about fetal development and reviews the birth process. During the exam, Carol and Jennifer notice several bruises on Jessica's abdomen. Carol has seen these types of injuries before on women who have been abused by their partners.

Carol asks Jessica how she got the bruises. Jessica says that she is very clumsy, and she ran into a table. She denies that anyone has hurt her and repeats that she is just clumsy. Carol makes a note of the injuries in Jessica's medical record. After she leaves, Jennifer asks Carol if they should report the abuse to the authorities. Carol explains the challenge this situation presents. Based on the state reporting laws, if Jessica denies abuse, it is premature for that level of action.

Episode 10

This week is Jennifer Porter's last week with Carol. Jennifer's nursing instructor, Debbie Koch, meets with Carol and Jennifer to learn if this rotation was an appropriate site to meet the learning objectives, and if Jennifer and Carol found the rotation of benefit. Both Carol and Jennifer agree it was a good clinical opportunity. Carol agrees to work with undergraduate nursing students in the future, but only when she is not precepting nurse midwifery students.

Episode 11

Carol sees Jessica Riley for her 36-week exam. Jessica is accompanied by her boyfriend Casey. Before she examines Jessica, Casey tells Carol that Jessica has bruises on her abdomen because she runs into things. When Casey leaves the room, Carol notices more bruises on Jessica's shoulder and arm. Carol tells Jessica that, if she needs help, there is information in the restroom about the local domestic abuse shelter for women and children who are being abused by a significant other ▶ ✉.

Episode 12

Carol sees Jessica Riley again this week. During the exam she notes that Jessica's cervix is thinning and dilating slightly. She knows Jessica will be having the baby in the next few weeks.

While working at the Community Health Department this week, Carol sees Terry Clark, a 16-year-old female who is concerned that she might be pregnant. Terry tells Carol that she has recently become sexually active with her boyfriend, Jeremy, and that she has not had a period "for a while." Terry cries when Carol confirms that she is pregnant, telling Carol that she doesn't know what to do, and that her parents will "kill her."

Carol talks with Terry about her options (having the baby, adoption, or abortion) and suggests that she talk with Jeremy and her parents so that she can make the best decision for herself. Terry tells Carol that she doesn't want a baby, but she can't have an abortion either. Carol refers Terry to Planned Parenthood and offers to provide prenatal care for Terry during her pregnancy ▶.

Episode 13

Carol receives a call from the Neighborhood Hospital Labor and Delivery unit, informing her that Jessica Riley delivered her baby. Carol goes to the hospital and learns of the circumstances of the delivery. When Carol talks with her, Jessica breaks down crying and tells Carol about the problems she has with Casey and their abusive relationship. Carol tells Jessica that she can call the police and press charges against Casey, but Jessica insists that Casey loves her and didn't mean to hurt her. Carol sets up a social work consultation for Jessica, explaining that it is standard procedure for social services to follow up any time there is a risk of intimate partner violence ✉.

Episode 14

Carol has a terrible week. The other midwife had unexpected emergency surgery for a ruptured appendix and will also be out for a few weeks. Carol reviews the patient list with the other physicians in the office and come up with a plan to see those who must be seen and cancels appointments among those who can wait. Carol hates to cancel appointments because she knows many people have to rearrange work schedules to be seen, but she has no other choice. As expected, Carol learns from the office manager that several patients are upset or angry about the canceled appointments. Carol reminds the practice manager and physicians that they are still down one provider and asks when they plan to hire ✉.

Episode 15

Jessica Riley comes to the clinic for a postpartum exam. Carol asks her how things are going at home, and Jessica tells her that Casey is being a wonderful father and is treating her and the children very well. Jessica tells Carol that she believes that Casey has changed. Carol encourages Jessica to get more iron in her diet and reminds her to keep taking vitamins. She notices that Jessica's breasts have reduced in size and asks her about breastfeeding. Jessica says she doesn't want to breastfeed, so Carol talks with her about formula feeding.

Carol Ramsey Season 3 Information

Episode 1

Carol Ramsey is a 52-year-old certified nurse midwife who works at Women's Health Services (WHS). She has been a midwife for 22 years

One of the obstetricians at the Women's Health Services practice resigned after his malpractice insurance premiums skyrocketed due to a pending lawsuit. Carol and the other nurse midwife now have even more patients to see. Carol is working 10–12 hours per day this week, trying to compensate for the increased patient load. The physician group places a national search for a new obstetrician and a new midwife. Carol feels further stressed because she had agreed to precept two undergraduate nursing students in the upcoming months. Ordinarily she does not mind working with students, but with everything else going on right now, it will be just another stressor. Carol thinks to herself, "At least they are both senior level students." The student in the first rotation is Kayla Sharif.

Carol and Kayla see Terry Clark, the 16-year-old pregnant teenager, in the office this week. Terry tells Carol that her parents want her to put the baby up for adoption. She is not sure she wants to, but she has pretty much decided it is for the best. She also tells Carol that her boyfriend wanted her to have an abortion, and when she refused to do this, he broke up with her. Carol can see that Terry and Kayla immediately form a connection in their short visit.

Episode 2

Nancy, a 40-year-old woman, sees Carol for prenatal care. She has a 9-year-old daughter named Lindsey. The woman tells Carol that she would like her daughter to be present and participate in the birth process. Carol is not against this but tells Nancy that she will need to clear it with the hospital first. Kayla, the student nurse, talks with Carol about the pros and cons of having a 9-year-old sibling present for a birth. The following day, Kayla brings to Carol a couple of research articles on the topic and tells Carol there is no evidence either for or against the practice, and such decisions are based on family preferences. Kayla also shares with Carol that institutional policies often create barriers for such requests. Carol is very impressed with Kayla. She does not remember being sophisticated enough as an undergraduate student to check the literature for evidence.

Episode 3

Carol, Kayla, and the nurse manager of the Labor and Delivery unit at Neighborhood Hospital meet with Carol's patient, Nancy, and her 9-year-old daughter, Lindsey, to discuss Lindsey's presence during the birth of her mother's baby. Carol tells Lindsey what birth is like and that she might feel frightened if she sees blood and or thinks that her mother is hurt. The girl says that she would like to be there when her little brother is born, and Nancy insists that Lindsey has been watching birth shows on television. Carol and the nurse manager approve Nancy's request to allow Lindsey to be present during the birth.

Episode 4

Kayla talks with Carol about her senior teaching project and proposes that she create an age-appropriate teaching plan for the 9-year-old girl who wishes to be present for the birth of her sibling. Carol thinks this is an excellent idea. As a senior nursing student, Kayla feels she is finally settling in on women's health and pediatric nursing as her preferred clinical interests ▼.

Episode 5

Kristina Martin comes into the Community Health Department to see Carol and Kayla this week. Carol remembers writing a prescription for birth control for Kristina several months ago. Kristina tells Carol and Kayla that her boyfriend told her to get tested for chlamydia, but she isn't sure what that is. Carol explains that chlamydia is a common sexually transmitted infection and then examines Kristina. Carol gives Kristina Azithromycin (Zithromax) 1 gram orally in a single dose. Kayla spends time with Kristina following the examination, talking with her about measures she can take to prevent sexually transmitted infections and reinforcing the need to take the birth control pills. As Carol observes this interaction, it occurs to her that Kayla may actually be more effective at delivering this message than if she were to do this. For whatever reason, Kayla seems to have a real gift for connecting with people.

Episode 6

Carol and Kayla see Terry Clark and her mother this week for a prenatal visit. Terry's mother tells Carol that there is no way Terry is old enough to raise a baby, and she is not interested in doing it either. The family has a friend who knows an attorney, and they are going to explore private adoption. Terry's mother hopes that they can get the adoptive family to help pay for Terry's medical bills. Terry turns to Kayla and tells her she is too embarrassed to go to school, so she is being home-schooled for the rest of the year. Kayla suggests to Terry that she stay connected with her close friends who know she is pregnant. She may find their support will be helpful during this time. Terry's mother, overhearing the conversation, makes an offhand remark: "Terry's friends are probably why she ended up pregnant."

Episode 7

A new certified nurse midwife is hired this week. Carol is thrilled to have another colleague in the office and agrees to orient her. Although having a nursing student while trying to orient a nurse midwife is stressful, Carol decides that this is the last thing she will complain about [NEWS].

Episode 8

This is Kayla's last week of clinical rotation and Carol meets with Kayla's clinical instructor, Debbie Koch, for her evaluation. It is the best clinical evaluation Kayla has ever earned. Carol encourages Kayla to consider working on a Doctor of Nursing Practice degree – either as a nurse practitioner or nurse midwife. Kayla is thrilled to hear that. During the entire time in nursing school, Kayla always felt her instructors did not think highly of her. Kayla loves the fact that Carol believes in her abilities [NEWS].

Episode 9

This week Carol has yet another student (Jacob McCain) completing a rotation with her – and is disappointed that the student is a man. "What am I going to do with a male student in this clinical rotation?" she thinks. "It is too bad Kayla can't just keep working with me."

Carol and Jacob see 16-year-old Terry Clark and her mother this week for a prenatal visit. Terry asks where Kayla is and is visibly disappointed when Carol tells her that Kayla has finished her clinical rotation and Jacob is now in her place. Terry's reaction to Jacob just reinforces to Carol her perspective about the problems of having male students in this clinical setting.

Carol learns that an adoptive family has been located, and Terry has agreed to give the baby up for adoption. Because Carol knows that this is what Terry's parents have been pushing for, she asks Terry how she is feeling about the decision. Terry tells Carol, "It is probably fine," and she is going to meet the adoptive family sometime in the next couple of weeks. She has been told they are really nice.

Episode 10

While on-call for the practice, Carol gets a phone call from Dr. Gordon, the ED physician, asking her to see a patient. Carol tells Jacob she is going to the ED and will be back in a while. Jacob annoys her when he replies, "Is there a reason I can't come with you?" Reluctantly, Carol takes Jacob along. When they arrive, they meet Reyna, a 13-year-old girl who presented to the ED with abdominal pain and heavy, bloody vaginal discharge. A pregnancy test ordered by Dr. Gordon is positive.

Carol tells Jacob to step out while she examines Reyna. After examining Reyna, Carol informs the girl and her mother that Reyna is pregnant and is having a miscarriage. The mother is in shock. Reyna denies that she is pregnant and tells Carol that she couldn't be pregnant because she's never had sex. When Carol comes out of the room she simply tells Jacob the patient was pregnant but does not elaborate further ▶.

Episode 11

Carol has a very busy week and sees multiple patients. She interacts with Jacob in between patients but does not include him with any of the patient interactions. Jacob spends the majority of his time for three straight clinical days sitting in the staff break room. Frustrated, he contacts his clinical instructor and asks what to do.

Jacob's clinical instructor, Debbie Koch, arranges to meet with Carol and Jacob to review the clinical objectives and expectations. During their meeting Jacob verbalizes his frustration with the experience and tells Carol he does not appreciate being left out of the patient interactions. Carol tells Debbie and Jacob this is really not an appropriate clinical rotation for an undergraduate student. Debbie reminds Carol that she recently had another senior student whom she included in the clinical experiences and praised highly. Recognizing her inconsistent message, Carol then admits that it is difficult to work with male students. In her experience, this population of patients prefers women providers.

Although Jacob had suspected Carol's issue with him was his being a man, he had tried to keep an open mind about it. Jacob also knew that reacting with anger would not resolve anything. Calmly he said to Carol, "It seems to me that if I could gain experience related to the unique health needs of women, I will be able to apply that to other clinical areas when I interact with women."

Carol feels a mixed set of emotions - both anger and embarrassment. She knows he is right, but she is angry

that an undergraduate student has made her look bad. She is also embarrassed about her overt discrimination. Carol apologizes for leaving Jacob out of the clinical activities and vows to include him more often, but she also reinforces the patient's right not to have a male involved if requested ▶ ▼.

Episode 12

Nancy, the patient who wants her 9-year-old daughter, Lindsey, present during her delivery, goes into labor. Carol tells Jacob about the daughter and asks him to keep an eye on her to be sure she is okay. During the birth process, Carol notices that Lindsey chooses not to watch the actual birth but stays in a corner of the room. She also sees Jacob interacting with her. He asks the girl if she wants to leave and the girl says no. Jacob stays with her and keeps talking with her to keep her calm while her mother delivers the baby. After the baby is born, Carol wraps him up in a receiving blanket and shows him to Nancy. Lindsey shyly comes to the bedside and peeks at her baby brother. She asks to hold him. Nancy thanks Carol for her flexibility and says she is glad Lindsey was allowed to witness her brother's birth. Nancy also thanks Jacob for being so good with Lindsey during the birth ▼.

Episode 13

Carol has a very busy week. She delivers seven babies within 4 days. Carol and the new midwife still have more patients asking for their services than they can accept, but they have added several new patients to their caseloads. Carol has become increasingly comfortable including Jacob in the care. Although it is still not her preference to have male students, she also recognizes that not one patient has requested that he leave. In fact, it has been her observation that many patients seem to appreciate his efforts.

Episode 14

Carol has a phone call with a nurse midwife who is interested in opening a new clinic for midwifery and gynecological care. The state allows certified nurse midwives to work independently of physicians, and Carol has full prescriptive authority. The two women talk for several hours about the benefits and challenges of stand-alone, nurse-run clinics ▼.

Episode 15

Terry Clark is in the office for her 39-week visit. Carol learns that Terry will not be giving the baby up for adoption after all. Terry tells Carol that her mother and father found out that the adoptive family was a same sex couple, and they could not stand the idea that their grandchild would be adopted and raised by a gay couple. Carol feels badly that Terry's parents control her life in this way and grieves for the two men who were anticipating adopting the baby ▶ ▼.

NEIGHBORHOOD NEWS

SEASON 1 NEWS

Episode 1

Free Immunizations Peak Interest

The Neighborhood Health Care Clinic is offering free immunizations today from 8:00 AM to 4:00 PM, provided that citizens bring a copy of their immunization records. "Our primary interest is a healthy community," said Jade Scott, MD, the physician organizing the immunization program. "Providing treatment at a fraction of a price is one thing, but providing it at no price is the best way to encourage people to get immunized," Dr. Scott added. The clinic's offering marks the second occurrence of an annual immunization program enabling individuals in the community to be immunized at no cost.

Immunizations Hit All-Time Low

According to local medical professionals, the number of individuals receiving immunizations is dwindling. "State immunizations have hit an all-time low," said Dan Sibray, MD, head of the immunization program at Neighborhood Hospital. The local hospital recently started discounting prices of routine physical examinations and immunizations, hoping to bring people back to the hospital. "Our worry is that if parents do not spend the time and money to bring their children into the hospital for routine procedures, they will end up spending more money on medicine, or worse, the emergency department," added Dr. Sibray. Statewide, medical professionals seem to agree with Sibray. "It's a real problem, and we hope that the discounts we're offering will encourage parents to bring their children in for immunizations. Our job is not to put a price on children's well-being, but with these new solutions, we hope to lessen the burden on citizens."

Medical Phobia Results in Tragedy

Last night, a 3-month old Ruralton boy died after a battle with pertussis. Thomas O'Brien was admitted to Neighborhood Hospital on Wednesday after being ill at home the previous day, and died on Friday while in the pediatric intensive care unit. Joseph Descloitres, MD, the attending physician to the infant, reported that the mother refused to vaccinate her child, citing personal opposition. "Her feelings toward immunization were not positive," said Dr. Descloitres. "She felt that certain immunizations could cause her child to develop autism, and despite the rapid deterioration of her son's health, we had to honor these wishes," he added. The hospital has the authority to overturn a parent's decisions, but according to medical reports and given the rapid progression of the illness, obtaining a court order would have been difficult.

Local Immunization Protest Ends in Arrest

Mark Bowie, head of a local group, People Against Injecting Sickness, or PAIS, was briefly taken into custody last night outside the free immunization clinic. Bowie blocked the door to the clinic while holding a "Don't Harm our Children!" sign and chanting, "Doctors make you sick! Nurses make you sicker!" He was charged with disorderly conduct and was released on bail.

While healthcare workers express concern that immunizations may be at an all-time low, PAIS sees that as a positive outcome. Members of PAIS believe that medical institutions are injecting patients with latent forms of various diseases in order to meet their high patient quotas. "Immunizations have led to many illnesses, such as autism, and sometimes they cause the very diseases they claim to prevent," said Mark Bowie, leader of PAIS.

Local physician, David Jackson, MD, thinks differently, "The idea that physicians immunize patients to get more business is preposterous. The goal of doctors and nurses is better health for the community. Claims about a link between autism and immunizations were long ago shown to be unsubstantiated. While every treatment has its side effects, the effects of immunization are undetectable in most people. Side effects in infants usually are mild and temporary, such as crankiness, soreness at the injection site, or perhaps a low-grade fever that lasts a few hours."

Episode 2

Can Blood Drive Eliminate Hospital's Shortage?

The Neighborhood Library will be holding a blood drive on Saturday from 8:00 AM to 4:00 PM. Last year's blood donation event at the library resulted in a record number of donations, and hospital officials are hoping for the same outcome this year. "It is good to know that the citizens care about other members of their community," Clancy Long, MD, a physician at Community Hospital, said during a meeting announcing the event. "While the supply intake last year was more than we could have hoped, the recent increase in traumatic injuries has caused the supply to dwindle once again," Dr. Long stated. He added that although publicly announced donation events always result in good turnout, people do not only have to donate when there is an event. Long added, "People should know that donations can be given at any time—even during a lunch hour." Statistically, donations throughout the year are scarce, leading to shortages when doctors need the blood most. Despite the substantial blood donations received during city-sponsored events, these events only supply one day of donations.

Low Blood Supplies Alarm Medical Professionals

The belief among many state and local medical professionals is that blood donations have hit an all-time low. Several members of the medical community have asserted that the cause of the low blood supply is the recent rise in traumatic injuries throughout the state. Erik Goldsmith, MD, a physician at Neighborhood Hospital, suggests that people make an effort to donate blood, regardless of when or the amount they donate. "The recent rise in traumatic injuries in the state is not something known to only the medical professionals," said Dr. Goldsmith. "People know that injuries are increasing because they are the people receiving the injuries," he asserted. The rise in the number of traumatic injuries has left health officials baffled as to why more people are not donating, since the problem affects the community directly.

Budget Cuts Increase Strike Concerns

Given the recent budget cuts in health-related fields, it appears that even companies that garnered awards are not permitted a saving grace. The local company Neighborhood Manufacturing, which won an award last year for the innovation of a workplace health promotion program, has been forced to shut down this promotion program. The closure came as a sudden shock to all, but no shock was greater than that of the employees. The president of the company, Albert Black, expressed his shock. "I came into work like any other day, and I received a conference call from the Financial-Handling Department and my bosses," Black stated. "While I cannot divulge the contents of that call, I can say that I was left with only one option—shutting down our health promotion program." Employees, on the other hand, do not believe that this was the only option and think that their superiors should have tried harder to keep the promotion program. These feelings have led to rumors and threats that soon the workers will begin to strike.

"Karate Kids Lack Discipline," Say Elders

The recent encouragement by local schools to have their students participate in more extracurricular and fitness activities has seemed to have a negative effect on the community, according to the elderly population. "I come outside in the morning and I find the boards on my fences either damaged or destroyed by kids who recently learned how to kick and hit in their violent program," said retired U.S. Army veteran Ross Webb. Police reports state that no children have been apprehended in relation to these allegations, but that law enforcement personnel are keeping a close eye on the issue. Master Nguyen of the local karate program High Kicks, Strong Discipline suggests that it is impossible that these labeled children are his students. "My program teaches defense and discipline. Just because there is a karate program in town does not mean that it should be the first to blame," said Nguyen. "The percentage of children who might have seen such an act on television is much higher than the chance that one of my students committed such a crime." Officer Wilson of the local police department.

Episode 3

Run–Not Swim–for Fish

While there may seem be some underlying irony in holding a running race to benefit aquatic creatures, enthusiasts suggest otherwise. "This event allows citizens of the Neighborhood to better themselves and their community," said head of the event, Kira Fort. The event Fort is referring to is the annual "Run for the Fish" fundraiser. The fundraiser's main objective is to clean up Neighborhood Lake, which has seen great deterioration and increased pollution since the recent growth of manufacturing in town. For an entry fee of $20.00, all participants receive a T-shirt and water bottle and the chance to participate in the run that spans the lake's 5-mile perimeter. Citizens are allowed to participate in the run even if they are not interested in donating $20.00 to the cause, and donations are welcome from those choosing not to participate. "We just want to gather support, and if we gather donations along the way, then that is twice as good," said Fort. Last year's run raised approximately $6,500 with around 294 participants. Fort added that people do not need to donate money in order to help the lake effort. "We are also hoping that each person interested will be an extra pair of hands when it comes to actually cleaning the lake."

Officials Confirm Pollution Worries

At last night's City Council meeting, Mayor Nathan Brice confirmed what many environmental activist groups have been proclaiming for months—Neighborhood Lake's concentration of pollutants has reached critical levels. Local resident Elton Bentley was quoted saying, "[The pollution] is too bad…I remember fishing here as a kid when the waters were pristine." Officials say that concerns that newer generations will be unable to enjoy the waters recreationally as Bentley did are the least of the community's worries. "Right now, our main concern is the town's water supply," said Councilman Richard Bradley. "This a concern because rather than affecting the newer generation's aesthetic view of the community, the severe pollution could affect their health and well-being". The mayor declined to comment directly to the press on the issue, but insisted that he was taking steps to correct it.

Police Report: Local Man Dies, Cause Unknown

"I assure you it wasn't the polluted water that killed him," joked Sheriff Mark Shuster. Local mechanic Jon Smith died in his home 2 nights ago of unknown causes, according to the initial police report. Shuster insists that jokes aside, the police department is taking this case very seriously. "While it may seem quick to jump to suspicions, there are too many variables to just toss this one aside to a death from natural cause," Shuster added. "The man was relatively young to die from natural causes, and although he was a smoker, his death came too suddenly to be blamed on either of these without further investigation." Police have questioned several neighbors of the Smith household, but their primary area of focus has been Smith's wife, Karen, who has been questioned several times since her husband's death. Shuster stated that "We do not want to jump to conclusions, and right now we're focusing on getting all the facts."

Episode 4

Hotline Puts Families at Ease

Recently, the state government passed a bill that opens up all cities to a convenience once enjoyed only by major cities-a poison hotline-and the Neighborhood is one of these towns that is now benefitting from this convenience. People can reach the hotline by dialing 1-800-POISONS on any model of phone. The hotline, which services the state 24 hours a day, 7 days a week, informs callers of how to deal with both foreign and domestic poisons. Local parent Sally Franken was put at ease, since the service provides her with a "comfort that is readily welcomed, especially given the rise of pollution in our community's most revered locations." Local physician Dan Sibray, MD, shared similar sentiments to Ms. Franken. "[The hotline] provides citizens with information that could save them a visit to the hospital and the bills involved with such a visit."

Terrorism Concerns Reach Community

In a recent press release, the U.S. Department of Homeland Security declared that chemical warfare has topped their list as the most serious threat to U.S. citizens following a string of terrorist threats against the nation. Local officials have declared that although the Neighborhood is smaller than neighboring cities, it is not immune to attacks. "The chances of an attack here are slim, but there is no harm in being prepared," said Councilman Richard Bradley.

In response to the Department of Homeland Security's press release, local officials have released this precaution and preparation list in the event of an attack, which they define as an inexpensive means to stay safe:

Ensure a sufficient supply of water and food (canned food is recommended due to its extended shelf-life)

Maintain a healthy diet and keep immunizations current

Organize an assortment of simple tools and mechanical supplies (hammer, screwdriver, duct tape, flashlight, etc.)

Create an evacuation plan or list of what to do in the event of a terrorist attack; a plan of action can sometimes eliminate indecisiveness and panic.

Police Report: Woman Arrested, Accused of Husband's Murder

"It is not the synopsis of a Hollywood film, nor creative, but sick and twisted," said Sheriff Mark Shuster during an interview announcing the arrest of Karen Smith in relation to the murder of her husband, Jon Smith. Shuster announced that his deputies apprehended Mrs. Smith late Thursday evening, after the autopsy of her husband revealed a concentration of arsenic so high that it could kill several people. Mrs. Smith's defense lawyer claims that his client was cleaning the kitchen that day and misplaced the arsenic in with an assortment of cooking spices. Scoffing at this defense, Shuster stated, "Given the concentration of poison found in Mr. Smith's body, there is no way this act was accidental. Such a defense is insulting to the memory of the deceased." Subsequent to the arrest of Mrs. Smith in suspicion of murder, police obtained a search warrant for her home, where they found an assortment of poisons in a shoebox under Mrs. Smith's bed. This assortment included several types of pesticides, but most prominently, arsenic. After this discovery, the Neighborhood Police Department officially charged Mrs. Smith with murder in the first degree (premeditated, with malice, and intent to kill).

Episode 5

Town Meeting Will Focus on Drunk Driving

"Statistically, with an increase in population, we see an increase in crime," said Neighborhood police officer John Capote. Although parents have been expressing a concern with this increase, no crime is more of a concern to both police and parents than drunk driving. The concern expressed will be the focus of this week's town meeting, which is scheduled for Thursday night at 7:00 PM. The discussion at the meeting will determine whether or not the local government pursues legislation against drunk driving—specifically, the imposing of harsher sentences and punishments if a person is convicted of drunk driving.

Accident Ends in Death of Two

An accident that occurred this past weekend claimed the lives of two of the Neighborhood's citizens-Myrna Ogdon, 24, and her son, Raymond Ogdon, 10 months. The crash took place Saturday night near Neighborhood Lake. Police report that the accident was apparently the result of drunk driving. The occupants of the other car, Amy Price, 16, and Carrie Rivera, 17, were declared drunk and arrested after Sheriff Mark Shuster administered a sobriety test that both young women reportedly failed. The Ogdons were struck head-on by Price's car, a sport utility vehicle, crumpling Ogdon's small sedan.

Police Report: Wife Denies Baking Poison Pie

A crime that seems more like the plot of a Hollywood movie is appearing to have its share of plot twists. Karen Smith, who was arrested recently in relation to the murder of her husband, Jon Smith, has reportedly changed her story, placing the blame on the local church. Smith delivered a new account of the crime at a press conference yesterday afternoon. This new account states that the pie was purchased from a bake sale at Neighborhood Church. Smith contended that someone at her church made the poison-laced pie and she bought it, not knowing its fatal contents. Initially, Smith claimed that while cleaning the kitchen, she misplaced a small container of arsenic among other spices, claiming that the similarity between the containers caused her to mistake arsenic for one of her many spices. Smith's defense attorney, Nicholas Ocoada, claims that this scenario was forced upon Smith in order for police to obtain a confession. "A woman whose husband has just been declared dead is not in the proper state of mind to make rational choices, and I motion that the police constructed a confession and in her emotional state, she accepted it," Ocoada said.

Episode 6

Mosey Down to the Rodeo Grounds

The annual Neighborhood Rodeo is taking place this week, every night from 7:00 PM to 11:00 PM. The Rodeo Daze competition is being held again as well. Entry into the competition is free, and every person who participates is guaranteed a prize-ranging from a free hat to a grand prize of $500. There is, however, an admission fee to the Rodeo, which is $10.00 for adults. Admission is free for children under 6 years of age. Other elements of the Rodeo event include amusement park rides, games, and an arts and crafts contest.

Shuster Rides Again

The Neighborhood's own Sheriff Mark Shuster will don his cowboy hat once again Thursday evening at 8:00 PM. Sheriff Shuster will be performing in a free concert as a fundraiser for the battered women's shelter. Shuster said, "By offering a free concert, we eliminate the barrier between who can afford it and those who can't. We hope that this benefit concert will encourage Neighborhood residents to give freely to others who need their help. The battered women's shelter is a valuable asset to our community and it needs our support." The concert will be accepting donations before and after the show. Sheriff Shuster added, "Most importantly, we want people to have a good time. If they can donate a dollar or two, we would be grateful, but we do not require it."

Police Report: Wife Formally Charged With Murder

As of last week, Karen Smith was being held on a $2 million bail but she now has been formally charged with murder in the first degree. At a press conference earlier this week, Sheriff Mark Shuster announced that the Neighborhood Police Department has officially charged Mrs. Smith with first-degree murder in the death of her husband Jon Smith, a skilled mechanic at the Neighborhood Toyota dealership. Jon Smith died after eating a pie laced with poison-specifically, arsenic. At her arraignment, Mrs. Smith contended that the pie was bought at a local church bake sale and that any poison contained in the pie was in the pie when she purchased it. Smith also cites that the relationship with her husband had a plethora of abuse problems lasting for more than 2 years. According to her attorney, Nicholas Ocoada, Smith constantly feared for her life, and her reaction to her husband's death was misinterpreted.

Episode 7

Health Fair Welcomes All

On Saturday, the Neighborhood Mall will be host to this year's Health Fair from 9:00 AM to 5:00 PM. The Health Fair will address a variety of issues, and all individuals are welcome. Programs at the fair are designed for individuals of every age group. Younger children can visit several information centers and participate in many programs, including one that helps inform the children how to avoid illness. The programs designed for teens and young adults focus specifically on sex education, including signs of sexually transmitted diseases and how to protect themselves. Programs for adults focus on health issues such as high cholesterol levels, elevated blood pressure, and obesity.

Emergency Department Sees Critical Capacities

Neighborhood Hospital is reportedly over capacity, and staffers are citing unsafe conditions. James Gordon, MD, physician director of the Neighborhood Hospital emergency department (ED), reports that the ED has become inundated with individuals seeking health care. Most of these individuals do not have emergency conditions but are unable to access health care through other means. Dr. Gordon stated that, "This city has a lack of adequate medical facilities, especially for low-income individuals or indigents." Gordon also suggested that people need to be educated about particular symptoms, because most of the time, an injury or sickness can be treated at home. Increasing hospital capacities force individuals to come to the ED for basic health care and a waiting period that can exceed 6 hours.

Cavities at All-Time Low, According to Dentists

Dental professionals say that recent advances in dental care have resulted in a decrease in the incidence of cavities in children and adolescents. Improvements such as sealants and fluoridated water have contributed to such successes, say dentists. Sealants have become routine, being found so effective that such treatments are now offered at no cost to children of low-income households. Individuals interested in having sealant treatments for their children should stop by the Health Fair on Saturday. A booth titled "Healthy Teeth for Tomorrow" will be present at the event, sponsored by the local chapter of the American Dental Association.

Episode 8

Health Career Fair This Weekend

Inspired by a recent interest of the general population in health care-related careers, there will be a Health Career Fair held at the Neighborhood High School on Saturday from 9:00 AM to 5:00 PM. The career fair is not only for students but also for the entire community. The careers that will be showcased during the fair include those in medicine, nursing, radiologic sciences, dentistry, and medical technologies, among others. Various local health care centers are sponsoring the event, including the Neighborhood Hospital Association, State Nursing Association, Ruralton College, and the local chapter of the American Dental Association.

Gun Scare at Elementary School Ends in Expulsion

Earlier this week, a young student was expelled from Neighborhood Elementary School for bringing a gun to school. The third-grader, whose name remains unreleased, claimed to be angry at another student after being teased at school. Being too young to own a firearm legally, the child claims he stole his father's handgun and brought it to school in order to scare the other student and not to hurt him. Police have yet to make an official announcement on the details of the case, and have only confirmed the information that other departments have released-essentially, that a child brought a gun to school and was expelled after being apprehended. Parents have expressed great concern with the age of the individual involved. An elementary teacher who asked to remain anonymous said, "The recent spate of school violence only increases the tension here among parents and staff."

HoLEP Procedure for Senior Men

If you are a man age 50 or older, you may have heard of a common condition of older men called benign prostatic hyperplasia, or BPH. BPH is not cancerous, but it causes urinary urgency, frequent urination (especially at night), diminished stream when urinating, and leaking of urine. These symptoms are caused by excessive growth of the prostate gland surrounding the urethra in men. Symptoms increase with age and can interfere with normal activities, social life, and sexuality.

Medications may relieve symptoms, but many men eventually have to undergo surgery. The traditional procedure called TURP involves an inpatient hospital stay of 1 to 4 days and recovery time of 4 to 6 weeks. Now a newer procedure is being offered called HoLEP. HoLEP, short for holmium laser enucleation of the prostate, uses laser to vaporize overgrown tissue, relieving pressure on the urethra and minimizing risk of damage to the surrounding area. Hospital discharge is same-day or next-day, depending on the setting. Symptom relief is rapid, and catheterization time is limited. Generally patients are able to void painlessly soon after surgery. HoLEP is now being introduced in major healthcare facilities. For Neighborhood residents, it may not be an immediate option, but it offers great promise for future treatment of BPH.

Nurses Leave Due to Poor Work Conditions

An increasing number of nurses are leaving health-related facilities across the Neighborhood, citing difficult working conditions and low wages. However, this is not only a local problem. Across the state, nurses have been leaving positions faster than the positions can be filled-a trend that has been maintained for the past 3 years. Although new nurses are hired, medical facilities have been unable to attract applicants at the same rate that positions are being vacated. Employment centers have said that over the past 3 years, the state has seen job openings in nursing positions rise by 8%. "This situation is completely unacceptable," stated lawmaker Howard Rome. "The people of our state deserve to be cared for by competent health care professionals, and something needs to be done." Locally, government and health care officials hope that the recent Health Career Fair will inspire more students to pursue a career in health care. However, considering the length of schooling required, such hopes would take years to be fulfilled.

Episode 9

Kicking the Habit

A group that meets weekly is offering more options for people trying to quit smoking. The Neighborhood Community Center will be host to the Smoking Cessation Class that will start meet every week (for 8 weeks) on

Wednesday evenings at 7:00 PM. Although the fee for the class is $30.00 per person, those organizing the class insist that the price is negligible compared with the price of cigarettes. "People should think of the cost over the long term," said program head Katherine Hirschfield. "The program costs about the same as six packs of cigarettes, and once the class concludes, the money saved from not having to buy cigarettes anymore will be a great benefit," she added.

Therapy Dogs: Fur Therapy in Assisted Living
A local assisted living center had two unusual guests visit the common room this week. Dr. Erin Spronk, a local veterinarian, brought Blackie, a 6-month-old Airedale, and Bulldozer, an 8-month-old wirehaired fox terrier, as therapy dogs. "I used to bring Blackie and Bulldozer to see my mother at Neighborhood Nursing Home," said Dr. Spronk. "After her death, these two just started to seem bored. It got me thinking how everybody used to pat them when we visited my mom. I wondered if they missed the attention!" Dr. Spronk contacted an administrator at the assisted living center, and she agreed to give the visit a try. Smiles filled the room as the therapy dogs accepted pats and loving words from residents and staff alike. Alice, age 91, was one of many residents who enjoyed the canine companions. She reported, "This was the best idea. I had so much fun watching the dogs play and petting them."

Trained therapy dogs have been shown to help people with depression and other mood disorders. In the assisted living setting, Blackie and Bulldozer's visit started a chain of reminiscences. Staff reported the canine experiment was a huge success and said that hours after Blackie and Bulldozer's departure, residents were still sharing stories about their own favorite pets. Administrators at the center said the response of residents to these two furry therapists was exciting. They hope to establish monthly "fur therapy days" as a part of their overall plan to provide a stimulating, mentally healthy environment. For more information on therapy dogs, contact Erin Spronk, DVM, at 605-690-1234.

Drug Use on the Rise
The Neighborhood Police Department claims that drug use in the Neighborhood is on the rise. This year the Neighborhood saw not only its first methamphetamine lab bust, but three subsequent lab busts succeeding the first. The elderly community is blaming the rise of drugs on changing values. "I do not know what has happened to this community. When I was young, drugs were nonexistent in this community," said Rayleen Cordova. The sheriff's office states that the increase of drug use is due to the rise in the general population.

Smoking Breaks a Thing of the Past?
Smoking bans at large companies around the country have continued to rise. Within the last decade, the majority of large U.S. companies have enacted policies to reduce smoking among workers. Most companies simply prohibit smoking indoors. In a few, however, employees who smoke can potentially lose their jobs if they refuse to quit smoking. A spokesperson for the National Work-Rights Association states that an overt ban on cigarette smoking is an infringement on workers' rights and that such a policy is illegal. They state that an employer cannot force its employees to quit smoking altogether, because employers do not have control of their workers outside the workplace. Supporters of the proposal say the bans are about the health and well-being of smokers and nonsmokers in the work environment. They also cite the rising cost on insurance for individuals who do choose to smoke, arguing that increased insurance costs are an infringement upon nonsmokers and smokers alike.

Episode 10
Express Yourself at Art Fair
Starting this Friday and lasting all weekend, the Neighborhood Community Center will be host to the Neighborhood Art Fair. The fair will feature a multitude of artistry works, including ceramics, water colors, oils, woodwork, and quilting, among others. Although the fair will feature works by several well-known artists, local artists are also encouraged to attend and display their own work. "Art is not limited to only those regarded with fame," said the art fair's host, Marvin Rourke. "[Art] is also not limited to painting, so we encourage people to bring in any of their works."

Pit Bull Attacks Child
A pit bull attack this week has placed a 3-year-old child in critical condition. In order to maintain the privacy of all individuals involved, police have not revealed the names of the victims or the owner of the dog, by the wishes of the latter party. The details that are available about the incident are that the child was attacked while playing in the backyard sandbox opposite the yard where the dog was kept. The dog's owner claims that the dog was gentle and has never been violent before, citing that the attack must have been provoked. James Gordon, MD, an emergency department physician at Neighborhood Hospital, was quoted saying that the incident was the worst he has ever seen and that the child will be lucky to recover without any facial scarring or lifelong trauma. The incident has ended tragically for both sides; when responding to the call, Sheriff Mark Shuster shot and killed the dog.

Trial Report: Smith Murder Trial Begins Next Week

Karen Smith's murder trial is scheduled to begin next week with opening arguments. She is charged with first-degree murder of her husband Jon Smith, and is entering a plea of not guilty. Many already feel the trial will be an open-and-shut case. The defense team's strategy for Mrs. Smith is to sway the jury with allegations that the defendant suffered great physical and emotional abuse from her husband prior to his death. The prosecution team believes they have a stronger case because the defense's entire case depends on Mrs. Smith's allegations but is not supported by hard evidence. Supporters of the defendant in this case suggest that Mrs. Smith should have pleaded temporary insanity, which would have yielded a lighter sentence if she is convicted.

Episode 11

Flu Shots Encouraged

This week, the Neighborhood Senior Center will offer flu shots daily from 1:00 PM to 4:00 PM. Health officials recommend citizens receive the vaccination while it is still early in the flu season. The price of the shot is $20.00; for adults older than age 65 and for children under 5, it is free. This year, health officials hope to see a high turnout for the event as part of a long string of health promotion events, including a healthcare careers night.

Flu Deaths Expected to Rise

Health officials are preparing for the worst this flu season, claiming that they expect flu-related deaths to increase. Officials state that the groups most at risk of contracting and dying from the flu are elderly individuals, those with chronic health conditions, and infants. Last year, numerous people died from the flu statewide, and five from this area alone. Health professionals have tried to increase immunizations through health fairs, but they fear it will not be enough to curb flu-related deaths.

Homeless Man Found Dead

"It is hard to believe anyone would hurt him," said director of the homeless shelter Carol Maddox. Yesterday, homeless man Lionel Daily, 62, was found dead next to a dumpster in the downtown Neighborhood area. According to the police report, Daily was found by a passerby around 7:00 AM, and an investigation is currently underway. Daily's death came as a shock for many of the homeless population in the Neighborhood. Daily was a well-known transient to the downtown area. "He frequented the homeless shelters and was very sociable," said Maddox.

Episode 12

Domestic Violence Hotline Established

A community-based project to protect citizens from domestic violence situations will enter its second phase starting next month with the establishment of a domestic violence hotline. The first phase of the project, a safe house, was completed last year, but the implementation of a hotline serves as a means for victims of violence to call in privacy and confidence. The operators are trained to detail clients with information on how to prevent domestic violence and what to do to escape an abusive relationship. The toll-free number for the service is 1-800-111-1112 and is initially opening with a total of 20 operators.

Citizens Seek Pit Bull Ban

In the wake of a near-fatal pit bull terrier attack on a 3-year-old Neighborhood boy, citizens are scouring the community for the necessary petition signatures to propose a ban on the dog breed. Those who are against the ban claim that the community is jumping the gun on banning an entire breed of dog based on one bad incident. However, supporters respond by saying that pit bull attacks are not isolated incidents, which is why several states maintain bans on ownership of these dogs. Nationwide, no dog breed is more legislated against than the pit bull (referring to American pit bull Terriers, American Staffordshire terriers, and Staffordshire bull terriers), and several states hold bans on owning pit bulls.

Trial Report: Defense Comes Out Strong

The second week of the Karen Smith trial began this week. Karen Smith stands charged for first-degree murder by serving and baking a poison-laced pie for her husband Jon Smith. This week, the defense presented a strong case for Mrs. Smith. According to the defense attorney, Nicholas Ocoada, Smith's action was solely based on self-defense. Jon Smith was portrayed as a controlling man with a vicious temperament. Karen Smith described years of abuse by his hand and allegedly killed him to escape the abuse. Prosecutors pointed out that the defendant never made attempts to seek help and believe her story to be made up simply to gain sympathy from the press, women's groups, and the jury. Police reports revealed, in favor of the prosecution, that Jon Smith did not have a criminal history.

Episode 13

Take Me Out to the Ball Game

This weekend, the Neighborhood Sports Stadium will sponsor a baseball tournament for any to attend. Several teams from across the state are expected to compete for a total of six games. All children aged 6 and younger, as well as individuals older than 65, will be allowed admittance free of charge. For those of all other ages, the price of admission is discounted to $5.00 per person, per game, or one can buy one ticket for the entire tournament at the discounted price of $30.00. The reason for the free admittance and discounted tickets (usual price is $8.00

per person, per game) is due to a slow sports season. Compared with previous seasons, the stadium has not been selling as many tickets as they would like, and the organizers of the tournament hope that attendance will inspire audiences to return to the sports pastime.

Officials Hopeful for Governor Award

The residents of the Neighborhood are being encouraged by their local officials to participate in the upcoming "America on the Move" beginning next month. "America on the Move" is a nationwide effort to increase activity levels of its citizens. Communities who make the most progress are eligible for a Governor's award at the completion of the activity. "Even if the town does not end up being eligible for the award, it still inspires people to become physically active, something that is very important in a time when obesity is becoming widespread," said Councilman Richard Bradley.

Childhood Obesity Rises

Proportional to the increase state and nationwide, the obesity rates continue to rise in the Neighborhood among children as well as adults. It is estimated that 15% of youth under the age of 18 are obese. State and local authorities have called for a reinstitution for mandated physical education programs and a ban of soda and candy machines in all state-funded K-12 schools. Health officials say that the lack of physical exercise coupled with changes in dietary habits of school children are obvious contributors to the obesity trend. Another issue that has developed—and a common excuse used by the obese—is that junk food is cheaper than healthy food, prompting a movement to put a "fat tax" on unhealthy foods. Parents are urged to consider foods eaten by their children and to get their children involved in regular physical activity.

Episode 14

Announcement: Directive Seminar This Week

The local Hospital Ethics Review Board of the Neighborhood will host an Advance Directive Seminar for community members on Friday at 7:00 PM in the Neighborhood Community Center.

Advance Directives Seminar Offered

The Hospital Ethics Review Board will be offering a seminar this month to assist people in planning for end-of-life care. Naturally, no one likes to think about dying, but making plans ahead of time ensures that your wishes about the level of care you receive will be considered whenever that time comes. These plans, called advance directives, are fairly simple tools that you can create in a couple of hours and that can be discussed with family and friends.

If you or someone close to you has been the victim of a debilitating stroke or accident, you probably already know how important advance directives can be. These legally binding documents allow you to state your preferences in many important areas, such as whether to perform CPR if your heart stops, or whether you wish to donate organs in the event of your death. If advance directives are not in place, decisions often fall on healthcare workers (in emergencies) or on family members who may have no idea what your desires would have been.

The Advance Directive Seminars will last 2 hours, and enrollment is on a first-come, first-served basis. There is a small fee of $5.00 per person to cover the cost of several advance directive forms. Contact the Neighborhood Community Center for details.

Family Sues Hospital

A local family has sued the Neighborhood Hospital over visitation rules in the intensive care unit. A Neighborhood man, Chad Winchester, has filed a lawsuit against the hospital over what has been labeled by some as a case of insensitivity. According to the affidavit, Winchester was not allowed into the intensive care unit to see his mother during what is described as the morning shift change. According to hospital policy, restrictions on the number of visitors and the hours of visitation are made in order to ensure quality of care for the patient. The allegation stated that Winchester left the hospital at that time and his mother, Mary Winchester, died unexpectedly later that day. Winchester contends that the nursing staff prevented him from seeing his mother one last time prior to her passing.

Trial Report: Murder Trial Ends in Conviction

Lasting a little less than 4 weeks, the trial of Karen Smith in relation to the murder of her husband Jon Smith could be considered an open-and-shut case. While the defense made a strong opening, its case depended greatly on emotional appeals, which in turn depend highly on the type of jury hearing the case. The trial ended this week with the jury delivering a guilty verdict for the first-degree murder charge against Karen Smith. Sentencing is scheduled for next week, and Smith has the possibility of being sentenced to a term of 50 years to life in prison. Prosecutors praised jurors for making the right decision in this case. "Individuals cannot take the law into their own hands," said lead prosecutor Jessie Corona.

Episode 15

Band Competition This Weekend

The Neighborhood high school will host the annual Regional Band Concert. Bands from all regions of the state will be competing, with participants ranging from grades K-12. The competition will be held on Friday and Saturday on the following schedule: Friday, 8:00 AM to 6:00 PM; Saturday, 8:00 AM to 3:00 PM. At 4:00 PM on Saturday, following the competition, an awards ceremony will commence. The event is available to all Neighborhood and state citizens free of charge. Last year, Neighborhood High School received the highest honor for performing a medley John Philip Sousa's works, interspersed with popular music.

Local Instructor Honored

This week, Ramona Rivera, a lifelong resident of the Neighborhood, will be honored for her undying devotion and instruction of the arts, specifically the piano. The local piano teacher has been revered for exposing the area's youth to music education. Rivera has taught piano lessons to children of the community for more than 30 years. Regarded as one of the best piano teachers in the area, Rivera explains that she loves what she does, believing that music is an important developmental component to reach children. Recent scientific studies appear to agree with Rivera's viewpoint, showing that children exposed to music education have greater academic success and critical thinking skills than those who are not exposed to music education.

New Treatment Facility Planned

State lawmakers recently approved a multimillion-dollar bond to be used in developing a modern treatment center for cancer in the Neighborhood. Plans are to build the facility adjacent to the Neighborhood Hospital. However, the facility will not be a subdivision of the hospital, as it is funded independently by several charities and philanthropists. The facility will branch off from several other cancer treatment centers nationally and internationally in order to conduct research related to finding a cure for the disease. Construction on this project is set to begin in about 3 months.

Letter to the Editor: Funding Cuts to Therapy Dogs

Dear Editor, Last week, you ran an article about the value of therapy dogs to older adults at the local Senior Center. Helping prevent depression in the elderly is just one of the benefits these specially trained dogs can provide. Therapy dogs used to be given as a benefit to selected veterans with post-traumatic stress disorder. (PTSD is a disorder that can cause victims of a traumatic event to relive the experience over and over again.) Therapy dogs were demonstrated to have a positive effect on the recovery of veterans with PTSD.

However, due to recent budget cuts, funds to provide therapy animals for veterans have been eliminated. One local man, a veteran of war in the Mideast, suffers from PTSD and is struggling to adjust. He would benefit from a therapy dog but is unable to afford one.

This veteran has PTSD as a result of serving our country. You have to ask yourself–How can we now serve him? *Shawn Jacobs, DNP Health Connections Clinic*

SEASON 2 NEWS

Episode 1

Alzheimer's Rising Statistics

The Neighborhood chapter of the Alzheimer's Association has released their annual report, showing the prevalence of the disease today. Deaths from Alzheimer's increased 68% over the past ten years, making Alzheimer's the sixth leading cause of death in the United States. More than 5 million Americans are currently living with the disease. The number of Americans with Alzheimer's disease will grow as the U.S. population age 65 and older continues to increase. "Although these statistics are startling, all is not lost!" said Richard Belzar, the president of the Neighborhood chapter of the Alzheimer's Association. "Alzheimer's research is a dynamic field, and momentum builds each year. Our association has been involved in every major advancement in Alzheimer's since the 1980s and plans to be a leader in the global fight for a world without Alzheimer's."

Childbirth Classes to Begin This Week

Are you or is someone you know expecting? The birth of a child is regarded as a joyous occasion by most, but the months before the delivery can be marked as an emotional rollercoaster. A new class hopes to dispel fears regarding adverse effects of pregnancy. The class covers the childbirth process as well as caring for an infant, including such topics as breastfeeding. Childbirth classes can ease the anxiety associated with childbirth, making the experience much more pleasurable for the mother, father, and infant. The organizers have informed that time is still available to sign up for the program before it starts this week. Classes will be held on Wednesday evenings from 7:00 PM to 9:00 PM for 6 weeks. To register, call the Neighborhood Hospital at 555-555-5555.

Child Seat Manufacturers Given a Crash Course in Safety

The National Highway Traffic Safety Administration's Ease of Use Ratings Program has delivered an ultimatum to child restraint device manufacturers—improve their products or incur legal action. These improvements are not just restricted to the realm of safety, but ease of use. Joel Zweick of the ratings program said, "An essential component in making a product truly safe is how easy it is to employ. One can make an infallible product, but its useless if the consumer does not know how to use it correctly." According to Neighborhood Sheriff Mark Shuster, the real benefit of the ratings program is to educate parents and caregivers about child safety seat features, and to assist them in finding the appropriate child safety seat for their needs. Under the new ratings system, child restraints are given an overall ease-of-use rating at defined levels of A, B, or C. The rating, however, does not apply to the performance of the restraint in the event of a crash. "Child restraints are most effective if the device is correctly installed," said the sheriff.

Domestic Violence Top Cause of Death for Pregnant Women

Pregnancy is usually associated with thoughts of a coming together of family and friends in the form of showers and well-wishes in eager anticipation of a new life. For many women, however, pregnancy is marked as the beginning of a violent time in their lives. Surfacing evidence reports that a pregnant woman is more likely to die at the hand of her partner than from complications associated with pregnancy and childbirth. According to Mira Roberts, director of the Neighborhood Women's Shelter, incidents of abuse are underreported, and it is estimated that one in five women are abused during the course of a pregnancy. "Pregnancy is often a time when physical abuse begins," said Roberts. "When the abuse begins, many women are in denial, having difficulty coming to terms with the dangers involved." Dangers to a battered women and child during pregnancy include blunt trauma to the abdomen leading to premature rupture of the membranes or uterine rupture, miscarriage, and preterm labor. Such statistics support the need for a greater emphasis on screening and prevention as part of prenatal care.

Episode 2

Members of Senior Center to Visit National Park

For a minimal fee, seniors can join the local Senior Center for a 3-day weekend trip, by bus, to one of the Neighborhood's many nearby National Parks. Karen Williams, the geriatric nurse specialist at the Senior Center, encourages those interested to attend. "Contrary to the image portrayed by the media, a large number of seniors are very active in the community but simply lack the means to travel," said Williams. Registration for the 3-day trip ends mid-week so it is recommended that seniors visit the Center earlier this week to ensure that they can attend.

Senior Center Visits on the Rise

According to Karen Williams, the nurse at the Senior Center Nursing Clinic, visits to the Center have been steadily increasing for the past years, making expansion of the Center a real need. Williams said that she has seen not only an increase in those using the facility, but also an increase in those seeking basic medical care. "It used to be that I might see a few people each day. Now I see at least one person every hour," said Williams. Williams has worked at the clinic for 5 years and says the increased use has been steady, but a recent surge in attendance may be related to the addition of a lunch program at the Senior Center.

Furry Friends, Healers?

Sometimes people can be healed by more than just medicine—or at least that's the mindset centers in the Neighborhood seem to be adopting with the incorporation of pet therapy into their respective programs. The therapeutic use of pets as companions has gained increasing attention in recent years and has made its way into health care. Studies have shown that pets are beneficial for a wide variety of patients—people with AIDS or cancer, the elderly, children with disabilities, and the mentally ill. Centers across the Neighborhood that are adopting pet therapy as a means of treatment include the Senior Center and Nursing Home.

Episode 3

Local Veteran Takes Steps to Raise PTSD Awareness

Willis Braverman, local Neighborhood hero and war veteran, is forming a weekly Wednesday night support group for those who suffer from post-traumatic stress disorder (PTSD). After being honorably discharged from the Army, Braverman earned his bachelor's degree in Psychology and a Trauma Counseling Certificate in order to better serve the community that helped him through his own struggle with PTSD. According to the Bureau of Veteran Affairs, PTSD is the most severe form of combat trauma. Nearly 1 in 5 recent combat veterans will suffer from PTSD, but less than 40% of veterans with this disorder will seek help from a doctor. Says Braverman, "Sometimes symptoms, like being jittery and having trouble sleeping, are easily disregarded, but they can change a person's whole life. I hope this PTSD support group will provide a safe environment for veterans to share and to heal from their experiences." Braverman's support group will start meeting this Wednesday in the Neighborhood Community Center at 7 p.m.

Cancer Awareness Fundraiser

Neighborhood residents are gearing up for the local "Walk for Life" fundraiser. The fundraiser will support efforts for the Neighborhood Cancer Treatment Facility, which was recently approved by the state. Participants for the event will walk a 10K course that begins and ends at the site of the future facility. Those who wish to participate can refer to any of the health-related centers in the Neighborhood for more information. Given the overwhelming support for the facility as well as the dire need for it, State lawmakers recently approved a multimillion-dollar bond to fund the facility, but organizers urge the community to contribute to the effort as well. The fundraiser will be held this weekend; free snacks beverages will be provided to those who participate in the walk.

Nursing Shortage Critical, Say Hospital Officials

If you have grown concerned about the apparent lack of nurses in Neighborhood Hospital, your fears are neither alone nor unfounded. In fact, communities are suffering from nursing shortages throughout the country–and the situation is only expected to get worse. According to Pam Lowell, Director of Nursing at the Neighborhood Hospital, healthcare professionals are bracing for an uncertain future. "It is like watching the destructive path of a hurricane coming right at you–there is nothing you can do to stop it, but you can only hope to ride out the storm," said Lowell. The number of unfilled positions at the Neighborhood Hospital has risen sharply, and shortages are seen on all patient care units. "The best we can do is try to minimize the damage," Lowell states.

Size Matters

Healthcare officials are concerned about the ever-increasing size of the college football athlete. The name of the game for front linemen is size and speed—but what are the long-term costs? Neighborhood fans were disappointed to see their beloved Maverick football team defeated by the top-ranked team in the conference this week. Johnny Sands, center for the Mavericks, lost more than just the game— he lost his mobility. A severe, career-ending knee injury sustained in the third quarter was made worse because of his 280-lb. frame. Sports nutritionist expert Tom Randall says scientific research concerning the nutritional needs of football players has been scant. Fortunately, new investigations are being conducted, and the up-to-date research suggests that football players should eat and drink like marathon runners, not like wrestlers.

Episode 4

Neighborhood School Strikes Back at Bullying

The distasteful phenomenon that is bullying has finally caught up with the Neighborhood. In the U.S. bullying has been on the rise in the past few years, with statistics from the American Justice Department suggesting that one in every four kids will be bullied mentally, verbally, or physically at some point during adolescence. With the growth of social media, 43% of students are now experiencing "cyberbullying" and each day 160,000 students miss school for fear of being bullied. One group of students in the Neighborhood is striking back against bullying. Inspired by the story of a local elementary student who was bullied mercilessly who wished every day he "could go to a school where the kids are nice," Neighborhood teacher Pam Dawes started the group Kids

Against Bullying (KAB). The group meets most days after school because bullies rarely target kids who are in tight-knit groups. "We even have these red rubber bracelets to wear with KAB on the front," said Dawes, showing off her bright bracelet. "This way we can recognize each other. If one of us is getting bullied in the halls, other members can step in and help. We also formed a public group on Facebook so that kids from all schools across the country can join!" KAB members hope that through this group they can eliminate the growing threat of bullying within schools.

"Two Green Thumbs Up" for Community Garden

Neighborhood City Council this week announced the dedication of roughly 2 acres for a community garden. The garden is to be maintained by individuals, not by the community. Individuals can apply for a plot within the garden and join others in learning how to grow nutritious foods. Focus will be on healthy eating and exercise. All are invited to participate, and parents with children are encouraged to make visiting the garden a weekly family activity. City counselors are hoping that the garden will forge closer ties within the community and teach Neighborhood residents more about the wide variety of foods that can be grown in this area.

Studies Show Inadequate Diets in Americans

It is no secret that American diets are commonly lacking in fruits and vegetables. The average person rarely eats recommended daily amounts of these foods. The common excuse is that dietary habits are hard to change and it's too hard to figure out exactly how much of each food to eat. Answering the need for simpler guidelines, the government has created a visual food guide called MyPlate. MyPlate illustrates the five food groups that are the building blocks of a healthy diet, shown in a simple, visual format. The government also offers fun online interactive tools that go with MyPlate. Tools like SuperTracker help people to plan, analyze, and track the balance of diet and physical activity.

Support Group Benefits Dieters

Whether the weight-gain culprit is food for comfort, the freshman fifteen, or holiday splurging, working together with another person who is interested in losing weight might improve your chances for weight loss. Recent research has shown that having the help of a support group may be beneficial to individuals participating in a weight-loss program. Results of this study showed that dieters who have the help of a support group experience less stress and less "brainpower drain" than those individuals who are undertaking a weight loss program alone. In the study, dieters who dieted alone had increases in the stress-associated hormone cortisol; those who attended weekly support-group sessions did not. Those dieting alone demonstrated lower working memory capacity than did those in support groups. These findings may be helpful in understanding the high incidence of diet failure among those who need to lose weight.

Episode 5

Announcement: Middle School to Host Science Fair

Join the community's best and brightest this weekend for an event that is sure to please, inspire, and educate. This weekend the Neighborhood Middle School will host the annual Science Fair. More than 50 children from the school will participate in the event, with projects ranging from theoretical to those that can be applied in everyday life. Prizes will also be awarded to those projects deemed the best of show by the judges. Prizes include gift certificates and the chance to enter projects into higher-level regional, statewide, or nationwide science fairs.

Forest Fire Continues to Burn

A forest fire that has been ravaging the forest west of the Neighborhood has still not been contained. For more than 5 days, the blaze has been destroying an uncalculated number of acres, and for each day the fire continues, it is causing irreversible damage. Initially, firefighters thought the fire would be easy to control, but the windy season has started earlier than expected, causing the fire to be less predictable and to spread rapidly. Although the fire is not contained, city officials stress that citizens are not in any direct danger and will be notified in advance if there is any chance the fire's direction will shift toward the town.

Smoky Air Fills Healthcare Facilities with Patients

While firefighters battle to bring the forest fire west of the Neighborhood under control, healthcare workers battle to keep patients breathing. "The smoky air conditions affect everyone, but especially those with pre-existing problems, such as chronic lung conditions," said Neighborhood Hospital Emergency Department (ED) physician James Gordon, MD. Increases in patient numbers can be seen in the ED and local physician offices. City officials have warned that while not life-threatening, the haze should still be regarded as a risk. They urge all citizens—particularly those with chronic respiratory conditions—to stay indoors unless a trip outside is absolutely necessary.

Episode 6

Mandatory Overtime Angers Nurses, Cite Unsafe Work Conditions

A recently proposed method to maintain adequate staffing at Neighborhood Hospital has angered many nurses. "The increasing shortage of nurses across the nation forces all hospitals to re-evaluate the way they operate," said Dan Packard, MD, a physician at the hospital. One of these re-evaluations resulted in the suggestion of mandatory overtime—the legality of which is currently under question. Nurse Janice Calgary said, "This is supposed to be a free country, not one where employers can dictate continuous and excessive work hours. If this measure is allowed, then the hospital is taking away a large portion of our private time. Hospital nurses manage patients who need acute care. It isn't safe to put overworked and exhausted nurses in charge of monitoring and caring for these patients." Hospital officials have claimed that mandatory overtime is only one of the proposed ideas; other alternatives include closing hospital beds. "We enjoy the prospect of overtime if we find ourselves strapped for cash, but forcing employees to work overtime is surely illegal," Nurse Calgary added.

The Myth of the Nursing Shortage?

Imagine going through nursing school hearing there is a critical shortage of nurses, then graduating and not being able to find work. This scenario is exactly what happened to Virginia Wade and her best friend Mila Tajen. Wade and Tajen, like many others, started nursing school when there was a loudly proclaimed nursing shortage. They expected to move quickly from school into permanent jobs. Instead, they are both working in temp nursing jobs while they seek fulltime employment. A recent survey of nursing grads found that more than a third had been unable to find fulltime work as registered nurses immediately after graduation. Economic factors played a large role in this shift. When the economy soured, nurses who had planned to retire early decided to hold onto their jobs. Many institutions scaled back staff and (some say) increased demands on their workers rather than hire more nurses. However, local ANA group representative Pam Bullock encourages new nurses not to give up hope. "Shortages and excesses occur in cycles and by region. Baby-boomers will retire and the demand for registered nurses will not go away." Bullock states that online employment sites and new-nurse support groups are good resources to use when looking for a job.

Task Force to Tackle Nursing Shortage

If you have noticed an apparent lack of nurses in the Neighborhood, you are not alone, This week, leaders from around the state will convene in the Neighborhood to address the alarming shortage of nurses available to meet the healthcare needs of area and state residents. The gathering is a response to the apparent scarcity of nurses not just statewide, but nationwide.

Laughing Away Alzheimer's

The Falling Down Funny Senior Improv Comedy Troupe, formed by participants at the Neighborhood Senior Center, is determined to laugh away Alzheimer's by practicing improvisational exercises to maintain their mental acuity. The group meets every week and has performed in assisted living facilities all around the Neighborhood. Vivian Greenwood, age 75, is just one of the many senior improv players who believes that this program has kept the disease at bay. But is she right in her belief? Dan Packard, a physician at the Neighborhood hospital explains. "While studies have shown that there is no sure way to prevent getting Alzheimer's disease, there is research suggesting that regular brain exercises help reduce brain loss and maintain cognitive abilities." Examples of brain exercises include crossword or Sudoku puzzles, drawing a map from memory, doing math in your head, or playing games that involve memorization. Dan continues, "Improvisational comedy games promote memorization and stimulate the brain, so Vivian's beliefs about exercise and Alzheimer's certainly have some truth to them."

Episode 7

City Hears From Parents on Proposed Music Ban

A public forum has been opened for parents to participate in response to the recently proposed ban on the use of personal music players on school grounds by students and faculty. The proposed ban comes in reaction to the increasing popularity of the devices among teens and reports that these players contribute to hearing loss. Students have protested the idea since its inception, arguing that the school should not be allowed to ban the devices. Neighborhood school officials cite a recent study indicating that a high percentage of young people have damaged their ears by playing devices too loudly. They say music devices placed directly in the ear lead to other dangers, such as distracted or impaired driving. School officials want to ban the players from school campuses. Students claim their "pursuit of happiness" would be violated by this ban.

Local Teen Pregnancy Numbers Down

While the state is seeing an ever-increasing rate of teen pregnancy, numbers of teen pregnancies in the Neighborhood have dropped significantly. Implementation of a school-based sex education class is cited for this difference. School nurse Connie Ruiz says, "If you want rates to drop even further, condoms should be made available to kids in the high school—free of charge." Many members of the community feel the same way and have tried to implement Ruiz's ideas to lower the pregnancy rate, but are met by opposition from parents. "Most parents are unable to admit that their children are sexually active, when in fact, a majority of them are," Ruiz added.

National Center on Elder Abuse Releases Warning Signs

The National Center on Elder Abuse (NCEA), a division of the Administration on Aging, has released their annual Warning Signs of Elder Abuse Report in the hopes of bringing attention to this important issue. The most common signs that point to an elder abuse problem are recurring bruises, pressure marks, broken bones, abrasions, and burns. Abused persons generally have evasive responses about their injuries and are reluctant to return to the abusive environment. In some cases of elder abuse, there is an unexplained withdrawal from normal activities or a sudden change in alertness. Behavior such as belittling, threats, and other uses of power and control by spouses are indicators of verbal or emotional abuse. "It's always important to remain alert," says Sally Ann, a representative of the NCEA. "Victims often suffer in silence, and abuse most often occurs in the home by a close family member. If you notice changes in an elder's personality, behavior, or physical condition, you should start to question what is going on. If you suspect elder abuse, report your suspicions to Adult Protective Services."

Signal to Noise

Neighborhood school and city officials are urging parents to reconsider buying portable audio devices for their children, in response to results of studies indicating that a high percentage of young people have damaged their ears by playing the devices too loudly. Further dangers suggested by studies include distraction during activities such as driving. School officials have made efforts to ban players from school campuses to reduce their potential liability in the event of an accident involving an audio device. "We are covering our own backs, that is true, but we also care about the well-being of students," said Principal Adam Hurwitz. Several lawsuits have been filed nationwide against audio device companies despite warnings printed in the device user manuals.

Episode 8

Rising Number of Elder Abuse Cases

Carol Bruno, director of the Elder Abuse Awareness Program, testified at a hearing of the Neighborhood Special Committee on Aging that agencies are seeing increasingly complex cases of elder abuse. Bruno stated that part of the increase in the number of cases has to do with the changes in population. The number of Americans 65 and over is projected to nearly double by 2030. The number of people over 85 is increasing at an even faster rate. Sadly, as many as 5.9 million seniors (a staggering 9.5% of the elderly population) are abused, exploited, or neglected each year, according to available statistics and surveys. There are two main types of elder abuse, domestic and institutional. Domestic elder abuse generally refers to mistreatment by anyone with whom the elder has a special relationship. Institutional abuse refers to mistreatment occurring in residential facilities. Roughly 60% of elderly abuse cases involve neglect, but the committee has also seen physical abuse, emotional abuse, sexual abuse, exploitation, and abandonment. The rising number of elder abuse cases could overwhelm local adult protective service agencies. Bruno is lobbying for further funding so that local protective services agency can be "on the front line in the fight against elder abuse."

Announcement: Campaign Puts Smiles on Faces

This weekend, children ages 5-11 will have the opportunity to receive a free dental screening at the Neighborhood Dental Office. The offer is in response to the statewide campaign, "Healthy Teeth," which was recently approved by the governor last month. The campaign is working with local dentists, schools, and parents to improve the overall dental health of the community.

Editorial: Gay and Lesbian Couples as Parents?

The question of gay or lesbian couples as parents has found its way into the national conversation and has even been popularized on mainstream television. In Congress, professional offices, and college campuses, the subject is discussed openly, but there is still a wide range of opinion. On the national front, there is a growing trend of extending adoption privileges to gay couples. Proponents say the trend cannot be harmful—what do children need but loving parents, regardless of sexual orientation? Opponents suggest that being raised by a gay person may encourage a child to be gay. Proponents say that such a statement is not logical, pointing to the fact that most gay or lesbian young people were raised by straight, not heterosexual, parents. Opponents often believe homosexuality to be immoral, and so object to placing a child in a morally "unhealthy" environment. Proponents often describe homosexual tendencies as innate. The debate will surely continue, but as people consider this complex topic, we hope they will think carefully about the children involved and ask themselves: What is better, a child with or without parents?

Think Twice About That Tan, Say Scientists

Skin cancer rates are on the rise. This comes as a shock to scientists, considering the multitude of warnings given every year regarding the risk of prolonged exposure to the sun. "Personally, I feel the disregard to the warnings is the obsession of vanity superseding one's health concern," says research scientist Steven Pearson, PhD. Doctors say exposure to the sun is not the threat, but exposure to the sun without protection is. Many individuals spend time outside without hats, sunglasses, sunscreen designed to protect against the risk of prolonged exposure to sunlight.

Episode 9

Changing Semantics

As the care-giving population has grown over the years, the definition of "caregiver" has taken on many meanings. The local Family Caregiver Alliance describes caregivers as, "family, friends, and neighbors who stand by those whom they love as they face chronic illness, disability, or death. Caregivers are a diverse group of people from all walks of life—some new to care-giving, some anticipating becoming caregivers, and others for whom providing care has become a way of life." In the United States alone, caregivers provide more than 20 hours of care each week, accounting for an estimated $257 billion in unpaid services annually. This is double the amount spent on nursing home placement and paid home-care combined.

Nursing Home Abuse and Neglect Widespread

According to results of new studies that have been surfacing over the past few months, a new epidemic has affected medical facilities. While the cause of this epidemic is neither bacteria nor virus, it is nevertheless deadly. Nursing home abuse and neglect has become a widespread, growing epidemic, affecting thousands of nursing home residents who are dependent on nursing homes for care. Abuse and neglect can be difficult to recognize and are often covered up by nursing home staff. It is suggested that individuals who have a relative in a nursing home should monitor for warning signs of nursing home abuse and neglect. It is estimated that as many as two million elderly patients are victims of nursing home abuse each year, a number that is projected to increase.

Announcement: Group Wants to Hear Your Troubles

Later this week, the Neighborhood will sponsor leadership training for formation of support groups. Support groups have been found to be an effective way to manage problems, whether these problems stem from divorce, coping with a chronic illness, anxiety, or other aspect. Support groups are more effective than trying to manage problems independently. The purpose of the leadership training is to teach individuals how to effectively lead a support group. The meeting will be held at the Neighborhood Community Center, Thursday evening at 7 p.m.

Episode 10

Hospital to Offer Life-Saving Course

The Neighborhood Hospital will host a series of 2-hour classes in cardiopulmonary resuscitation, or CPR, at 7PM over the next five days. Completion of a 2-hour class will result in qualification to administer CPR. The class is free to all Neighborhood residents and Hospital staff hope that the classes will fit everyone's schedule. Training in CPR saves lives. You don't know when you or a loved one will need emergency CPR. For more information call 555-555-5555.

Local Pathologist Dies

Pathologist Danilo Ocampo, MD, PhD, died suddenly this week after an apparent heart attack. Dr. Ocampo is best known for his contributions to law enforcement agencies during his career as the medical investigator for the Neighborhood County. In recent years, Dr. Ocampo assisted in gathering the evidence that was a key factor in the conviction of Harlan Randolph for the crime of murdering his wife with arsenic; a crime many believe was an influencing factor in the recent Karen Smith case. "His ability to determine specific details involving the deaths of crime victims was astounding and invaluable to our department," said Sheriff Mark Shuster following the announcement of the pathologist's death. "The amount of attention he gave to even the most minute detail of a case is only one of remarkable qualities of this man, and he will be sorely missed."

Profile Sites Appeal to Teens

To say that internet use is pervasive is an understatement—if internet use were a virus, we would all be doomed. One of the most popular features of the internet, the personal website, is overwhelmingly popular among teens. Personal profiles are often established well before high school, and millions if not billions of postings occur every day via computer and mobile device. Parents as well as youth enjoy these pages, but grown-ups tend to be more cautious in the personal information they divulge. Although these sites do promote socialization, they also allow invasion of personal space. Two serious ways this impacts young people is through sexual predation and cyberbullying. Sexual predators and pedophiles have been documented using sites to attract young, unassuming victims. Several suicides have occurred in which teens, besieged by insults via the internet, ended by taking their own lives.

Episode 11

Announcement: Event May Make People Play a Different Tune

Musicians from across the city are coming together in conjunction with the local Neighborhood Community Arts Program to sponsor a music appreciation workshop, open to children and adults. The workshop will be held each afternoon and evening through Saturday and will cover subjects both vocal and instrumental. Event organizer Ramona Rivera, well known to the community through her tireless efforts as a piano teacher, says that "Not enough children are given an opportunity to explore music has a hobby." The event marks the first exclusively oriented music workshop staged for the community in what Mrs. Rivera hopes to be a "recurring, if not continuous, event."

Sleep Deprivation Is No Dream

Have trouble sleeping at night? You are not alone. In a recent national report, health experts seem to agree that most adults do not obtain enough sleep each night and are indeed suffering from sleep deprivation. Sleep deprivation is a rising cause of concern among the health community due to the adverse effects it can have on all levels of society. Health officials say that in order to prevent sleep deprivation, one must get at least 8 hours of sleep per night. Symptoms of sleep deprivation include irritability, blurred vision, slurred speech, memory lapses, and even hallucinations.

Road Construction Woes

Residents of the west side of the Neighborhood are complaining about the continuous, bombarding sounds coming from an ongoing construction project. Construction superintendent Stephen Morton claims his company and workers are not violating any sound ordinance, as the Neighborhood has yet to sign any such legislation. Issues have been raised with the construction crews about working at night, but the company states they are doing this to avoid problems with daytime traffic. Local resident Joseph Marrs says, "The noise is bad enough, but I've got bright, halogen construction lights shining into my bedroom every night. I can't get any sleep, just because the city said they wanted to avoid traffic congestion".

Episode 12

Cancer Center Construction Halted

In what appears to be one in a series of setbacks, the future site of the regional Cancer Center has once again been halted, with planners blocking proposed changes. City engineers and traffic experts say the current plan will create traffic flow problems within a 2-mile radius of the construction site. The problem of traffic does not seem to be a primary concern with the citizens who will be traveling these routes, however. Many area residents are angered by the ongoing delays to begin construction, citing the center is desperately needed by the community.

Cutting Through the Smoke

Neighborhood Council members are meeting this week to deliberate on the recently proposed citywide smoking ban. The gray area in the decision is whether to maintain the current ban on smoking in public areas, such as restaurants and city buildings. Those against the ban claim that limiting smoking to private residences is restricting freedom, making those who smoke less equal than nonsmokers. Anti-smoking advocates support the ban and assert that the general health of the community is at stake when people are allowed to smoke in public.

Announcement: Adopt a Pet

Everyone wants a loving family, and family is not limited to those who walk on two feet. The local animal shelter is offering a free pet adoption clinic to individuals 18 and older each day this week from 9:00 AM to 3:00 PM. Types of pets that can be adopted include birds, cats, and especially dogs. Dogs remain the most-abandoned pets in the Neighborhood. Staff at the animal shelter try to ensure that their animals end up in the hands of a loving family so they are not abandoned again. All the animals available for adoption will have the appropriate vaccinations at no extra cost to the patrons.

Episode 13

Announcement: Special Olympics Golf Tournament Next Week

Late next week, the Neighborhood Golf Course will play host to a statewide Special Olympics golf tournament. The event organizers expect anywhere between 50 and 75 participants for the tournament and over 100 spectators. Admission is free, as is participation. Due to this event, the golf course will be closed to the public between 7:00 AM and 3:00 PM on Saturday and Sunday.

Exposing Fears

This week, a local college experienced a crime that is making female students wary of their walks to class. According to a police report, two female students were walking to class on campus when they spotted a man lying naked on the grass. Claiming they had no idea what the man's intentions were, whether he was injured or planning to attack them, the women called the campus police, who arrested 18-year-old Anthony Martin for indecent exposure. Martin reportedly became combative when officers arrived on the scene, although no one was hurt during the incident. Martin was transported to a local hospital for a psychiatric evaluation.

Nest Eggs Hardly "Grade-A"

How well have you prepared for your golden years? This question was addressed in a recent national survey—and as it turns out, the most common answers to the question did not bode well. The report showed that only 25% of Americans believe they will have enough money to pay for long-term care when they are elderly. The concern about inadequate finances increases with age. Those who are between 50 and 65 years of age have far greater concerns than do younger adults. Adding to this, less than half of all adults have taken steps to prepare for retirement. Many middle-aged adults are concerned about financing their own long-term care as well caring for their aging parents.

Episode 14

Announcement: Neighborhood to Host State Arts and Crafts Fair

The Neighborhood Community Center will hold its very first statewide Arts and Crafts Fair next Saturday. "We expect a huge crowd as it is the first time our state chose the Neighborhood as host." Tara Andrews, chairperson of the Arts and Crafts Committee, said. "This fair will be a passionate celebration of the arts. There will be a quilt competition, a glass blowing demonstration, an art lesson by the Neighborhood's local landscape artist Giovanna Marti, and much more. We couldn't be more thrilled with the exposure!" A few of the events taking place at the Arts and Crafts Fair will require preregistration. RSVP to those events by calling Tara Andrews at 666-666-6666 or by visiting the Neighborhood Community Center website.

Pedaling to Safety

The Neighborhood Elementary School will be the host of an annual Bicycle Safety Awareness Fair this weekend for children ages 6-12. The purpose of the fair is to ensure that children are educated in riding safety. Bicycle professionals will be attending the fair and will be offering free bike checkups. Nationally known biker Lars Yurtsen will teach children right techniques and equipment for lifelong biking success. Lectures on bicycle safety, agility tests, and games will be conducted to reinforce safe riding practices and use of helmets. Prizes will be awarded for the best riders in various age categories.

Angered Golfers Hit Back at Olympics

Many area golfers were angered this week when no tee times were available because the golf course had chosen to sponsor the Special Olympics rather than remain open on its regular schedule. "It amazes me that event organizers were not sensitive to the routines of the serious golfers in this community—to give the Special Olympics the preferred tee times on the busiest golf days of the week was poor planning on the part of the golf club," says Neighborhood Golf Association (NGA) president Lee Malcoeur. "These individuals can play anytime, and the ones who support this golf course should always be given priority over others—after all, we're paying members." The recent Special Olympics event drew over 60 participants and over 100 spectators.

Vending Frustration

A recent school-board decision about the Neighborhood High School vending machines has angered many parents and students. Citing the national obesity trend and the rise in type 2 diabetes among youngsters, the board determined that "junk food" would no longer be served in the school's vending machines. Parents and students of the high school are claiming that, by limiting what the students can purchase, the school is limiting the teenager's freedom of choice. Parents and students assert that high schoolers are capable of making food choices, and the school system should not be making decisions about what is appropriate to eat and what is unhealthy for students.

Episode 15

Announcement: Vending Viewpoints

This week, parents who are against the recent School Board decision to ban "junk food" from high school vending machines will be given a chance to voice their concerns. The school was compelled to offer a public forum to debate the issue after the decision was met with such outrage the previous week. The event will be held Wednesday at 7:00 PM in the Neighborhood High School auditorium.

Theft, Narcotics Use on the Rise

The recent string of unsolved car thefts has prompted fears and apprehension in the Neighborhood. Many believe the thefts are a result of drug-related activity in the community. The series of thefts began around the residential and apartment district of the downtown area of the Neighborhood, but has since moved into the wealthier and seemingly more protected areas of town. While theft of the vehicles seems the common thread among these crimes, other reports that cars are also being vandalized, and car stereos are being stolen. Sheriff Mark Shuster believes the thefts are related to the recent rise in drug-related activity in the town, a view shared by a majority of the Neighborhood. "Statistically, high school and college students are the most frequent perpetrators of these crimes. At this stage of the investigation, they remain our primary focus," said Shuster at a recent press conference.

Crafting a Community

Like a quilt is a combination of many types of fabric, this past weekend's state-sponsored Arts and Crafts Fair drew a diverse population as well. Drawing hundreds from around the state, the fair, held at the Neighborhood Community Center, drew both competition and spectators. Neighborhood resident Pam Allen won the grand prize for the best quilt, which was sold to local businessman Greg Ross for $2,500. The opinion of many quilt experts was that the quilt was well inspired and worth the cost.

SEASON 3 NEWS

Episode 1

Seminar Offers Closure

Death symbolizes the final transition in life, but this transition does not just affect one life—the grief inflicted by a loved one's death can affect many. A Neighborhood nurse hopes to change the long-term effects of death by offering a Grief and Bereavement Seminar titled, "Don't Let Death Ruin Your Life: Reclaim Happiness After the Death of Your Loved One." The seminar will take place every night this week at 7:00 PM. Admission is free. Call 555-947-6341 for more information.

Local Man Dies in "Freak Accident"

"It happened so fast," commented assembly-line worker Adam Delpy on the death of his coworker, James Palmer. Palmer met a tragic end 3 days ago in an accident at a local automobile production annex. The reports gathered indicate that Palmer died while moving a set of car doors that were suspended from the roof by several chains. "We were behind on production, and we thought the chains could support the extra weight," stated Palmer's supervisor Alan Sharp. The chains, however, did not support the added weight. They snapped, and falling parts caused severe head trauma to Palmer, killing him before the ambulance could arrive. The Occupational Safety and Health Administration (OSHA) is investigating the incident. Sharp has been put on paid administrative leave during the investigation. A closed memorial service and mass, said by Fr. John Olivia, will be held at the Neighborhood Catholic Church on Saturday.

'Roid Ruckus

Nathan Roberts, widely held as Neighborhood's star high school football player, was accused last week of use and possession of steroids. The 17-year-old football player admitted to steroid use, stating he wanted to get a full-paid scholarship to a prestigious university and knew he would be overlooked by Division I scouts without the enhancement. Roberts, a linebacker, was known for his ability to hold a strong defense in any situation and was a standout athlete this past season. "It is too bad," says Coach Anderson. "Kids these days have just gotten so competitive," he added. Roberts did not disclose the source of the steroids, but it is speculated that his father, Randall Roberts, not only knew about his son's steroid use but was also the supplier. Nathan denies the former allegation. Steroid use is known to be harmful because it causes high blood pressure, edema, unwanted hair growth, hormonal disruption.

Episode 2

Changing Eating Habits

Starting next week, the Neighborhood Community Center will be offering a cooking class for individuals aged 15-18. The class is designed to modify current diets with healthier alternatives. The class is being offered in response to the growing obesity trend in the Neighborhood and nationwide. "Our children need to learn what they are putting into their bodies. We want to them to know that eating healthily does not mean just eating rabbit food," said class sponsor Damien Nichols. The course will focus on nutrition, risk assessment, dietary modification, and meal preparation using all four food groups.

Tragedy Strikes Family, Community

Yesterday morning, the body of Allison Bloom was found in a field near the outskirts of the Neighborhood following an extensive all-night search. The 6-year-old girl was reported missing the preceding morning after Bloom's playmate reported seeing her leave with an adult white man from the front yard of Bloom's household. The report was corroborated by a neighbor, who said he saw the two entering a white sedan. Initial findings showed the girl had been raped before being killed and was dropped in the field where she was found. Sheriff Mark Shuster reported that a manhunt is in progress and that there are no concrete suspects as of yet.

Food Fight

Kentucky Fried Chicken, the nation's largest fried chicken restaurant, has again been put in the deep fryer by food activists' complaints regarding the chain's use of unhealthy trans-fatty acids in food preparation. "Americans are demanding healthier eating conditions," said food activist Gene Westchester. "It is fast food businesses such as KFC that benefits from obesity. They don't care what they feed us; they are only out to make a buck," added activist Jaren Dolland. KFC company spokesperson Gerald Rossum said that the company was "willing to adopt and explore alternative cooking preparation, but not at the expense of changing the recipe." Neighborhood customers continue to gobble (no pun intended) the fried chicken during the lunch and evening hours. "I don't want some political dude telling me that I can't eat KFC-I happen to like it," says local citizen Emma Barrowman.

Episode 3

Local Vet Dies Outside Bar

A local man was found bleeding and unconscious in an alley behind the Late Sunsets Bar on the west side of Southend last night. The victim, 29-year-old Matt Nolan, was pronounced dead on arrival at the Emergency Department of Neighborhood Hospital. According to a hospital statement, death was the result of traumatic injuries, and police are investigating the death as a homicide. Witnesses say Nolan, a recently discharged veteran, had been drinking heavily and was seen accosting a customer shortly before leaving the bar. Anyone with information about this incident is urged to contact the police.

Announcement: Conference Focuses on Substance Abuse

This weekend, the Neighborhood Community Center and Neighborhood Medical Association are coming together to host an event titled, "Multidisciplinary Health Providers Conference: Approaches to Treating Substance Abuse." Approved by the National Association of Substance Abuse Treatment, the conference will focus primarily on drug abuse, with a secondary focus on alcoholism. The event will be held at the Neighborhood Community Center on Saturday from 1:00 to 4:00 p.m.

Drug Use Rise Continues

There has been an alarming rise in the rate of drug use and addiction in the Neighborhood. The culprit? Methamphetamines, otherwise known as "meth." Communities nationwide have seen a sharp increase in meth houses, and an increase has also been seen in use among youth attending Neighborhood schools. It has become commonplace for students to know someone who uses in the school setting, where drug deals are being conducted in classes, between classes, and during lunch breaks under the eyes of teachers and administration. "It has become as frequent as passing a note in class," said a student from the high school.

Suspect in Rape Case Injured During Chase

Alvin Cromwell, suspected child rapist and murderer, was injured following a brief chase with police. Cromwell, who was wanted in connection with the rape and murder of 6-year-old Allison Bloom last week, was the target of a 7-day manhunt. Police began to associate the 38-year-old Cromwell with the rape and murder of Bloom after a DNA test returned with Cromwell's profile based on samples taken from previous crimes. The chase began when Cromwell saw police approaching his one-bedroom apartment downtown, and he escaped out a back window of the apartment. While running from police, Cromwell broke his femur and sustained internal injuries when he jumped from a 30-foot cliff in attempts to elude authorities. Currently conscious and in the Neighborhood Hospital for treatment, Cromwell has been undergoing questioning by Sheriff Mark Shuster and other members of law enforcement.

Episode 4

Announcement: Run, Neighborhood, Run!

Why walk when you can run? The Neighborhood is forming a running club for its residents. An information and organizational meeting for the runners club will be held next week at the Neighborhood Community Center. "Most communities our size have running clubs," says event organizer Ron Williams. The purpose of the club is to motivate individuals to improve their health through running, and to provide a mechanism for individuals with mutual interests to meet. In order to kindle social interaction, the primary location where the running club will meet for their runs is the Neighborhood Community Garden. The club is welcome for individuals of all ages at no cost. "We just want people to be healthy and have a fun time achieving that goal," concluded Williams.

Suspected Rapist Complains of Poor Medical Treatment

In what appears to be an ethical battle waiting to boil over, Alvin Cromwell, a suspect in the brutal rape and murder of 6-year-old Allison Bloom, is claiming he received poor and substandard treatment at Neighborhood Hospital while recovering from injuries sustained when he tried to escape arrest. According to hospital officials, Cromwell, 38, claims that nurses at Neighborhood Hospital withheld pain medications from him as punishment for the crime of which he is accused. Cromwell also cited rude comments and being referred to as a child killer by some of the nurses. Neighborhood Hospital spokeswoman Elizabeth Blanchett did not comment, other than to say that an investigation is currently underway and that any incidence of confirmed abuse or neglect would be disclosed.

Auto Accident Leaves Local Man in Critical Condition; Nursing Staff Insensitive

Last night, local Mark Martin rolled his vehicle after failing to negotiate a turn. Martin was taken to Neighborhood Hospital, where he remains in critical condition with spinal cord injuries. According to bystanders and those who interacted with him before the crash, Martin had been drinking heavily all evening and was drunk when the accident occurred. Martin will not face jail time, since the only person he hurt was himself and there was no property damage. "In a way, given his current state, he has already received punishment for his actions. We are just happy no one else was hurt," said Sheriff Mark Shuster. Martin's father, Gil Martin, has accused the Neighborhood Hospital emergency department nursing staff of being insensitive and uncaring because they refused to allow family members to see Mark while he was being treated in the emergency department. Hospital spokesperson Beverly Mayer refused to comment on the situation.

Episode 5

Announcement: Senior Center Set to Host Talk

Medication management can be a problem even for the young, and needless to say, the hassle of managing medications increases as individuals age and as the number of required medications increases. Karen Williams, local gerontology nurse, hopes to change this fact of life. This Thursday afternoon at 1:00 PM, Williams will present a local talk on "Medication Management for Seniors." The talk will be presented in the Neighborhood Senior Center. "We chose this location because older adults are accustomed to visiting here, and a comfortable locale provides a better atmosphere to help people change," said Williams. The presentation will focus on issues older adults face when taking medications. The talk is free and will be open to the public.

Nursing Strike Imminent?

Can it get any worse? In the midst of a nursing shortage, now there is the possibility of a Neighborhood nursing strike. The nursing union announced demands for better working conditions, citing insufficient staffing and mandatory overtime as two major concerns. They also are challenging a new administration guideline that Hospital nurses obtain advanced degrees. "Ultimately this is about quality of care for patients," said nurse Marie Weldon. One of the leaders of the nursing union in the Neighborhood added, "The public needs to know this is not about wanting to be paid more. It is about allowing nurses to provide the level of care we have an obligation to provide." Community members have found themselves in an impossible situation—accepting a tax increase to fund the nurses, or trying to cope with potentially substandard care. Hospitals and healthcare agencies are searching hard for alternatives, but a clear answer has yet to emerge.

7-Year-Old Hit by Car, Remains in Hospital

"Speed and inattention were the leading causes of the accident," said Sheriff Mark Shuster in response to the accident. Yesterday, a car struck 7-year-old Marcus Young while he was riding his bike near home. The car, driven by 16-year-old Charles Dirk, was traveling at a high rate of speed through a residential neighborhood. The car hit Young after he swerved into the street to avoid an aggressive dog. The boy was flung 30 feet through the air and landed on a grassy median, "a fact that may have saved his life," said Shuster. Young suffered multiple fractures and laceration and remains at the Neighborhood Hospital.

Episode 6

Announcement: Forum Open to Discuss Proposed Community

Next Tuesday, discussion will be open on the topic of a recently proposed large-scale retirement community. The meeting, hosted at the Community Center, will begin with a focus on the common questions regarding the proposed construction-cost to townspeople and the effects it will have on the community. The proposed community, referred to as The Mature Oasis, expects to break ground on a 17-acre facility in the northwest part of the city late this season.

Water Supply Breached–Broken Water Line?

When a natural resource is a basic necessity for life, one would expect pandemonium and chaos to erupt in its absence. Such has not appeared to be the case with the Neighborhood's recent water crisis. Many Neighborhood residents have no access to water due to a broken water line. Affected residents are expected to be without water for at least the next 48 hours. Officials have jumped on the issue immediately, by having the National Guard dispense water bottles to all citizens in need. Residents are also urged to use water conservatively if they have a separate supply of water. Facilities such as the Neighborhood Hospital have assured patients that the current situation will not affect their care. The hospital keeps large caches of water in reserve for emergencies.

March MADDness

This week, the group Mothers Against Drunk Driving, or MADD, marched outside of City Hall calling for tougher laws in the Neighborhood for drunk driving offenses. The catalyst for this march was an alcohol-related crash involving Mark Martin of the Neighborhood a few weeks ago. While the members of MADD admit that no one but Martin was hurt in the accident, drunk-driving accidents very often involve people who happen to be in the way. In addition, MADD holds the position that since Martin himself was hurt, it was not a victimless crime. "We must protect the drunk drivers from themselves as well as innocent bystanders," said a member of MADD.

Episode 7

Local Hospice Offers Home Care

With rehabilitation facilities becoming overcrowded, a brand new Hospice, Life Caring Solutions, opened its doors this week in The Neighborhood. They have a multidisciplinary team of physicians, nurses, certified home health aides, companion caregivers, bereavement counselors and social workers to attend to the emotional and physical needs of patients and families. The hospice team at Life Caring Solutions enables patients to live out their days in the comfort of their own home. They offer a wide range of services including a complete management of all medical issues and nurses who are available at all times for questions and consultations. "Life Caring Solutions is a hospice that helps patients live with dignity and respect," says Rachel Polson, president and founder of Life Caring Solutions. "We use advanced medications and therapies lessen suffering and control distressing symptoms. We do all we can to help the dying be in control of the last chapter of their life."

Announcement: Anti-violence Organization Holds Festival

Starting Friday, and lasting until the end of the weekend, the organization Safe Haven will be sponsoring its second annual River Jazz Fest. The statewide organization is one that speaks out against domestic violence. Proceeds from the festival will support shelters and counseling for battered women and children. Individuals who attend the event will find music, food, arts and crafts, and carnival games. The event is scheduled to start Friday, and Safe Haven is looking for anyone who would offer a hand in setting up for the festival. Hours for the festival will be Friday and Saturday, 12:00 PM to 11:00 PM, and Sunday, 12:00 PM to 5:00 PM.

Negligence Cited in Amputation Mishap

Earlier this week, 62-year-old Joseph Benson underwent an amputation of his leg just below the left knee and suffered a horrible complication—the wrong leg was amputated. Benson, a diabetic who has suffered from poor circulation for the past 5 years, was shocked to wake up after his surgery and learn of the mishap. "I hoped that I was just dreaming, but I keep waking up to the same thing," said Benson. Staff at Neighborhood Hospital have not officially commented on the case, but this incident comes at a dire time for the hospital, which has experienced an assortment of problems lately, including complaints of poor treatment, union problems, and nursing shortages.

Teenage Girls Lead in Smoking, Drug Use

According to a recently released health report, teenage girls have surpassed their male counterparts in smoking and prescription drug abuse. In the past 2 years, more young women than men started using marijuana, alcohol, and cigarettes. In support of these findings, Sheriff Mark Shuster reported that most of the recent drug violations at the local high school have involved female suspects. Given the recent rise in methamphetamines in Neighborhood schools, the sheriff only sees this number rising. High school student Tara Pritchet told reporters, "Girls want to do what older guys are doing—they want to be cool." Pritchet denied using drugs herself, but admits that some of her friends do. Carol Ramsey, a nurse midwife who also works at the Neighborhood

Community Health Department, finds the results disturbing. "Adolescent girls who consume illicit substances are at a higher risk for depression, addiction, and stunted growth," said Ramsey. Those who were surveyed reported that they felt peer pressure was more common among female cliques than male ones, stating that the chances of becoming an outcast are more likely for female students than for male students. "Because substance abuse goes hand-in-hand with risky sexual behavior, these females are more likely to contract a sexually transmitted disease or become pregnant," warned Ramsey. The surveys that led to the reported results canvassed over 70,000 households in the nation.

Episode 8

Announcement: Lecture to Help People See Danger

Peter Raush, MD, a Neighborhood ophthalmologist, will present a lecture, "Things You Should Know About Macular Degeneration," on Thursday at 7:00 P.M. at the Neighborhood Community Center. Raush explains that the purpose of the lecture is to inform individuals of a relatively common and significant eye disorder among elderly individuals. Macular degeneration is a disease of the eye in which the light-sensing cells of the macula mysteriously malfunction and cease to work over time. While the lecture does not offer ways of preventing the disease, early signs and symptoms will be discussed with the hopes that individuals will recognize a need for medical treatment. Macular degeneration occurs most often in people older than 60 years of age. Estimates indicate that one in six Americans between the ages of 55 and 64 are afflicted with the disease; the incidence rises to one in four Americans between ages 64 and 74, and one in three over the age of 75. It is also estimated that about 1.2 million of the estimated 12 million people with macular degeneration suffer severe central vision loss each year-200,000 individuals will lose all central vision in one or both eyes. The talk is open to the public, and individuals of all ages.

Nurses Walk Out, Cite Poor Working Conditions

In what seems to be a series of unfortunate events, nurses at the Neighborhood Hospital staged a walkout yesterday. Although the hospital responded immediately by recruiting nurses from several other communities, the impact on the Neighborhood is not easily mended. Several nursing units have been closed, and only the sickest of patients are being kept for treatment. Patients involved in trauma cases have been diverted to other hospitals until the strike is resolved. James Gordon, MD, an emergency department (ED) physician at Neighborhood Hospital, says that the effects of the strike will be devastating. Dr. Gordon states that only a few nurses in his department are involved in the strike, but that his department is not immune from its effects. "Even if we keep our nurses from walking off the job in the ED, we have no place to send patients who then need to be admitted," says Gordon.

Teen Charged With Murder of Infant

This week, Reyna Clarkson was formally charged with murder after leaving a newborn infant in a toilet at Neighborhood High School. Clarkson, a junior, first claimed she did not know she was pregnant and thought she was simply having bad menstrual cramping and heavy bleeding-stating that she did not know the infant was in the toilet. The story garnered her a great deal of sympathy in the community, but with each retelling, her story changed, and the truth finally emerged. Clarkson later admitted that she had the baby and attempted to dispose of it by flushing the infant down the toilet. Sheriff Mark Shuster took the teen into custody following the confession Tuesday night. Her parents posted the $100,000 bail.

Episode 9

Announcement: Meditation Group Forming

Do you often feel irritable? Do you have trouble sleeping? Do you have difficulty focusing? No, this is not an advertisement for pills or products, but if you have answered yes to any of these questions, you might be experiencing stress. Meditation has been shown to be an effective way to manage and curb stress levels. A meditation group is forming in the Neighborhood, and if you or someone you know might be interested in joining, come to the information meeting at the Neighborhood Community Center, Wednesday night at 7:00 P.M.

Local Woman Loses Battle With Cancer

The Neighborhood lost one of their finest residents this week. Pam Allen, a woman known for her highly sought-after homemade quilts, died this week following a long battle with cancer. Allen leaves behind a husband, Clifford, and son, Gary. "One cannot say that she merely left a family behind, she left a legacy. Everyone in the community got some sense of comfort by owning or even looking at one of her quilts," said Greg Ross, who owns this year's first-prize quilt made by Allen. Father John Olivas will lead a funeral mass in dedication to Allen this Friday, with a private memorial service the night before.

Nursing Strike Enters Second Week

Neighborhood Hospital administrators and nurses remain in a deadlock over the ongoing nursing strike. "The hospital is still open and serving patients," says hospital spokesperson Raymond Fletcher. "It is true, however, that the number of inpatients is significantly down, and we are not admitting any new patients." Fletcher says new admissions are being diverted to other hospitals in nearby communities, and currently hospitalized patients are being cared for by a temporary workforce of nurses from other locales. Meanwhile, strike organizers say hospital administrators are not cooperating in talks to bring closure to the dispute as the strike enters its second week. "We are striking to ensure safe conditions for our patients," reports nurse Cheryl Keller. "The media is trying to make us look like the bad guys," she added.

Episode 10

"Queen of Roses" Dies

Lydia Ocampo, long-time resident of the Neighborhood, died quietly in bed this week at a local nursing home. Her death was attributed to Alzheimer's disease. Lydia was predeceased by her husband of 51 years, the late Dr. Danilo Ocampo, a highly regarded Neighborhood pathologist. Originally from the Philippines, Ocampo was 70 years old and lived a long and fulfilling life. For years, Lydia and Danilo Ocampo were well known in this community for their prize-winning roses. Fondly referred to as the "king and queen of roses," neighbors remember Lydia for her laughter and the Ocampos, for their lifelong devotion to each other. She leaves a great niece, Kristina Ocampo, and extended family in the Philippines. In lieu of flowers, the family asks that a donation be made to the Alzheimer's Association in memory of Lydia.

Announcement: Swimming Classes to Be Offered

The local pool will begin to offer swimming classes to young children early next week. The Neighborhood Community Parks and Recreation is offering free swimming classes to Neighborhood children in three age-separated classes: 4-6, 7-9, 10-12. Classes will be available on a first-come, first-served basis. Signups begin this weekend at the Community Center.

Sexual Predator Apprehended in Sting

As social networking sites become as large as societies themselves, it is obvious that the indecency that exists in society will migrate into these digital media. Such was the case last weekend when a sting operation lead to the arrest of a 42-year-old man in his attempt to meet with an underage female. The man, Bryan Phillips, was apprehended when he used a popular online communication site to arrange a meeting with a girl he thought was 13 years old. The person he contacted was in fact an undercover police officer posing as a girl.

Hospital Strike Ends

To the relief of Neighborhood residents, the nursing strike at the Neighborhood Hospital has come to an end, and nurses have returned to their jobs in full force. In the agreement to end the strike, Hospital Administrators agreed to reduce the patient load and hire more nurses, as opposed to non-licensed staff. "This is a victory for patients as much as it is for nurses," says local nurse Cheryl Keller. Nurses who had been pulled from other communities to assist in maintaining during the strike have returned to their local areas. Patients who were redirected to outlying communities are glad to be moved back to Neighborhood Hospital so they can be nearer their families and be seen by doctors they know.

Episode 11

Announcement: Bin Burning Ban to Begin

Local government officials want to remind citizens of the new trash burning ban that is set to begin this week following a 6 to 2 vote in favor of the ban at the last City Council meeting. The council was quick to approve the ban in light of the negative effects on the air quality in the city from the recent forest fire. Councilman Ray Santori stated that if production of manmade pollutants could be curbed, the adverse effects of things such as forest fires would be slightly less severe.

Robbing Spree Ends in Deadly Crash

What started as a robbery ended in a death this weekend in the Neighborhood when two individuals, Casey Holmes and Robert Bandish, caused a collision with another vehicle while fleeing the scene of a robbery they had committed. The names of the two victims have not been released, but it is known that one was an honor student at Neighborhood High School. Holmes and Bandish have been arrested and charged with armed robbery and vehicular homicide. Current reports state that the robbery was conducted in support of a long-standing drug habit.

Bumping Up Safety

A local woman is circulating a petition to install speed bumps around residential areas. Angie Young, whose son Marcus was seriously injured several months ago by a speeding car, is attempting to get enough signatures on a petition for a proposal to install speed bumps in most of the residential areas around the Neighborhood. It is Young's opinion that the streets are unsafe for children because speed limits are not enforced by the local police. If she is able to collect enough signatures, Young plans to take up the issue with city officials.

Episode 12

Announcement: Scout Food Drive

Girl and Boy Scouts in the area are joining forces to increase food donations for the Neighborhood homeless shelter. Boy Scout official Gary Eddy states the combined efforts of Girl and Boy Scouts within the community are expected to yield large donations desperately needed by the shelters. Scouts will be going door-to-door asking for donations. Alternatively, food donations can be dropped off at any of the four local Stanley Food Market locations.

Black Widow Outbreak Worries Residents

Residents of certain areas of the Neighborhood are reporting large number of black widow spiders in recent weeks. James Gordon, MD, director of the Neighborhood Hospital emergency department, confirmed there have been several individuals treated in recent weeks following an alleged black widow bite. According to Dr. Gordon, the female black widow spider is the most venomous spider in North America, although it rarely causes death to humans. The male black widow spider is relatively tame by comparison and will not bite unless intensively provoked—the female is far more territorial and vicious. National statistics indicate that human mortality is less than 1% from black widow spider bites. The bite itself is often not painful and may go unnoticed, but the poison can cause abdominal pain similar to that associated with appendicitis as well as pain to muscles or the soles of the feet. Other symptoms include alternating salivation and dry-mouth, paralysis of the diaphragm, profuse sweating, and swollen eyelids. If bitten, a person should apply ice to the bite and contact a local poison control center.

Homeless Shelters Running at Critical Capacity

The city homeless shelter manager cannot explain the increase in the homeless population, but the numbers are expected to increase further as winter approaches. Many of those staying in shelters are mentally ill or suffering from severe drug and alcohol dependencies. Sheriff Mark Shuster confirms that along with the increases in shelter guests, there has also been a sharp increase in local area crime rates.

Episode 13

Encouraging the Elderly to Exercise

When thinking of old age, some people still envision the cliche of an elderly person in a rocking chair, waiting for the inevitable end. Fitness Guru Jack Blaine hopes to change this image. Blaine, 78, who has performed endurance feats such as participating in a triathlon and the Tour de France, has been well known throughout the country as an expert in exercise regimens for older adults. Blaine will be hosting a free seminar at the Neighborhood Senior Center this coming week. The seminar will focus on exercise, fitness, and aging, although all ages are welcome. Call the Neighborhood Senior Center at 260-4400 for more information.

Safety Crusader Met With Mixed Reception

This week at city hall, a local woman was greeted with both praise and complaints regarding her movement to install speed bumps into all residential areas. The woman, Angie Young, took her petition with 500 signatures to the City Council meeting this week. Although there were many people at the meeting complaining about speeding, few spoke in favor of installing speed bumps on all the streets. Those opposed to the idea cited possible damage to the suspension of vehicles and huge impairment of traffic flow. City counselors voted down the motion in order to appease the majority against the speed bumps. Others claim, however, that the movement is not over, stating that Young inspired them to pursue action at higher levels of government.

Breast Cancer Mortality Rates

The National Cancer Institute reports that more than 200,000 new cases of invasive cancer will be diagnosed in women in the US this year, along with close to 65,000 new cases of noninvasive breast cancer. The lifetime risk of breast cancer has almost tripled in the United States; currently, a woman has a one-in-eight lifetime risk of being diagnosed with breast cancer. However, after increasing for more than two decades, female breast cancer incidence rates began decreasing about ten years ago, then dropped by about 7%. Death rates from breast cancer have also been declining in recent years, with larger decreases in women younger than 50.

Screening and treatment rates vary. Hispanic women have lower breast cancer screening rates than do non-Hispanic White women, and they tend to seek and obtain healthcare services less frequently than individuals of other ethnicities. The report also indicates some disparities among cultures. Although the lifetime risk of developing breast cancer is higher for White women than for African American and Hispanic women, African American women and subgroups of Hispanic women continue to have a lower breast cancer survival rate. At this time there are an estimated 2.9 million breast cancer survivors in the United States.

Episode 14

Announcement: Pride Parade Addresses Inequities

Local chapters are sponsoring a GLBT (gay, lesbian, bisexual, and transgender) Awareness Parade Saturday in the Neighborhood Community Garden. The parade will begin in the Neighborhood's downtown district, at the city government offices, and then work its way up to the garden, where there will be a multitude of booths available to attendees to provide information on equality groups, safe sex, and disease prevention. Event sponsors say the goal of the parade is to raise awareness of the societal inequities experienced by nonheterosexual citizens. The event will begin at 9:00 AM Saturday, and attendance is free. All are encouraged to participate in the parade.

Hospital to Go Under the Microscope

The Joint Commission, formerly the Joint Commission on Accreditation of Healthcare Organizations or JCAHO, will be making an accreditation site visit next week to Neighborhood Hospital. The organization sets standards for healthcare organizations to meet for accreditation purposes. The accreditation essentially serves as a nationwide "seal of approval" that indicates a hospital meets high performance standards for patient care. Many are concerned about the visit, given the recent controversies that the hospital has endured, including the nursing strike that was only recently resolved. However, hospital spokeswoman Mimi Patterson is optimistic, and shared with reporters that the hospital is more than ready for the visit, despite setbacks to planning in recent months.

School Field Trips Increase Knowledge Retention

To counter the constant pressure of preparing students for standardized tests, teachers are looking for ways to get their students engaged and excited about the process of learning. A new study has been released suggesting that field trips are an important tool in giving students real-world experience while providing a fun and interactive environment. The experience-based learning that field trips provide can actually get students to retain knowledge more completely than traditional in-class learning methods. "What could be better than watching your students figure out how abstract theories apply to real life?" said Sebastian Stills, a member of the Neighborhood Board of Education. "As long as field trips are scheduled around what students are learning in class and attention is taken to point out the connections, field trips can be a stimulating learning tool; by creating more excitement about learning, they may even be an aid in increasing Neighborhood test scores."

Student Nurse Selected to Aid in Alleviating Nursing Shortage

This week, a student nurse was selected to the Governor's Task Force charge with increasing the number of nurses in the state. State Governor Joe Desmedt named local student nurse Jill Harris to participate on the task force, stating that he hopes she might offer insight into the student view of nursing in the state. The goal is to increase the number of students who are accepted to and who graduate from nursing programs. Said Desmedt, "Adding a student to the task force will provide a unique perspective on the benefits and shortcomings of particular nursing programs. We must know what areas to address in order to remedy the shortage."

Episode 15

Strike Ends Hospital Hiring Woes

The Neighborhood Hospital has hit the ground running, having fully recovered from the controversial strike. Previously postponed surgeries are back on schedule and the ER is running more smoothly than it has in years, according to sources inside the hospital. In a surprising turn of events, the strike may have actually helped improve the quality of staffing. "The number of applicants who are applying for jobs and who have advanced nursing degrees has increased dramatically," said Pat Richman, a nursing administrator at Neighborhood Hospital. "The quality of applicants is a win not only for the hospital but also, and more importantly, for our patients."

Letter to the Editor: Adoption Woes for Gay Parents

Last week you published an op-ed piece about the negative effects that extending adoption privileges to same-sex parents could have. This article hit very close to home, as I and my long-time partner recently lost the opportunity to adopt the child we intended to love and raise as our own, simply because of a prejudice against our sexual orientation. What does this say? That women and men can only be loving parents and nurturing caregivers if there is one of each of them in a household? How can loving and nurturing a child be confined to a single gender? Shouldn't fostering a healthy and supportive environment be the most important consideration in rearing a child? Certainly sexual orientation will have no lasting negative effect on your child as long as you love your child with all your heart. Only through educating our community can we avoid prejudices against gay parenting. It is my hope that your readers will take time to think about this issue, instead of relying on fears or skewed studies. What is truly better for our society: for a child to have loving and healthy parents of whatever gender, or for a child to have no parents at all?

Yours Sincerely,
Benito Jaramillo

ILLUSTRATED TEACHING TOOLS

FIGURE 1 CASE STUDY PAM ALLEN

This case study follows Pam Allen and her family through the trajectory of her cancer diagnosis and eventual death. Refer to the Allen family stories in *The Neighborhood* (Seasons 1–3) and Pam Allen's medical records to complete this work.

- In Season 1, Pam is diagnosed with colorectal cancer (CA). Complete the following tables regarding an analysis of risk factors and recommended screenings in relationship to what we know about Pam.

Textbook Risk Factors for Colorectal CA	Screening Recommendations for Colorectal CA	Pam's Personal Risk Factors for Colorectal CA	Screenings Performed on Pam (if Any Known)

- What are the classic signs and symptoms of colorectal CA? What signs and symptoms does Pam have in Season 1?

Classic Signs and Symptoms According to Text	Pam's Signs and Symptoms

In episodes 13 and 14, Pam sees her physician. What assessment findings does the physician notice, and what diagnostic tests are done? What is the relationship of some of her symptoms to the findings?

- Assessment findings:

- Diagnostic tests performed and results:

- What is the relationship of Pam's symptoms to her clinical findings?

At the end of Season 1 and beginning of Season 2, Pam has surgery and begins adjuvant therapy.

- Which of the following best describes the goal of Pam's treatment plan at this point? (Circle one)   Cure   Control   Palliation

- What does adjuvant therapy mean, and what is it in Pam's case?

  _____

- What agents does Pam receive? _____

- Which agents are classified as chemotherapy, and which are considered biotherapy?

  _____

  _____

- What are the actions of the drugs?

  _____

  _____

  _____

- Describe the schedule for administration of her treatment. Explain the purpose of this schedule. Does this follow national recommendations? (Hint: Consult the National Comprehensive Cancer Network Web site at NCCN.org)

  _____

  _____

  _____

  _____

- What are the *major* side effects of these agents, and what would you include in your patient education?

  _____

  _____

  _____

  _____

- What is a central line port, why is it inserted, and what would you need to teach Pam or Clifford about caring for it at home?

  _____

  _____

  _____

  _____

- In the following table, link Pam's experiences to concepts and nursing diagnoses. What do you consider the top six problems Pam experiences during this time? What concepts do these represent? If you were developing a care plan for Pam, what do you believe are the nursing diagnoses with highest priority?

Top Six Problems	Concepts Represented	Priority Nursing Diagnoses

- Up to this point, what impact has Pam's illness had on Clifford and Gary?

Clifford	Gary

At the beginning of Season 3, Pam suffers a setback. She experiences discomfort to the right upper quadrant of her abdomen, decreased appetite, yellowish tint to her sclera, and dark urine. She learns that the cancer has metastasized to her liver.

- Explain the physiologic causes of the symptoms.

Symptom	Physiologic Explanation
Discomfort in upper right abdomen	
Decrease in appetite	
Yellow sclera	
Dark urine	

- Pam has conflicting thoughts about beginning chemotherapy because of the side effects. Her physician and Clifford talk Pam into starting chemotherapy again. At this point, which of the following best describes the goal for Pam's treatment plan? (Circle one)   Cure   Control   Palliation

In Season 3, Episode 4, Pam's treatment is withheld. Refer to the story and Pam's medical record.

- What is her white blood cell count? _____
  - What problem does this represent? _____
- What is her platelet count? _____
  - What problem does this represent? _____
- What is the specific cause of these problems?

  _____

- If you were the nurse in the chemotherapy clinic, what nursing interventions and education would you provide to Pam and Clifford?

  _____

  _____

  _____

Tension exists between Clifford and Pam regarding her treatment wishes, representing concepts of family dynamics and ethics. Analyze the interactions between the nurse, Pam, and Clifford in Season 3, Episode 6.

- In what ways do you think this was handled well by the nurse? What could have been said or done differently?

- The goal of Pam's treatment shifts to palliation in Season 3, Episode 7. What are the specific goals and nursing interventions for Pam, Clifford, and Gary during this end-of-life care?

FIGURE 2 ROLE-PLAY JESSICA RILEY AND CAROL RAMSEY

Preparation and Briefing:

Divide students into groups of three to four individuals each. Select roles:

1. Jessica Riley

2. Carol Ramsey, CNM

3. Observer

4. Observer

Explain to students that the objective of the activity is to role-play an interview involving a nurse and patient who is possibly the victim of domestic violence. For five to ten minutes, students in the roles of Jessica and Carol should role-play the situation described next; observers should take notes about the nonverbal and verbal exchanges and provide feedback. (Consider videotaping the role-play if possible.)

Situation:

Jessica Riley from The Neighborhood *presents for a routine prenatal visit with Carol Ramsey, the Certified Nurse Midwife. Carol notices that Jessica has some bruises on her upper arms and an older bruise under her right eye. Jessica's boyfriend is waiting for her in the waiting room.*

Debriefing:

Following the five- to ten-minute role-play, lead the entire class in a discussion of the following questions:

1. What questions should Carol have asked, and how should they have been asked?

2. What information should be documented on Jessica's record?

3. What information should Carol share with Jessica before she leaves the clinic?

4. What is Carol's legal responsibility in this situation?

FIGURE 3 SIMULATION LEARNING ACTIVITY

Topic: Patient following outpatient colonoscopy with conscious sedation

Target Concepts: Assessment, oxygenation, medication management, communication, safety

Neighborhood Characters/Season Featured: Greg Ross and Benito Jaramillio— Season 1, Episode 14 (and after)

Learning Objectives:

1. Assess patient condition.
2. Recognize abnormal findings.
3. Implement appropriate interventions related to scenario.
4. Demonstrate appropriate therapeutic communication skills during scenario.
5. Reflect on scenario during debriefing; identify missed opportunities related to interventions and communication strategies.

Total Time Allotment for Simulation Activity:	1 hour
• briefing for all students	10 minutes
• data gathering	5 minutes
• exchange of report	5 minutes
• assessment of vital signs	5 minutes
• intervention related to vital signs	3 minutes
• response for help	2 minutes
• debriefing	30 minutes

Setting of Simulation Interaction:

• Outpatient procedures unit

Equipment and Props Needed:

• Hospital bed with bedside table and call light
• Blood pressure cuff
• Stethoscope
• Oxygen saturation probe
• Assortment of oxygen delivery devices, including Ambu bag.
• Medication cart (assortment of medications, including Narcan and Romazicon)
• Medical record from procedure
• Drug book
• IV fluid 0.9% NaCL to gravity, TKO rate

Active Participants Needed:

- Student Nurse #1 (to be played by student)
- Student Nurse #2 (to be played by student)
- Primary Nurse (to be played by instructor)
- Ben Jaramillio (to be played by student)

NEIGHBORHOOD LINK: GREG ROSS—SEASON 1, EPISODE 14

Actual Story: Greg continues to have pain and diarrhea and recognizes that he is having an acute exacerbation of colitis. He makes an appointment with the gastroenterologist, who gives Greg a prescription for oral prednisone and sulfasalazine and advises him to drink plenty of fluids. The physician also comments that Greg's blood pressure is 146/96 mm Hg. The gastroenterologist explains that his blood pressure is higher than it should be, and his abdominal pain might have something to do with it. Greg is told to have his blood pressure rechecked when he is feeling better.

What-If Scenario: *What if the gastroenterologist wanted to do a colonoscopy?* Greg's gastroenterologist recommends that he undergo a colonoscopy procedure. Greg goes to the outpatient gastrointestinal lab at Neighborhood Hospital. He has been NPO since breakfast and should tolerate conscious sedation for the procedure. Greg asks Ben to take a break from his intense training to pick him up at the hospital after the procedure. The primary focus of this scenario is communication and appropriate intervention.

Situation:

- Greg has just been transferred from the procedure room to the recovery area following a colonoscopy with conscious sedation.
- Two nursing students are assigned to care for Greg during the recovery period. A primary nurse is working with them. The students receive the report from the primary nurse, who tells them that during the procedure Greg received 10 mg Versed, and 4 mg morphine. The procedure occurred without incident, and Greg is in stable condition. The primary nurse instructs the students to assess Greg and provide post-procedure care.
- Ben is at Greg's bedside. It is expected that Greg will be discharged home within a few hours.

Roles:

Student Nurses: Receive assignment and the patient's chart with the patient history, conscious sedation medications given, and procedure that was completed. The student nurses are expected to get the report from the primary nurse before caring for the patient. The student nurses will have five minutes to review the chart and obtain the report from the primary nurse prior to starting the simulation (accepting care of the patient).

Primary Nurse: Give students their assignment and Greg's medical record to review. Ask students to review chart before getting report. The primary nurse will give report to the students before they begin caring for Greg.

Ben Jaramillio: When student nurses go in to assess Greg, Ben has pushed the call light on and tells the students he thinks something is wrong with Greg. However, he is unable to say what is wrong, other than that Greg just does not seem right. Ben becomes very loud and disruptive the longer it takes for the problem to be determined and action taken.

Scenario Data and Expected Student Behavior:

1. Assess and evaluate Greg's vital signs and level of sedation.
   - Respiratory: respiratory rate of 4 breaths/min, room air SP02 = 80%, decreased breath sounds at the bases; patient will continue to decompensate until reversal agent is given.
   - Neurological: patient is excessively sedated and will continue to become less responsive as time progresses until he receives reversal agent.

2. Assess Safety
   - Safety: side rails of bed will be down x4, and bed will be completely elevated.

3. Therapeutic Communication
   - Ben becomes concerned, overly anxious, and subsequently interferes with care.

4. Expected Student Actions
   - Raise side rails/lower bed.
   - Take a set of vitals.
   - Recognize sedation level and inadequate oxygen exchange.
   - Attempt to arouse patient.
   - Encourage deep breathing and administer proper oxygen delivery system.
   - Review medical record for medications given during procedure and critically think of reversal agent(s).
   - Obtain help from primary nurse if patient remains excessively sedated or there is no improvement in respiratory status.
   - Primary nurse may guide students to the use of a reversal agent for patient.
   - Calm Ben down and communicate they are getting help for Greg.

FIGURE 4 CONCEPT ANALYSIS PAPER

Choose one of the following *Neighborhood* characters—Anthony Martin, Jimmy Bley, or Ryan Riley—and identify three concepts best represented by that character. The following table contains a list of potential concepts.

Examples of Concepts

• Nutrition	• Acid–base balance	• Sleep
• Fluid electrolyte balance	• Metabolism	• Cellular regulation
• Thermoregulation	• Perfusion	• Intracranial regulation
• Oxygenation	• Reproduction	• Safety
• Inflammation	• Motion	• Sexuality
• Infection	• Pain	• Immunity
• Tissue integrity	• Fatigue	• Developmental delay
• Elimination	• Nausea and vomiting	• Addiction
• Communication	• Family dynamics	• Interpersonal violence
• Coping	• Mood and affect	• Cognitive impairment
• Stress	• Anxiety	• Altered thought process

For each concept, describe the concept (based on the literature) and how the character exemplifies or exemplified the concept (currently or in the past). Comment on the interventions described in the stories, including whether they are consistent with recommended nursing and collaborative care in the literature.

Your paper should not exceed ten double-spaced pages (not including your title page or references). Follow APA style for your citations. You can use your textbooks as references, but you should also use nursing journals. Do not cite lecture notes, PowerPoint presentations, and so on; they are not a substitute for the nursing literature. The idea is that you read, reflect, and then write. Also, you do not need to cite *The Neighborhood* when you include specific examples from the stories.

This paper is worth _____% of your final course grade. Your project will be graded on the following criteria:

Character introduction (_____ points)

Concepts exemplified (_____ points)

Grammar, APA formatting, quality of presentation/references (_____ points)

This project can be done individually or in small groups (no more than four students per group). If you decide to work in a group, be aware that all group members will earn the same grade. Also be aware that after everyone contributes their sections, your group must read each other's work for clarity, use of references, and so on.

HEADINGS TO USE FOR YOUR PAPER

Introduction of Character

Provide a general overview of the character's story. (Pretend your reader does not know the character.) In this overview, you must mention the applicable featured concepts.

Featured Concepts Exemplified

Concept

Description of the concept
How character exemplifies/exemplified this concept

- *Risk factors*
- *Onset of problem*
- *Impact of problem on the character and family*

Interventions done for the character

Concept

Description of the concept
How character exemplifies/exemplified this concept

- *Risk factors*
- *Onset of problem*
- *Impact of problem on the character and family*

Interventions done for the character

Concept

Description of the concept
How character exemplifies/exemplified this concept

- *Risk factors*
- *Onset of problem*
- *Impact of problem on the character and family*

Interventions done for the character

Summary

FIGURE 5 NEIGHBORHOOD JEOPARDY

The basic game of Jeopardy requires that teams/players alternate in the selection of a category and points (e.g., "'Teach Me Something' for 400"). They are given an answer, and the team/player must state the question. Correct responses win the corresponding points, and the team/player with the most points at the end of the game wins. If a team/player is unable to answer a question, the opposite team/player gets the opportunity to answer the question and receive the points.

The five categories are linked to *Neighborhood* characters or stories. This can be done with multiple teams competing at the same time in one game or multiple simultaneous games in small groups. Categories can be changed depending on the specific course or class.

In the following example, the table illustrates categories that could be created for a game at any level. The instructor writes the questions/answers for each of the categories (total of 30); questions should get successively more difficult as the point values increase. The sample questions listed at the end of this section could be used as an early Level 1 game as a way to introduce the characters.

Who's Who	Teach Me Something	Name That Concept	Interventions	Drugs
100	100	100	100	100
200	200	200	200	200
300	300	300	300	300
400	400	400	400	400
500	500	500	500	500
600	600	600	600	600

SAMPLE QUESTIONS FOR DRUGS CATEGORY

Drugs 100	**Clue:** Clifford Allen takes this drug as conservative treatment for benign prostatic hyperplasia.
	Answer: What is Proscar?
Drugs 200	**Clue:** Gil Martin takes Atorvastin as a treatment measure for this condition.
	Answer: What is hyperlipidemia?
Drugs 300	**Clue:** Angelo Reyes anticipates long-acting glycemic control with this agent.
	Answer: What is NPH insulin?
Drugs 500	**Clue:** Failure to take this drug places Mrs. James at a very high risk for stroke.
	Answer: What is Coumadin?
Drugs 600	**Clue:** This drug, taken by Danilo Ocampo, is known to reduce mortality following acute myocardial infarction.
	Answer: What is metoprolol?

FIGURE 6 COMPARE AND CONTRAST: SUBSTANCE ABUSE (ALCOHOL) LEARNING ACTIVITY

With your learning group, compare and contrast the stories of *The Neighborhood* characters Casey Holmes, Mark Martin, and Bobby Schofield on several aspects of substance abuse.

	Casey Holmes	Mark Martin	Bobby Schofield
Risk factors for alcohol abuse			
Impact of alcohol on their lives			
Impact of alcohol on lives of others			
How is this typical or not typical of presentation in class or in textbooks?			
What interrelated concepts apply?			

Developed by Jean Giddens

FIGURE 7 LINKING POLICY TO CLINICAL APPLICATION

1. Go to the Healthy People 2020 Web site (www.healthypeople.gov), and review "Injury and Violence Protection." Which objectives link to preventing problems associated with head injury? For each of these, what supporting information and recommendations are made? (Organize your information using a table like the following example.)

Healthy People 2020 Objective	Information/Recommendations

2. Making links to *The Neighborhood*: Consider the stories of *The Neighborhood* characters and community events depicted in the Neighborhood News. List all examples of evidence in which head injury (from prevention to tertiary care) is represented in *The Neighborhood*. List the character or site, season and episode, and situation. (Organize your information using a table like the following examples.)

Character	Season and Episode	Situation

Neighborhood News	Season and Episode	Situation

Developed by Jean Giddens

FIGURE 8 FAMILY HISTORY FOR ANTHONY AND KRISTINA MARTIN

Consider the Martin family in *The Neighborhood*. Using character information from *The Neighborhood*, along with the following supplemental information, draw a genogram for Anthony Martin and Kristina Martin. After drawing the genogram, list any risk factors that Anthony and Kristina have.

- Mary Martin (age 75) is the youngest of three children. She is in good health, with the exception of having glaucoma and cataracts. She was married for 52 years to Dominic Martin, who died last year at age 80 of prostate cancer. Mary and Dominic had three children: Gilbert (age 52), Isaac (died in a car accident—DUI at age 20), and Julia (age 49). Julia is a recovering alcoholic and has hypertension.

- Gilbert Martin married Jennifer Sanchez 28 years ago, and they had one son, Mark Martin (age 27). They divorced when Mark was 5 years old. Jennifer has severe asthma; she has not remarried or had other children. Gilbert married Helen Wilson Martin (age 48) 18 years ago. They had two children together: Anthony Martin (age 17) and Kristina Martin (age 16). Helen was previously married to Rick Ames and had one daughter, Tracie Ames (age 20). They divorced soon after Tracie was born.

- Helen has one older brother, Sean Wilson (age 52), who has schizophrenia. Her parents, Jerry and Ruth Wilson, are both deceased. Jerry was an alcoholic and died at age 57 from liver cancer. Ruth died from breast cancer when she was 66.

Adapted from an assignment developed by Mary Wright, RN, MSN College of Nursing, University of New Mexico

FIGURE 9 CONCEPT MAP: PAM ALLEN

Consider the story of Pam Allen from *The Neighborhood*. Pam has colorectal cancer and has undergone a colectomy with colostomy; she is also receiving chemotherapy and radiation therapy. Using the following table, identify what you consider the most significant problems Pam experiences as a result of each of these treatments.

Colectomy and Colostomy	Chemotherapy	Radiation Therapy

Next, draw a concept map that reflects the problems you identified previously. Following is the beginning of a concept map. Add to this map, using the information you identified in the preceding section. Be sure to show the interrelationship of concepts and problems to one another, as well as collaborative interventions that are described in the story or could be applied.

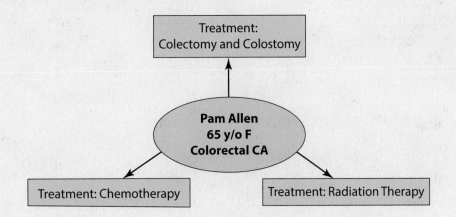

Developed by Jean Giddens

FIGURE 10 CARING IN *THE NEIGHBORHOOD*: GROUP DISCUSSION AND LEARNING ACTIVITY

Reading assignment as preparation for class:

1. Ocampo family story—Season 1
2. Brilowski, G. & Wendler, C. (2005). An evolutionary concept analysis of caring. *Journal of Advanced Nursing, 50*(6), 641–650.

With your learning group, complete the following activities:

1. Discuss examples of caring behaviors that Danilo displays toward Lydia.
2. Categorize the caring behaviors by the attributes of caring (i.e., relationship, action, attitude, acceptance, and variability) that are identified in Brilowski and Wendler's article. Give the rationale for the categorization of each behavior.
3. Discuss the care Lydia experienced from Bobby (Lydia's primary nurse) when she was hospitalized in Episode 10. Does Bobby exhibit caring behavior? Why or why not?
4. Develop a plan of care that displays caring for Lydia using the attributes identified by Brilowski and Wendler.
5. Select one member of your learning group to present a summary of your work during the class wrap-up session.

Adopted from an assignment developed by Debra Brady, PhD, Associate Professor College of Nursing, University of New Mexico

FIGURE 11 GARY ALLEN AND COGNITIVE IMPAIRMENT:
SMALL GROUP DISCUSSION

Gary Allen (from *The Neighborhood*) has Down syndrome. In your learning groups, engage in a discussion related to Gary and how he exemplifies impaired cognition.

1. Gary Allen has innate cognitive impairment. What does this term mean?

2. Based on Gary's story, how would you characterize his level of intellectual disability? Base your answer on specific examples from Gary's story.

3. *Gary presents to the emergency department of Neighborhood Hospital after work and tells you it hurts to pee.*

   What questions would you typically ask a male who presented with these symptoms? How would you elicit the same information from Gary?

4. *Gary is diagnosed with a urinary tract infection. The physician prescribes Bactrim for five days.*

   What specific discharge instructions would you write, and how would you explain to Gary how to take his medicine?

Developed by Jean Giddens

FIGURE 12 CARE PLAN ASSIGNMENT

Develop a care plan for Mrs. James of *The Neighborhood*, focusing on her visit to Karen Williams at the Senior Center in Season 1, Episode 3.

Start by completing the database on the first two pages. This information can be found in her weekly stories and the biographical information.

Biographical Data

Name:	Gender: M F	Age:	Race/Ethnicity:
LMP:	Marital Status:	Occupation:	Source/Reliability:

History

Presenting Problem/Chief Complaint:

History of Presenting Problem (Symptom Analysis):

Past Medical and Surgical History (from Biographical Information):

Current Medications (include dose and frequency from Biographical Information):

Allergies:

Family History:

Social History:

Examination Findings

Vital Signs: T   BP   HR   RR

General Survey (overall appearance, gait, level of orientation, etc):

Lower Extremities:

Problem List (Nursing Diagnoses)

NURSING CARE PLAN

CLIENT ID (INITIALS): _____ SETTING: _____ STUDENT: _____ DATE: _____

Assessment Data	Nursing Diagnosis	Expected Client Outcome(s) or Client Goals	Nursing Interventions and Activities	Evaluation

FIGURE 13 DEVELOPING A TEACHING PLAN: GROUP PROJECT

This is a two-part assignment that involves developing a teaching plan and presenting it to the class. You should complete this assignment with your learning group. Your final grade for this assignment will be the average of points for Parts 1 and 2.

Part 1: Developing a Teaching Plan

With your learning group, design a teaching plan for one of the following *Neighborhood* characters. Base all of your work on the character as he or she appears during any point of time during Episodes 1–7, focusing on the identified stage of change.

- Jimmy Bley (preparation stage of change)
- Norma James (precontemplation stage of change)
- Casey Holmes (precontemplation stage of change)
- Jenna Riley (precontemplation stage of change)

For the teaching plan, include all of the following:

1. What data do you need to formulate a comprehensive teaching plan for a client? List the data needed and why. Cite your references.
2. What assessment data do you have that might affect your teaching plan for this individual?
3. Develop five objectives that may be appropriate for your teaching plan.
4. Identify four subjects that you will teach and the methods you will use. State your rationale for the chosen methods and include your references.
5. How would you determine that your teaching plan was effective? What methods would you use to evaluate your teaching?

Part 1 will be graded on the following criteria:

• Assessment data needed with rationale	15 points
• Assessment data you have for your client	15 points
• Objectives and planning	20 points
• Interventions with rationales	20 points
• Evaluation	20 points
• Grammar, spelling, sentence structure, APA format	10 points
Total Points Possible	100 points

Part 2: Student Presentations

After developing the teaching plan, present it to the class, as if you are teaching *The Neighborhood* character. The group may provide a lecture, demonstration, group discussion, gaming application, video, CD, or any other method appropriate to the material being taught to the selected *Neighborhood* character. Each group will have 20 minutes for the presentation.

Part 2 will be graded on the following criteria:

• Presentation is well organized, clear, and effectively structured. Information is presented in a logical, interesting sequence that the audience can follow.	8 points
• Presentation begins with a clear purpose. Objectives are reviewed at the beginning of the presentation and met by the end.	10 points
• Learning objectives, content, and teaching strategies are consistent.	15 points
• The content presented is comprehensive, accurate, and believable.	10 points
• Approach is creative.	10 points
• Conclusion is clear.	5 points
• Class is included in the learning process.	10 points
• There is evidence of balanced group participation in the presentation.	9 points
• Class evaluation of the teaching effectiveness*	15 points
• Self and group analysis*	8 points
Total Points Possible	**100 points**

* Note: Each student will complete an evaluation of teaching effectiveness and evaluate each group member using forms provided by the instructor.

REFERENCES

Aebersold, M. Tschannen, D. & Sculli, G. Improving nursing student's communication skills through utilization of crew resource management strategies. (2013). *Journal of Nursing Education*, 52(3),125-130.

Benner, P. & Sutphen, M. (2007). Learning across the professions: The clergy, a case in point. *Journal of Nursing Education, 46,*103–108.

Benner, P., Sutphen, M., Leonard, V. & Day, L. (2010). *Educating Nurses: a Call for Radical Transformation*. Washington D.C.: Carnegie Foundation.

Berns, R. G., & Erickson, P. M. (2001). Contextual teaching and learning: Preparing students for the new economy. *The Highlight Zone: Research @ Work, 5,* 2-9. (ERIC Document Reproduction Service No. ED452376)

Brilowski, G., & Wendler, M. (2005). An evolutionary concept analysis of caring. *Journal of Advanced Nursing*, 50, 641–650.

Carlson-Sabelli, L. L., Giddens, J., Fogg, L., & Fiedler, R. A. (2011). Challenges and Benefits of Using a Virtual Community to Explore Nursing Concepts Among Baccalaureate Nursing Students. *International Journal of Nursing Education Scholarship,* 8(1), 1-14.

Charon, R. (2004). Narrative and medicine. *New England Journal of Medicine, 350*(9), 862–864.

Cronenwett, L., Sherwood, G., Barnsteiner, J., et al. (2007). Quality and safety education for nurses. *Nursing Outlook*, 55(3), 122-131. doi: 10.1016/j.outlook.2007.02.006.

Daly, W. (2001). The development of an alternative method in the assessment of critical thinking as an outcome of nursing education. *Journal of Advanced Nursing,* 36(1), 120-130.

Davidhizar, R. & Lonser, G. (2003). Storytelling as a teaching technique. *Nurse Educator, 28*(5), 217–221.

Diekelmann, N. (2005). Engaging the students and the teacher: Co-creating substantive reform with narrative pedagogy. *Journal of Nursing Education, 44*(6), 249–252.

Diekelmann, N., & Lampe, S. (2004). Student-Centered Pedagogies: Co-Creating Compelling Experiences Using the New Pedagogies. *Journal of Nursing Education*, 43(6), 245-247.

Durgahee, T. (1997). Reflective practice: Nursing ethics through story telling. *Nursing Ethics, 4*(2), 135–146.

Ebbert, D. W. & Connors, H. (2004). Standardized patient experiences: Evaluation of clinical performance and nurse practitioner satisfaction. *Nursing Education Perspectives, 25*, 12–15.

Giddens, J. (2007). The Neighborhood: A web-based platform to support conceptual teaching and learning. *Nursing Education Perspectives, 28*(5), 251-256.

Giddens, J., Fogg, L. & Carlson-Sibelli, L. (2010). Learning and engagement with a virtual community by undergraduate nursing students. *Nursing Outlook*, 58, 261-167. doi: 10.1016/j.outlook.2010.08.001

Giddens, J., Shuster G.,& Roehrig N., (2010). Early student outcomes associated with a virtual community for learning. *Journal of Nursing Education*, 46(6), 355-359.

Giddens, J. & Walsh, M. (2010). Collaborating Across the Pond: The Diffusion of Virtual Communities for Nursing Education. *Journal of Nursing Education,* 49(8), 449-454.

Heims, M., & Boyd, S. (1990). Concept-Based Learning Activities in clinical nursing education. *Journal of Nursing Education*, 29(6), 249-254.

Hodge, F. S., Pasqua, A., Marquez, C. A., & Geishirt-Cantrell, B. (2002). Utilizing traditional storytelling to promote wellness in American Indian communities. *Journal of Transcultural Nursing, 13*(1), 6–11.

Ibarra, R. (2001). *Beyond Affirmative Action: Reframing the Context of Higher Education.* Madison, WI: University of Wisconsin Press.

Ironside, P. M. (2005). Teaching thinking and reaching the limits of memorization: Enacting new pedagogies. *Journal of Nursing Education, 44*(10), 441–449.

Lasater, K., & Nielsen, A. (2009). The influence of concept-based learning activities on students' clinical judgment development. *The Journal Of Nursing Education,* 48(8), 441-446.

Milton, C. L. (2004). Stories: Implications for nursing ethics and respect for another. *Nursing Science Quarterly, 17*(3), 208–211.

Nielsen, A. (2009). Concept-based learning activities using the clinical judgment model as a foundation for clinical learning. *The Journal of Nursing Education,* 48(6), 350-354.

Rutledge, C. M., Garzon, L., Scott, M., & Karlowicz, K. (2004). Using standardized patients to teach and evaluate nurse practitioner students on cultural competency. *International Journal of Nursing Education Scholarship,* 1. Article 17.

Shawler, C. (2008). Standardized patients: A creative teaching strategy for psychiatric mental-health nurse practitioner students. *Journal of Nursing Education, 47*(11), 528–531.

Siebert, D. C., Guthrie, J. T., & Adamo, G. (2004). Improving learning outcomes: Integration of standardized patients and telemedicine technology. *Nursing Education Perspectives, 25,* 232–237.

Thomas, M. D., O'Conner, F. W., Albert, M. L., Boutain, D., & Brandt, P. A. (2001). Case-based teaching and learning experiences. *Issues in Mental Health Nursing, 22,* 517–531.

Ulrich, J. & Karvonen, M. (2011) Faculty instructional attitudes, interest, and intention: Predictors of Web 2.0 use in online courses, Internet and Higher Education, 14, 201-206

Vessey, J. A. & Huss, K. (2002). Using standardized patients in advanced practice nursing education. *Journal of Professional Nursing, 18,* 29–35.

Zander, P. (2007). Ways of knowing in nursing: The historical evolution of a concept. Journal of Theory Construction and Testing, 11(1), 7–11.

INDEX

Note: '*f*' denotes figure

A

Acid base disturbances, 25
Acute myocardial infarction (AMI), 20, 22
ADHD (attention deficit hyperactivity disorder), 187–188, 195, 197, 200, 201
Adult health nursing, 21–26
Adoption, 31, 95, 98, 170, 175–176, 226, 228–233, 235–237, 320–322, 336, 338, 347
Alden, Mr., 50, 280, 287, 293, 306–311
Allen, Clifford
benign prostatic hyperplasia (BPH), 14, 24
colorectal cancer, 24
depression, 34, 37
family and social issues, 39
Foley catheter, 19
holmium laser enucleation of the prostrate (HoLEP), 14
intravenous (IV) therapy, 20
postoperative pain/care, 17, 20
story, 59–65
substance abuse, 36
Allen, Gary
cognitive impairment, small group discussion, 365*f*
community events, 43
Special Olympics, 43
story, 72–77
Allen, Pam
anemia, 22
anorexia, 14
colorectal cancer, 24
elimination, 13
end of life/death, 15, 41
fatigue, 15
nasogastric (NG) tube, 20
nausea/vomiting, 15
Neighborhood hospital links, 25
pain, 17
story, 66–72
Allergic reaction, 29, 152, 154
Alzheimer's disease, 18, 34, 37, 39, 48, 157, 158, 162, 164, 166, 285, 332, 335, 344
Ames, Tracie
dental screening, 48
family and social issues, 31
story, 143–147
Anemia, 19, 22, 23, 27, 37, 38, 68, 69, 106, 162, 164
Angina, 157–158, 160–161
Anorexia, 14, 17

Anxiety, 35, 84, 119, 122–124, 142, 230, 268, 273, 292, 332, 337
Aphasia, 14, 92, 96
Asthma, 17, 29, 32, 172, 240, 244, 245, 248, 251, 252, 255, 256, 287, 300, 308
Atrial fibrillation, 22, 37, 92
Auditory system, 26

B

Basic nursing skills, 14–21
Benign prostatic hyperplasia (BPH), 14, 24, 327
Bley, Cecelia
family and social issues, 39, 40
osteoarthritis, 17, 23, 38
story, 85–90
Bley, Jimmy
emphysema, 21, 38
environmental issues, 44
family and social issues, 40
fatigue, 15
health promotion, 48, 49
influenza, immunization, 25
IV therapy, 20
oxygenation, 17, 20
pneumonia, 22, 38
respiratory failure, 22, 25, 38
sensory perpetual, 18, 26, 38
septic shock, 22, 39
story, 79–84
Brinkworth, Violet
death news, patients, 42
diabetes type 2, articles on fast food, 25
health related problems, students, 29
hearing and vision screening, 29, 48
junk food ban, 46
medical records, keeping, 51
nutrition information, monitoring, 17, 24, 49
professional practice issues, 50, 51, 52
role as a nurse, 53, 54
school nursing responsibilities, 53, 54, 296–304
school nursing topics, 32, 33
sex education in schools, 28, 49
story, 296–304

C

Cancer, 14, 15, 22, 24, 26, 42, 43, 44, 59, 61, 63, 65, 66, 68, 69, 70, 76, 82, 88, 125, 127, 129, 230, 241, 279, 281, 292, 308, 313, 316, 318, 327, 331, 333, 336, 338, 344, 346

Cardiovascular system, 22
Care plan, 11, 366*f*–368*f*
Caregiver, 15, 18, 34, 37, 39, 44, 96, 124, 131, 157, 162,
    165–166, 217, 219, 274, 332, 337, 342, 347
Case study, 8, 9, 349*f*–352*f*
Cataract, 26, 37, 41, 117, 125–130, 306, 309, 312
Chemotherapy, 14, 16, 17, 20, 59, 61–64, 66, 68–71
Childbirth classes, 27, 48, 53, 54, 173, 178–179, 207,
    242, 248, 317, 318, 332
Chlamydia, 28, 30, 137, 141–142, 147, 176, 316, 321
Cholecystitis, 119
Cholelithiasis, 16, 18, 24, 119, 120
Chronic back pain, 18, 23, 113, 115
Chronic obstructive pulmonary disease (COPD), 15, 17,
    20–22, 25, 38
Clark, Terry, 5, 6*f*, 31, 231–232, 237–238, 316, 320–322
Colitis, 15, 18, 226, 228, 231, 237
Colorectal cancer, 14, 22, 24, 42, 59, 63, 66, 68, 70
Community health topics, 42–47
Community services, 43, 53, 54, 318
Comparing and contrasting, 10, 360*f*
Concept map, 11, 363*f*
Concept or topic analysis, 10, 357*f*–358*f*
Conjunctivitis, 16, 29, 32, 247, 258
Crohn's disease, 24

D

Decubitus ulcer, 18, 21, 23, 148, 151, 152, 162, 166
Dehydration, 25, 29, 172, 206, 217, 218, 219, 285
Dental caries, 29, 152, 154
Depression, 23, 34, 37, 39, 59, 61–64, 69, 84, 92, 136,
    148, 151–152, 242, 249, 266, 270, 273–274,
    300–301, 328, 331, 343
Diabetes, 25, 30, 37, 41, 92–93, 95, 98, 169–170,
    172–173, 176, 184, 189–190, 195, 196, 197, 202,
    299, 303, 306, 307, 339
Diarrhea, 15, 18, 29, 30, 66, 67, 69, 71, 81, 96, 228, 231,
    234, 250, 262, 263, 264
Diversion program, 36, 50, 281–282, 290, 294–295
Domestic violence, 27, 31, 35, 36, 46, 204, 211, 212,
    231, 237, 329, 332, 343
Down syndrome, 59, 63, 66, 67, 70, 72, 75, 230, 232, 273
Drunk driving, 36, 42, 47, 213, 298, 325–326, 342

E

Eating habits, 17, 25, 32, 121, 194, 340
Elder abuse, 39, 40, 45, 47, 50–51, 280, 293, 306, 309,
    311, 336
Emphysema, 21, 22, 25, 38, 79–81, 83, 285, 287, 288,
    292, 307, 310
End of life, 15, 24, 66
Erectile dysfunction, 229
Ethics, 50, 330

F

Failure to thrive, 16, 30, 206, 217–220
Family history, 11, 362*f*
Family nursing
    health promotion, 28–29
    health related problems, 29–31
    wellness, 28–29
Family and social issues, 31, 39–40
Fatigue, 15, 24, 66, 69, 70, 89, 100, 102, 104, 105, 106,
    157, 159, 161, 172, 178, 205, 206, 229, 283, 285,
    286, 319
Featured characters, *see* Pedagogical tools
Fluid electrolyte disturbances, 25

G

Gastrointestinal system, 24
Geriatric nursing
    family and social issues, 39–40
    health-related conditions, 37–39
    senior center, topics, 40–41
Gordon, Dr, 80, 84, 89, 95, 102, 151, 154, 161, 172, 210,
    218, 223, 231, 322, 326, 328, 334, 343, 345

H

Hardin, Amanda, 36, 266–270, 272
Health promotion, nurses' role in, 47–49
Hearing loss, 26, 38, 79, 81, 83, 85, 88, 335
Heart failure, 15, 18, 22, 37, 38, 157, 161
HELLP syndrome, 26, 175, 179
Hidalgo, Aaron, 36, 266, 271
Hip fracture, 16, 17, 23, 26, 38, 160, 163, 285
Holmes, Casey
    domestic violence, 31, 35
    fatal crash, 42
    hearing and vision screening, 48
    story, 212–216
    substance abuse, 36, 47
Holmes, Carrie
    diarrhea, infant pain, 18
    domestic violence, victim, 31
    family and social issues, 31
    health promotion and wellness, 29
    new born care, 28
    otitis media, 16, 30
    professional practice issues, 52
    story, 222–224
Holmium laser enucleation of the prostrate (HoLEP), 14,
    19, 20, 24, 60, 61, 327
Homelessness, 15, 33, 34, 42, 44, 75, 89, 118, 125, 131,
    267, 272, 329, 345
Homosexuality, 236, 238, 336
Household information. *see* Story, *specific entries in
    characters*

Hyperkalemia, 25
Hypertension, 22, 25, 37, 38, 92, 157, 288, 311

I

Immune system, 25
Immunizations, 19, 28, 32, 43, 45, 48, 149–150, 152, 154,
    181, 182, 185, 205–206, 217, 219, 223–224, 243,
    249–252, 255, 257, 263, 264, 300, 303, 323, 325, 339
Infertility, 27, 169–171, 175–178
Influenza, 22, 25
Instructional tips and techniques, 7–8
Internet, 31, 33, 47, 79, 82, 83, 100, 104–106, 169, 175,
    196, 229, 248, 289, 309, 337

J

Jackson, Robert, 1 27, 93, 96, 285–288, 292, 294,
    306–312, 314, 323
Jacobe, Dr, 5, 134–136, 267
Jacobs, Shawn
    group therapy, 49
    health connections clinic, 266–275
    mental health patients, 35, 36, 37
    mood disorders, 34
    patient's death, 15, 42
    professional practice issues, 50, 52
    psychotic disorders, 33
    role as a nurse, 54, 55
    story, 265–275
James, Norma
    atrial fibrillation, 22, 37
    catheter insertion, 15, 19, 24
    comments on, 15–20, 22–24, 34, 37–39
    depression, 34, 37
    diabetes, 18, 25, 37
    feeding tube, 17, 19
    hypertension, 22, 38
    Intravenous (IV) therapy, 20
    mobility issues, 16, 18, 20
    story, 92–98
    stroke, 14, 23, 39
Jaramillo, Benito
    gay parenting, 31
    mobility issues, 16
    post-traumatic disorder (PTSD), 36
    story, 233–238
    stress fracture, 23
"Jeopardy" game, 10, 359f
Johnson, Randall
    family and social issues, 31
    health promotion and wellness, 29
    story, 107–111
Johnson, Yvonne
    anemia, 22

family and social issues, 31, 50
fatigue, 15, 17, 18
renal failure, 24
story, 99–106
systemic lupus erythematosus (SLE), 25

K

Kattan, Zainah
    documentation timing, difficulties, 19
    health promotion activities, 48
    hospital responsibilities, 26, 283–290
    immunization clinic volunteer, 32
    mental health issues, handling, 35
    professional practice issues, 49, 50, 51, 52, 53
    role as a nurse, 54, 55
    smoky air fills healthcare facilities, patients, 17
    story, 283–290
Ketoacidosis, 20, 25, 169, 172, 178
Koch, Debbie, 55, 277–281, 284, 286, 291, 319, 321, 322

L

Larson, Mr., 278, 284, 291

M

Mandatory overtime, 51, 52, 277, 279, 280, 287–288,
    293, 334–335, 342
Marquette, Carolyn, 5, 28, 180, 248, 254, 264
Martin, Anthony
    family and social issues, 31
    injury and suicide risk, 18
    psychotic disorder, 21, 33, 34
    story, 131–137
Martin, Gilbert
    chronic back pain, 18, 23
    family and social issues, 31
    story, 113–118
    substance abuse, 36, 39, 50
Martin, Helen
    anxiety, 35
    cholelithiasis, pain, 18, 24
    family and social issues, 31
    IV therapy, 20
    menopause, 27
    nausea and vomiting, 16
    obesity, 25
    postoperative care, 20
    story, 119–125
Martin, Kristina
    community health, 43
    contraception, 27
    eating disorder, 30, 35
    health promotion, 49
    sexually transmitted infection, 28, 30
    story, 137–142

Martin, Mark
  community health department's service, 43
  dental screening, 48
  mobility issues, 16, 20
  mood disorder, 34
  paraplegia complication, 18, 21
  spinal cord injury, 23
  story, 148–152
  substance abuse, 36, 47
Martin, Mary
  cataracts, 26, 37
  community services, 43, 44
  dental caries, 29
  family and social issues, 39, 40
  glaucoma, 26, 38
  health promotion, 48
  osteoporosis, 23, 38
  professional practice issues, 50
  senior center nurse topics, 41
  sensory perpetual, 18
  spirituality, 19
  story, 125–131
Martin, Tyler
  allergic reaction, 29
  community health department's service, 152–155
  dental caries, 29
  family and social issues, 31
  health promotion and wellness, 28
  story, 152–155
Maternity. see Women's health
Matsui, Vincent, 286–287
McCain, Jacob, 39, 40, 41, 48, 50, 127, 280, 290, 293,
    297–298, 306, 308–310, 316, 321
Medication management, 41, 48, 306, 313, 342
Mental health nursing
  cognitive disorders, 34
  mood disorders, 34
  other disorders, 33–37
  psychotic disorders, 33
Metabolism, 24–25

N
Nausea
  and abdominal fullness, 95
  and diarrhea, 71
  and fatigue, 172, 205
  and vomitting, 17, 24, 71
Neighborhood, The
  caring analysis, 364f
  community facts, 5
  description, 2
  interpretative pedagogy, 3

longitudinal case studies, 3
  news, 5
  standardized patients, 3–4
  story telling, 3
  supporting characters, 5
  teaching strategies, 2
  visual map, 5–6
  See also Pedagogical tools
Neighborhood hospital links, 26
Neighborhood News
  adult health care topics, 21
  community health, 42
  health promotion, 47
  geriatric nursing, 37
  learning activities, 49
  mental health nursing, 33
  pediatric and family nursing, 28
  policy analysis, 10
  season 1, 323–331
  season 2, 332–339
  season 3, 340–347
  women's issues, 26
Neurologic system, 23
Nolan, Matt, 5, 6f, 15, 36, 42, 266–270, 272, 341
Nursing fundamentals
  additional assets, 14–19
  character season/episodes, 14–19
  comments, 14–19
  concept focus, 14–19
Nursing skills
  additional assets, 19–21
  character season/episodes, 19–21
  comments, 19–21
  featured skill/equipment, 19–21
Nursing shortage, 51, 279, 281, 286, 288, 333, 335,
    342, 343
Nursing strike, 51, 89, 282, 289, 295, 342, 344, 346
Nutrition, 16, 17, 18, 24–25, 30, 32, 38, 49, 84, 162,
    164–165, 167, 182, 196, 219, 233, 235, 237,
    245–246, 298, 301, 303, 333, 340

O
Obesity, 16, 17, 25, 30, 32, 44, 195, 298, 299, 303, 326,
    330, 339, 340
Ocampo, Danilo
  acute myocardial infarction (AMI), 22, 37
  death news, 42
  dementia, 34, 37
  end of life, 15
  family and social issues, 39, 40
  fatigue, 15
  health care issues, 44

heart failure, 22, 38
hypertension, 22, 38
IV therapy, 20
professional practice issues, 51
self-care, 18
sleeping problem, 18
story, 157–161
Ocampo, Lydia
  Alzheimer's disease, 18
  anemia, 37
  blood transfusion, 19
  death news, 42
  decubitus ulcer, 21
  end of life, 15
  family and social issues, 40
  health promotion, 48
  infection (open reduction with internal fixation (ORIF), 16
  injury risk, 18
  mobility issues, 16
  Neighborhood Hospital care, 26
  nutrition problems, 17, 25, 38
  post-operative complications, ORIF, 19, 20, 21, 23, 38
  professional practice issues, 50, 51
  psychotic disorder, 33, 34, 37
  self-care, 18
  sleep disorder, 18
  story, 162–167
Osteoarthritis, 17, 23, 38, 85, 86, 87, 88
Osteoporosis, 23, 38, 40, 41, 86, 125, 126, 127, 129, 309
Otitis media, 16, 30, 222, 223

P

Pain
  abdominal, 115, 121, 145, 228, 231, 234, 312, 313, 322, 345
  chest, 117, 124, 158
  joint, 85–88, 90, 103–105
  postoperative, 17, 24
Patterson, Blake, 6f, 33, 36, 241
Patterson, Rebecca, 5, 7f, 241, 242, 246, 247, 248, 250, 300, 301, 302, 303
Patterson, Victoria, 245, 247, 254–255, 259, 299, 301, 304
Pedagogical tools
  biographies, 4
  case studies, 8, 9, 349f–352f
  content links, 4
  health records, 4–5
  Neighborhood connections, 4
  photographs, 4
  related news, 5
  stories, 4
  video vignettes, 4

Pediatric nursing. *see* Family nursing
Pelvic fracture, 23, 260
Pneumonia, 22, 38, 39, 62, 70, 84, 127, 285, 287, 292, 310, 311
Poisoning, 134, 302
Policy analysis, 10, 361f
Porter, Jennifer, 14, 41, 48, 98, 159, 283–285, 291–292, 306, 312, 316, 319, 329, 343, 346
Power of attorney, 40, 158, 165, 166
Preeclampsia, 26, 30, 175, 179, 181, 316, 319
Pregnancy, 15, 16, 26, 27, 35, 45, 140, 169, 171–173, 175, 177–179, 206–208, 215, 229, 235, 238, 241, 246–247, 303, 316–317, 319–320, 322, 332, 335
Prematurity, 30, 182
Professional concepts, nursing
  nurses' roles, 53–55
  practical issues, 49–53

R

Ramsey, Carol
  childbirth classes, 48
  gay and lesbian parenting, 31
  health issues, women, 27, 28
  mental health issues, women, 35
  multiple patient issues, 27
  nursing skills, 19, 51
  professional practice issues, 52
  role as a nurse, 53, 54, 55
  role-play, 353f
  safe sex education, 49
  sexually transmitted infection, 30
  shelter information, 42
  story, 315–322
  teen pregnancy, handling, 27
  Women's Health Service responsibilities, 315–322
Reactive airway disease, 248, 252, 254
Renal insufficiency, 100, 104–105
Respiratory acidosis, 25, 38
Respiratory failure, 17, 20, 22, 25, 38, 39, 79, 84, 280
Respiratory syncytial virus (RSV), 16, 180, 206, 218, 219
Respiratory system, 21–22
Restraints, 18, 21, 49, 159, 332
Reyes, Angelo
  child birth classes, 48
  diabetes, type 1, 25
  diabetic retinopathy, 26
  electrolyte disturbances, 25
  infertility, 27
  IV therapy, 20
  sensory perceptual, 18
  story, 169–174

Reyes, Marissa
  health promotion and wellness, 29
  hyperbilirubinemia, 30
  newborn care, 28
  prematurity complication, 30
  story, 181–182
Reyes, Peter
  health promotion and wellness, 29
  hyperbilirubinemia, 30
  Infant respiratory distress syndrome, 30
  newborn care, 28
  prematurity complication, 30
  story, 181–182
Reyes, Rachel
  childbirth classes, 48
  high risk pregnancy (Cesarean section), 26
  infertility, 27
  newborn care, 28
  story, 175–181
Richman, Patrick
  hospital responsibilities, 277–282
  professional practice issues, 49, 50, 51, 52, 53
  role as a nurse, 54, 55
Riley, Evelyn
  attention deficit hyperactivity disorder (ADHD), 34
  domestic violence, 35
  parenting stress, 31
  spirituality, 19
  story, 184–191
Riley, Jason
  attention deficit hyperactivity disorder (ADHD),
    29, 34
  hearing and vision screening, 32, 48
  learning problem, 32
  school bullying, 33
  story, 197–203
Riley, Jenna
  adolescent obesity, 16, 30
  diabetes, type 2, 25, 30
  family and social issues, 31
  story, 191–197
  violence, Internet predator, 33, 46, 47
Riley, Jessica
  constipation associated with pregnancy, 15
  contraception, 27
  domestic violence, 27, 35
  nausea, 16
  professional practice issue, 50, 52
  shelter information, 42
  sleep disorder, 19
  story, 204–211
  teen pregnancy, 27

Riley, Ryan
  colic pain, infant, 17, 29
  domestic violence, 31
  family and social issues, 31
  health promotion and wellness, 29
  nutrition problem, 16, 30
  professional practice issues, 52
  respiratory syncytial virus (RSV), 16, 17, 29, 30
  story, 217–221
Role-play, 9, 353f
Rollins, Joyce, 267
Ross, Greg
  colitis exacerbation, 15, 18
  Crohn's disease, 24
  gay parenting, 31
  hypertension, 22
  post-traumatic stress disorder (PTSD), 36
  story, 226–232
Rowe, Dr, 5, 17, 18, 67–68, 70, 73, 80, 82,
    86–89, 100–104, 120–121, 127, 144,
    186, 188–189, 195, 199, 201, 229, 236, 270,
    300, 302, 309

S
Saunders, Eloise, 41, 50, 306, 310–313
Schizophrenia, 33, 34, 117, 131, 135
Schofield, Bobby
  family and social issues, geriatric nursing, 39
  handling mental health issues, 36
  hospital responsibilities, 26, 290–295
  nursing skills, 21
  professional practice issues, 50, 51
  role as a nurse, 53, 54, 55
  smoking ban links, 46
  story, 290–295
School nursing, 32–33
Septic shock, 22
Sex education, 28, 33, 49, 54, 326, 335
Sharif, Kayla, 32, 40, 41, 55, 93, 127, 283, 286, 290,
    292, 298, 297, 301, 302, 306, 308, 320–321
Spinal cord injury, 23, 39, 117, 148, 151,
    260, 273
Stroke, 14, 15, 16, 17, 19, 20, 22, 23, 25, 34, 37, 39, 92,
    95, 97, 306, 311, 313, 330
Simulation activities, 9-10, 354f
Sleep deprivation, 19, 268, 338
Small group discussion, 11, 364f–365f
Smoking cessation, 48, 49, 80–81, 86, 241,
    246, 327
Substance abuse, 32, 36, 46, 47, 212, 213, 266–272, 290,
    294, 297–298, 341, 343, 360f
Systemic lupus erythematosus (SLE), 15, 104, 105

T

Teaching strategy
  care plan, 12, 366*f*–368*f*
  case study, 9, 349*f*–352*f*
  comparing and contrasting, 10, 360*f*
  concept map, 11, 363*f*
  concept or topic analysis, 10, 357*f*–358*f*
  family history, 10, 362*f*
  "jeopardy" game, 10, 359*f*
  policy analysis, 10, 361*f*
  role-play, 9, 353*f*
  simulation, 9, 354*f*–356*f*
  small group discussion, 11, 364*f*–365*f*
  teaching plan, 11, 369*f*–370*f*
Transitional care, 38, 40, 54
Trauma, 27, 30, 117, 170, 209, 222–223, 244, 250, 257, 286, 328, 332–333, 340, 343

U

Urinary tract infection, 15, 24, 96
Urologic system, 24

V

Visual system, 26
Vitreous hemorrhage, 18, 26, 169, 171

W

Williams, Karen
  caregiving issues, 23
  family and social issues, handling, 39
  health promotion activities, 48
  health related conditions, seniors, 38, 39
  professional practice issues, 49, 50, 51, 52, 53
  role as a nurse, 54, 55
  senior center responsibilities, 15, 18, 40–41, 43, 305–314
  story, 305–314
  supervising nursing students, 19

Women's health
  issues, 27–28
  pregnancy and, 26–27

Y

Young, Angie
  childbirth classes, 48
  community health service, 46
  oxygenation, 17
  planned pregnancy, 27
  story, 245–251
Young, Eric
  diarrhea, infant, 15, 29, 30
  health promotion and wellness, 29
  newborn care, 28
  story, 262–264
  upper respiratory infection, 30
Young, Kelsey
  asthma, 29, 32
  influenza, 22, 25
  oxygenation, 17
  story, 252–257
Young, Marcus
  conjunctivitis, 16, 29, 32
  influenza, 22, 25
  mobility issues, 16, 30
  pelvic fracture, 23
  safety issues, 32
  story, 257–262
Young, Steve
  childbirth classes, 48
  post-traumatic stress disorder (PTSD), 36
  smoking cessation, 49
  story, 240–245